Ebersole and Hess'

Gerontological Nursing

& Healthy Aging

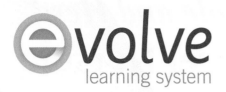
learning system

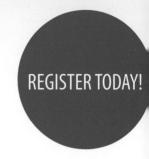
To access your Student Resources, visit:

http://evolve.elsevier.com/
Ebersole/gerontological

Register today and gain access to:

Evolve® Student Resources for *Touhy, Jett: Ebersole & Hess' Gerontological Nursing & Healthy Aging,* **Third Edition** offer the following features:

Student Resources

- ## Dermatological Photos
  Vivid, full-color photographs of the most common dermatological problems seen in older adults are presented to aid in identifying and clarifying these problems.

- ## Additional Resources
  Print, electronic, and visual resources are included to help in further research, study, and understanding of the material presented in each chapter.

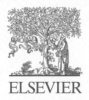
ELSEVIER

Ebersole and Hess'
Gerontological Nursing
& Healthy Aging

THIRD EDITION

THERIS A. TOUHY, DNP, GCNS-BC
Professor
Christine E. Lynn College of Nursing
Florida Atlantic University
Boca Raton, Florida

KATHLEEN F. JETT, PhD, GNP-BC
Gerontological Nurse Practitioner
Gaithersburg, Maryland

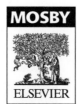

MOSBY

ELSEVIER

MOSBY
ELSEVIER

11830 Westline Industrial Drive
St. Louis, Missouri 63146

EBERSOLE & HESS' GERONTOLOGICAL
NURSING & HEALTHY AGING, THIRD EDITION

ISBN: 978-0-323-05701-1

Notice

Knowledge and best practice in this field are constantly changing. As new research and experience broaden our knowledge, changes in practice, treatment and drug therapy may become necessary or appropriate. Readers are advised to check the most current information provided (i) on procedures featured or (ii) by the manufacturer of each product to be administered, to verify the recommended dose or formula, the method and duration of administration, and contraindications. It is the responsibility of the practitioner, relying on their own experience and knowledge of the patient, to make diagnoses, to determine dosages and the best treatment for each individual patient, and to take all appropriate safety precautions. To the fullest extent of the law, neither the Publisher nor the Authors assumes any liability for any injury and/or damage to persons or property arising out of or related to any use of the material contained in this book.

The Publisher

Library of Congress Cataloging-in-Publication Data
Touhy, Theris A.
  Ebersole & Hess' gerontological nursing & healthy aging/Theris A. Touhy, Kathleen F. Jett.—3rd ed
   p. ; cm.
  Rev. ed. of: Gerontological nursing & healthy aging. 2nd ed. c2005.
  Includes bibliographical references and index.
  ISBN 978-0-323-05701-1 (pbk. : alk. paper)
  1. Geriatric nursing. 2. Aging. 3. Older people—Health and hygiene. I. Ebersole, Priscilla. II. Jett, Kathleen Freudenberger. III. Hess, Patrica A., 1938-IV. Gerontological nursing & healthy aging. V. Title. VI. Title: Gerontological nursing & healthy aging.
  [DNLM: 1. Geriatric Nursing. 2. Aged. 3. Aging. 4. Health Promotion. 5. Holistic Nursing. WY 152 T722e 2010]
  RC954.G455 2010
  618.97'0231—dc22

                                                                                    2009003577

Managing Editor: Michele Hayden
Developmental Editor: Heather Bays
Publishing Services Manager: Jeff Patterson
Project Manager: Amy Rickles
Design Direction: Paula Catalano
Cover Designer: Paula Catalano

Printed in Canada

Last digit is the print number: 9 8 7 6 5 4 3 2 1

Dedication

To my beautiful grandchildren, Colin and Molly Touhy.
Thanks for merry-go-round rides, tea parties, Barney, cannonballs in the pool,
scuba divers, and Twinkle Twinkle Little Star. Being your Gramma TT makes
growing older the best time of my life and I love you.

To the older people I have been privileged to nurse, and their caregivers,
like Peggy Bennett and Joan Belton, thanks for making the words
in this book a reality for the elders you care for and for teaching me
how to be a gerontological nurse.

To Pat and Priscilla, thanks for entrusting us with the care
of this very special book.

Theris Touhy

To my husband Steve, who is a source of never-ending support.
Without his willingness to keep me supplied with food,
the long hours sitting in front of the computer and writing
would not have been possible.

To the older adults who have opened their lives to me so that I may learn.

To our four children and four wonderful grandchildren, Haley, Amelia, Emory and
Logan, who always remind me that the best part of life is the time we spend
together and that the older we get, the more we have loved
and the more adventures we have shared.

Kathleen Jett

Reviewers

Patricia Burbank, DNSc, RN
Professor, College of Nursing
University of Rhode Island
Kingston, Rhode Island

Vickie Ann Grosso, PhD, RN
Professor, Department of Nursing
Essex County College
Newark, New Jersey

Colleen J. Hewes, RN, MSN, DC
Instructor of Nursing
Lake Washington Technical College
Kirkland, Washington

Laurie Kennedy-Malone, PhD, APRN-BC, FAAN
Professor, School of Nursing
University of North Carolina at Greensboro
Greensboro, North Carolina

Marie Messier, BSN, MSN, MEd
Associate Professor of Nursing
Germanna Community College
Locust Grove, Virginia

Carmella M. Mikol, PhD, MN, BSN
Professor, Nursing Program
College of Lake County
Grayslake, Illinois

Claudia Mitchell, RN, MSN
Assistant Professor of Clinical Nursing
College of Nursing
University of Cincinnati
Cincinnati, Ohio

Margaret Moriarty-Litz, BSN, MNA
Instructor/Coordinator
St. Joseph School of Nursing
Nashua, New Hampshire

Lillian A. Rafeldt, RN, MA, CNE
Assistant Professor of Nursing
Three Rivers Community College
Norwich, Connecticut

Janine Ray, RN, MSN
Instructor, Nursing Program
Cisco Junior College
Abilene, Texas

Judith Townsend Rocchiccioli, PhD, RN
Professor of Nursing
James Madison University
Harrisonburg, Virginia

Tracy A. Szirony, PhD, RNC, CHPN
Associate Professor of Nursing
College of Nursing
University of Toledo
Toledo, Ohio

Anne Viviano, RN, MSN
Nursing Faculty
Baker College
Clinton Township, Michigan

Loretta Wack, RN, MSN
Associate Professor of Nursing
Blue Ridge Community College
Weyers Cave, Virginia

Tricia Wickers, RN, MSN
Associate Professor of Nursing
Los Angeles Harbor College
Wilmington, California

Preface

This text is about health, wellness, and aging. It is designed to provide nurses, faculty, and students with the most current information on evidence-based gerontological nursing, an area often neglected in basic nursing education and nursing texts. This totally revised and updated 3rd edition provides content consistent with the *AACN Older Adults: Recommended Competencies for Geriatric Nursing Care* developed by AACN in collaboration with the John A. Hartford Foundation Institute for Geriatric Nursing at New York University. The goals set forth by *Healthy People 2010* provide the framework for the study of healthy aging. Although Maslow's Hierarcy of Needs is the organizing framework, it includes additional frameworks for a range of situations. Enhanced content on the roles of gerontological nurses, care issues across the continuum, communicating with elders, genetic influences, spirituality, and sexuality has been added.

In Section I, the foundations of healthy aging are explored, from the origins of gerontological nursing and the impact of culture and health disparities to the importance of skillful documentation. In Section II, the many changes associated with normal aging are presented, along with specific implications for nursing and working with the older adult to respond and adapt to the changes with the goal of maintaining or restoring optimal wellness. Section III focuses on common health problems seen in older adults and what nurses can do to help elders living with chronic illness. This section does not provide the in-depth coverage of the topics that one would find in a medical-surgical nursing textbook, but highlights the key aspects of the problems as they relate specifically to older adults. In Section IV, we present discussions of the global topics that affect all of us as we age: economic and legal issues; relationships; roles and transitions; mental health and wellness; coping with grief, loss, dying and death, and care across the continuum.

The text is organized for optimal student learning experiences. Each chapter begins with the phenomenological consideration of the lived experience of an elder. Key concepts, glossaries, learning activities, and discussion questions summarize the important points presented and relate directly to the objectives of the chapter. Resources, including teaching materials, films, and websites, are provided at the end of each chapter and at evolve.elsevier.com/Ebersole/gerontological for the reader who may wish to seek additional information or referral sources.

Gerontological nurses have always assumed a leadership role in improving care for elders, insuring fulfillment of all levels on Maslow's Hierarchy of Needs, and promoting healthy aging. Since the first edition of this text, there has been an explosion of knowledge, research, interest, and resources in gerontological nursing. The specialty continues to grow in importance and gerontological nursing competencies are now recognized as basic education requirements for nurses in all specialties. It would be hard to imagine a nursing student graduating without content in pediatrics, medical-surgical nursing, or mental health nursing. Today, the expectation is that all nurses will also be prepared to care for the growing numbers of diverse older adults and have the knowledge and skills to promote healthy aging for people of all ages around the globe. We can look forward to the coming years when aging in health will be the norm and we hope this text will provide the knowledge nurses need to play a key role in making this happen.

Ancillaries (available at http://evolve.elsevier.com/Ebersole/gerontological)

For Instructors
- **Instructor's Electronic Resource:** Includes learning objectives, chapter summaries, suggested classroom activities, and clinical activities that can be used for classroom discussion, projects, and further study
- **PowerPoint Presentations:** PowerPoint slide presentations to accompany each chapter (approximately 700 total)
- **Test Bank:** Approximately 500 questions in the latest NCLEX examination formats
- **Image Collection:** Over 25 illustrations and photos that can be used in a presentation or as visual aids.

For Students
- **Dermatological Photos:** Full-color photographs of common dermatological problems.
- **Resources:** Additional resources organized by chapter are included for further study of concepts presented in the chapter

Theris A. Touhy
Kathleen F. Jett

Acknowledgements

We would like to thank Priscilla Ebersole and Patricia Hess for the opportunity to author this book and to share their beautiful words and passion for gerontological nursing. We hope that our work honors them and the specialty we all love. It has been a real privilege for us to be a part of the work of two gerontological nurses from whom we have learned how to care for older people.

Theris Touhy
Kathleen Jett

Contents

Introduction to Healthy Aging

LEARNING OBJECTIVES

Upon completion of this chapter, the reader will be able to:

- Identify at least three factors that influence the aging experience.
- Define health and wellness within the context of aging and chronic illness.
- Describe the trends seen in global aging today.
- Apply Maslow's Hierarchy of Needs to gerontological nursing.

GLOSSARY

Cohort Group where members share some common experience

Wellness A state of health which is optimal for the individual person at any point in time

Centenarian A person who is at least 100 years old

Holistic health care That which considers the whole person and the interaction with and between the parts

THE LIVED EXPERIENCE

I believe a human life is like a river, meandering through its course, rushing through rapids, flowing placidly over the plains, twisting and turning through countless bends until it spends itself. It is the same river; yet it looks very different from one place to another. So it is with our lives; circumstances vary from one time to another in the course of a life, but I think each stage has its own value.

Georgia, a 35-year-old

Providing nursing care to older persons is a rewarding, life-affirming vocation. Through this textbook we hope to provide students with the basics to begin a career as a gerontological nurse or simply care for older adults with more skill and sensitivity. We present an overview of aging, the health care needs of older adults, and the vital and exciting role of the nurse in facilitating healthy aging.

AGING IN THE UNITED STATES

Although all of us begin aging at birth, both the meaning of aging and those who are identified as elders are determined by society and culture and influenced by history and gender. In the early American Puritan community of the 1600s, the process of aging was considered a sacred pilgrimage to God, and as such, persons in late life were revered. However, by the late 1800s, aging was devalued as youth became the symbol of growth and expansion. In 1935, with the establishment of Social Security, the time when one became "old" was set at 65.

Psychologists have divided the "old" into three groups: the young-old, roughly 65 to 74 years old; the middle-old, 75 to 84 years old; and the old-old, or those over 85. A fourth group of persons, 100 years old and older (centenarians) is growing rapidly (Box 1-1). Currently about 3.1% of the population in the United States are at least 100 years old, compared with 0.1% in 1901. The total number is expected to increase by more than 400% by 2030. The majority of these centenarians will be women (U.S. Census Bureau, 2004; NIA, 2007).

Box 1-1	Super-Centenarian Extraordinaire: Jeanne Louise Calment

Jeanne Louise Calment died in France at age 122. At that time she was believed to be the longest-lived person in the world. She outlived her husband, her daughter, her only grandson, and her lawyer. Her husband died in 1942, just four years before their 50th anniversary. Her daughter died in 1936 and her grandson in 1963. She was four when the Eiffel tower was built and reportedly once sold art supplies to Vincent Van Gogh. Not only did she live a long life, but did so with vigor. Madame Calment took up fencing at 85 and was still riding a bike at 107. She smoked until she was 117 and ate a lifelong diet rich in olive oil. Her longevity remains a mystery to experts and researchers.

Dollemore D: *Aging under the microscope: A biological quest*, Bethesda, MD, 2006, National Institute of Aging, National Institutes of Health, Publication #02-2756.

Those born within the same decade and country may share a common historical context and are usually referred to as a cohort. For example, men born between 1920 and 1930 were very likely to have been active participants in World War II and the Korean War. In comparison, men born between 1940 and 1950 were likely to have been involved in the Vietnam conflict, an entirely different experience. It is not surprising that these two groups of men have different perspectives and different health problems. Likewise, privileged women born between 1920 and 1930 were raised with what are known as traditional values and roles and may have either never worked outside the home or been limited to what was considered "women's work," such as housekeeping, teaching, and nursing. In contrast, similar women born between 1940 and 1950 had pressure to work outside the home and also had considerably more opportunities, partially as a result of the feminist revolution of the 1960s and 1970s.

Gender can have a significant effect on various aspects of aging. Women usually live longer than men and live alone after widowhood. Men who survive their wives often remarry and live alone significantly less often. Women usually have larger social networks outside the work environment than men, which could potentially reduce social isolation after the death of a spouse or companion.

Finally, the United States is experiencing a "gerontological explosion" of ethnically diverse older adults, primarily those persons of color and persons who self-identify as Hispanic or Latino, regardless of race. Persons comprising groups that have been considered statistical minorities in the late 1900s can now be considered an emerging majority as the relative percentage of their numbers rises rapidly. See Figure 1-1 for the projected changes in the demographics of older adults by ethnicity and race by the year 2030.

Although the health status of racial and ethnic groups has improved over the past century, disparities in major health indicators between white and nonwhite groups are growing (www.nia.gov). Increasing the numbers of health care providers from different cultures as well as ensuring cultural competence of all providers is essential to meet the needs of a rapidly growing, ethnically diverse elderly population. One of the two major goals of *Healthy People 2010* is to eliminate health disparities. The other goal is that of increasing the span of healthy life (USDHHS, 2000). Gerontological nurses have a special responsibility for helping the nation achieve these goals related to the lives of those already in late life.

Global Aging

For the first time in recorded history, the number of persons 60 years and older worldwide is likely to exceed those younger than 15 years by the year 2045 (see Figure 1-2). This occurred in Europe in 1995 but will not occur in North America until 2015. Those older than 60 years will not surpass children until 2040 in Asia, Latin American, and the Caribbean (UN, 2007a). However in 2007, Japan had the highest percentage of persons 60 years and older at 27.9% (UN, 2007b). These changes pose major challenges in meeting the needs of the aging global community.

Africa stands out as the only major region whose population is still relatively young and where the number of elderly, although increasing, will still be far below the number of those aged 0 to 59 in 2050. Those between 15 and 59 years of age in Africa is projected to rise from half a billion in 2005 to over 1.2 billion in 2050 (UN, 2007a), while those older than 60 will only increase from 0.05 billion to 0.2 billion in the same period.

HEALTH, WELLNESS, AND AGING

The definitions of health vary greatly and are influenced by culture and where one is on the life span. The strong emergence of the holistic health movement has resulted in even broader definitions of health and wellness. Wellness involves one's whole being—physical, emotional, mental, and spiritual—all of which are vital components

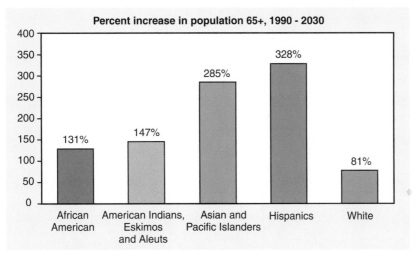

Fig. 1-1   Percent increase in population ages 65 and older by race and ethnicity, 1990-2030. *(From U.S. Census Bureau, January 2000.)*

(Figure 1-3). In a classic work, Dunn (1961) defined the holistic approach to health as "an integrated method of functioning which is oriented toward maximizing the potential of which the individual is capable within the environment where he is functioning." A holistic view of health incorporates the components in Figure 1-3. Wellness involves achieving a balance between one's internal and external environment and one's emotional, spiritual, social, cultural, and physical processes.

Wellness is a state of being and feeling that one strives to achieve through effective health practices. An individual must work hard to achieve wellness. In working toward wellness, an individual may reach plateaus in his or her ascension to higher-level wellness. The person may also regress because of an illness or acute event or crisis, but these events can be a potential stimulus for growth and a return to moving along the wellness continuum (Figure 1-4).

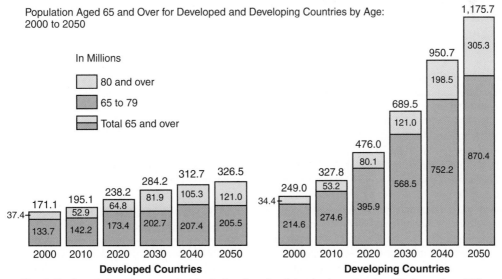

Fig. 1-2   Population 65 years and older in developed and developing countries. *(Redrawn from U.S. Census Bureau, 2004.)*

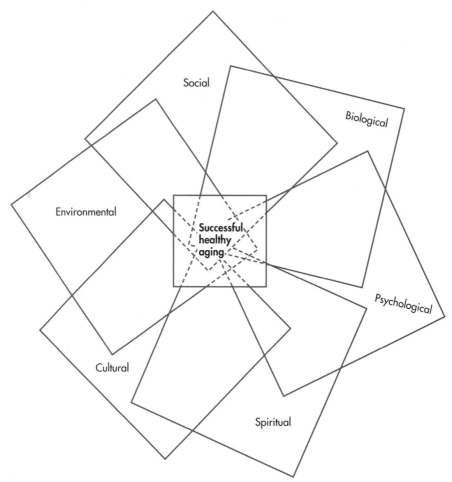

Fig. 1-3   Healthy aging. *(Developed by Patricia Hess.)*

Consistent with Dunn (1961), health in later life is often thought of in terms of functional ability rather that the absence of disease, that is, the ability to do what is important to a given person. This may mean the person's ability to live independently or the ability to enjoy great-grandchildren when they visit at the nursing home, but it is always individually determined. Well-being for those older than 60 years is strongly related to functional status but is affected also by socioeconomic factors, degree of social interaction, marital status, and aspects of one's living situation and environment.

Approaching aging from a viewpoint of health emphasizes strengths, resilience, resources, and capabilities rather than focusing on existing pathological conditions. A wellness perspective is based on the belief that every person has an optimal level of health independent of his or her situation or functional ability. Even in the presence of chronic illness or multiple disabilities or while dying, movement toward higher wellness is possible if the emphasis of care is placed on the promotion of well-being in the least restrictive environment, with support and encouragement for the person to find meaning in the situation, whatever it is.

MASLOW'S HIERARCHY OF HUMAN NEEDS

Maslow's theories of the hierarchy of human needs provide an organizing framework for this text and for understanding individuals and their concerns at any

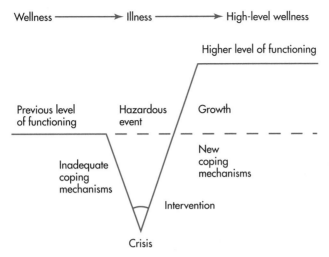

Fig. 1-4   Growth potential: crisis as a challenge.

particular time or situation (Figure 1-5). It also can serve as a guide for prioritizing nursing interventions to promote healthy aging and as a framework for this text. The hierarchy ranks needs from the most basic, related to the maintenance of biological integrity, to the most complex, associated with self-actualization. According to this theory the needs of higher levels cannot be met without first meeting those of lower levels. In other words, moving toward healthy aging is an evolving and developing process. As basic-level needs are met, the satisfaction of higher-level needs is possible, with ever deepening richness to life, regardless of one's age. The nurse prioritizes care from the most essential to those things thought of as quality of life.

As far back as Hippocrates and Galen, the necessities of all living people were recognized as the need for air, fluids, nutrition, hygiene, elimination, activity, and skin integrity. More recently these needs have become identified as self-care requirements (Box 1-2). Along with those listed in the box is the need for comfort or relief from suffering. The gerontological nurse works to ensure that these needs are met for older adults and realizes that as this is accomplished, higher levels of wellness are possible. The person with dementia may begin to wander or become agitated because of the need to find a toilet and not knowing where to look. Until toileting needs are met, the nurse's attempt to comfort may be ineffective. As people's basic needs are met they will feel safe and secure (second level). They will likely sleep better and feel more comfortable interacting with others. While interacting with others, people often begin

to meet their needs of belonging (third level). Participation in church, synagogue, or mosque activities, civic or social organizations and the maintenance of ties to family and friends all are ways people fulfill belonging needs. After retirement a member of a work organization may instead become involved in special interest groups. Involvement is an opportunity to form new alliances and associations and to create environments in which meaningful relationships and activities can remain a part of life regardless of the setting.

A person whose basic needs are met, who feels safe and secure, and who has a sense of belonging will also develop self-esteem and a belief in self-efficacy (fourth level). In other words, people will accept and honor who they are and feel that they have some personal power and self-confidence; they will know that they are important as people and that they inherently have value. Self-esteem is not something that can be given. It is, however, something that others can negatively influence through ageist attitudes and behavior. For example, a nurse who assumes that a patient cannot do something based solely on the person's age is being ageist and is actually belittling the individual. Unfortunately this is common, but it can be challenged by the knowledgeable and sensitive gerontological nurse.

Finally, some people reach Maslow's highest level of wellness, that of self-actualization. Self-actualization is seen as people reaching out beyond themselves and finding meaning and a sense of fulfillment. This may not seem possible for all, but the nurse can foster this in unique and important ways. One of the authors (KJ) was

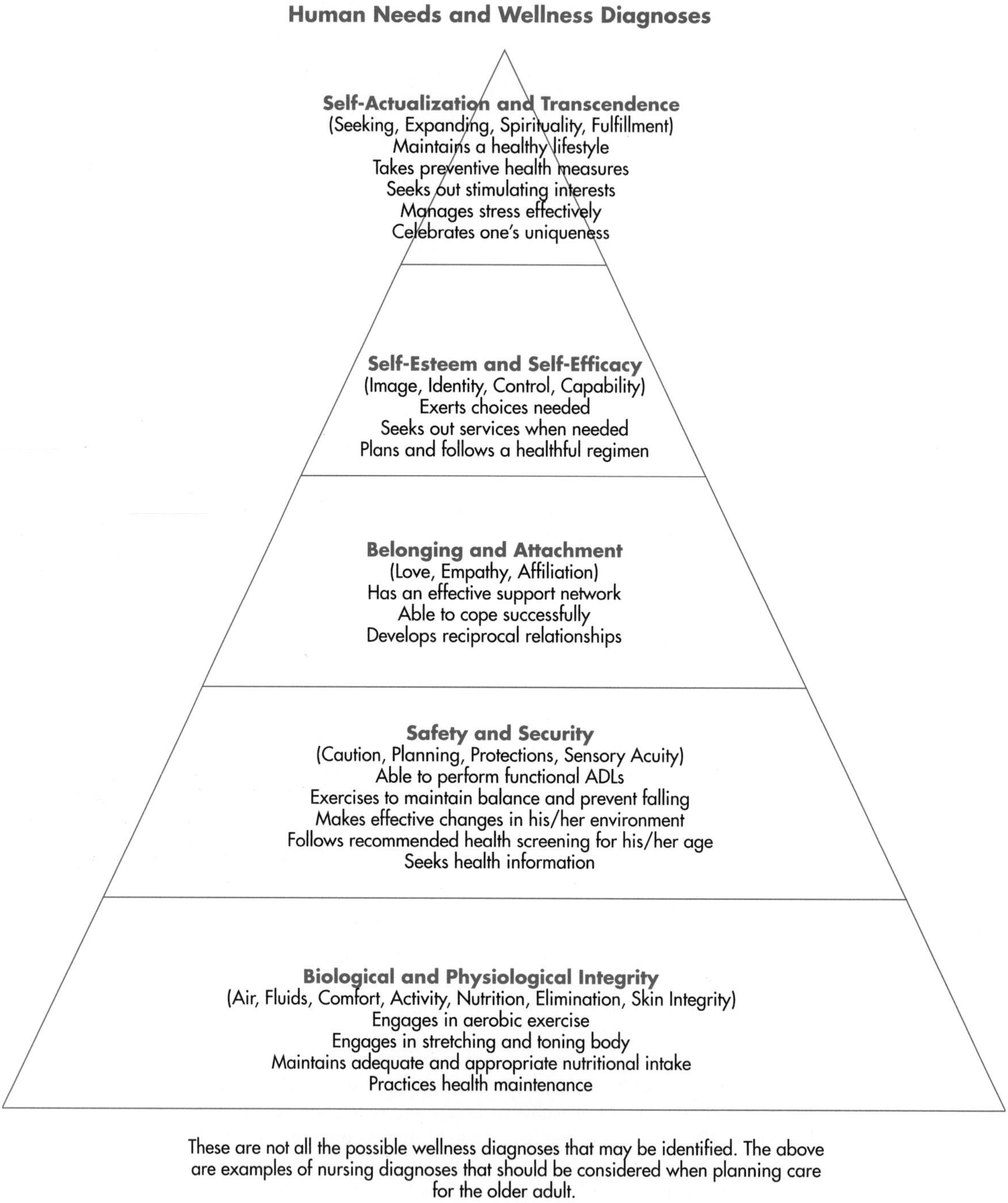

Human Needs and Wellness Diagnoses

Self-Actualization and Transcendence
(Seeking, Expanding, Spirituality, Fulfillment)
Maintains a healthy lifestyle
Takes preventive health measures
Seeks out stimulating interests
Manages stress effectively
Celebrates one's uniqueness

Self-Esteem and Self-Efficacy
(Image, Identity, Control, Capability)
Exerts choices needed
Seeks out services when needed
Plans and follows a healthful regimen

Belonging and Attachment
(Love, Empathy, Affiliation)
Has an effective support network
Able to cope successfully
Develops reciprocal relationships

Safety and Security
(Caution, Planning, Protections, Sensory Acuity)
Able to perform functional ADLs
Exercises to maintain balance and prevent falling
Makes effective changes in his/her environment
Follows recommended health screening for his/her age
Seeks health information

Biological and Physiological Integrity
(Air, Fluids, Comfort, Activity, Nutrition, Elimination, Skin Integrity)
Engages in aerobic exercise
Engages in stretching and toning body
Maintains adequate and appropriate nutritional intake
Practices health maintenance

These are not all the possible wellness diagnoses that may be identified. The above
are examples of nursing diagnoses that should be considered when planning care
for the older adult.

Fig. 1-5 Human needs and wellness diagnoses using Maslow's Hierarchy framework. *ADLs*,
Activities of daily living.

Box 1-2	Orem's Universal Self-Care Requirements

1. Maintaining sufficient intake of air, water, food
   a. Taking in the quantity required for normal functioning
   b. Preserving the integrity of associated anatomic structures and physiologic processes
2. Maintaining satisfactory elimination function
   a. Preserving the integrity of associated anatomic structures and physiologic processes
   b. Providing hygienic care of body surfaces and parts to the extent necessary to prevent injury or exposure to infection
   c. Maintaining adequate and sanitary disposal systems
3. Maintaining a balance between activity and rest
   a. Selecting activities that stimulate, engage, and keep in balance physical movement and rest adequate for health
   b. Responding to manifestations of needs for rest and activity
   c. Using personal capabilities, interests, and values as well as culturally prescribed norms as bases for development of a rest-activity pattern
4. Maintaining a balance between solitude and social interaction
   a. Maintaining the ability and interest necessary for the development of personal autonomy and enduring social relations
   b. Fostering bonds of affection, love, and friendship
   c. Participating in situations of social warmth and closeness
   d. Pursuing opportunities for satisfying group interactions

Based on the work of Dorothea Orem. See Hartweg, D: *Dorothea Orem: self-care deficit theory*, Newbury Park, CA, 1991, SAGE.

asked to speak to a group in a nursing home about death and dying. To her surprise the room was not filled with staff, as she had expected, but with the frailest of elders in wheelchairs. Instead of the usual lecture, she spoke of legacies and asked the silent audience, "What do you want people to remember about you? What made your life worthwhile?" Without exception each member of the audience had something to say, from "I had a beautiful garden" to "I was a good mother" to "I helped design a bridge." Meaning can be found for life everywhere—you just have to ask.

IMPLICATIONS FOR GERONTOLOGICAL NURSING AND HEALTHY AGING

It is the responsibility of the nurse to assist elders to achieve the highest level of wellness in relation to whatever situation exists. The nurse can, through knowledge and affirmation, empower, enhance, and support the person's movement toward the highest level of wellness possible. The nurse assesses and can help explore the underlying situation that may be interfering with the achievement of wellness, and work with the person and significant others to develop affirming and appropriate plans of care. The nurse and the elder collaboratively implement interventions to achieve individual goals and evaluate their effectiveness. The goals of the nurse are to care and comfort always, to cure sometimes, and to prevent that which can be prevented.

▶ KEY CONCEPTS

▶ Gerontological nursing is an opportunity to make a significant difference in the lives of older adults.

▶ The meaning of aging is influenced by many factors.

▶ Nurses have a responsibility to contribute to the nation's goals of increasing the quality of life lived and to reduce health disparities.

▶ Health, history, and gender are among the major factors influencing the aging experience.

▶ In some ways each age cohort is distinctly different from others.

▶ Individual persons become more unique the longer they live. Thus one must be cautious in attributing any specific characteristics of older adults to "old age."

▶ All persons, regardless of age or life and/or health situation, can be helped to achieve a higher level of wellness, which is uniquely and personally defined.

▶ Maslow's Hierarchy of Needs can be used as an organizing framework for health promotion, regardless of age or situation.

▶ Gerontological nurses have key roles in the provision of the highest quality of care to older adults in a wide range of settings and situations.

ACTIVITIES AND DISCUSSION QUESTIONS

1. Discuss the ways in which elders contribute to society today.
2. Interview an older person, and ask how he or she has changed since being 25 years old.
3. Discuss health and wellness with your peers. Develop a definition of aging.
4. Discuss the dimensions of wellness and which you think may be most important.
5. Explain wellness in the context of chronic illness.
6. Discuss how you seek wellness in your own life.
7. Discuss what you can do to enhance the quality of life for the persons to whom you provide care.
8. Draw a picture of yourself at 80. Compare your drawing to those of others who have done the same and discuss the implications of the representation.
9. Discuss how older adults are portrayed in popular TV shows, commercials, and movies.

RESOURCES

Websites

Administration on Aging
website: www.aoa.gov

Gerontological Society of America
website: www.geron.org

Nurse Competency in Aging Project
website: www.geronurseonline.org

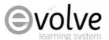
learning system

For additional resources, please visit evolve.elsevier.com/Ebersole/gerontological.

REFERENCES

National Institute on Aging, National Institutes of Health: Why population aging matters: a global perspective. March 5, 2007. Accessed September 22, 2008 from http://www.nia.nih.gov/NR/rdonlyres/C13CE0FA-59E4-49CA-BAC2-10E35297BDFD/6580/WPAM.txt.

Dunn HL: *High-level wellness,* Arlington, VA, 1961, Beatty.

NIA: Review of minority aging research at the NIA 2008. Accessed November 24, 2008 from http://www.nia.gov/AboutNIA/minorityagingresearch.htm.

Redberg R: Gender, race, and cardiac care, *J Am Coll Cardiol* 46 (7):1852-1854, 2005.

United Nations: Department of Economic and Social Affairs, Population Division, Fact sheet, Series A, 7 March 2007a. Accessed September 22, 2008 from http://www.un.org/esa/population/publications/wpp2006/FS_ageing.pdf.

United Nations: World population ageing. NY: United Nations Publications 2007b. Accessed September 22, 2008 from http://www.un.org/esa/population/publications/WPA2007/wpp2007.htm.

U.S. Department of Health and Human Services (USDHHS): *Healthy people 2010,* Washington, DC, 2000, US Government Printing Office, USDHHS.

Gerontological Nursing History, Education, and Roles

2

LEARNING OBJECTIVES

Upon completion of this chapter, the reader will be able to:

- Discuss the history of gerontological nursing and the factors influencing the development of this specialty practice.
- Identify elements of the American Nurses Association (ANA) *Scope and Standards of Practice for Gerontological Nursing.*
- Examine the recommended competencies for gerontological nursing practice.
- Recognize and discuss the importance of certification.
- Discuss the professional nursing leadership role in the care of older people across the continuum.
- Describe several gerontological nursing roles and the educational preparation for practicing them.
- Discuss formal gerontological organizations and their significance to the gerontological nurse.

THE LIVED EXPERIENCE

I don't think I will work in gerontological nursing; it seems depressing. I don't know many older people, but they are all sick without much hope to get better. I'll probably go into labor and delivery or the emergency room where I can really make a difference.

Student nurse, age 24

To know that I have made them feel they are human, that they're loved . . . that someone still cares about them. I believe that lots of times they feel ignored and as if they have no value. It's very important to me that they feel valued and they know that they still contribute not only to society but to the personal growth of everyone that comes into interaction with them.

Gerontological nurse, age 35, working in a nursing home

This chapter examines the foundations of the specialty practice of gerontological nursing, and the education, roles, organizations, communication, and leadership attributes that contribute to competent and satisfying practice in the care of older adults.

Geriatric nursing, the first name given to the nursing specialty, was replaced by *gerontological nursing* in 1976 to reflect nursing's emphasis on health rather than disease. Burnside (1988) noted that there is ambivalence abut the choice of terminology because both terms are in common usage in nursing. *Gerontic nursing* was another term coined by Laurie Gunter and Carmen Estes (1979) to describe the specialty, but it is rarely seen in the literature today. Gerontological nursing will be used throughout this book, reflecting the newer terminology and broader scope of the specialty.

GERONTOLOGICAL NURSING: GROWTH OF A SPECIALTY

The world population is aging. By 2050, 20% of the American population will be over the age of 65, with those over 85 showing the greatest increase in numbers. Older people today are healthier, better educated, and expect a much higher quality of life as they age than did their elders. As the number of older people continues to increase and the need for specialized knowledge becomes even more critical in every specialty and every health care setting, nurses prepared to care for older people will be in great demand (Ebersole and Touhy, 2006). "Whether in the home, hospital, or various community and long-term care agencies, the older adult requires comprehensive care that focuses on individualized health promotion and disease prevention, ongoing assessment of functional and cognitive status, rapid identification of acute problems, rehabilitation and restorative care, ongoing education, and appropriate referrals" (ANA, 2001, pp. 7-8).

Although interest in the specialty and the numbers of nurses prepared academically are increasing, there remains a critical need for gerontological nurses to meet the needs of a rapidly aging population. Most nurses will care for older people during the course of their careers. In addition, the public will look to nurses to have the knowledge and skills to assist people to age in health and to provide guidance to individuals and families facing the social and health challenges that often accompany aging. Positive interactions with older people over the course of a nurse's life, faculty role models, a deep commitment to caring, and an appreciation of the significant contribution of a nursing model of care to the well-being of older people, are often the motivating factors that draw nurses to the specialty. Box 2-1 presents the views of some of the geriatric nursing pioneers, as well as of current leaders, on the practice of gerontological nursing and what draws them to the specialty.

History of Gerontological Nursing

Historically, nurses have always been in the frontlines of caring for older people. They have provided hands-on care, supervision, administration, program development, teaching, and research and are, to a great extent, responsible for the rapid advance of gerontology as a profession. Nurses have been, and continue to be, the mainstay of care of older adults (Mezey and Fulmer, 2002). Gerontological nurses have made substantial

contributions to the body of knowledge guiding best practice in care of older people. In examining the history of gerontological nursing, one must marvel at the advocacy and perseverance of nurses who have remained deeply committed to the care of older adults despite struggling against insurmountable odds over the years. We are proud to be the standard-bearers of excellence in care of older people. Box 2-2 presents a timeline of significant accomplishments in the history of gerontological nursing.

The origins of gerontological nursing go back to when Florence Nightingale, the founder of modern nursing, accepted a position as superintendent in an institution comparable to today's nursing home, the Institution for the Care of Sick Gentlewomen in Distressed Circumstances. Patients at this institution were primarily governesses and ladies' maids from wealthy English families (Wykle and McDonald, 1997). Awareness of the need for education in gerontological nursing, as well as the need for improvement in the care of institutionalized older adults, was first noted in the American nursing literature in the early 1900s. In 1908, Lavinia Dock, editor of the *American Journal of Nursing*, discussed the findings of a scathing report on conditions in almshouses (early nursing homes) and supported the need for trained nurses to work in these institutions and for student education in almshouses (Dock, 1908). Another editorial in the *American Journal of Nursing* in 1925 called for nurses to consider a specialty in nursing care of the aged. Again, in 1943, an article describing nursing care of the aged recommended that nurses with special aptitude care for the aged and that nursing and medical schools include geriatric education (Geldbach, 1943). The first book on gerontological nursing was written by Newton and Anderson in 1950 and in 1966, the Division of Geriatric Nursing Practice was established within the ANA, giving the nursing care of older people specialty status along with maternal-child, medical-surgical, psychiatric, and community health.

In 1965, establishment of nationalized health care for older people in the form of Medicare and Medicaid and passage of The Older Americans Act brought major changes in the way health care for the elderly was financed. All older people over the age of 65 were provided assurance of access to health care. Care for older adults shifted away from the family to the federal government, and the growth of the nursing home industry began. The study of aging accelerated with more research and development of the scientific basis for much of the modern perspective on aging. Federal funding for

Box 2-1   Reflections on Gerontological Nursing From Gerontological Nursing Pioneers and Current Leaders in the Field

Doris Schwartz, Gerontological Nursing Pioneer

"We need to remind ourselves constantly that the purpose of gerontic nursing is to prevent untimely death and needless suffering, always with the focus of doing *with* as well as doing *for*, and in every instance to attempt to preserve personhood as long as life continues." (From interview data collected by Priscilla Ebersole between 1990 and 2001.)

Mary Opal Wolanin, Gerontological Nursing Pioneer

"I believe that one of the most valuable lessons I have learned from those who are older is that I must start with looking inside at my own thinking. I was very guilty of ageism. I believed every myth in the book, was sure that I would never live past my seventieth birthday, and made no plan for my seventies. Probably the most productive years of my career have been since that dreaded birthday and I now realize that it is very difficult, if not impossible, to think of our own aging." (From interview data collected by Priscilla Ebersole between 1990 and 2001.)

Terry Fulmer, Dean, College of Nursing, New York University and Co-Director, John A. Hartford Institute for Geriatric Nursing

"I soon realized that in the arena of caring for the aged, I could have an autonomous nursing practice that would make a real difference in medical outcomes. I could practice the full scope of nursing. It gave me a sense of freedom and accomplishment. With older patients, the most important component of care, by far, is nursing care. It's very motivating." (Ebersole P, Touhy T: *Geriatric nursing: growth of a specialty*, New York, 2006, Springer, p. 129.)

Neville Strumpf, Edith Clement Chair in Gerontological Nursing, University of Pennsylvania, Director of the Hartford Center of Geriatric Nursing Excellence and Center for Gerontological Nursing Science

"My philosophy remains deeply rooted in individual choice, comfort and dignity, especially for frail, older adults. I fervently hope that the future will be characterized by a health care system capable of supporting these values throughout a person's life, and that we shall someday see the routine application of evidence based practice to the care of all older adults, whether they are in the community, a hospital, or the nursing home. We have not yet achieved that dream." (Ebersole P, Touhy T: *Geriatric nursing: growth of a specialty*, New York, 2006, Springer, p. 145.)

Mathy Mezey, Independence Foundation Professor of Nursing Education, Division of Nursing, Steinhardt School of Education at New York University and Director, John A. Hartford Foundation Institute for Geriatric Nursing at New York University

"Because geriatric nursing especially offers nurses the unique opportunity to dramatically impact people's lives for the better and for the worst, it demands the best that you have to offer. I am very optimistic about the future of geriatric nursing. Increasing numbers of older adults are interested in marching into old age as healthy and involved. Geriatric nursing offers a unique opportunity to help older adults meet these aspirations while at the same time maintaining a commitment to the oldest and frailest in our society." (Ebersole P, Touhy T: *Geriatric nursing: growth of a specialty*, New York, 2006, Springer, p. 142.)

Jennifer Lingler PhD, FNP

"When I was in high school, a nurse I knew helped me find a nursing assistant position at the residential care facility where she worked. That experience sparked my interest in older adults that continues today. I realized that caring for frail elders could be incredibly gratifying, and I felt privileged to play a role, however small, in people's lives. At the same time, I became increasingly curious about what it means to age successfully. I questioned why some people seemed to age so gracefully, while others succumbed to physical illness, mental decline, or both. As a Building Academic Geriatric Nursing Capacity (BAGNC) alumnus, I now divide my time serving as a nurse practitioner at a memory disorders clinic, teaching an ethics course in a gerontology program, and conducting research on family caregiving. I am encouraged by the realization that as current students contemplate the array of opportunities before them, seek counsel from trusted mentors, and gain exposure to various clinical populations, the next generation of geriatric nurses will emerge. And, I am confident that in doing so, they will set their own course for affecting change in the lives of society's most vulnerable members." (Jennifer Lingler as cited in Fagin C, Franklin P: Why choose geriatric nursing? Six nursing scholars tell their stories, *Imprint*, September/October, 2005, p. 74.)

Box 2-2	Professionalization of Gerontological Nursing: A Timeline

1906	First article published in *American Journal of Nursing* (*AJN*) on care of the aged
1925	*AJN* considers geriatric nursing a possible specialty in nursing
1950	Newton and Anderson publish first geriatric nursing textbook
	Geriatrics becomes a specialization in nursing
1962	American Nurses Association (ANA) forms a national geriatric nursing group
1966	ANA creates the Division of Geriatric Nursing
	First master's program for clinical nurse specialists in geriatric nursing developed by Virginia Stone at Duke University
1970	ANA establishes Standards of Practice for Geriatric Nursing committee, chaired by Dorothy Moses; included Lois Knowles and Mary Shaunnessey
1973	ANA defines *Standards of Practice for Geriatric Nursing*
1974	Certification in geriatric nursing practice offered through ANA; process implemented by Laurie Gunter and Virginia Stone
1975	*Journal of Gerontological Nursing* published by Slack; first editor, Edna Stilwell
1976	ANA renames Geriatric Division "Gerontological" to reflect a health promotion emphasis
	ANA publishes *Standards for Gerontological Nursing Practice*, a revision of the 1973 *Standards of Practice for Geriatric Nursing;* committee chaired by Barbara Allen Davis
	ANA begins certifying geriatric nurse practitioners
	Nursing and the Aged edited by Irene Burnside and published by McGraw-Hill
1977	First gerontological nursing track funded by Division of Nursing and established by Sr. Rose Therese Bahr at University of Kansas School of Nursing
1979	*Education for Gerontic Nursing* written by Gunter and Estes; suggested curricula for all levels of nursing education
	ANA Council of Long Term Care Nurses established; group first chaired by Ella Kick
1980	*Geriatric Nursing* first published by *AJN*; Cynthia Kelly, editor
1981	ANA Division of Gerontological Nursing issues statement regarding scope of practice
1983	Florence Cellar Endowed Gerontological Nursing Chair established at Case Western Reserve University, first in the nation; Doreen Norton, first scholar to occupy chair
	National Conference of Gerontological Nurse Practitioners established
1984	National Gerontological Nurses Association established
	Division of Gerontological Nursing Practice becomes Council on Gerontological Nursing (councils established for all practice specialties)
1986	ANA publishes survey of gerontological nurses in clinical practice
1987	ANA issues *Scope and Standards of Gerontological Nursing Practice,* a revision of the 1973 and 1976 documents
1989	ANA certifies gerontological clinical nurse specialists
1990	ANA establishes a Division of Long-Term Care within the Council of Gerontological Nursing
1992	ANA redefines long-term care to include life-span approach
	John A. Hartford Foundation funds a major initiative to improve care of hospitalized older patients: Nurses Providing Care for Health System Elders (NICHE)
1993	National Institute of Nursing Research established as separate entity
1994	ANA redefines *Scope and Standards of Gerontological Nursing Practice*
1996	John A. Hartford Foundation establishes the Institute for Geriatric Nursing at New York University under the direction of Mathy Mezey
2000	Recommended baccalaureate competencies and curricular guidelines for geriatric nursing care published by the American Association of Colleges of Nursing and the John A. Hartford Foundation Institute for Geriatric Nursing
2001	ANA, in collaboration with the National Gerontological Nursing Association, National Association of Directors of Nursing Administration in Long Term Care, and the National Conference of Gerontological Nurse Practitioners, publishes revised *Scope and Standards of Gerontological Nursing Practice* and reaffirms the need for competent gerontological nursing

Box 2-2	Professionalization of Gerontological Nursing: A Timeline—cont'd

2003	Nurse Competence in Aging (funded by Atlantic Philanthropies) initiative to improve the quality of health care to older adults by enhancing the geriatric competence of nurses who are members of specialty nursing associations (ANA, American Nurses Credentialing Center [ANCC], John A. Hartford Foundation Institute for Geriatric Nursing)
2004	*Nurse Practitioner and Clinical Nurse Specialist Competencies for Older Adult Care* published by the American Association of Colleges of Nursing and the Hartford Geriatric Nursing Initiative
	ANA Scope and Standards of Practice for all registered nurses referenced to include care of older adults
	Terry Fulmer becomes the first nursing president of the Gerontological Society of America
	"A New Look at the Old," a collaborative effort between the *AJN* and the Gerontological Society of America, supported with funding from Atlantic Philanthropies available to nurses and other providers in either print format or streaming video. This series details best practices around issues in the care of older adults. All materials available at no cost and can be found at www.nursingcenter.com
2005	Fifth White House Conference on Aging
2007	Atlantic Philanthropies provides a grant to the American Academy of Nursing of $500,000 to improve care of older adults in nursing homes by improving the clinical skills of professional nurses
2008	Four new Centers of Geriatric Nursing Excellence (CGNE) are funded by the John A. Hartford Foundation. The new centers at Arizona State University, Pennsylvania State University, the University of Minnesota, and the University of Utah will each receive $1 million to prepare over 500 nursing faculty with expertise in geriatrics
	Research in Gerontological Nursing launched by Slack; Dr. Kitty Buckwalter, Editor
	"How to Try This" series developed to build geriatric assessment skills (www.hartfordign.org/trythis) available as a cost-free, web-based resource including demonstration videos and a corresponding print series, available in *AJN*

nursing education also increased, particularly at the master's and doctoral levels.

The first master's program to prepare nurses as clinical nurse specialists in gerontological nursing was developed in 1966 by Virginia Stone at Duke University. In 1973, the ANA's Division of Geriatric Nursing Practice was the first to publish standards of practice. The standards were revised in 1976 and reissued as *Standards for Gerontological Nursing Practice,* and the name of the division was changed to Gerontological Nursing Practice. In 1974, geriatric nursing was the first certification program offered by the ANA and nursing was the first professional group to develop standards of care and certification in the field of gerontology. In the mid 1970s, certificate and master's programs to prepare gerontological nurse practitioners were begun with funding from the Department of Health, Education, and Welfare. Whereas most specialties in nursing practice developed from those identified in medicine, this was not the case with the specialty of gerontological nursing since health care of the elderly was traditionally considered to fall within the domain of nursing (Davis, 1984).

Gerontological nurse educators, scholars, and clinicians continue their commitment to and advocacy for older people. Gerontological nursing research has provided a solid knowledge base for important clinical issues such as restraint reduction, incontinence, care of people with Alzheimer's disease, informal caregiving, nutrition, health promotion, care environments, physical and emotional health, transitional care, and reminiscence therapy (Fitzpatrick and Fulmer, 2000).

Gerontological nursing research has gained wide acceptance in the scientific community and has made significant contributions to improved patient care and to policy decisions that influence care outcomes, particularly in the long-term care setting. Gerontological nurses have taken their place as vital members of the interdisciplinary community of gerontology professionals. Advanced-practice gerontological nurses have demonstrated positive outcomes as well as cost-effectiveness across a variety of settings. Research has shown that better care for older adults is possible and should be expected. The task before us now is to communicate the knowledge to all nurses who care for older adults in all settings (Mezey and Fulmer, 2002). May Wykle and Ruth Tappen, gerontological nursing scholars, educators, and researchers, provided suggestions for future research (see Box 2-3).

Box 2-3	Future Directions for Gerontological Nursing Research as Suggested by Wykle and Tappen

- Staffing patterns and the most appropriate mix to improve care outcomes in long-term care settings
- The influence of culture, diversity, and ethnicity on aging
- Health disparities and health literacy
- Factors contributing to successful aging, health promotion, and wellness in the upcoming Baby Boomer generation
- Retirement decisions of the Baby Boomers: how they are made and how they are changing
- Dementia as a chronic illness and staying well in the presence of the disease
- Caregiving, particularly intergenerational
- Values and attitudes of the current generation toward aging and expectations of its members
- Interventions to assist with the increasing prevalence of drug and alcohol abuse and other mental health problems of the current and future generations of older adults
- Integration of current best practice protocols into settings across the continuum in cost-effective and care-efficient models
- Models of acute care designed to prevent negative outcomes in elders
- Strategies to increase preparation in gerontological nursing and increased recruitment of the brightest and best into gerontological nursing
- Models of interdisciplinary practice
- Health promotion and illness management interventions in the assisted living setting; role of professional nurses and advanced-practice nurses in this setting; aging in place
- Development of models for end-of-life care in home and nursing home

From Ebersole P, Touhy T: *Geriatric nursing: growth of a specialty,* New York, 2006, Springer.

ANA and the *Scope and Standards of Gerontological Nursing Practice*

To develop accurate and informed attitudes, gerontological nursing organizations have established standards, legitimized the specialty, upgraded the knowledge base, enhanced the image of gerontological nurses, and identified the benefits of working with older adults. In 1995 and 2001, the ANA updated the *Scope and Standards of Gerontological Nursing Practice,* and revision was again begun in 2008.

The 2001 edition of the scope and standards was published jointly with the National Gerontological Nursing Association, the National Conference of Gerontological Nurse Practitioners, and the National Association of Directors of Nursing Administration in Long-Term Care. The 2001 document emphasizes the need for competence in the care of older adults so that professional nurses will be prepared to "meet the special needs of the increasing numbers of older adults, particularly those over 85 years of age, minorities, and those with decreased financial and social resources" (ANA, 2001, p. 7). The scope of practice for gerontological nursing, levels of gerontological nursing practice (basic and advanced), standards of

clinical gerontological nursing care, and gerontological nursing performance are discussed in the document (Box 2-4). The 2004 ANA *Scope and Standards of Practice* for all registered nurses now also includes specific reference to care of older adults recognizing that this population comprises the majority of patients in acute, home and long-term care facilities.

Certification is a means of assuring the public that the certified individual has pursued some specialized study in a given area, has successfully demonstrated the requisite knowledge, and has been awarded recognition of this achievement. ANA certification in gerontological nursing is one way to verify professional competency and assures nursing colleagues, the public, and employers that the nurse has specialized skills and knowledge in providing care to older people. A nurse with a diploma or an associate or baccalaureate education can be certified as a gerontological nurse. Nurses with master's degrees (clinical nurse specialists and nurse practitioners) can become certified at the advanced level. For additional information on certification, see the following websites: www.nursingworld.org/ and www.nursingworld.org/ancc/.

Box 2-4	Knowledge and Skills for Basic Gerontological Nursing

- Recognize the right of competent older adults to make their own care decisions and assist them in making informed choices.
- Establish a therapeutic relationship with the older adult to facilitate development of the plan of care, which may include family participation as needed.
- Use current gerontological standards to initiate, develop, and adapt the older adult's plan of care while involving the patient, family, and other providers as needed.
- Recognize age-related changes based on an understanding of physiological, emotional, cultural, social, psychological, economic, and spiritual functioning.
- Collect data to determine health status and functional abilities to plan, implement, and evaluate care.
- Participate and collaborate with members of the interdisciplinary team.
- Participate with older adults, their families if needed, and other health professionals in ethical decision making that is centered on the older adult, empathetic, and humane.
- Serve as an advocate for older adults and their families.
- Teach older adults and families about measures that promote, maintain, and restore health and functional performance; promote comfort; foster independence; and preserve dignity.
- Refer older adults to other professionals or community resources for assistance as necessary.
- Identify common chronic and/or acute physical and mental health processes and problems that affect older adults.
- Apply the existing body of knowledge in gerontology to nursing practice and intervention.
- Exercise accountability to older adults by protecting their rights and autonomy, recognizing and respecting their decisions about advance directives.
- Facilitate palliative care and comfort during the dying process to preserve dignity.
- Support the surviving spouse and family members, providing strength, comfort, and hope.
- Use the standards of gerontological nursing practice and collaborate with other health care professionals to improve the quality of care and the quality of life of older adults.
- Engage in professional development through participation in continuing education, involvement in state and national professional organizations, and certification.

From American Nurses Association: *Scope and standards of gerontological nursing practice*, Washington, DC, 2001, ANA, pp 8-9.

GERONTOLOGICAL NURSING EDUCATION

Ensuring gerontological nursing competency in all students graduating from a nursing program is imperative for the improvement of health care to older adults. Yet, schools of nursing have only recently begun to include gerontological nursing content in their curricula, and most still do not have freestanding courses in the specialty similar to courses in maternal-child or psychiatric nursing. Often the content, difficult to promote, has met with resistance on the part of faculty. Reasons posed for this include the following: faculty may not have the expertise or enthusiasm, it is regarded as an extra requirement that overloads the already extensive informational requirements of the accrediting organizations, it is thought to be "integrated" throughout the program, and students tend to be most interested in critical care and maternity. Some of this is because of age identification and some

because more highly technical care is intriguing and challenging in a specific and concrete way that is not true of the subtle complexities of geriatric care. Still, many educational institutions have incorporated dynamic courses in aging into their curricula. Content issues that are sorely neglected and need to be included are health promotion, mental health, elder abuse, atypical presentation of illness, geriatric syndromes, acute care of older adults, long-term and palliative care, and aging in minority and rural populations.

The John A. Hartford Foundation has been responsible for some of the most significant advances in gerontological nursing, education, and research. In the past decade, the foundation has granted $40.7 million in various educational and clinical demonstrations of effective programmatic changes in the provision of care to older people (www.hartfordign.org). These initiatives include the Institute for Geriatric Nursing at New York University and the Centers for Geriatric Nursing Excellence at the University of Iowa, University of Arkansas,

University of Pennsylvania, University of California at San Francisco, Oregon Health Sciences University, Arizona State University, Pennsylvania State University, University of Minnesota, and University of Utah. The John A. Hartford Foundation Institute for Geriatric Nursing, under the direction of Mathy Mezey and Terry Fulmer, is the only nurse-led organization in the country seeking to shape the quality of the nation's health care for older Americans by promoting geriatric nursing excellence to the nursing profession and to the larger health care community.

The Hartford Institute for Geriatric Nursing and the American Association of Colleges of Nursing (AACN) partnered to develop gerontological nursing competencies and curriculum materials for baccalaureate programs (www.aacn.nche.edu/Education/gercomp.htm). Nationally recognized competencies in gerontological nursing have also been developed for graduate programs preparing advanced-practice nurses in specialties other than gerontological nursing who will work with older adults (www.aacn.nche.edu/Education/Hartford/OlderAdultCare.htm). An additional resource for faculty is *Caring for an Aging America: A Guide for Nursing Faculty* (Thornlow et al, 2006). Those in the field of nursing education must seriously consider specific minimum requirements in care of older adults at each level of education to fulfill the responsibility of nurses to the public and the profession and to meet accreditation criteria.

Another significant program is the Nurse Competence in Aging initiative (NCA), funded by the Atlantic Philanthropies and implemented through a strategic alliance between the ANA and the Hartford Institute for Geriatric Nursing. The initiative provides grant and technical assistance to 55 specialty nursing organizations to enhance the gerontological competence of their more than 400,000 members. A gerontological nursing resource center (ConsultGeriRN.org) and a national gerontological nursing certification outreach are components of this project. Goals and descriptions of these projects are described by Stierle et al (2006); in November/December 2007, *Geriatric Nursing* featured a special supplement on the results of the NCA initiative (Kancelbaum, 2007).

ROLES IN GERONTOLOGICAL NURSING

Gerontological nursing roles encompass every imaginable venue and circumstance. The opportunities are limitless because we are a rapidly aging society. Older adults are the largest consumers of health care services

in all settings (www.ConsultGeriRN.org). "Nurses have the potential to improve elder care across settings through effective screening and comprehensive assessment, facilitating access to programs and services, educating and empowering older adults and their families to improve their health and manage chronic conditions, leading and coordinating the efforts of members of the health care team, conducting and applying research, and influencing policy" (Young, 2003, p. 9).

A gerontological nurse may be a generalist or a specialist. The generalist provides care according to various models and draws on the expertise of the specialist in planning and evaluating care. To prepare nurse generalists, it is important to provide nursing practice experiences with elders across the continuum of care. For clinical practice sites one is not limited in gerontological nursing education to the acute care setting or the nursing home. Creative faculty members consider sites such as retirement homes, assisted living facilities, private practice with families, nutrition centers, home care agencies, adult day health programs, and senior housing complexes. Experiences with well elders in the community and opportunities to focus on health promotion should be the first experiences for students. This will assist them to develop more positive attitudes toward older people, understand the full scope of nursing practice in the specialty, and learn nursing responses to enhance health and wellness for older people. Rehabilitation centers, subacute and skilled nursing facilities, and hospice settings provide opportunities for leadership training, nursing management of complex problems, interdisciplinary teamwork, and research application for more advanced students.

The gerontological nursing specialist has advanced preparation at the master's level and performs all of the functions of the generalist but has developed advanced clinical expertise, as well as an understanding of health and social policy and proficiency in planning, implementing, and evaluating health programs. With shortages in nursing faculty prepared in gerontological nursing, there is a critical need for nurses to assume faculty roles who have master's and doctoral preparation and expertise in care of older adults.

One of the most important roles emerging in the past few decades is that of advanced-practice gerontological nurses (APGNs) as major service providers. APGNs include geriatric nurse practitioners (GNPs) and gerontological nursing clinical specialists (CNSs). The educational and training programs arose from evident need, particularly in long-term care settings. Beginning with a mentorship and continuing education model, the requirements now include a master's degree. APGNs practice in the full range of settings in which older adults can be found including nursing homes, acute care and subacute care facilities, assisted living and retirement complexes, health maintenance organizations, adult day health programs, community clinics, physicians' offices, independent practices, and any situation requiring expert nursing in combination with midlevel medical practitioner skills. There are at present a full range of opportunities and roles to be filled. Practice privileges vary from state to state, but the federal Medicaid and Medicare programs allow for individual provider numbers and direct reimbursement for nationally certified APGNs.

Advanced-practice nurses have demonstrated their skill in improving health outcomes as well as cost-effectiveness. The role of APGNs in nursing homes is well established, and the positive outcomes for care include increased patient and family satisfaction, decreased costs, less frequent hospitalizations and emergency room visits, and improved quality of care (Ryden et al, 2000; Bourbonniere and Evans, 2002; Kane et al, 2004; Mezey et al, 2004a; Stolee et al, 2006; Ryden et al, 2000). Currently, fewer than 6% of all advanced-practice nurses are certified as GNPs and gerontological clinical nurse specialists. These numbers are far short of the current and projected need for advanced-practice nurses specializing in the care of older adults. Family and adult nurse practitioner programs often attract more students, and many of these students go on to practices that include a large number of older adults. Some have had intensive attention in their curricula to gerontological nursing care, but some have not and must learn on the job. Major problems are the lack of faculty with the necessary level of gerontological nursing expertise, sparse attention to gerontological nursing in basic nursing programs, and the routing of federal grants for education in medicine and nursing to family practice. Mezey and Fulmer (2002) suggest that all graduate programs should be "gerontologized" and all nurse practitioner graduates should have gerontological nursing competencies to meet the health care needs of an aging population.

Generalist Roles Across the Continuum of Care

Acute Care

Older adults often enter the health care system with admissions to acute care settings. Older adults comprise 60% of medical-surgical patients and 46% of critical care patients (Mezey et al, 2007). Kagan (2008) reminds us that "older adults are the work of hospitals but most nurses practicing in hospitals do not say they specialize in geriatrics…We, as a profession and a force in an aging society, must make the transformation to understanding care of older adults is acute care nursing…Care of older adults would be the rule instead of the exception" (2008, p. 103). Kagan goes on to suggest that such a transformation would mean that acute care nurses would proudly describe themselves as geriatric nurses with subspecialities (geriatric vascular nurses, geriatric radiology nurses) and, along with geriatric nurse generalists, would populate hospital nursing services across the country.

Exacerbations of chronic illnesses and injuries are often the cause of hospitalizations for older adults. Acutely ill older adults frequently have multiple chronic conditions and comorbidities and present many care challenges (Benedict, Robinson & Holder, 2006). Hospitals are dangerous places for elders: 34% experience functional decline, and iatrogenic complications occur in as many as 29% to 38%, a rate 3 to 5 times higher than in younger patients (Inouye et al, 2000; Kleinpell, 2007). Common iatrogenic complications include functional decline, new-onset incontinence, malnutrition, pressure ulcers, medication reactions, and falls.

Recognizing the impact of iatrogenesis, both on patient outcomes and cost of care, CMS has instituted changes to the inpatient prospective payment system that will reduce payment to hospitals relative to poor care. Many of these conditions are directly related to nursing care and reinforce the need for hospital nurses to be competent in the care of older adults. "These changes target conditions that have a high cost or high volume and result in higher payment when present as a secondary diagnosis, are not present on admission, and could have reasonably been prevented through the application of evidence-based guidelines" (Welton, 2008, p. 325). Targeted conditions include catheter-associated urinary track infections, pressure ulcers, and falls. In 2009, additional targeted conditions may include delirium, deep vein thrombosis, and clostridium difficile-associated disease, conditions that are very common in older hospitalized patients.

Nurses caring for older adults in hospitals may function in the direct care provider role, as well as in leadership and management positions. Most nurses who work in hospitals are caring for older patients, and many have not had gerontological nursing content in their basic nursing education programs. In a recent survey of hospital nurses, only 37% reported participating in a hospital in-service training program on care of older adults (Mezey et al, 2007). "Few of the country's approximately 6000 hospitals have institutional practice guidelines, educational resources, and administrative practices that support best practices care of older adults" (Boltz et al, 2008, p. 176).

The Nurse Competence in Aging initiative, described earlier in this chapter, is an effort to enhance the knowledge of practicing nurses in gerontological nursing. "Nurses who care for older critically ill patients must have a rehabilitation and restorative philosophy that values such basic care interventions as ensuring a safe environment and providing good nutrition, meticulous skin and oral care, and bladder retraining as much as the importance of more highly technical tasks, as they strive to prevent functional decline" (Kaplow and Hardin, 2007, p. 86).

Recognizing the need for models of nursing practice to prevent iatrogenesis and improve outcomes for older hospitalized patients, the Hartford Geriatric Nursing Institute developed the Nurses Improving Care for Health System Elders (NICHE) program. More than 200 hospitals in more than 40 states, as well as parts of Canada, are involved in NICHE projects. NICHE units of various types have been developed including the geriatric resource nurse (GRN) model and the acute care of the elderly (ACE) unit (www.nicheprogram. org/about).

In the GRN model, staff nurses are trained by advanced-practice gerontological nurses, and then they function as clinical resource experts on geriatric issues to other nurses on their unit. This is an innovative role for a hospital staff nurse interested in care of older adults. Outcomes in hospitals using NICHE models include enhanced nursing knowledge and skills related to treatment of common geriatric syndromes, improved patient satisfaction, decreased length of stay, reductions in admission rates, and reductions in hospital costs (Fulmer et al, 2002; Mezey et al, 2004b; Boltz et al, 2008).

Community- and Home-Based Care

Nurses will care for older adults in hospitals and long-term care but the majority of older adults live in the community. Only about 6% of older adults at any given time reside in nursing homes, although a greater percentage can expect to spend some time in the setting, often recovering from acute illness or accidents. Community-based care settings include home care, independent senior housing, retirement communities, adult day health programs, primary care clinics, and public health departments. The growth in home- and community-based health care is expected to continue since older people prefer to age in place. Nurses in the home setting provide comprehensive assessments and may provide and supervise care for older people with a variety of care needs including chronic wounds, intravenous therapy, tube feedings, unstable medical conditions, and complex medication regimens, and for those receiving rehabilitation services. Advances in technology for remote monitoring of health status, as well as safety, show promise in improving outcomes for elders who want to age in place. These technologies present exciting opportunities for nurses in the management and evaluation of care (see Chapter 15). Gerontological nurses will find opportunities to create practices in community-based settings with a focus not only on care for those who are ill but also on health promotion.

Long-Term Care

When long-term care is discussed, many nurses, as well as the general public, may think only of the nursing home. In reality, long-term care comprises a variety of health, social, and personal care that is provided during an extended period to persons of all ages who need help managing chronic illness or functional and cognitive deficits. Older people comprise the majority of those needing long-term care. It is important to note that the majority of long-term care is provided by family, not agencies and institutions. Discussion of the varying levels of long-term care and family caregiving issues are discussed in more depth in Chapters 23 and 26.

Nursing homes have evolved into a significant location where health care is provided across the continuum. Nursing homes today are complex health care settings that are a mix of hospital, rehabilitation facility, hospice, and dementia-specific units, and are for many elders a final home. Nurses accustomed to practice in an acute care hospital will find many differences in subacute and skilled nursing facilities. Differences in focus of care and goals between acute and long-term care are presented in Boxes 2-5 and 2-6. In addition, stringent federal regulations governing care practices, the interdisciplinary team model, greater use of licensed practical nurses (LPNs) and nursing assistants, and the more limited presence of medical providers on site influence the role of professional nursing in this setting. Excellent assessment skills; ability to work in partnership with other team members and families; skills in acute, rehabilitative, and palliative care; and leadership, management, and delegation skills are essential. Box 2-7 presents suggested resources related to leadership in long-term care.

Box 2-5	Focus of Acute and Long-Term Care

Acute Care Orientation
- Illness
- High technology
- Short term
- Episodic
- One-dimensional
- Professional
- Medical model
- Cure

Long-Term Care Orientation
- Function
- High touch
- Extended
- Interdisciplinary model
- Ongoing
- Multidimensional
- Paraprofessional and family
- Care

Adapted from Ouslander J, Osterweil D, Morley J: *Medical care in the nursing home*, New York, 1997, McGraw-Hill.

Box 2-7	Resources for Leadership in Long-Term Care

- Sullivan-Marx E, Gray-Micelli D: *Leadership and Management Skills for Long-Term Care,* New York, 2008, Springer.
- Long-Term Care Nursing Leadership and Management, University of Minnesota Center for Gerontological Nursing. Available at www.nursing.umn.edu/CGN/LTCNurseLeader/LeadershipResources/home.html.
- American College of Health Care Administrators: *Effective Leadership in Long-Term Care: The Need and the Opportunity,* 2008. Available at http://www.achca.org/content/pdf/achca_leadership_need_and_opportunity_paper_dana-olson.pdf
- Association of Homes & Services for the Aging and the Institute for the Future of Aging: *The Long-Term Care Workforce: Can the Crisis be Fixed?,* 2007. Available at: http://www.futureofaging.org/publications/pub_documents/LTCCommissionReport2007.pdf.
- Institute of Medicine: *Retooling for an Aging America: Building the Health Care Workforce,* 2008. Available at: http://www.iom.edu/?ID=53452.

Box 2-6	Goals of Long-Term Care

1. Provide a safe and supportive environment for chronically ill and functionally dependent people.
2. Restore and maintain highest practicable level of functional independence.
3. Preserve individual autonomy.
4. Maximize quality of life, well-being, and satisfaction with care.
5. Provide comfort and dignity at the end of life for residents and their families.
6. Provide coordinated interdisciplinary care to subacutely ill residents who plan to return to home or a less restrictive level of care.
7. Stabilize and delay progression, when possible, of chronic medical conditions.
8. Prevent acute medical and iatrogenic illnesses and identify and treat them rapidly when they do occur.
9. Create a homelike environment that respects dignity of each resident.

Adapted from Ouslander J, Osterweil D, Morley J: *Medical care in the nursing home*, New York, 1997, McGraw-Hill.

Professional nurses in nursing homes must be highly skilled and often practice much more independently because there are fewer physicians in the nursing home setting. This setting provides significant opportunities for independent decision making, nursing leadership, and evaluation of nursing models of care on patient outcomes. Roles may include nursing administrator, manager, supervisor, educator, Minimum Data Set (MDS) coordinator, case manager, quality improvement coordinator, and direct care provider.

Many nursing homes offer subacute care units that function much like the general medical-surgical hospital units of the past. Subacute care is more intensive than traditional nursing home care and several times more costly, but far less costly than care in an acute-care hospital. The expectation is that the patient will be discharged home or to a less intensive settings. Length of stay is usually less than 1 month and is largely reimbursed by Medicare. Patients in subacute units are usually younger and less likely to be cognitively impaired than those in traditional nursing home care. Generally, higher levels of professional nurse staffing are found in the subacute setting than in the traditional nursing home because of the acuity of the patients' condition.

Nursing homes also care for patients who need skilled nursing care but who may not need the intense care that is given in subacute units. Persons in skilled care may include those with severe stroke, dementia, Parkinson's disease, and those receiving hospice care. More than 50% of the residents in nursing homes are cognitively impaired, and nursing homes are increasingly caring for people at the end of life (Alzheimer's Association, 2007). Twenty-three percent of Americans die in nursing homes, and this figure is expected to increase 40% by 2040 (Carlson, 2007). Nursing home residents represent the most frail of the older adult population; their needs for 24-hour care could not be met in the home or residential care setting, or may have exceeded what the family was able to provide.

Predictions of a more than threefold increase in the numbers of older people residing in nursing homes by 2030, and critical shortages of all levels of nursing personnel in the nursing home setting, make a compelling case for increased education and recruitment of gerontological nurses as well as creation of new models of care. Those who live to the age of 85 will have one in two chances of spending some time in a nursing home (Teno, 2002). A growing concern is the lack of adequate staffing of professional nurses in nursing homes (Mezey and Harrington, 2005). Despite increases in the acuity level of nursing-home patients' conditions and the positive relationship between nurse staffing and quality of care, the care provided in U.S. nursing homes continues to be almost devoid of the participation of professional nurses.

A study by the Centers for Medicare and Medicaid Services (CMS) revealed that registered nurse (RN) staffing levels below 0.75 hours/resident day can jeopardize health and safety, and yet approximately 97% of nursing homes do not meet these standards (Mezey and Harrington, 2005). Current federal standards require only one RN in the nursing home for 8 hours a day—a figure quite shocking considering the ratio of RNs to patients in acute care, even in the face of shortages in that setting. More RN direct-care time per resident in nursing homes is associated with fewer pressure ulcers, fewer hospitalizations, fewer urinary tract infections, less weight loss, fewer catheterizations, and less deterioration in the ability to perform activities of daily living (ADLs) (Horn et al, 2005).

An expert panel on nursing home care convened by the John A. Hartford Institute for Geriatric Nursing (Harrington et al, 2000) provided comprehensive recommendations for improved RN staffing, increased gerontological nursing education requirements for all staff, including a bachelor of science in nursing (BSN) degree for directors of nursing, and increased staffing ratios for RNs, LPNs, and nursing assistants. Additional recommendations were that most nursing homes should have a full-time CNS or GNP on staff. Many groups dealing with issues of the aging as well as the ANA have supported the critical need for adequate staffing in nursing homes, but to date the federal government has not acted to mandate increases in minimum staffing requirements.

For those of us committed to quality care for the most frail of our elders, the lack of professional nurse staffing in nursing homes is reason for grave concern. We urge our readers to join with the professional nursing organizations and consumer advocacy groups to lobby for adequate nurse staffing with funding to support it, improved education in gerontological nursing, and an increasing presence of professional nurses in nursing homes. The culture change movement, discussed in Chapter 26, provides many exciting opportunities for professional nurses to lead the change from an institution-centered to a person-centered culture in the nursing home setting. We agree with Eliopoulos (2001, pp. 533-537): "The increased demands and complexities of long-term care facilities necessitate that highly competent nurses be employed in this setting...gerontological nurses can cast a new vision for long-term care that can enable residents of nursing facilities to experience the highest possible quality of life for the time remaining in their lives."

Certified Nursing Assistants and Nurse Aides

Although it is important to promote professional nursing care for all elders, certified nursing assistants (CNAs) provide the majority of direct care in nursing homes and significantly contribute to the quality of life for nursing home residents. Critical shortages of CNAs exist now in both skilled care and home care, and these shortages will worsen in the future. "Difficulty recruiting and retaining these long-term care workers continues to plague nursing homes, as turnover rates approach 100%" (Carpenter and Thompson, 2008). Several recent studies have investigated the relationship of factors such as turnover, work satisfaction, staffing, and power relations to quality of care and positive outcomes in nursing homes. Results support the importance of developing a culture of respect in which the work of CNAs is understood and valued at all levels of the organization. Research findings also indicate that the most influential factor in turnover among CNAs was the perception that they were not appreciated or valued by the organization (Bowers, Esmond et al, 2003).

Results of several studies confirm the deep committment and passion that nursing assistants bring to their jobs as they "struggle to find and maintain a balance between the task-oriented needs of residents (e.g. bathing, toileting, feeding) and developing relationships and building community" (Carpenter and Thompson, 2008, p. 31). The significance and importance of close personal relationships between nursing assistants and residents, often described as "like family," is emerging as a central dimension of quality of care and postive outcomes (Bowers, Esmond et al, 2000, 2003; Carpenter and Thompson, 2008; Ersek, Kraybill and Hansberry, 2000; Parsons et al, 2003; Sikma, 2006; Touhy, Strews and Brown, 2005).

One of the most important components of the culture change movement is the creation of models of care that value and honor the important work of nursing assistants. Culture change must be equally concerned about the needs of residents and the well-being of staff (Thomas and Johnson, 2003). "An organization that learns to give love, respect, dignity, tenderness, and tolerance to all members of the staff will soon find these same virtues being practiced by the staff" (Thomas and Johnson, 2003, p. 3). Until we health care professionals and our society make a real commitment to providing adequate wages, individual supports (e.g., health insurance, education, career ladders), and an appreciation of their significant contribution to quality of nursing home care, these neglected workers cannot be expected to have the energy or incentive to extend themselves to the elders in their care (Kash et al, 2007). Chapter 26 discusses the culture change movement in more depth.

An important organization for nursing assistants in nursing homes is the National Association of Geriatric Nursing Assistants (NAGNA). NAGNA was established in 1995 as a professional association of CNAs. The purpose of NAGNA is to ensure that the highest quality of care is provided to our elders living in nursing homes, achieved by elevating the professional standing and performance of the caregivers. With a membership of more than 30,000 CNAs representing more than 500 nursing homes, the organization provides recognition for outstanding achievements, development training for CNAs, mentoring programs to reduce CNA turnover, and advocacy for issues important to long-term care and CNAs.

Another organization, the National Clearinghouse on the Direct Care Workforce, supports efforts to improve the quality of jobs for frontline workers who assist people who are elderly and/or living with disabilities. This organization provides information resources needed to effect change in industry practice, public policy, and public opinion. The clearinghouse is also working with the Paraprofessional Healthcare Institute to improve understanding for the direct care workforce crisis through research and analysis funded by the U.S. Department of Health and Human Services and the Center for Medicare and Medicaid Services.

GERONTOLOGICAL NURSING AND GERONTOLOGY ORGANIZATIONS

The Gerontological Society of America (GSA) demonstrates the need for interdisciplinary collaboration in research and practice. The divisions of Biological Sciences, Health Sciences, Behavioral and Social Sciences, Social Research, and Policy and Practice include individuals from myriad backgrounds and many disciplines who affiliate with a section based on their particular function rather than their educational or professional credentials. Nurses can be found in all sections and occupy important positions as officers and committee chairs in the GSA. The nurses' special interest group is the most rapidly growing membership contingent.

This mingling of the disciplines based on practice interests is also characteristic of the American Society on Aging (ASA). Other interdisciplinary organizations have joined forces to strengthen the field. The Association for Gerontology in Higher Education (AGHE) has partnered with GSA, and the National Council on Aging (NCOA) is affiliated with ASA. These organizations and others have encouraged the blending of ideas and functions, furthering our understanding of aging and of the integration necessary for optimum care. International gerontology associations such as the International Federation on Aging and the International Association of Gerontology and Geriatrics also have interdisciplinary membership and offer the opportunity to study aging internationally.

The American Medical Directors Association is a professional association of medical directors, physicians, and nurse practitioners practicing in the long-term care continuum, dedicated to obtaining excellence in patient care by providing education, advocacy, information, and professional development. The American Geriatrics Society is a professional organization of health care providers dedicated to improving the health and well-being of older adults. Both of these organizations have monthly journals and practice protocols for the care of older adults. These excellent evidence-based practice protocols are available on their websites.

Organizations specific to gerontological nursing include the National Gerontological Nursing Association (NGNA), the National Conference of Gerontological Nurse Practitioners (NCGNP), the National Association Directors of Nursing Administration in Long Term Care (NADONA/LTC) (also includes assisted living RNs and LPNs/LVNs as associate members), and the Canadian Gerontological Nursing Association (CGNA). The CGNA, founded in 1985, addresses the health needs of older Canadians and the nurses who care for them. The CGNA has developed *Scope and Standards of Practice for Gerontological Nursing*. In 2003 the CGNA and the NGNA formed an alliance to exchange information and share mutual goals and opportunities for the advancement of both groups (Mantle, 2005).

IMPLICATIONS FOR GERONTOLOGICAL NURSING AND HEALTHY AGING

Nursing is a vital aspect of the health care of older people, and the practice of gerontological nursing provides a unique vantage point from which to make an impact on it. Nurses attracted to this specialized field recognize that expertise in caring for older adults can make a significant difference in the quality of life of the persons served. In times of illness and rehabilitation and end of life care, outcomes for the older person more often than not depend on the nursing care received. Through research, gerontological nurses have made substantial contributions to the body of knowledge of best practices in the care of elders, and they are recognized as leaders in aging care.

Gerontological nurses have opportunities to provide care across the continuum of aging services, caring for everyone from the most ill and frail elders to those who are active and independent. As phrased by Mezey and Fulmer (2002), the commitment of gerontological nurses to "tackle difficult but exceptionally meaningful issues that impact profoundly on the health and quality of life for older adults, the opportunities for decision making, independent action, innovation, and the significant contribution of geriatric nursing research to improved patient outcomes and health policy position the specialty for continued growth, recognition, contribution and value to society" (Mezey & Fulmer, 2002, p. 440). Gerontological nursing may be the most needed specialty in nursing, both now and in the future (Ebersole and Touhy, 2006). As Mezey and Fulmer (2002) suggested, we need to ensure that in the future, all older adults will be cared for by a nurse who has received special preparation in gerontological nursing.

▶ KEY CONCEPTS

▶ Certification assures the public of nurses' commitment to specialized education and qualification for the care of the aged.

▶ All students graduating from nursing programs and all practicing nurses working with older adults should have competency in gerontological nursing.

▶ The major changes in health care delivery and the increasing numbers of older adults have resulted in numerous revised, refined, and emergent roles for nurses in the field of gerontological nursing. There is a critical shortage of competent and compassionate gerontological nurses.

▶ Advanced-practice nurses may have either nurse practitioner qualifications or clinical nurse specialist education or a combination of both.

▶ Advanced-practice role opportunities for nurses are numerous and offer more independence, are cost-effective, and facilitate more holistic health care and improved outcomes for patients.

▶ ACTIVITIES AND DISCUSSION QUESTIONS

1. Identify factors that have influenced the progress of gerontological nursing as a specialty practice.
2. Consider and discuss with classmates the various gerontological nursing roles that you find most interesting and stimulating.
3. Discuss what you consider the most important elements of the 2001 American Nurses Association *Scope and Standards of Practice for Gerontological Nursing.*
4. Discuss the gerontological organizations of today and their significance to the practicing nurse.
5. Why do you think more students do not choose gerontological nursing as a specialty? What would increase interest in this area of nursing?
6. What do you think are the most important issues in gerontological nursing education at this time?

▶ RESOURCES

Organizations

Hartford Institute for Geriatric Nursing
New York University, Steinhardt School of Education
Division of Nursing, John A. Hartford Foundation Institute for Geriatric Nursing

246 Greene Street
New York, NY 10003
(212) 998-9018; (212) 995-4561 (fax)
website: www.hartfordign.org

National Conference of Gerontological Nurse Practitioners
7794 Grow Drive
Pensacola, FL 32514
(866) 355-1392
website: www.ncgnp.org

National Gerontological Nursing Association (NGNA)
7794 Grow Drive
Pensacola, FL 32514-7072
(800) 723-0560
website: www.ngna.org

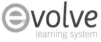

For additional resources, please visit evolve.elsevier.com/Ebersole/gerontological.

REFERENCES

Alzheimer's Association: *Dementia care practice recommendations for assisted living residences and nursing homes,* Chicago, IL, 2007, The Association.

American Nurses Association: *Scope and standards of gerontological nursing practice,* Washington, DC, 2001, The Association.

Benedict L, Robinson K, Holder C: Clinical nurse specialist practice within the acute care for elders interdisciplinary team model, *Clin Nurse Spec* 20(5):248-252, 2006.

Boltz M, Capezuti E, Bower-Ferres S, et al: Changes in the geriatric care environment associated with NICHE (Nurses Improving Care for Health System Elders), *Ger Nurs* 29(3):176-185, 2008.

Bourbonniere M, Evans L: Advanced practice nursing in the care of frail older adults, *J Am Geriatr Soc* 50(12):2062-2076, 2002.

Bowers B, Esmond S, Jacobson N: The relationship between staffing and quality in long-term care facilities: exploring the views of nurses aides, *Jour Nurs Care Quality* 14(4):55-64, 2000.

Bowers B, Esmond S, Jacobson N: Turnover reinterpreted: CNAs talk about why they leave, *Jour Gerontol Nurs* 29(3):36-43, 2003.

Burnside IM: *Nursing and the aged,* New York, 1988, McGraw-Hill.

Carlson A: Death in the nursing home: resident, family and staff perspectives, *J Gerontol Nurs* 33(4):32-41, 2007.

Carpenter J, Thompson SA: CNAs experience in the nursing home: "It's in my soul," *Jour Gerontol Nurs* 34(9):25-32, 2008.

Davis B: Nursing care of the aged: historical evolution. In Fondmiller S, editor: *Conference proceedings. Historical*

basis of clinical nursing practice in the United States. New Orleans, LA, Jun 26, 1984. Chicago, 1984, American Association for the History of Nursing.

Dock L: The crusade for almshouse nursing, *Am J Nurs* 8(7):520, 1908.

Ebersole P, Touhy T: *Geriatric nursing: growth of a specialty,* New York, 2006, Springer.

Editorial, *Am J Nurs,* 25, 394, May 1925

Editorial: A neglected field of nursing—the county almshouse, *Am J Nurs* 493-4, May 1906

Eliopoulos C: *Gerontological nursing,* Philadelphia, 2001, Lippincott Williams & Wilkins.

Ersek M, Kraybill B, Hansberry J: Educational needs and concerns of nursing home staff, *Jour Gerontol Nurs* 26(10):91-99, 2000.

Fitzpatrick JJ, Fulmer T, editors: *Geriatric nursing research digest,* New York, 2000, Springer.

Fulmer T et al: Nurses improving care for health system elders (NICHE): using outcomes and benchmarks for evidence-based practice, *Geriatr Nurs* 23(3):121-127, 2002.

Geldbach S: Nursing care of the aged, *Am J Nurs* 43(12):1113, 1943.

Gunter L, Estes C: *Education for gerontic nursing,* New York, 1979, Springer.

Harrington C et al: Experts recommend minimum nurse staffing standards for nursing facilities in the United States, *Gerontologist* 40(1):5-15, 2000.

Horn S, Buerhaus P, Bergstrom N, Smout R: RN staffing time and outcomes of long-stay nursing home residents, *Am J Nurs* 105(11):58-70, 2005.

Inouye S, Baker DI, Leo-Summers L: The hospital elder life progress: a model of care to prevent cognitive and functional decline in older hospitalized patients, *J Am Geriatr Soc* 48(12):1657-1706, 2000.

Kagan S: Moving from achievement to transformation, *Geriatr Nurs* 203:102-104, 2008.

Kane R, Flood S, Bershadsky B, Keckhafer F: Effect of an innovative Medicare managed care program on the quality of care for nursing home residents, *Gerontologist* 44(1):95-103, 2004.

Kancelbaum B, (2007) (ed.). *Enhancing care to older adults: specialty association efforts and achievements.* 28(6 Suppl), 1-40.

Kaplow R, Hardin S: *Critical care nursing: synergy for optimal outcomes,* Sudbury, MA, 2007, Jones and Bartlett.

Kash B, Castle N, Phillips C: Nursing home spending, staffing and turnover, *Health Care Manage Rev* 32(3):253-262, 2007.

Kleinpell R: Supporting independence in hospitalized elders in acute care, *Crit Care Nurs Clin N Am* 19:242-252, 2007.

Mantle JH: Personal correspondence, March 2, 2005.

Mezey MD, Fulmer TT: The future history of gerontological nursing, *J Gerontol* 57A(7): M438-M441, 2002.

Mezey M, Harrington C: Addressing the dramatic decline in RN staffing in nursing homes, *Am J Nurs* 105(9):25, 2005.

Mezey M, Harrington C, Kluger M: NPs in nursing homes: an issue of quality, *Am J Nurs* 104(9):71, 2004a.

Mezey M, Kobayashi M, Grossman S: Nurses improving care to health system elders (NICHE): implementation of best practice models, *J Nurs Adm* 34(10):451-457, 2004b.

Mezey M, Stierle L, Huba G, Esterson JM, et al: Ensuring competence of specialty nurses in care of older adults, *Geriatr Nurs* 28(6S): 9-13, 2007.

Newton K, Anderson H: *Geriatric nursing,* St. Louis, 1950, Mosby.

Parsons S, Simmons W, Penn K, Furlough M: Determinants of satisfaction and turnover among nursing assistants: results of a statewide survey, *Jour Gerontol Nurs* 29(3):51-60, 2003.

Ryden M, Snyder M, Gross C, et al: Value-added outcomes: the use of advanced practice nurses in long term care facilities, *Gerontologist* 40(6):654-662, 2000.

Sikma S: Staff perceptions of caring: the importance of a supportive environment, *Jour Gerontol Nurs* 32(6):22-29, 2006.

Stierle L, Mezez M, Schumann M, et al: Professional development: the nurse competence in aging initiative: encouraging expertise in the care of older adults, *Am J Nurs* 106(9):93-96, 2006.

Stolee P, Hillier L, Esbaugh N, et al: Examining the nurse practitioner in long-term care, *J Geron Nurs* 32(10):28-36, 2006.

Teno J: Now is the time to embrace nursing homes as a place of care for dying persons, *Innovations in End-of-Life Care* 4(2), 2002. Retrieved July 12, 2008 from www.edc.org/lastacts.

Thomas W, Johnson C: Elderhood in Eden, *Top Geriatr Rehabil* 19(4):282-289, 2003.

Thornlow D, Latimer D, Kingsborough J, Arietta L: *Caring for an aging America: a guide for nursing faculty,* 2006, American Association of Colleges of Nursing/John A. Hartford Foundation.

Touhy T, Strews W, Brown C: Staff perceptions of caring as lived by nursing home staff, residents and families, *Int J Hum Car* 9(3):31-36, 2005.

Welton J: Implications of medicare reimbursement changes related to inpatient nursing care quality, *JONA* 38(7/8):325-330, 2008.

Wykle M, McDonald P: The past, present, and future of gerontological nursing. In Klein S, editor: *A national agenda for geriatric education,* New York, 1997, Springer.

Young H: Challenges and solutions for care of frail older adults, *Online J Issues Nurs* 8(2):1-13, 2003.

Communicating with Elders

3

> ▶ **LEARNING OBJECTIVES**

Upon completion of this chapter, the reader will be able to:

- Describe the importance of communication to the lives of older adults.
- Discuss how ageist attitudes affect communication with older adults.
- Describe interventions that facilitate communication individually and in groups.
- Understand the significance of the life story of an elder.
- Discuss the modalities of reminiscence and life review.
- Identify effective communication strategies for older adults with speech, language, hearing, vision, and cognitive impairment.

> ▶ **GLOSSARY**

Ageism Discrimination against older people.
Aphasia A communication disorder that affects the ability to use and understand spoken or written words.
Apraxia An impairment in the ability to manipulate objects or perform purposeful acts, including speech.
Dysarthria A speech disorder caused by a weakness or incoordination of the muscles used for speech.

Elderspeak A common speech style used by younger people when talking to older people that communicates messages of dependence, incompetence, and control. Includes baby talk, using terms like "honey" and "dear," and speaking louder and more slowly.
Life review A critical analysis of one's past life with the goal of facilitating integrity.

> ▶ **THE LIVED EXPERIENCE**

Listen to the aged for they will tell you about living and dying.

Listen to the aged for they will enlighten you about problem-solving, sexuality, grief, sensory deprivation, and survival.

Listen to the aged for they will teach you how to be courageous, loving, and generous.

They are a distinguished faculty without formal classrooms, tenure, sabbaticals. They teach not from books but from long experience in living.

From Burnside IM: Listen to the aged, Am J Nurs 75(10):1801, 1975.

COMMUNICATING WITH ELDERS: GENERAL PRINCIPLES

Communication is the single most important capacity of human beings, the ability that gives us a special place in the animal kingdom. Little is more dehumanizing than the inability to reach out to others verbally. Maslow's hierarchy places the human need for affiliation second only to the need for safety and survival. The need to communicate, to be listened to, and to be heard, does not change with age or impairment. Meaningful communication and active involvement in society contributes to healthy aging, improves older adults' chances of living longer, responding better to health care interventions, and maintaining optimal function (Kiely et al, 2000; Rowe and Kahn, 1998; Williams, 2006).

Older people may have fewer opportunities for social interaction as a result of loss of family and friends, illnesses, and hearing, vision, and cognitive impairment. The ageist attitudes of the public, as well as health professionals, also present barriers to communicating effectively with older people. Good communication skills are the basis for accurate assessment, care planning, and the development of therapeutic relationships between the nurse and the older person.

This chapter discusses the effect of health professionals' attitudes toward aging on their communication with older people, communication skills essential to therapeutic interactions with older adults, and adaptation of communication for elders with vision and hearing impairments, speech and language disorders, and cognitive impairment. The significance of the life story, reminiscence, and life review, and communication with groups of elders is also included in this chapter. A discussion of age-related changes in hearing and vision is presented in Chapter 6; assessment of hearing, vision, and cognition in Chapter 13; diseases of the eye and the ear in Chapter 19; and care of elders with cognitive impairment in Chapter 21.

Ageism and Communication

Belief in myths and stereotypes about older adults and ageist attitudes can interfere with the ability to communicate with them effectively. For example, if the nurse believes that all older people have memory problems, or are unable to learn and process information, he or she will be less likely to engage in conversation, provide appropriate health information, or treat the person with respect and dignity. Ageism is a term used to express prejudice toward older adults through attitudes and behavior. Similar to other prejudices (racism, anti-Semitism, sexism), ageism will affect us all if we live long enough. Although ageism is found cross-culturally, it is essentially prevalent in the United States where aging is viewed with depression, fear, and anxiety (Nelson, 2004). It is important for nurses who care for older people to be aware of their own attitudes toward aging and recognize how their beliefs may influence communication. Evaluating and enhancing one's interpersonal communication skills is the foundation for therapeutic interactions with older adults.

Elderspeak is a form of ageism in which younger people alter their speech based on the assumption that all older people have difficulty understanding and

comprehending (Touhy and Williams, 2008). It is especially common in communication between health care professionals and older adults in hospitals and nursing homes, but occurs in non-health care settings as well (Williams, Kemper and Hummert, 2003, 2004; Williams, 2006). Elderspeak is similar to "baby talk" that is often used to talk to very young children (Box 3-1).

Nurses may not be aware that they are using elderspeak but research has shown that use of this form of speech is patronizing and conveys messages of dependence, incompetence, and control (Williams, 2006). Some features of elderspeak (speaking more slowly, repeating, or paraphrasing) may be beneficial in communication with older people with dementia, and further research is needed. Other examples of communication that conveys ageist attitudes are ignoring the older person and talking to family and friends as if the person is not present, and limiting interaction to task-focused communication only (Touhy and Williams, 2008).

Therapeutic Communication with Older Adults

Basic communication strategies that apply to all situations in nursing, such as attentive listening, authentic presence, non-judgmental attitude, cultural competence, clarifying, giving information, seeking validation of understanding, keeping focus, and using open-ended questions, are all applicable in communicating with

Box 3-1	Characteristics of Elderspeak

- Using a singsong voice, changing pitch and tone, and exaggerating words
- Using short and simple sentences
- Speaking more slowly
- Using limited vocabulary
- Repeating or paraphrasing what has just been said
- Using pet names (diminutives) such as "honey" or "dear" or "grandma"
- Using collective pronouns such as "we"—for instance, "Would we like to take a bath now?"
- Using statements that sound like questions

Modified from: Williams K, Kemper S, Hummert L: Enhancing communication with older adults: overcoming elderspeak, *J Gerontol Nurs* 30(10):17-25, 2004; and Williams K: Improving outcomes of nursing home interactions, *Res Nurs and Health* 29(2):121-133, 2006.

older adults. Basically, elders may need more time to give information or answer questions simply because they have a larger life experience to draw from. Sorting through thoughts requires intervals of silence, and therefore listening carefully without rushing the elder is very important. Word retrieval may be slower, particularly for nouns and names.

Open-ended questions are useful but difficult for some elders. Those who wish to please, especially when feeling vulnerable or somewhat dependent, may wonder what it is you want to hear rather than what it is they would like to say. Communication that is most productive will initially focus on the issue of major concern to the elder, regardless of the priority of the nursing assessment. When using closed questioning to obtain specific information, be aware that the elder may feel on the spot and thus the appropriate information may not be immediately forthcoming. This is especially true when asking questions to determine mental status. The elder may develop a mental block because of anxiety or feel threatened if questions are asked in a quizzing or demeaning manner (see Chapter 21). Older people may be reluctant to disclose information for fear of the consequences. For example, if they are having problems remembering things or are experiencing frequent falls, sharing this information may mean that they might have to leave their home and move to a more protective setting.

When communicating with individuals in a bed or wheelchair, position yourself at their level rather than talking over a side rail or standing above them. Pay attention to their gaze, gestures, and body language, and the pitch, volume, and tone of their voice to help you understand what they are trying to communicate. Thoughts unstated are often as important as those that are verbalized. You may ask, "What are you thinking about right now?" Clarification is essential to ensure that you and the elder have the same framework of understanding. Many generational, cultural, and regional differences in speech patterns and idioms exist. Frequently seek validation of whatever you think you heard. If you tend to speak quickly, particularly if your accent is different from the elder's, try to slow down and give the person time to process what you are saying (National Institute on Aging, 2008).

IMPLICATIONS FOR GERONTOLOGICAL NURSING AND HEALTHY AGING

Every time nurses communicate with someone, their words and actions affect the relationship in either positive or negative ways depending on their own attitude and skills (Buckwalter et al, 1995). Enhancing communication with older adults is an important skill in gerontological nursing that has rewards for both the nurse and the older person. Communication with older adults provides the nurse with the opportunity to share in their wisdom and gain insight on life.

COMMUNICATION WITH ELDERS WITH SENSORY IMPAIRMENTS

Sensory impairments, such as hearing and vision deficits, place older people at risk for communication difficulties. We rely on our senses to perceive the environment and to enjoy the pleasures of life. Gerontological nurses need to have special knowledge and skills to promote effective communication with older people who have these deficits. This section describes adaptations to enhance communication with elders with hearing and vision impairments.

Hearing Impairment

While both vision and hearing impairment significantly affect all aspects of life, Oliver Sacks (1989), in his book *Seeing Voices,* presents a view that blindness may in fact be less serious than loss of hearing. Hearing loss interferes with communication with others and the interactional input that is so necessary to stimulate and validate. Helen Keller was most profound in her expression: "Never to see the face of a loved one nor witness a summer sunset is indeed a handicap. But I can touch a face and feel the warmth of the sun. But to be deprived of hearing the song of the first spring robin and the laughter of children provides me with a long and dreadful sadness" (Keller, 1902).

Hearing loss is the third most prevalent chronic condition in older Americans and the number one communicative disorder of older adults. Today in the United States, between 25% and 40% of people over the age of 65 are hearing-impaired, and the incidence increases with age. Up to 65% of nursing home residents have serious hearing loss (Cohen-Mansfield and Taylor, 2004; American Speech-Language-Hearing Association, 2008; Wallhagen and Pettengill, 2008). In all age-groups, men are more likely than women to be hearing-impaired.

Hearing loss diminishes quality of life and is associated with multiple negative outcomes including decreased function, miscommunication, depression, falls, loss of self-esteem, safety risks, and cognitive decline (Wallhagen and Pettengill, 2008). Hearing impairment increases feelings of isolation and may cause older adults to become suspicious or distrustful or to display feelings of paranoia. Because older persons with a hearing loss may not understand or respond appropriately to conversation, they may be inappropriately diagnosed with dementia. Older people may be initially unaware of hearing loss because of the gradual manner in which it develops (Box 3-2). The Hartford Institute for Geriatric Nursing's "Try This" series provides guidelines for hearing screening (www.hartfordign.org/publications/trythis/issue_12.pdf). The Better Hearing Institute provides a Quick Hearing Check for older adults who want to check their own hearing (www.betterhearing.org/hearing_loss/quickHearingCheck.cfm). An evidence-based guideline for nursing management of hearing impairment in nursing facility residents is also available (Adams-Windling and Pimple, 2008). Additional information about hearing assessment can be found in Chapter 13.

Hearing impairment is underdiagnosed and undertreated in older people. Although screening for hearing impairment and appropriate treatment is considered an essential part of primary care for older adults and one of the goals of *Healthy People 2010* (U.S. Department of Health and Human Services [USDHHS], 2002) (Box 3-3), it is rarely done. Screening rates for hearing impairment among older adults is estimated to be as low as 12.9%, and only 25% of persons with hearing impairments receive hearing aids (Ham et al, 2007;

Box 3-2   Do I Have a Hearing Problem?

- Do I have a problem hearing on the telephone?
- Do I have trouble hearing when there is noise in the background?
- Is it hard to me to follow a conversation when two or more people talk at once?
- Do I have to strain to understand a conversation?
- Do many people I talk to seem to mumble (or not speak clearly)?
- Do I misunderstand what others are saying and respond inappropriately?
- Do I have trouble understanding the speech of women and children?
- Do people complain that I turn the TV volume up too high?
- Do I hear a ringing, roaring, or hissing sound a lot?
- Do some sounds seem too loud?

Source: National Institute on Deafness and Other Communication Disorders. Retrieved 7/10/04 from www.nidcd.gov/health/hearing/older.asp.

Box 3-3   *Healthy People 2010* Goals and Objectives: Hearing

- Increase the number of persons who have a hearing examination on schedule
- Increase the number of persons who are referred to their primary care physician for hearing evaluation and treatment
- Increase the use of appropriate ear protection devices, equipment, and practices
- Increase access by hearing-impaired persons to hearing rehabilitation services and adaptive devices, including hearing aids, cochlear implants, or tactile or other assistive or augmentative devices

U.S. Department of Health and Human Services (USDHHS): *Healthy People 2010: Vision and hearing, 2002.* Accessed July 3, 2008 from www.health.gov/healthypeople/document/html/volume2/28vision.htm.

Wallhagen and Pettengill, 2008). The cost of hearing aids are not covered under Medicare and other health plans, but screening for hearing loss is recommended as part of the comprehensive physical for older adults joining Medicare for the first time.

Findings of a recent study (Box 3-4) suggest that hearing loss is "an overlooked geriatric syndrome in primary care settings—an assessment gap that can have significant negative consequences" (Wallhagen and Pettengill, 2008, p. 41). Lack of assessment and treatment of hearing loss in nursing homes is even more of a concern since a majority of the residents have hearing impairment. A recent study of hearing-aid use in nursing homes (Cohen-Mansfield and Taylor, 2004) reported that 65% of the residents had a serious hearing loss but staff members were aware of fewer than 50% of the problems. Of the 279 residents who participated in the study, 39% had been treated for excessive cerumen, but 81% had neither cerumen removal nor a hearing test. Murphy et al (2005, p. 96) estimate that nearly half of nursing home residents never talk to other residents because of hearing and speech difficulties.

The two major forms of hearing loss are conductive and sensorineural. Sensorineural hearing loss results from damage to any part of the inner ear or the neural pathways to the brain. Presbycusis is a form of sensorineural hearing loss that is related to aging. It is the most common form of hearing loss in the United States (see Chapter 13). To gain a better understanding of hearing loss, take the

| Box 3-4 | Evidence-Based Practice: Hearing Impairment: Significant but Underassessed in Primary Care Settings |

Purpose
The study explored whether primary care providers ever screened older adults for or asked about hearing loss and what effects the lack of inquiry or follow-up may have had on the older adults and their communication partners.

Sample/Setting
Ninety-one older adults (over 60 years) with currently untreated hearing impairment were recruited from 19 different sites—clinics or centers that performed hearing evaluations or provided seminars on hearing loss.

Method
Longitudinal qualitative-quantitative study using interviews, assessment of subjective hearing impairment utilizing the Hearing Handicap Inventory for the Elderly (HHIE), and subjective rating of the emotional and social impact of hearing loss. Audiograms were also performed during the study period.

Results
Of participants, 85% reported that their primary care provider had never asked about their hearing or provided screening for hearing loss. In fact, 33% had mild hearing loss and 58% had moderate hearing loss. If the provider did ask about hearing loss, the participants were the ones to bring it up in order to obtain a referral for hearing evaluation. Samples of the narrative data revealed how several providers discounted the importance of hearing loss, and other narratives demonstrated the detrimental effects of unrecognized hearing loss on the affected individuals and their communication partners.

Implications
Hearing loss is an overlooked geriatric syndrome—a gap in assessment that can have significant negative consequences. Authors recommend that nurses take a leadership role in making hearing assessment a regular part of nursing assessment and providing educational information and referrals as appropriate. The HHIE-S is an easy-to-administer screening instrument; a single-item, self-report question about hearing such as "Do you have a hearing problem now?" or "Would you say you have any hearing difficulty" would be useful in suggesting a referral for additional testing.

Wallhagen M, Pettengill E: Hearing impairment significant but underassessed in primary care settings, *J Gerontol Nurs* 34(2):36-42, 2008.

Unfair Hearing Test, available at www.irrd.ca/education/presentation.asp?refname=e2c1. Sensorineural hearing loss is treated with hearing aids and, in some cases, cochlear implants. Conductive hearing loss usually involves abnormalities of the external and middle ear that reduce the ability of sound to be transmitted to the middle ear. Otosclerosis, infection, perforated eardrum, fluid in the middle ear, or cerumen accumulations cause conductive hearing loss. Cerumen impaction treatment is discussed later in this chapter.

Hearing Aids

A hearing aid is a personal amplifying system that includes a microphone, an amplifier, and a loudspeaker. The appearance and effectiveness of hearing aids has greatly improved in recent years, and many can be programmed to meet specific needs. Most individuals can obtain some hearing enhancement with a hearing aid. While hearing aids generally improve hearing by about 50%, they do not correct hearing deficits. It is important that hearing-impaired elders understand that the goal of hearing aid use is to improve communication and quality of life, not to restore normal hearing.

Hearing aids necessitate a period of adjustment and training in correct use. In most states, the purchase of a hearing aid comes with a 30-day trial during which the purchase price is totally refundable. The investment in a good hearing aid is considerable, and a good fit is critical. Before a hearing aid can be purchased, medical clearance must be obtained from a physician. Hearing aids can range in price from about $500 to several thousand dollars, depending on the technology. Batteries are changed every 1 to 2 weeks, adding to overall costs. The cost of hearing aids is not usually covered by health insurance or Medicare. It is important for nurses in hospitals and nursing homes to be knowledgeable about the care and maintenance of hearing aids. Many older people experience unnecessary communication problems when in the hospital or nursing home because their hearing aids are not inserted and working properly, or are lost. Box 3-5 presents suggestions for the use and care of hearing aids.

Cochlear Implants

Cochlear implants are increasingly being used for older adults who are profoundly deaf as a result of sensorineural hearing loss. Unlike hearing aids that magnify sounds, the cochlear implant converts sound waves into electrical impulses and transmits them to the inner ear. A cochlear implant is surgically implanted in the mastoid bone behind the ear and electrically stimulates the cochlea, setting the cilia in motion and transmitting impulses along the auditory nerve to the brain's hearing center. For persons whose hearing loss is so severe that amplification is of little or no benefit, the cochlear implant is a safe and effective method of auditory rehabilitation. Most insurance plans cover the cochlear implant procedure. The transplant carries some risk

because the surgery destroys any residual hearing that remains. Therefore, cochlear implant users can never revert to using a hearing aid. Individuals with cochlear implants need to be advised not to undergo magnetic resonance imaging (MRI), and the Food and Drug Administration advises "not to even be close to a MRI unit since it may dislodge the implant or demagnetize its internal magnet" (Wallhagen et al, 2006, p. 47).

Assistive Listening and Adaptive Devices

Assistive listening devices (also called personal listening systems) should be considered as an adjunct to hearing aids or used in place of hearing aids for people with hearing impairment. These devices are available commercially and can be used to enhance face-to-face communication and to better understand speech in large rooms such as theaters, use the telephone, and listen to television. Examples of assistive listening and adaptive devices include text messaging devices for telephones and closed-caption television,

Box 3-5	The Use and Care of Hearing Aids

Hearing Aid Use
- Initially, wear the aid 15 to 20 minutes a day
- Gradually increase wearing time to 10 to 12 hours
- Be patient and realize that the process of adaptation is difficult but ultimately will be rewarding
- Make sure fingers are dry and clean before handling hearing aids. Use a soft dry cloth to wipe your hearing aids.
- Each day, remove any earwax that has built up on the hearing aids. Use a soft brush to clean difficult-to-reach areas
- Insert aid with the canal portion pointing into the ear; press and twist until snug
- Turn aid slowly to one-third to one-half volume
- A whistling sound indicates incorrect ear-mold insertion or that aid is in wrong ear
- Adjust volume to a level for talking at a distance of 1 yard
- Do not wear aid when using hair dryer or when swimming or taking a shower or bath
- Note that fine particles of hair spray or make-up can obstruct the microphone component of the hearing aid

Care of the Hearing Aid
- Insert and remove your hearing aid over a soft surface. When inserting or removing battery, work over a table or countertop or soft surface
- Insert battery when hearing aid is turned off
- Store hearing aid in a marked container in a safe place when not in use; remove batteries
- Batteries last 1 week with daily wearing of 10 to 12 hours
- Common problems include switch turned off, clogged ear mold, dislodged battery, twisted tubing between ear mold and aid
- Ear molds need replacement every 2 or 3 years
- Check ear molds for rough spots that will irritate ear
- If sound is not loud enough, check for the following: need new battery? sound channel blocked? aid turned off? volume set too low? battery door not closed? hearing aid loose?

now required on all televisions with screens 13 inches and larger. Alerting devices, such as vibrating alarm clocks that shake the bed or activate a flashing light, and sound lamps that respond with lights to sounds such as doorbells and telephones, are also available. Assistive devices, such as pocket-talkers, that amplify sound and send it to the user's ears through earphones, clips or headphones, are helpful in healthcare situations in which accurate communication and privacy are essential. Any facility that receives financial aid from Medicare is required by the Americans with Disabilities Act to provide equal access to public accommodations. This includes access to sign language interpreters, telecommunication devices for the deaf (TDDs), and flashing alarm systems. Nurses working in these facilities should be able to obtain appropriate devices to improve communication with hearing-impaired individuals. See the Resources section and evolve.elsevier.com/Ebersole/gerontological for additional information.

A program called Hearing Dogs for the Deaf has gained recognition with seventeen locations in the United States that train hearing dogs. Hearing dogs serve to warn the hearing-impaired of impending danger, audible signals, phones ringing, fire and smoke alarms, emergencies, and intruders. Although other electronic means are available for dealing with these concerns, persons who have hearing dogs consistently comment on the alleviation of the sense of isolation that often accompanies hearing impairment. With a hearing-dog companion, elders may experience renewed courage, confidence, and freedom, as well as reduction of tension, anxiety, and depression (Guest et al, 2006).

Cerumen Impaction

Cerumen impaction is the most common and easily corrected of all interferences in the hearing of older people. Cerumen interferes with the conduction of sound through air in the eardrum. The reduction in the number and activity of cerumen-producing glands results in a tendency toward cerumen impaction. Long-standing impactions become hard, dry, and dark brown. Individuals at particular risk of impaction are African Americans, individuals who wear hearing aids, and older men with large amounts of ear canal tragi (hairs in the ear) that tend to become entangled with the cerumen. When a hearing loss is suspected, or a person with existing hearing loss experiences increasing difficulty, it is important to first check for cerumen impaction as a possible cause. Box 3-6 presents a protocol for cerumen removal.

Box 3-6	**Protocol for Cerumen Removal**

- Assess for ear pain, traumas, abnormalities, drainage, surgeries, or perforations. These or any other unusual findings should be referred to an otolaryngologist.
- When aural examination reveals cerumen impaction with no other abnormalities, the nurse may irrigate for cerumen removal using the following techniques.
  NOTE: Do not use a water pick for cerumen removal since water pressure is too high and may damage the ear.
  1. Carefully clip and remove hairs in ear canal.
  2. Instill a softening agent such as slightly warm mineral oil 0.5 to 1 ml twice daily or ear drops such as Cerumenex, Debrox, or Murine ear drops for several days until wax becomes softened. Allergic reactions to Cerumenex have been noted if used for longer than 24 hours.
  3. Protect clothing and linens from drainage of oil or wax by placing small cotton ball in each external ear canal.
  4. When irrigating the ear, use hand-held bulb syringe, 2- to 4-ounce plastic syringe, or otologic syringe (20- to 50-ml syringe equipped with an Angiocath or Jelso catheter rather than a needle) with emesis basin under ear to catch drainage; tip head to side being drained.
  5. Use solution of 3 ounces of 3% hydrogen peroxide in quart of water warmed to 98° to 100° F; if client is sensitive to hydrogen peroxide, use sterile normal saline.
  6. Place towels around neck; empty emesis basin frequently, observing for residue from ear; keep client dry and comfortable; do not inject air into client's ear or use high pressure when injecting fluid.
  7. If the cerumen is not successfully washed out, begin the process again of instilling a softening agent for several days.

Modified from Meador JA: Cerumen impaction in the elderly, *J Gerontol Nurs* 21(12):43-45, 1995.

IMPLICATIONS FOR GERONTOLOGICAL NURSING AND HEALTHY AGING

Hearing impairment is very common among older adults and significantly affects communication, function, safety, and quality of life. Inadequate communication with older adults with hearing impairment can also lead to misdiagnosis and affect adherence to the medical regimen. The gerontological nurse must be able to assess hearing ability and utilize appropriate communication skills and devices to help older adults minimize or even avoid problems. Box 3-7 presents communication strategies for elders with hearing impairment.

Vision Impairment

Vision decline occurs normally with age (Chapter 6) but the major causes of visual impairment and blindness among older adults are cataracts, macular degeneration, glaucoma, and diabetic retinopathy (Chapter 19). Blindness and visual impairment are among the 10 most common causes of disability in the United States and are associated with shorter life expectancy and lower quality of life (Centers for Disease Control and Prevention [CDC], 2006). Visual impair-

ment (low vision) is generally defined as a Snellen reading of worse than 20/40 but better then 20/200. Legal blindness is a reading equal to or worse than 20/200 (Whiteside et al, 2006). Vision loss is becoming a major public health problem and is projected to increase substantially with the aging of the population. Goals of *Healthy People 2010* (USDHHS, 2002) related to vision are presented in Box 3-8.

Some 1.8 million community-dwelling elders report difficulties with activities of daily living because of visual impairment, and 2.7 million older people have severe visual impairment (CDC, 2002). African Americans are twice as likely to be visually impaired as whites of comparable socioeconomic status, and Hispanics also have a higher risk of visual complications than whites (USDHHS, 2002). It is estimated that 40% of blindness and visual impairment is treatable or preventable (Rowe et al, 2004). However, many older people, particularly ethnically and racially diverse elders, do not receive necessary care.

Estimates of visual impairment among nursing home residents is anywhere from 3 to 15 times higher than adults of the same age living in the community (Owsley et al, 2007). A recent study examining the effect of visual impairment among nursing home residents with Alzheimer's disease reported that 1 in 3 were not using

---

Box 3-7	Communication Strategies for Elders with Hearing Impairment

- Never assume hearing loss is from age until other causes are ruled out (infection, cerumen buildup).
- Inappropriate responses, inattentiveness, and apathy may be symptoms of a hearing loss.
- Face the individual, and stand or sit on the same level and don't turn away to face a computer when speaking.
- Gain the individual's attention before beginning to speak.
- Determine if hearing is better in one ear than another, and position yourself appropriately
- If hearing aid is used, make sure it is in place and batteries are functioning.
- Ask patient or family what helps the person to hear best.
- Keep hands away from your mouth and project voice by controlled diaphragmatic breathing.
- Avoid conversations in which the speaker's face is in glare or darkness; orient the light on the speaker's face.
- Careful articulation and moderate speed of speech are helpful.
- Lower your tone of voice, use a moderate speed of speech, and articulate clearly.
- Label the chart, note on the intercom button, and inform all caregivers that the patient has a hearing impairment
- Use nonverbal approaches: gestures, demonstrations, visual aids, and written materials.
- Pause between sentences or phrases to confirm understanding.
- Restate with different words when you are not understood.
- When changing topics, preface the change by stating the topic.
- Reduce background noise (e.g., turn off television, close door).
- Utilize assistive listening devices such as pocket talker.
- Verify that the information being given has been clearly understood.
- Share resources for the hearing-impaired and refer as appropriate.

| Box 3-8 | *Healthy People 2010* Goals and Objectives: Vision |

- Increase the number of persons who have dilated eye examinations at appropriate intervals
- Reduce visual impairment due to diabetic retinopathy, glaucoma, and cataracts
- Increase vision rehabilitation

U.S. Department of Health and Human Services (USDHHS): *Healthy People 2010: Vision and hearing, 2002.* Accessed July 3, 2008 from www.health.gov/healthypeople/document/html/volume2/28vision.htm.

or did not have glasses that were strong enough to correct their vision. They had either lost their glasses or broken them, had prescriptions that were no longer adequate, or were too cognitively impaired to ask for help (Koch et al, 2005). Routine eye care is sorely lacking in nursing homes and is related to functional decline, decreased quality of life, and depression (Owsley et al, 2007).

Low-Vision Assistive Devices

Technology advances in the past decade have produced some low-vision devices that may be used successfully in the care of the visually impaired elder. Persons with severe visual impairment may qualify for disability and financial and social services assistance through government and private programs including vision rehabilitation programs. An array of low-vision assistive devices are now available, including insulin delivery systems, talking clocks and watches, large-print books, magnifiers, telescopes (handheld or mounted on eyeglasses), electronic magnification through closed circuit television or computer software, and software that converts text into artificial voice output. Because individual needs are unique, it is recommended that before investing in vision aids, the client consult with a low-vision center or low-vision specialist. See the Resources section and evolve.elsevier.com/Ebersole/gerontological for additional information.

IMPLICATIONS FOR GERONTOLOGICAL NURSING AND HEALTHY AGING

Vision impairment is common among older adults in connection with aging changes and eye diseases and can significantly affect communication, functional ability, safety, and quality of life. To promote healthy aging and quality of life, nurses who care for elders in all settings can improve outcomes for visually impaired elders by assessing for vision changes and providing appropriate health teaching and referrals for prevention and treatment. Suggestions to improve communication and care for visually impaired elders are presented in Box 3-9.

COMMUNICATION WITH ELDERS WITH NEUROLOGICAL DISORDERS

Three major categories of impaired verbal communication arise from neurological disturbances: (1) reception, (2) perception, and (3) articulation. Reception is impaired by anxiety or is related to a specific disorder, hearing deficits, and altered levels of consciousness. Perception is distorted by stroke, dementia, and delirium. Articulation is hampered by mechanical difficulties such as dysarthria, respiratory disease, destruction of the larynx, and cerebral infarction with neuromuscular effects. Specific difficulties include the following:

▶ Anomia: Word retrieval difficulties during spontaneous speech and naming tasks.

▶ Aphasia: A communication disorder that can affect a person's ability to use and understand spoken or written words. It results from damage to the side of the brain dominant for language. For most people, this is the left side. Aphasia usually occurs suddenly and often results from a stroke or head injury, but it can also develop slowly because of a brain tumor, an infection, or dementia.

▶ Dysarthria: Impairment in the ability to articulate words as the result of damage to the central or peripheral nervous system that affects the speech mechanism.

Aphasia

The most commonly occurring language disorder after a cerebral vascular accident is aphasia. Cerebral vascular accidents are discussed in Chapter 21. Aphasia, in varying degrees, affects a person's ability to communicate in one or more ways, including speaking, understanding, reading, writing, and gesturing. Depending on the type and severity of the aphasia, there may be little or no speech, speech that is fragmented or broken, or speech that is fluent but empty in content. When a cerebral vascular accident damages the dominant half of the brain, some disruption will occur in the "word factory." Broca's area and Wernicke's area in the cerebral cortex are integral to the expression and understanding of language. The National Aphasia Association categorizes

Box 3-9	Strategies for Communicating with Elders with Visual Impairment

- Make sure you have the person's attention before you start talking.
- Always speak promptly and clearly identify yourself and others with you. State when you are leaving to make sure the person is aware of your departure.
- Get down to the person's level and face them when speaking.
- Speak normally but not from a distance; do not raise or lower your voice and continue to use gestures if that is natural to your communication.
- When others are present, address the visually impaired person by prefacing remarks with his or her name or a light touch on the arm.
- Use the analogy of a clock face to help locate objects (e.g., describe positions of food on a plate in relation to clock positions such as meat at 3 o'clock, dessert at 6 o'clock).
- Ensure adequate lighting on your face and eliminate glare.
- Select colors for paint, furniture, pictures with rich intensity (red, orange).
- Use large, dark, evenly spaced printing.
- Use contrast in printed material (e.g., black marker on white paper).
- Do not change the room arrangement or the arrangement of personal items without explanation.
- Use some means to identify patients who are visually impaired, and include visual impairment in the plan of care.
- Screen for vision loss, and recommend annual eye exams for older people.
- If the person is institutionalized, label glasses and have a spare pair if possible.
- Be aware of low-vision assistive devices such as talking watches, talking books, and facilitate access to these resources
- If the person is blind, offer your arm while walking. Pause before stairs or curbs and alert the person. When seating the person, place his or her hand on the back of the chair. Always let the person know his or her position in relation to objects. Never play with or distract a seeing-eye dog.

the two major types of aphasia as fluent and nonfluent. Following is a description of several types of aphasia that the nurse may encounter with older adults:

▶ *Fluent aphasia* is the result of a lesion in the superior temporal gyrus, an area adjacent to the primary auditory cortex (Wernicke's area). This type is also known as sensory, posterior, or Wernicke's aphasia. Persons with fluent aphasia speak easily with many long runs of words, but the content does not make sense. There are word-finding problems and errors of word and sound substitution. Often the speech of persons with fluent aphasia sounds like "jabberwocky." Unrelated words may be strung together or syllables repeated. These persons also have difficulty understanding spoken language and may be unaware of their speech difficulties.

▶ *Nonfluent aphasia* typically involves damage to the posteroinferior portions of the dominant frontal lobe (Broca's area). This type is also called motor, anterior, or Broca's aphasia. Persons with nonfluent aphasia usually understand others but speak very slowly and use minimal numbers of words. They often struggle to articulate a word and seem to have lost the ability to voluntarily control the movements of speech. Difficulties are experienced in communicating orally and in writing.

▶ *Verbal apraxia* or *apraxia of speech* is a motor speech disorder that affects the ability to plan and sequence voluntary muscle movements. The muscles of speech are not paralyzed; instead there is a disruption in the brain's transmission of signals to the muscles. When thinking about what to say, the person may be unable to speak at all or may struggle to say words. In contrast, the person may be able to say many words or sentences correctly when not thinking about the words. Apraxia frequently occurs with aphasia.

▶ *Anomic aphasia* is associated with lesions of the dominant temporoparietal regions of the brain, although no single locus has been identified. Persons with anomic aphasia understand and speak readily but may have severe word-finding difficulty. They may be unable to remember crucial content words. This is a frequent form of aphasia characterized by the inability to name objects. The individual struggles to come forth with the correct noun and often becomes frustrated at his or her inability to do so.

▶ *Global aphasia* is the result of large left hemisphere lesions and affects most of the language areas of the brain. Persons with global aphasia cannot understand words or speak intelligibly. They may use meaningless syllables repetitiously.

A speech language pathologist (SLP) should be consulted for each type of aphasia to develop appropriate rehabilitative plans as soon as the individual is physiologically stabilized. SLPs bring expertise in all types of communication disorders and are an essential part of the interdisciplinary team. The SLP can identify the areas of language that remain relatively unimpaired and can capitalize on the remaining strengths. Much can be done in aggressive speech-retraining programs to regain intelligible conversational ability. For those who do not regain meaningful speech, assistive and augmentative communication devices can be most helpful. Happ and Paull (2008) note the importance of consulting with the SLP in acute and critical care settings, as well as in rehabilitation and long-term care, and describe a program to improve communication with ICU patients who are unable to speak (The Study of Patient-Nurse Effectiveness with Assisted Communication Strategies [SPEACS]).

Alternative and Augmentative Speech Aids

Alternative or augmentative systems are frequently used, and communication tools exist for every imaginable type of language disability. These can be low tech or high tech. An example of a low-tech system would be an alphabet or picture board that the individual uses to point to letters to spell out messages or point to pictures of common objects and situations. High-tech systems include electronic boards and computers. Studies have shown that computer-assisted therapy can help people with aphasia improve speech. An example is speech-therapy software that displays a word or picture, speaks the word (using prerecorded human speech), records the user speaking it, and plays back the user's speech. Murphy et al (2005) report on research with frail elders experiencing communication difficulties using a "talking mat" to enhance communication and sharing of ideas and feelings. The "talking mat" is a visual framework using picture symbols to aid in expression of feelings about activities, the environment, people in their lives, and their own personal views and interests.

For individuals with hemiplegic or paraplegic conditions, electronic devices and computers can be voice-activated or have specially designed switches that can be activated by just one finger or by slight contact with the ear, nose, or chin. In addition to speech therapy, some experimental studies indicate that drugs may help improve aphasia in the acute phase of stroke and assist after the acute situation and in chronic aphasia.

IMPLICATIONS FOR GERONTOLOGICAL NURSING AND HEALTHY AGING

Nurses are responsible for accurately observing and recording the speech and word recognition patterns of the person and for consistently implementing the recommendations of the SLP. Communication with the older adult experiencing aphasia can be frustrating for both the affected person and the nurse as they struggle to understand each other. It is important to remember that in most cases of aphasia, the person retains normal intellectual ability. Therefore communication must always occur at an adult level but with special modifications. Hearing and vision losses can further contribute to communication difficulties for older adults with aphasia. Sensitivity and patience are essential to promote effective communication. It is most helpful if staff caring for the person remain consistent so that they can come to know and understand the needs of the person and communicate these to others. It is exhausting for the person to have to continually try to communicate needs and desires to an array of different people. Plans of care should include specific communication strategies that are helpful for the individual person so that all staff, as well as families and significant others, know the most effective way to enhance communication. Suggestions for communicating with patients with aphasia are presented in Box 3-10.

Dysarthria

Dysarthria is a speech disorder caused by a weakness or incoordination of the speech muscles. It occurs as a result of central or peripheral neuromuscular disorders that interfere with the clarity of speech and pronunciation. Dysarthria is second in incidence only to aphasia as a communication disorder of older adults and may be the result of stroke, head injury, Parkinson's disease, multiple sclerosis, and other neurological conditions. Dysarthria is characterized by weakness, slow movement, and a lack of coordination of the muscles associated with speech. Speech may be slow, jerky, slurred, quiet, lacking in expression, and difficult to understand. It may involve several mechanisms of speech, such as respiration, phonation, resonance, articulation, and prosody (the meter, or rhythm of speech). A weakness or lack of coordination in

Box 3-10	Communicating with Individuals Experiencing Aphasia

- Explain situations, treatments, and anything else that is pertinent to the person. Treat the person as an adult, and avoid patronizing and childish phrases. Talk as if the person understands.
- Be patient, and allow plenty of time to communicate in a quiet environment.
- Speak slowly, ask one question at a time, and wait for a response. Repeat and rephrase as needed.
- Create an environment in which the person is encouraged to make decisions, offer comments, and communicate thoughts and desires.
- Ask questions in a way that can be answered with a nod or the blink of an eye; if the person cannot verbally respond, instruct him or her in nonverbal responses.
- Be honest with the person. Let him or her know if you cannot quite understand what he or she is telling you but that you will keep trying.
- When you have not understood what the person said, it helps to repeat the part that you did not understand as a question so that the person only has to repeat the part that you did not understand. For example, if you hear "I would like an XX," rather than saying pardon and getting a repetition that may sound the same, try asking "You would like a ...?"
- Speak of things familiar to and of interest to the person.
- Use visual cues, objects, pictures, gestures, and touch as well as words. Have paper and pencil available so you can write down key words or even sketch a picture.
- If the person has fluent aphasia, listen and watch for the bits of information that emerge from the words, facial expressions, and gestures. Ignore the nonwords.
- Encourage all speech. Allow the person to try to complete his or her thoughts and to struggle with words. Avoid being too quick to guess what the person is trying to express.
- Use augmentative communication devices, such as a picture board. These are useful to "fill in" answers to requests such as "I need" or "I want." The person merely points to the appropriate picture.
- Try to keep staff caring for the person with aphasia consistent, and make the care plan specific to the most helpful communication techniques.

any one of the systems can result in dysarthria. If the respiratory system is weak, then speech may be too quiet and be produced one word at a time. If the laryngeal system is weak, speech may be breathy, quiet, and slow. If the articulatory system is affected, speech may sound slurred and be slow and labored.

Treatment of dysarthria depends on the cause, the type, and the severity of the symptoms. An SLP works with the individual to improve communication abilities. Therapy for dysarthria focuses on maximizing the function of all systems. In progressive neurological disease it is important to begin treatment early and continue throughout the course of the disease, with the goal of maintaining speech as long as possible.

IMPLICATIONS FOR GERONTOLOGICAL NURSING AND HEALTHY AGING

The gerontological nurse needs to be familiar with techniques that facilitate communication with persons with dysarthria as well as strategies that can be taught to the person to improve communication. Boxes 3-11 and 3-12 present suggestions for the person with dysar-

thria and the listener to improve communication. The nurse may encounter older people in the acute or long-term phase of an illness that affects communication. Although early intensive rehabilitation efforts are the most effective, all older adults with communication deficits should have access to state-of-the-art techniques and devices that enhance communication, a basic human need. In addition to being knowledgeable about appropriate communication techniques, it is important for the nurse to be aware of equipment and resources available to the person with aphasia or dysarthria so that hope can be offered. Teaching families and significant others effective communication strategies is also an important nursing role. Several resources for people with aphasia and dysarthria are presented at evolve.elsevier.com/Ebersole/gerontological.

COMMUNICATION WITH ELDERS WITH COGNITIVE IMPAIRMENT

The experience of losing cognitive and expressive abilities is both frightening and frustrating. One type of cognitive impairment that affects memory, speech, and

Box 3-11	Tips for the Person with Dysarthria

Explain to people that you have difficulty with your speech.
Try to limit conversations when you feel tired.
Speak slowly and loudly and in a quiet place.
Pace out one word at a time while speaking.
Take a deep breath before speaking so that there is enough breath for speech.
Speak out as soon as you breathe out to make full use of the breaths.
Open the mouth more when speaking; exaggerate tongue movements.
Make sure you are sitting or standing in an upright posture. This will improve your breathing and speech.
If you become frustrated, try to use other methods, such as pointing, gesturing, or writing, or take a rest and try again later.
Practice facial exercises (blowing kisses, frowning, smiling), and massage your facial muscles.

Adapted from Dysarthria and coping with dysarthria. Accessed 7/3/04 from www.rcslt.org and www.asha.org.

Box 3-12	Tips for Communicating with Individuals Experiencing Dysarthria

Pay attention to the speaker; watch the speaker as he or she talks.
Allow more time for conversation, and conduct conversations in a quiet place.
Be honest, and let the speaker know when you have difficulty understanding.
If speech is very difficult to understand, repeat back what the person has said to make sure you understand.
Repeat the part of the message you did not understand so that the speaker does not have to repeat the entire message.
Remember that dysarthria does not affect a person's intelligence.
Check with the person for ways in which you can help, such as guessing or finishing sentences or writing.

Adapted from Dysarthria and coping with dysarthria. Accessed 7/3/04 from www.rcslt.org and www.asha.org.

communication is dementia (Chapter 21). Older adults experiencing dementia have difficulty expressing their personhood in ways easily understood by others. However, the need to communicate and the need to be treated as a person remain despite memory and communication impairments. No group of patients is more in need of supportive relationships with skilled, caring health care providers. People with cognitive and communication impairments "depend on their relationship with and trust of others to provide emotional support, solve problems, and coordinate complex activities" (Buckwalter et al, 1995, p. 15).

Communication with elders experiencing cognitive impairment requires special skills and patience. "Caregivers are subject to frustration and anxiety when their attempts to communicate with the person who has cognitive limitations are unsuccessful" (Williams and Tappen, 2008).

Dementia affects both receptive and expressive communication components and alters the way people speak. Early in the disease, word finding is difficult (anomia), and remembering the exact facts of a conversation is challenging. The following reflection from a man with dementia illustrates (Snyder, 2001, pp. 8, 11, 16):

I'm aware that I'm losing larger and larger chunks of memory...I lose one word and then I can't come up with the rest of the sentence. I just stop talking and people think something is really wrong with me. For awhile, I'll search for a word and I can see it walking away from me. It just gets littler and littler. It always comes back, but at the wrong time. You just can't be spontaneous.

As the disease progresses, there is difficulty expressing thoughts and emotions and understanding verbal messages. In later stages, verbalizations may be limited. Williams and Tappen (2008) remind us that even in the later stages of dementia, the person may understand more than you realize and still needs opportunities for interaction and caring communication, both verbal and nonverbal. Often, health care providers do not communicate with older adults with cognitive impairment, or they limit communication to only the task-focused.

To effectively communicate with a person experiencing cognitive impairment, it is essential to believe that the person is trying to communicate something; it is just as essential for nurses to believe that what the person is trying to communicate is important enough to make the effort to understand. The best thing we can do is to treat everything the person says, however jumbled it may seem, as important and an attempt to tell us something. It is our responsibility as professionals to know how to understand and respond. The person with cognitive impairment cannot change his or her communication; we must change ours (Box 3-13).

Research conducted by Ruth Tappen of Florida Atlantic University and her colleagues (Tappen et al, 1997, 1999) provided insight into communication strategies that were helpful in creating and maintaining a therapeutic relationship with people in the moderate to later stages of dementia. The research challenged some of the commonly held beliefs about communication with persons with cognitive impairment, for example, avoiding the use of open-ended questions and keeping communication focused only on simple topics, task-oriented topics, and questions that can be answered with *yes* or *no*. Research findings provided suggestions for specific communication strategies effective in various nursing situations as well as hope for nurses to establish meaningful relationships that nurture the personhood of people with cognitive impairments. "Approaches to communication must be adapted not only to the person's ability to understand but to the purpose of the interaction. What is appropriate for assessment may be a barrier to conversation that is designed to facilitate expression of concerns and feelings" (Williams and Tappen, 2008, p. 93).

The Hartford Institute for Geriatric Nursing "Try This" series (www.hartfordign.org) provides an evidence-based practice guide for communicating with hospitalized older adults with dementia. Box 3-14 presents suggestions for communication with persons experiencing cognitive impairment.

IMPLICATIONS FOR GERONTOLOGICAL NURSING AND HEALTHY AGING

Care and communication that respect and value the dignity and worth of every person nursed, including those with cognitive impairment, and use of research-based communication techniques, will enhance communication and personhood. "Gerontological nurses who are sensitive to communication and interaction patterns can assist both formal and informal caregivers in using more personal verbal and nonverbal communication strategies which are humanizing and show respect for the person. Similarly, they can monitor and try to change object-oriented communication approaches, which are not only insensitive and dehumanizing, but also often lead to diminished self-image and angry, agitated responses on the part of the patient with cognitive impairment" (Buckwalter et al, 1995, p. 15).

THE LIFE STORY

Older people bring us complex stories derived from long years of living. In caring for older adults, listening to life stories is an important component of communication. The life story can tell us a great deal about the person and is an important part of the assessment process. Stories are "critical sources of information about etiology, diagnosis, treatment, and prognosis from the patient's point of view" (Sandelowski, 1994, p. 25). Listening to memories and life stories requires time and patience and a belief that the story and the person are valuable and meaningful. A memory is an incredible gift given to the nurse, a sharing of a part of oneself when one may have little else to give. The more personal memories are

Box 3-13	Communicating Effectively with Persons with Dementia

Envision a tennis game: the caregiver is like the tennis coach, and whenever the coach plays the ball, he or she seems to be able to put the ball where the person on the other side of the net can return it. The coach also returns the ball in such a way as to keep the rally going; he or she does not return it to score a point or win the match, but rather returns the ball so that the other player is able to reach it and, with encouragement, hit it back over the net again. Similarly, in our communication with people with dementia, our conversation and words must be put into play in a way such that the person can respond effectively and share thoughts and feelings.

Source: Kitwood T: *Dementia reconsidered: the person comes first,* Bristol, Pa, 1999, Open University Press.

Box 3-14   Four Useful Strategies for Communicating with Individuals Experiencing Cognitive Impairment

Simplification Strategies (Useful with ADLs)
- Give one-step directions.
- Speak slowly.
- Allow time for response.
- Reduce distractions.
- Interact with one person at a time.
- Give clues and cues as to what you want the person to do. Use gestures or pantomime to demonstrate what it is you want the person to do—for example, put the chair in front of the person, point to it, pat the seat, and say, "Sit here."

Facilitation Strategies (Useful in Encouraging Expression of Thoughts and Feelings)
- Establish commonalities.
- Share self.
- Allow the person to choose subjects to discuss.
- Speak as if to an equal.
- Use broad openings, such as "How are you today?"
- Employ appropriate use of humor.
- Follow the person's lead.

Comprehension Strategies (Useful in Assisting with Understanding of Communication)
- Identify time confusion (*in what time frame is the person operating at the moment?*).
- Find the theme (*what connection is there between apparently disparate topics?*). Recognize an important theme, such as fear, loss, or happiness.
- Recognize the hidden meanings (*what did the person mean to say?*).

Supportive Strategies (Useful in Encouraging Continued Communication and Supporting Personhood)
- Introduce yourself, and explain why you are there. Reach out to shake hands, and note the response to touch.
- If the person does not want to talk, go away and return later. Do not push or force.
- Sit closely, and face the person at eye level.
- Limit corrections.
- Assume meaningfulness.
- Use multiple ways of communicating (gestures, touch).
- Search for meaning.
- Know the person's past life history as well as daily life experiences and events.
- Recognize feelings, and respond.
- Treat the person with respect and dignity.
- Show interest through body posture, facial expression, nodding, and eye contact. Assume a pleasant, relaxed attitude.
- Attend to vision and hearing losses.
- Do not try to bring the person to the present or use reality orientation. Go to where the person is, and enjoy the conversation.
- When leaving, thank the person for his or her time and attention as well as information.
- Remember that the quality, not the content or quantity, of the interaction is basic to therapeutic communication.

ADLs, Activities of daily living.

saved for persons who will patiently wait for their un-veiling and who will treasure them. Stories are impor-tant, as Robert Coles states (1989, p. 7): "The people who come to see us bring us their stories. They hope that we will tell them well enough so that we understand the truth of their lives. They hope we understand how to interpret their stories correctly."

The life story as constructed through reminiscing, journaling, life review, or guided autobiography has held great fascination for gerontologists in the last quarter-century. The universal appeal of the life story as a vehicle of culture, a demonstration of caring and generational continuity, and an easily stimulated ac-tivity has held allure for many professionals. The most exciting aspect of working with older adults is being a part of the emergence of the life story: the shifting and blending patterns. When we are young, it is important for our emotional health and growth to look forward and plan for the future. As one ages, it becomes more important to look back, talk over experiences, review and make sense of it all, and end with a feeling of satisfaction with the life lived. This is very important work and the major developmental task of older adult-hood that Erik Erikson called *ego integrity versus self despair*. Ego integrity is achieved when the person has accepted both the triumphs and disappointments of life and is at peace and satisfied with the life lived (Erikson, 1963).

Reminiscing

Reminiscing is an umbrella term that can include any recall of the past. Reminiscing occurs from child-hood onward, particularly at life's junctures and transi-tions. Reminiscing cultivates a sense of security through recounting of comforting memories, belong-ing through sharing, and self-esteem through confir-mation of uniqueness. Robert Butler (2002) pointed out that 50 years ago, reminiscing was thought to be a sign of senility or what we now call Alzheimer's dis-ease. Older people who talked about the past and told the same stories again and again were said to be boring and living in the past. From Butler's seminal research (1963), we now know that reminiscence is the most important psychological task of older people. For the nurse, reminiscing is a therapeutic intervention impor-tant in assessment and understanding. The work of several gerontological nursing leaders, including Irene Burnside, Priscilla Ebersole, and Barbara Haight, has contributed to the body of knowledge about reminis-cence and its importance in nursing.

Reminiscence can have many goals. It not only provides a pleasurable experience that improves quality of life, but also increases socialization and connectedness with others, provides cognitive stimu-lation, improves communication, and can be an ef-fective therapy for depressive symptoms (Haight and Burnside, 1993; Bohlmeijer et al, 2003). The thera-peutic implications of reminiscence can be seen in Box 3-15. The process of reminiscence can occur in individual conversations with older people, be struc-tured as in a nursing history, or can occur in a group where each person shares his or her memories and listens to others sharing theirs. Group work is dis-cussed later in this chapter.

The nurse can learn much about a resident's history, communication style, relationships, coping mecha-nisms, strengths, fears, affect, and adaptive capacity by listening thoughtfully as the life story is constructed. Box 3-16 provides some suggestions for encouraging reminiscence.

Life Review

Robert Butler (1963) first noted and brought to public attention the review process that normally occurs in the older person as the realization of his or her approach-ing death creates a resurgence of unresolved conflicts. Butler called this process life review. Life review oc-curs quite naturally for many persons during periods of crisis and transition; however, Butler (2002) noted that in old age, the process of putting one's life in order increases in intensity and emphasis. Life review occurs most frequently as an internal review of memories, an intensely private, soul-searching activity.

Box 3-15	Uses of Reminiscence as a Developmental and Therapeutic Strategy

Maintain continuity
Extract meaning
Define and develop personal philosophy
Identify cycles and themes
Recapitulate learning and growth
Enhance self-worth and feeling of accomplishment
Evolve identity
Provide insight and growth
Integrate and accept regrets and disappointments
Perceive universality

Box 3-16	Suggestions for Encouraging Reminiscence

- Listen without correction or criticism. Older adults are presenting their version of their reality; our version belongs to another generation.
- Encourage older adults to cover various ages and stages. Use questions such as "What was it like growing up on that farm?" "What did teenagers do for fun when you were young?" "What was WWII like for you?"
- Be patient with repetition. Sometimes people need to tell the same story often to come to terms with the experience, especially if it was very meaningful to them. If they have a memory loss, it may be the only story they can remember, and it is important for them to be a member of the group and contribute. If group members seem bothered by repetition, be sure to acknowledge the person's contribution and then direct conversation to include others.
- Be attuned to signs of depression in conversation (dwelling on sad topics) or changes in physical status or behavior, and provide appropriate assessment and intervention.
- If a topic arises that the person does not want to discuss, change to another topic.
- If individuals are reluctant to share because they don't feel their life was interesting, reassure them that everyone's life is valuable and interesting and tell them how important their memories are to you and others.
- Keep in mind that reminiscing is not an orderly process. One memory triggers another in a way that may not seem related; it is not important to keep things in order or verify accuracy.
- Keep the conversation focused on the person reminiscing, but do not hesitate to share some of your own memories that relate to the situation being discussed. Participate as equals, and enjoy each other's contributions.
- Listen actively, maintain eye contact, and do not interrupt.
- Respond positively and give feedback by making caring, appropriate comments that encourage the person to continue.
- Use props and triggers such as photographs, memorabilia (e.g., a childhood toy or antique), short stories or poems about the past, and favorite foods.
- Use open-ended questions to encourage reminiscing. You can prepare questions ahead of time, or you can ask the group members to pick a topic that interests them. One question or topic may be enough for an entire group session. Consider using questions such as the following:
  How did your parents meet?
  What do you remember most about your mother? father? grandmother? grandfather?
  What are some of your favorite memories from childhood?
  What was the first house you remember?
  What were your favorite foods as a child?
  Did you have a pet as a child?
  What do you remember about your first job?
  How did you celebrate birthdays or other holidays?
  What do you remember about your wedding day?
  What was your greatest accomplishment or joy in your life?
  What advice did your parents give you? What advice did you give your children? What advice would you give to young people today?

Life review is considered more of a formal therapy technique than reminiscence and takes a person through his or her life in a structured and chronological order. Life review therapy (Butler and Lewis, 1983), guided autobiography (Birren and Deutchman, 1991), and structured life review (Haight and Webster, 1995) are psychotherapeutic techniques based on the concept of life review. Gerontological nurses participate with older adults in both reminiscence and life review, and it is important to acquire the skills to be effective in achieving the purposes of both. Life review may be especially important for older people

facing death. The Hospice Foundation of America provides a "Guide for Recalling and Telling Your Life Story" (www.hospicefoundation.org) that nurses and families may find helpful.

Life review should occur not only when we are old or facing death but also frequently throughout our lives. This process can assist us to examine where we are in life and change our course or set new goals. Butler (2002) commented that one might avoid the overwhelming feelings of despair that may surface when there is no time left to make changes if life review was conducted throughout our lives.

IMPLICATIONS FOR GERONTOLOGICAL NURSING AND HEALTHY AGING

One of the greatest privileges of nursing elders is to accompany them in the final journey of life. As each person confronts mortality, there is a need to integrate events and to then transcend the self. The human experience, the person's contributions, and the poignant anecdotes within the life story bind generations together, validate the uniqueness of each brief journey in this level of awareness, and provide the assurance that one will not be forgotten. When the nurse takes the time to listen to an older person share memories and life stories, it communicates respect and valuing of the individual. What more can one ask at the end of life than to know that who one is and what one has accomplished holds personal meaning and meaning for others as well? This is the essence of life's final tasks—achieving ego integrity and self-actualization.

Communication with Groups of Elders

Group work with older adults has been used extensively in institutional settings to meet myriad needs in an economical manner. Nurses have led groups of older people for a variety of therapeutic reasons, and expert gerontological nurses such as Irene Burnside and Priscilla Ebersole have extensively discussed advantages of group work for both older people and group leaders and have

provided in-depth guidelines for conducting groups. Box 3-17 presents some of the benefits of group work.

Many groups can be managed effectively by staff with clear goals and guidance and training. Skills important to effective group leadership were reported by Cook (2004) (Box 3-18). Volunteers, nursing assistants, and recreation staff can be taught to conduct many types of groups, but groups with a psychotherapy focus require a trained and skilled leader. Some basic considerations for group work are presented in this chapter, but nurses interested in working with groups of older people should consult a text on group work for more in-depth information.

Groups can be implemented in many settings, including adult day health programs, retirement communities, assisted living facilities, nutrition sites, and nursing homes. Examples of groups include reminiscence groups, psychoeducational groups, caregiver support groups, and groups for people with memory impairment or other conditions such as Parkinson's disease or stroke. Groups can be organized to meet any level of human need; some meet multiple needs (Figure 3-1).

Group Structure and Special Considerations for Groups of Older Adults

Implementing a group intervention follows a thorough assessment of environment, needs, and the potential for various group strategies. Major decisions regarding goals will influence the strategy selected. For instance, several older people with diabetes in an acute care setting may

---

Box 3-17	**Benefits of Group Work With Elders**

- Group experiences provide older adults with an opportunity to try new roles—those of teacher, expert, storyteller, or even clown.
- Groups may improve communication skills for lonely, shy, or withdrawn older people as well as those with communication disorders or memory impairment.
- Groups provide peer support and opportunities to share common experiences, and they may foster the development of warm friendships that endure long after the group has ended.
- The group may be of interest to other residents, staff, and relatives and may improve satisfaction and morale. Staff, in particular, may come to see their patients in a different light—not just as persons needing care but as persons.
- Active listening and interest in what older people have to say may improve self-esteem and help them feel like worthwhile persons whose wisdom is valued.
- Group work offers the opportunity for leaders to be creative and use many modalities, such as music, art, dance, poetry, exercise, and current events.
- Groups provide an opportunity for the leader to assess the person's mood, cognitive abilities, and functional level on a weekly basis.

Adapted from: Burnside IM: Group work with older persons, *J Gerontol Nurs* 20(1):43, 1994.

Box 3-18 | **Group Leadership Skills**

- Attend to group participants
- Reflect group and members feelings
- Link members to each other
- Guide group discussion
  a. Use open-ended questions
  b. Shift the focus as needed
  c. Hold the focus to complete a discussion
- Scan the group to pick up nonverbal communication
- Assist the group in processing the group experience

From Linton AD, Lach HW: *Matteson & McConnell's gerontological nursing: concepts and practice,* ed 3, Philadelphia, 2007, Saunders.

---

need health care teaching regarding diabetes. The nurse sees the major goal as education and restoring order (or control) in each individual's lifestyle. The strategy best suited for that would be motivational or educational. A group of people experiencing early-stage Alzheimer's disease may benefit from a support group to express feelings or a group that teaches memory-enhancing strategies. Successful group work depends on organization, attention to details, agency support, assessment and consideration of the older person's needs and status, and caring, sensitive, and skillful leadership.

Group work with older people is different from that with younger age groups; and there are some unique aspects that require special skills and training and an extraordinary commitment on the part of the leader. Although these unique aspects may not apply to all types of groups of older adults, some of the differences and particularities of group work are presented in Box 3-19.

Reminiscing and Storytelling with Individuals Experiencing Cognitive Impairment

Cognitive impairment does not necessarily preclude older adults from participating in reminiscence or storytelling groups. Opportunities for telling the life story, enjoying memories, and achieving ego integrity

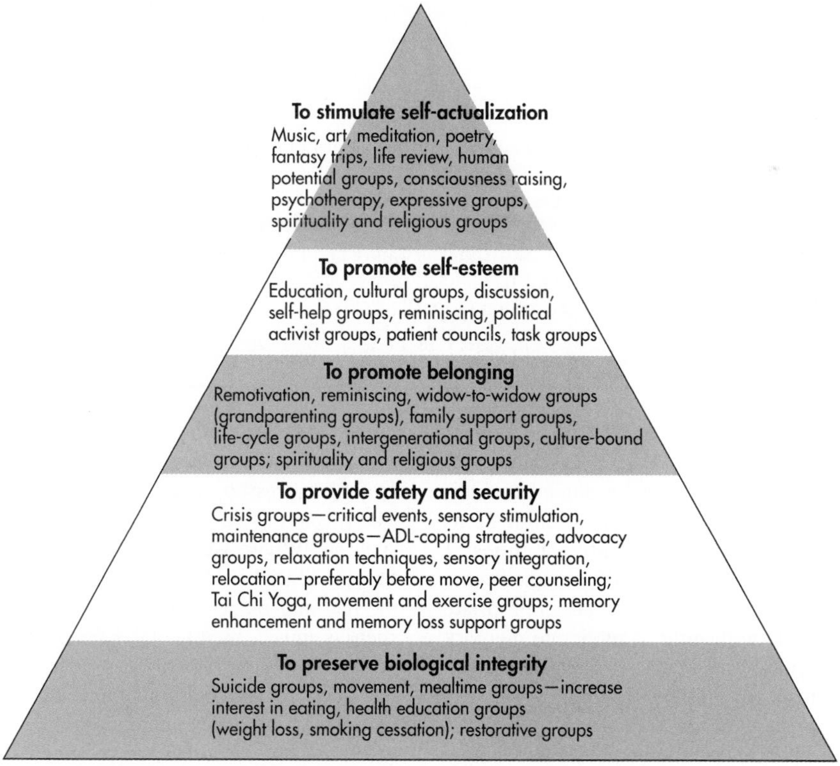

To stimulate self-actualization
Music, art, meditation, poetry, fantasy trips, life review, human potential groups, consciousness raising, psychotherapy, expressive groups, spirituality and religious groups

To promote self-esteem
Education, cultural groups, discussion, self-help groups, reminiscing, political activist groups, patient councils, task groups

To promote belonging
Remotivation, reminiscing, widow-to-widow groups (grandparenting groups), family support groups, life-cycle groups, intergenerational groups, culture-bound groups; spirituality and religious groups

To provide safety and security
Crisis groups—critical events, sensory stimulation, maintenance groups—ADL-coping strategies, advocacy groups, relaxation techniques, sensory integration, relocation—preferably before move, peer counseling; Tai Chi Yoga, movement and exercise groups; memory enhancement and memory loss support groups

To preserve biological integrity
Suicide groups, movement, mealtime groups—increase interest in eating, health education groups (weight loss, smoking cessation); restorative groups

Fig. 3-1   Hierarchical needs met in group work with older adults.

Box 3-19	Special Considerations in Group Work with Elders

1. The leader must pay special attention to sensory losses and compensate for vision and hearing loss.
2. Pacing is different, and group leaders must slow down in both physical and psychological actions.
3. Group members often need assistance or transportation to the group, and adequate time must be allowed for assembling the members and assisting them to return to their homes or rooms.
4. Time of day a group is scheduled is important. Meeting time should not conflict with bathing and eating schedules, and evening groups may not be good for older people who may be tired by then. For community-based older people, transportation logistics may become complicated in the evening.
5. A warm and friendly climate of acceptance of each member and showing appreciation and enjoyment of the group and each member's contribution are important. As a result of ageist attitudes in society, older people's wisdom and contributions are not often valued, making them feel useless or a bother.
6. Older adults may need more stimulation and be less self-motivating. (This is, of course, not true of self-help and senior activist groups such as the Gray Panthers.)
7. Groups generally should include people with similar levels of cognitive ability. Mixing very intact elders with those who have memory and communication impairments calls for special skills. Burnside* suggests that in groups of people with varying abilities, alert persons tend to ask, "Will I become like them?" whereas the people with memory and communication impairments may become anxious when they are aware that they cannot perform as well as the other members.
8. Many older people likely to be in need of groups may be depressed or have experienced a number of losses (health, friends, spouse). Discussion of losses and sad feelings can be difficult for group leaders. A leader prone to depression would not be appropriate.
9. Leaders must be prepared for some members to become ill, deteriorate, and die. Plans regarding recognition of missing members will need to be clear. The following, which occurred during a reminiscence group conducted by one of the authors (TT), illustrates: "As I arrived at the nursing home for the weekly reminiscence group meeting, I was told by the nursing home staff that one of our members had died. One of the members had been a priest so we asked him to say a prayer for our deceased group member. He did so beautifully, and the group was grateful. The next week, to our surprise, the supposedly deceased member showed up for the group (she had been in the hospital). We didn't know how to handle the situation, but the other members came to our rescue by saying, 'Father's prayers really worked this time.'" Older people's wisdom and humor can teach us a lot.
10. Leaders are continually confronted with their own aging and attitudes toward it. Co-leaders are ideal and can support each other. It is important to share thoughts and feelings, recapitulate group sessions, and modify approaches as needed. If leading the group alone, try to have someone with expertise in group work with elders who can discuss the group experiences with you and provide support and direction. Students generally should work in pairs and will need supervision. Skills in developing and implementing groups for older adults improve with experience. Burnside* reminds us that "all new group leaders should have guidance from an experienced leader to help them weather the difficult times" (p. 43).

*Burnside I: Group work with older persons, *J Gerontol Nurs* 20(1):43, 1994.

and self-actualization should not be denied to individuals based on their cognitive status. Modifications must be made according to the cognitive abilities of the person, and although individual life review from a psychotherapeutic approach is not an appropriate modality, individuals with mild to moderate memory impairment can enjoy and benefit from group work focused on reminiscence and storytelling.

When the nurse is working with a group of cognitively impaired older adults, the emphasis in reminiscence groups is on sharing memories, however they

may be expressed, rather than specific recall of events. There should be no pressure to answer questions such as "Where were you born?" or "What was your first job?" Rather, discussions may center on jobs people had and places they have lived. Additional props, such as music, pictures, and familiar objects (e.g., an American flag, an old coffee grinder), can prompt many recollections and sharing. The leader of a group with participants who have memory problems must be more active. Many resources are available to guide these groups, including books such as *I Remember When*

(Thorsheim and Roberts, 2000), that offer numerous ways to adapt the reminiscing process for those with cognitive impairment. StoryCorps Memory Loss Initiative (www.storycorps.net/special-initiatives/mli) is an innovative program featuring the stories of people with memory loss. Other helpful resources are listed at the end of the chapter and at evolve.elsevier.com/Ebersole/gerontological.

Bastings (2003, 2006) (www.timeslips.org) has described a storytelling modality designed for individuals with cognitive impairment called Time Slips. Group members, looking at a picture, are encouraged to create a story about the picture. The pictures can be fantastical and funny, such as from greeting cards, or more nostalgic, such as Norman Rockwell paintings. All contributions are encouraged and welcomed, there are no right or wrong answers, and everything that the individuals say is included in the story and written down by the scribe. Stories are read back to the participants during the session, using their names to identify their contributions. At the beginning of each session, the story from the last session is read to the participants. Care is taken to compliment each member for his or her contribution to the wonderful story. The stories that emerge are full of humor and creativity and often include discussions of memories and reminiscing. John Killick (1999, p. 49), writer in residence at a nursing home in Scotland, stated: "Having their words written down is empowering for people with dementia. It affirms their dignity and gives an assurance that their words still have value . . . One woman said, 'Anything you can tell people about how things are for me is important. It's a rum do, this growing ancient . . . The brilliance of my brain has slipped away when I wasn't looking.'"

One of the authors (TT) has used the storytelling modality extensively with mild to moderately impaired older people with great success as part of a research study on the effect of therapeutic activities for persons with memory loss. Potential outcomes include increased verbalization and communication, socialization, alleviation of depression, and enhanced quality of life. Qualitative responses from group participants and families indicate their enjoyment with the process. At the end of the 16-week group, the stories are bound into a book and given to the participants with a picture of the group and each member's name listed. Many of the participants and their families have commented on the pride they feel at their "book" and have even shared them with grandchildren and great-grandchildren. In Basting's work (Bastings, 2003), some of the stories were presented as a play. Although further research is indicated in relation to the outcomes of this intervention, it seems to have potential as a beneficial and cost-effective therapeutic intervention in many settings.

IMPLICATIONS FOR GERONTOLOGICAL NURSING AND HEALTHY AGING

Throughout this chapter we have tried to convey the potential for honest and hopeful communication regardless of the impairment the elder may be experiencing. Communicating with older people calls for special skills, patience, and respect. We must break through the barriers and continue to reach toward the humanity of the individual with the belief that communication is the most vital service we offer. This is the heart of nursing.

APPLICATION OF MASLOW'S HIERARCHY

Skilled, sensitive, and caring individual and group communication strategies with elders are essential to meeting needs for elders at all levels of Maslow's hierarchy. Elders with communication difficulties may have difficulty expressing basic needs for food, water, toileting, sleep, nutrition, and safety and security. Adapting communication to enhance understanding and satisfaction of basic needs not only assists in preserving biological integrity, but is also the basis for the establishment of therapeutic nursing relationships that help individuals grow toward self-actualization. Just as all people have the need to communicate and have their basic needs met, they also have the right to experiences that are meaningful and fulfilling. Age, language impairment, or mental status do not change these needs.

Creation of care environments that are rich with pleasant experiences—a good cup of coffee, a meal shared with friends, a sunrise, beautiful music, learning something interesting, or sharing experiences from the life one has lived—is as important as getting enough to eat. Our nursing care with older people experiencing cognitive and communication impairments must be more than keeping their bodies alive, safe, and clean, or preventing injury. The unique contribution that nursing brings to the care of people is the intimate, personal knowing of the person behind the disease and the creation of relationships and environments of care that support, validate, and celebrate the person as someone of value and worth (Touhy, 2004). Within this framework, gerontological nurses assist in the meeting of needs at all levels.

KEY CONCEPTS

▶ Communication is a basic need regardless of age or communication or cognitive impairment. Respect for the person and knowledge of therapeutic communication techniques are essential skills for gerontological nurses.

▶ Group work can meet many needs at all levels of Maslow's hierarchy and is satisfying and rewarding for both the older adult and the group leader.

▶ In a rapidly changing society, the shared life histories of elders provide a sense of continuity among the generations.

▶ The life history of an individual is a story to be developed and treasured. This is particularly important toward the end of life.

▶ Gerontological nursing responses related to communication are focused mainly on using therapeutic communication techniques, providing necessary information, encouraging individuals to express personal interests and preferences and, when function is impeded, ensuring that basic needs are recognized by all, discussed, and met to the greatest extent possible.

ACTIVITIES AND DISCUSSION QUESTIONS

1. Using ear plugs or glasses with the lens covered in Vaseline, try performing some of your daily activities or engage in conversation with your peers.
2. Discuss how you might provide medication instruction to a client with a hearing or vision loss.
3. Discuss adaptations to communication for individuals with aphasia or dysarthria.
4. Discuss ways in which you might respond to a person with cognitive impairment who has difficulty expressing thoughts and feelings.
5. Role-play a simulated interaction with an older adult experiencing communication or cognitive impairments such as aphasia, dysarthria, or memory loss.
6. With a partner, plan and discuss an activity that would be appropriate for an individual with cognitive impairment.
7. Rent the movie *Iris, The Notebook,* or *Away from Her,* and discuss effective and ineffective communication strategies you observed with persons experiencing cognitive impairment.
8. With your peers, form a small group and share memories about a type of event all have experienced in their lives (e.g., first date, first day of school).
9. Interview an elder and ask to hear his or her life story.

RESOURCES

Communication
Organizations

National Eye Institute
31 Center Drive, MSC 2510, Building 31, Room 6A32
Bethesda, MD 20892-2510
(301) 496-5248
website: www.nei.nih.gov

National Institute on Deafness and Other Communication Disorders
National Institutes of Health
31 Center Drive, MSC 2320
Bethesda, MD 20892-2320
e-mail: nidcdinfo@nidcd.nih.gov
website: www.nidcd.nih.gov

Unfair Hearing Test
website: www.irrd.ca/education/presentation.asp?refname=e2c1

Vision Simulator (*to experience visual impairments*)
website: visionsimulator.com

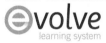

For additional resources, please visit evolve.elsevier.com/Ebersole/gerontological.

REFERENCES

Adams-Wendling L, Pimple C: Evidence-based guideline: nursing management of hearing impairment in nursing facility residents, *J Gerontol Nurs* 34(11):9-17, 2008.

American Speech-Language-Hearing Association: Incidence and prevalence of hearing loss and hearing aid use in the United States, 2008 edition. Accessed March 6, 2008 from www.asha.org/members/research/reports/hearing.htm.

Bastings A: Reading the story behind the story: context and content in stories by people with dementia, *Generations* 27(3):25-29, 2003.

Bastings A: Arts in dementia care: "This is not the end . . . it's the end of this chapter," *Generations* 30(1):16-20, 2006.

Beck CT: Nursing students' experience caring for cognitively impaired elderly people, *J Adv Nursing* 23(5):992-998, 1996.

Birren JE, Deutchman DE: *Guiding autobiography groups for older adults: exploring the fabric of life,* Baltimore, 1991, Johns Hopkins University Press.

Bohlmeijer E, Smit F, Cuijpers P: Effects of reminiscence and life review on late-life depression: a meta-analysis, *Int J Geriatr Psychiatry* 18(12):1088-1094, 2003.

Buckwalter KC, Gerdner LA, Hall GR et al: Shining through: the humor and individuality of persons with Alzheimer's disease, *J Gerontol Nurs* 21(3):11-16, 1995.

Burnside IM: Listen to the aged, *Am J Nurs* 75(10):1800-1803, 1975.

Butler R: The life review: an interpretation of reminiscence in the aged, *Psychiatry* 26:65-76, 1963.

Butler R: Age, death and life review, 2002. Available at www. hospicefoundation.org. Accessed June 24, 2004.

Butler R, Lewis M: *Aging and mental health: positive psycho-social approaches,* ed 3, St. Louis, 1983, Mosby.

Centers for Disease Control and Prevention (CDC): *Trends in vision and hearing among older Americans,* March 2002. Accessed June 24, 2006 from www.cdc.gov.

Clark DJ: Older adults living through and with their computers, *Comput Inform Nurs* 20(3):117-124, 2002.

Cohen-Mansfield J, Taylor J: Hearing aid use in nursing homes, *J Am Med Dir Assoc* 5(5):283-296, 2004.

Coles R: *The call of stories,* Boston, 1989, Houghton Mifflin Co.

Erikson EH: *Childhood and society,* ed 2, New York, 1963, WW Norton.

Fazio S: Person-centered language is an essential part of person-centered care, *Alzheimer Care Q* 2(2):87-90, 2001.

Guest C, Collis G, McNicholas J: Hearing dogs: a longitudinal study of social and psychological effects on deaf and hard-of-hearing recipients, *J Deaf Stud Deaf Educ* 11(2):252-261, 2006.

Haight B, Burnside IM: Reminiscence and life review: explaining the differences, *Arch Psychiatr Nurs* 7(2):91-98, 1993.

Haight B, Webster J: *Critical advances in reminiscence work: from theory to application,* New York, 2002, Springer.

Ham R, Sloane P, Warshaw G et al: *Primary care geriatrics,* ed 5, St. Louis, 2007, Mosby.

Happ M, Paull B: Silence is not golden, *Geriatr Nurs* 29(3):166-167, 2008.

Keller H: *The story of my life,* Garden City, NY, 1902, Doubleday.

Kiely DK, Simon MA, Jones RN, Morris JN: The protective effect of social engagement on mortality in long-term care, *J Am Geriatr Soc* 48(11):1367-1372, 2000.

Killick J: "What are we like here?" Eliciting experiences of people with dementia, *Generations* 13(3):46-49, 1999.

Koch J, Datta G, Makhdoom S, Grossberg G: Unmet visual needs of Alzheimers patients in long-term care facilities, *J Am Med Dir Assoc* 6(4):233-237, 2005.

Moore T, Hollett J: Giving voice to persons living with dementia: the researcher's opportunities and challenges, *Nurs Sci Q* 16(2):164-167, 2003.

Murphy J, Tester S, Hubbard G, Downs M: Enabling frail older people with communication difficulties to express views: the use of talking mats as an intervention tool, *Health Soc Care Community* 13(2):95-107, 2005.

National Institute on Aging: Chapter 2: Listening to older people. Accessed March 6, 2008 from www.nia.nih.gov.

Nelson T: *Ageism,* Cambridge MA, 2004, MIT Press.

Owsley C, Ball K, McGwin G et al: Effect of refractive error correction on health-related quality of life and depression in older nursing home residents, *Arch Opthalmol* 125(11):1471-1477, 2007

Rowe JW, Kahn RL: *Successful aging,* New York, 1998, Pantheon-Random House.

Rowe S, MacLean C, Shekelle P: Preventing vision loss from chronic eye disease in primary care: scientific reviews, *JAMA* 291(12):1487-1495, 2004.

Sacks O: *Seeing voices: a journey into the world of the deaf,* Berkeley, 1989, University of California Press.

Sandelowski M: We are the stories we tell, *J Holistic Nurs* 12(1):23-33, 1994.

Snyder L: The lived experience of Alzheimer's - understanding the feeling and subjective accounts of persons with the disease, *Alzheimer Care Q* 2(2):8-22, 2001.

Talarico K, Evans L: Making sense of aggressive/protective behavior in persons with dementia, *Alzheimer's Care Q* 1(4):77-88, 2000.

Tappen RM, Williams-Burgess C, Edelstein J et al: Communicating with individuals with Alzheimer's disease: examination of recommended strategies, *Arch Psychiatr Nurs* 11(5):249-256, 1997.

Tappen RM, Williams C, Fishman S et al: Persistence of self in advanced Alzheimer's disease, *Image J Nurs Sch* 31(2): 121-125, 1999.

Thorsheim H, Roberts B: *I remember when: activity ideas to help people reminisce,* Forest Knolls, CA, 2000, Elder Books.

Touhy T, Williams C: Communicating with older adults. In Williams C: *Therapeutic interaction in nursing,* ed 2, Boston, 2008, Jones and Bartlett.

Touhy TA: Dementia, personhood, and nursing: learning from a nursing situation, *Nurs Sci Q* 17(1):43-49, 2004.

U.S. Department of Health and Human Services (USDHHS): *Healthy People* 2010. *Vision and hearing,* 2002. Accessed July 3, 2008 from www.health.gov/healthypeople/document/html/volume2/28vision.htm.

Wallhagen M, Pettengill E: Hearing impairment significant but underassessed in primary care settings, *J Gerontol Nurs* 34(2):36-42, 2008.

Wallhagen M, Pettengill E, Whiteside M: Sensory impairment in older adults: Part 1: hearing loss, *AJN* 106(10):40-8, 2006.

Whiteside M, Wallhagen M, Pettengill E: Sensory impairment in older adults. Part 2: vision loss, *Am J Nurs* 106(11):52-61, 2006. Accessed July 3, 2008 from www.nursingcenter.com/ajnolderadults.

Williams K: Improving outcomes of nursing home interactions, *Res Nurs and Health* 29(2):121-133, 2006.

Williams K, Kemper S, Hummert L: Improving nursing home communication: an intervention to reduce elderspeak, *Gerontologist* 43(2):242-247, 2003.

Williams K, Kemper S, Hummert L: Enhancing communication with older adults: overcoming elderspeak, *J Gerontol Nurs* 30(10):17-25, 2004.

Williams C, Tappen R: Communicating with cognitively impaired persons, In Williams C: *Therapeutic interaction in nursing,* ed 2, Boston, 2008, Jones and Bartlett.

Woods B: The person in dementia care, *Generations* 13(3): 35-39, 1999.

Culture and Aging

4

LEARNING OBJECTIVES

Upon completion of this chapter, the reader will be able to:

- Identify factors contributing to the nurse's cultural sensitivity.
- Discuss approaches that facilitate an appreciation of diverse cultural and ethnic experiences.
- Explain the prominent health care belief systems.
- Identify nursing care interventions appropriate for ethnically diverse elders.
- Formulate a plan of care incorporating ethnically sensitive interventions.

GLOSSARY

Culture Beliefs, customs, and values that are shared by a group and passed on from one generation to the next

Ethnicity Belonging to or deriving from the cultural, racial, religious, or linguistic traditions of a people or country.

Ethnocentrism The belief in the inherent superiority of one's ethnic group, accompanied by devaluation of other groups.

Folk medicine Healing methods originating among the people of a given culture and primarily transmitted from person to person.

Interpreter A person who transmits the meaning of what is spoken in one language in another spoken language.

Stereotype Belief applied to a group of persons based on actual or assumed knowledge of an individual member of the group.

Translator A person who converts written materials from one language to another.

THE LIVED EXPERIENCE

I feel so out of place here. If my children weren't so busy, I suppose I could live with them, but they seemed so relieved when this retirement home would accept me. I wonder if they knew I was the only Chinese person in this place. A sweet young Chinese student tried to talk with me, but she only spoke Mandarin and I speak Cantonese. She had never lived in China. I want so much to talk to someone my age who lived in China and speaks my language.

Shin, a 75-year-old woman

Interest in and attention to culture and health care are increasing. In the field of gerontology, this interest is stimulated to a great extent by two major issues: the realization of a "gerontological explosion" and the recognition of the significant health disparities in the Unites States. The *gerontological explosion* refers both to the rapid increases in the total numbers of older adults, especially those over the age of 85, and to the relative proportion of older adults in most countries across the globe (see Chapter 1). *Health disparities* refers to the differences in disease burden between people. Those found to be especially vulnerable to health disparities are men and women from ethnically distinct groups.

Today's nurse is expected to provide competent care to persons with different life experiences, cultural perspectives, values, and styles of communication than their own. The nurse may need to effectively communicate with people regardless of the languages being spoken. In doing so, the nurse depends on limited verbal exchanges and attends more to facial and body expressions, postures, gestures, and touching. However, these forms of communication are heavily influenced by culture and ethnicity and easily may be misunderstood. To be able to skillfully assess and intervene, nurses must first develop cultural sensitivity through awareness of their own ethnocentrism. Effective nurses develop cultural competence through new cultural knowledge about ethnicity, culture, language, and health belief systems, and develop the skills needed to optimize intercultural communication.

Knowing how to provide culturally competent care is especially important in gerontological nursing since many older adults are just now immigrating to the United States. Many others have spent their lives in self-contained, homogenous communities and may not have become acculturated to a Western model of care. This situation is likely to result in cultural conflict and in the health care setting.

This chapter provides an overview of culture and aging, as well as strategies that gerontological nurses can use to best respond to the changing face of aging and in doing so, help reduce health disparities. These strategies include increasing cultural sensitivity, knowledge, and skills in working with diverse groups of older adults.

THE GERONTOLOGICAL EXPLOSION

The population of the United States is rapidly becoming more diverse. Persons of color, who have long been classified as those from "minority groups," will come to represent about 50% of the population in the next 50 years. Among those over 65 years of age, the numbers are not as dramatic, but the effect of the growth is being seen in all aspects of gerontological nursing and long-term care. It would not be unusual for nurses working in states with the greatest number of immigrant elders (California, Nevada, Florida, Texas, New Jersey, and Illinois) to care for persons from a variety of backgrounds in the same day (Gelfand, 2003). The greatest increase in the number

of ethnically diverse elders in the United States will be those who identify themselves as Hispanic, followed by Asian and Pacific Islanders (Figure 4-1). It must be noted, however, that these and many of the figures available today are drawn from the U.S. Census, in which persons of color are often underrepresented and those who reside illegally are not included at all. In reality, the numbers of elders from diverse backgrounds in the United States may be and may become substantially higher.

HEALTH DISPARITIES

In 2003 the Institute of Medicine (IOM) prepared the landmark analysis of the state of the science on health disparities. It began with the acknowledgement that persons of color had difficulty accessing the same care as their white counterparts. The researchers were to determine the state of care while controlling for access issues. The study showed that health care treatment in the United States in and of itself was unequal (Smedley et al, 2002) (Box 4-1). The barriers to quality care were found to be wide, ranging from those related to geographical location to age, sex, race, ethnicity, and sexual orientation. Disparities were consistently found across a wide range of disease areas and clinical services.

Reducing Health Disparities

The IOM study also provided a number of recommendations for reducing health disparities. However, before change can occur, health care providers must become more culturally competent. The objective is not just to become competent but to become culturally proficient, that is, able to move smoothly between the world of the nurse and the world of the patient (in this case, the world of the elder). Moving toward culturally proficient gerontological nursing care is one of the major strategies to reduce health disparities.

INCREASING CULTURAL COMPETENCE

As nurses move toward cultural competence, they increase their cultural awareness, knowledge, and skills. Nurses can learn of their personal biases, prejudices, attitudes, and behaviors toward persons different from themselves in race, ethnicity, age, gender, sexual orientation, social class, economic situations, and many other factors. Through increased knowledge, nurses can better assess the strengths and weaknesses of the older

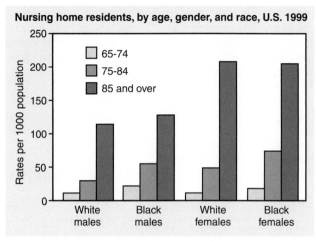

Fig. 4-1   Nursing home residents, by age, sex, and race—United States, 1999. *(From The National Nursing Home Survey.)*

adult within the context of their culture and know when and how to effectively intervene to support rather than hinder cultural patterns that enhance wellness and coping. Cultural competence means having the skills to put cultural knowledge to use in assessment, communication, negotiation, and intervention.

Box 4-1	Examples of Health Disparities Relevant to Older Adults

African Americans
African American women are twice as likely to die from cervical cancer than white women and more likely to die to breast cancer than any other women
When compared to whites, African American men and women are:
- 29% more likely to die from heart disese
- 40% more likely to die from stroke
- Two times more likely to have diabetes
African Americans account for 66% of all adults with HIV

American Indians and Alskan Natives
2.6 times more likely to have diagnoses diabetes than non-Hispanic whites

Source: CDC Office of Minority Health Disparities: Disease burden and risk factors, 2007. Accessed November 24, 2008 from http://www.cdc.gov/omhd/AMH/dbrf.htm.

Cultural Awareness

Increased awareness calls for openness and self-reflection. If the nurse is white, it is realizing that this whiteness means special privilege and freedoms in a predominantly white society. Older adults of color may not have had the same advantages or experiences as the nurse (McIntosh, 1989). For example, in many regions of the United States, especially in the South, the current cohort of African Americans was limited to a fourth-grade education, with far-reaching implications. African Americans who are elderly today lived during the time of Jim Crow laws which legalized discrimination and segregation and significantly restricted their lives. Events of the time included numerous murders by lynching (Box 4-2) (see www.jimcrowhistory.org). These elders are also aware of the Tuskegee Experiment, in which black men with syphilis were purposely deceived and not treated so scientists could study its effect over time (see www.cdc.gov/tuskegee/timeline.html). For some, this has left a continuing distrust of the health care system and a reluctance to become involved in research.

Cultural awareness means recognizing the presence of the "isms" such as the racism just described. It is imperative to understand how these affect not only the pursuit and receipt of health care, but also the quality of life for older adults (Smedley et al, 2002). Moreover, as older adults they may have to face ageism, in addition to racism, sexism, classism, and so on.

Box 4-2	Racism in the Boston Naming Test*

During a study to evaluate the cultural applicability of several standard psychological tools sometimes administered by nurses, an 82-year-old African American woman reluctantly agreed to take what is called the Boston Naming Test. This measure of verbal fluency used in the diagnosis of dementia comprises a packet of pictures. The patient is asked to name the pictures. After doing so the volunteer shared, "Did you know that one of the pictures is a hangman's noose? Do you have any idea what that means to a black person to look at that picture!" Indeed, none of the white researchers had noticed this.

*Personal experience of Kathleen Jett.

Ageism is a term coined by Robert Butler, the first director of the National Institute on Aging, to describe the discrimination and negative stereotypes that are based solely on age. Cole (1997) examined the historic roots of ageism in America. At one time, power in the United States was held almost exclusively by older white males. With the shift to urban industrialism and a growing emphasis on productivity and the ability to withstand the rigors of factory work, power and influence shifted from older to younger white men. We now know that ageism is not universal but is most often reflective of the Euro-American culture. In many other cultures, especially those outside of the United States, elders are treated with special respect and honor. For example, African American elders are respected. They often provide wisdom and insight to younger members of the family. Owing to a number of factors, African American grandparents are increasingly assuming the role of parent, for grandchildren and other teenage and younger relatives (Caminha-Bacote, 2008) (see Chapter 23).

Some health care professionals demonstrate ageism, undoubtedly in part because providers tend to see many frail older persons and fewer of those who are healthy and active. The impact of these perceptions has largely been ignored but almost certainly negatively affects health outcomes.

Before the gerontological nurse provides quality care to elders from ethnic groups that are different from their own, it is useful to self-reflect and consider whether one holds any personal beliefs about such persons and whether these beliefs are negative or positive,

how they affect care delivery, and if they are based on facts rather than anecdotal experiences.

Cultural Knowledge

Cultural knowledge is both what the nurse brings to the caring situation and what the nurse learns about older adults, their families, their communities, their behaviors, and their expectations. Essential knowledge includes the elder's way of life (ways of thinking, believing, and acting). This knowledge is obtained formally and informally through the individual's professional experience of nursing.

Some nurses prefer to use what can be called an "encyclopedic" approach to details of a particular culture or ethnic group, such as proper name usage, touch, greeting, eye contact, gender roles, foods, and beliefs about relevant topics such as health promoting practices, pain expression, death rituals, or caregiving. This information is available in many compendiums of cross-cultural information (see Resources section at the end of this chapter and at evolve.elsevier.com/Ebersole/gerontological). When working with elders from specific cultures, knowledge about attitudes toward caregiving, decision making, and death rituals are especially important.

Although cultural knowledge is helpful and essential, caution must be used with regard to the potential for stereotyping. Stereotyping is the application of limited knowledge about one person with specific characteristics to other persons with the same characteristics; negative characteristics are especially prone to this treatment. Stereotyping limits the recognition of the heterogeneity of the group. Relying on knowledge of a positive stereotype can be useful as a starting point in understanding, but it too can be used to limit understanding of the uniqueness of the individual and impose unrealistic expectations. For example, a common way to stereotype older African Americans is to assume that the church is a source of support to them. The nurse's assumption can easily have a negative outcome, such as fewer referrals for other forms of support (e.g., home-delivered meals). On the other hand, this stereotype can be used to shortcut the discharge planning. In discussing discharge plans with an African American elder, the nurse may say, "I understand that the church is often a source of support in the African American community. Is this one of the resources you will be able to depend on when you return home?"

Persons from a specific ethnic group may share a common geographical origin, migratory status, race, language or dialect, or religion. Traditions, symbols, literature, folklore, food preferences, and dress are expressions of ethnicity that are often adopted. This may be particularly true for older adults who have had no need to leave their culture-specific neighborhoods such as Chinatowns in the major cities, or the barrios of the Southwest. Persons who identify with the same ethnic group may or may not share a common race. For example, persons who consider themselves Hispanic are members of the most diverse ethnic group in the United States and may be from any race and from any one of a number of countries. However, those who consider themselves Hispanics usually have the Catholic religion and the Spanish language in common.

Health beliefs and practices are usually a mixed expression of life experience and cultural knowledge. In most cultures, older adults are likely to treat themselves for familiar or chronic conditions in ways they have found successful in the past, practices that are referred to as domestic medicine, folk medicine, or folk healing. The basis for much folk medicine was and remains making the most of whatever is available. When self-treatment fails, a person will consult with others known to be knowledgeable or experienced with the problem, such as a community or indigenous healer, often an elder in the community. Only when this, too, fails do people seek help within the formal health care system.

The culture of nursing and health care in the United States is one that advocates what is called the Western or biomedical system with its own set of beliefs about the cause of illness, the choice of treatments, and so on. In most settings this belief system is considered superior to all others, an ethnocentric viewpoint. However, many of the world's people have different beliefs, such as those of the personalistic (magicoreligious) system or the naturalistic (holistic) system. Each system is complete with beliefs about disease causation and recommendations for prevention and treatment. Nurses who are familiar with the range of health beliefs and realize their importance to the followers will be able to provide more sensitive and appropriate care. In the absence of understanding there is great potential for conflict. This is especially important to remember when working with ethnic immigrants or those who have lived in culturally homogeneous communities.

Western or Biomedical System

In the Western or biomedical belief system, disease is thought to be the result of abnormalities in the structure and function of body organs and systems, often caused by an invasion of germs. The terms *disease* and *illness*

are subjective; they are used by care providers and not always understood by others. In the biomedical system, assessment and diagnosis are directed at identifying the pathogen or the process causing the abnormality by using laboratory and other procedures. Treatment is based on removing or destroying the invading organism or repairing, modifying, or removing the affected body part. Prevention, in this belief system, involves the avoidance of pathogens, chemicals, activities, and dietary agents known to cause abnormalities. Health is often considered the absence of disease (see Chapter 1).

Personalistic or Magicoreligious System

Those who follow the beliefs of the personalistic or magicoreligious system believe that illness is caused by the actions of the supernatural, such as gods, deities, or nonhuman beings, such as ghosts, ancestors, or spirits. Health is viewed as a blessing or reward of God and illness as a punishment for a breach of rules, breaking a taboo, or displeasing or failing to please the source of power. Beliefs about illness and disease being caused by the wrath of God are prevalent among members of the Holiness, Pentecostal, and Fundamentalist Baptist churches. Examples of magical causes that illness can be attributed to are voodoo, especially among persons from the Caribbean; root work among southern African Americans; hexing among Mexican Americans and African Americans; and Gaba among Filipino Americans. Treatments may include religious practices, such as praying, meditating, fasting, wearing amulets, burning candles, and establishing family altars. Making sure that social networks with their fellow humans are in good working order is viewed as the essence of prevention. It is therefore important to avoid angering family, friends, neighbors, ancestors, and gods. This belief system can be traced back to the ancient Egyptians, thousands of years before the common era, and persists in its entirety or in parts in many groups. Current practices that would be included in this group include rituals such as "laying of the hands" and prayer circles. It is not uncommon to hear an older adult pray for a cure or lament, "What did I do to cause this?"

Naturalistic or Holistic Health System

The naturalistic or holistic health belief system is based on the concept of balance and stems from the ancient civilizations of China, India, and Greece (Wang and Paulanka, 2008). Many people throughout the world view health as a sign of balance—of the right amount of exercise, food, sleep, evacuation, interpersonal relationships, or the geophysical and metaphysical forces in the universe, such as *chi*. Disturbances in this balance result in disharmony and subsequent illness. Diagnosis calls for the determination of the type and extent of imbalance. The appropriate interventions, therefore, are methods of restoring balance and harmony.

Traditional Chinese medicine is based on this belief, on the balance between *yin* and *yang*, darkness and light, hot and cold. Older adults who were raised in one of the countries on the Pacific Rim (especially in Asia and the Pacific Islands) or in a traditional American Indian community frequently rely on these beliefs. The naturalistic system practiced in India and some of its neighboring countries is known as ayurvedic.

Another variation is seen in those who follow the hot-cold beliefs, apart from traditional Chinese medicine. Illness is believed to be the result of an excess of heat or cold that has entered the body and caused an imbalance. Hot and cold are generally metaphoric, although at times actual temperature is an aspect. Various foods, medicines, environmental conditions, emotions, and body conditions, such as menopause, may possess the characteristics of either hot or cold (Spector, 2006). Selecting an appropriate treatment requires the identification of disease type, either hot or cold; treatments are likewise divided. Treatment is focused on using the opposite element; if the disease is the result of excess heat, treatment will be with something that has cold properties, and vice versa. The treatments may take the form of teas, herbs, food, dietary restrictions, techniques, or medications from Western medicine that have hot and cold properties, such as antibiotics, massage, poultices, or other therapies.

Naturalistic healers can also be advanced practice nurses, physicians, or herbalists who specialize in symptomatic treatment and know which medicines will restore the body's equilibrium. In the American Indian culture, the healer is referred to as a medicine man or woman who combines naturalistic and magicoreligious systems. Prevention is directed at protecting oneself from imbalance.

Cultural Skills

Skillful cross-cultural nursing means developing a sense of mutual respect between the nurse and the elder. It is working "with" the client rather than "on" the client. Providing the highest quality of care for ethnically diverse elders and enhancing healthy aging calls for a new or refined set of skills. These skills include listening carefully to the person, especially for his or her perception of the situation, and attending not just to the words but to the nonverbal communication and the meaning behind the stories. It is a skill to be able to listen to the elder's perception of the situation, desired goals, and ideas for treatment. Cultural skills include the ability to explain your (the nurse's) perceptions clearly and without judgment, acknowledging that there are both similarities and differences between your perceptions and goals and those of the elder. Finally, cross-cultural skills include the ability to develop a plan of action that takes both perspectives into account and negotiate an outcome that is mutually acceptable (Berlin and Fowkes, 1983).

Working with Interpreters

Working with persons in the cross-cultural nursing situation often includes working with an interpreter. Interpretation is the process of rendering oral expressions made in one language system into another in a manner that preserves the meaning and tone of the original without adding or deleting anything. The job of the interpreter is to work with two different linguistic codes in a way that will produce equivalent messages. The interpreter tells the elder what the nurse has said and the nurse what the elder has said without adding meaning or opinion but in a way in which communication is as accurate as possible. This is often confused with translation (when interpreters are called "translators"), which instead deals with the written word.

Respectful communication is called for at all times; it is essential, however, with older adults from cultures in which this is the expectation and for those with limited or no English proficiency. Respectful communication includes addressing the person in the appropriate manner (surname unless otherwise instructed by the elder) and using acceptable body language. For example in most cultures other than those of northern Europe (including Euro-Americans) direct eye contact is considered disrespectful. To press eye contact with an elder may be particularly rude.

An interpreter is needed any time the nurse and the elder speak different languages, when the elder has limited English proficiency, or when cultural tradition prevents the elder from speaking directly to the nurse, for example as a result of the nurse's being a man or woman. The more complex the decision that must be made, the more important the skills of the interpreter are, such as when determining the elder's wishes regarding life-prolonging measures or the family's plan for caregiving.

It is ideal to engage persons who are trained in medical interpretation and who are of the same age, sex, and social status as the elder whenever possible. Unfortunately it is usually necessary to call upon younger interpreters; the effectiveness of the exchange may be hampered by the presence of intergenerational boundaries. Children and grandchildren are often called on to act as interpreters. In such a situation the nurse may realize that the child or the elder is "editing" comments because of cultural restrictions about the sharing of certain information (i.e., what is or is not considered appropriate to speak of to an elder or a child).

When working with an interpreter the nurse first introduces herself or himself to the client and the interpreter and sets guidelines for the interview. Sentences should be short, employ the active voice, and avoid metaphors because they may be impossible to convert from one language to another. The nurse asks the interpreter to articulate exactly what is being said, and all conversation is addressed directly to the client.

For more information, see Box 4-3 and refer to the detailed guidelines and protocols available from Enslein and colleagues at the University of Iowa (Enslein et al, 2001, 2002).

IMPLICATIONS FOR GERONTOLOGICAL NURSING AND HEALTHY AGING

The contact between elders and gerontological nurses often begins with assessment. During that process, the nurse and the elder have an opportunity to come to know each other. Listening is the key to the assessment; the nurse tries to understand the meaning of the situation and the person's perceptions. A thorough assessment includes a cultural assessment. A comprehensive assessment takes time, and listening is the key. It is clear that not all situations allow for this, but even if it must be done bit by bit over time, it will give the caregiver a better understanding of how to work with and within the culture of the client.

Several tools or instruments can assist the nurse to elicit health care beliefs and at the same time identify to the nurse his or her own perceptions of alternative beliefs. Although Leininger's Sunrise Model (Shen, 2004; Schim et al, 2007) is often recommended, alternative models may be more useful in the fast-paced health care situations of today. The explanatory model developed by Kleinman and associates (1978) has become a classic and has helped nurses and other health care professionals obtain the basic information needed in a culturally sensitive manner. An adaptation of this model for use in obtaining a meaningful cultural health

---

Box 4-3	Working with Interpreters

- Before an interview or session with a client, meet with the interpreter to explain the purpose of the session.
- Encourage the interpreter to meet with the client before the session to identify the client's educational level and attitudes toward health and health care and to determine the depth and type of information and explanation needed.
- Look and speak directly to the client, not the interpreter.
- Be patient. Interpreted interviews take more time because long, explanatory phrases are often needed.
- Use short units of speech. Long, involved sentences or complex discussions create confusion.
- Use simple language. Avoid technical terms, professional jargon, slang, abbreviations, abstractions, metaphors, or idiomatic expressions.
- Encourage interpretation of the client's own words rather than paraphrased professional jargon to get a better sense of the client's ideas and emotional state.
- Request that the interpreter avoids inserting his or her own ideas and to avoid omitting information.
- Listen to the client and watch nonverbal communication (facial expression, voice intonation, body movement) to learn about emotions regarding a specific topic.
- Clarify the client's understanding and the accuracy of the interpretation by asking the client to tell you in his or her own words what he or she understands, facilitated by the interpreter.

Reference: Enslein J, Tripp-Reimer T, Kelley LS et al: Evidence-based protocol: interpreter facilitation for individuals with limited English proficiency, *J Gerontol Nurs* 28(7):5-13, 2002. Available on-line from http://www.nursing.uiowa.edu/products_services/documents/June07Catalog.pdf. Accessed September 22, 2008.

---

assessment appears in Box 4-4. The LEARN Model (Berlin and Fowkes, 1983) can be used to increase the effectiveness of nursing interventions. It is a useful guide for the nurse in the clinical setting. Through it, the nurse will increase his or her cultural sensitivity and in doing so will be instrumental in providing more culturally competent care, thus helping reduce health disparities (Box 4-5).

With an understanding of the basics, the nurse can negotiate a clear understanding of problems and solutions with the person or with the identified support figure in his or her life. Once an understanding is reached, the nurse may need to include consultation or collaboration with traditional or alternative healers if the patient believes this is important. Priests, monks, rabbis, ministers, or indigenous healers may provide essential consultation, support, and interventions of their own. A sense of caring is conveyed in giving support to cultural beliefs and practices. Unbiased caring can surmount cultural differences.

Also critical to the cultural assessment is to determine the person's health beliefs, as discussed earlier. Most people (nurses and patients alike) subscribe to more than one belief system, combining Western biomedical approaches with those that may be considered more traditional. People choose among the health belief systems or include aspects of several of them in their attempt to make sense of health, illness, and treatments. To optimize the healthy aging of the person who depends on the nurse for intervention and caring, the nurse must be sensitive to the possibility that the person may hold one or more of these beliefs.

When a patient refuses biomedical treatments because the health problem is viewed as God's will or destiny, this is often particularly difficult for the nurse

---

Box 4-5	The LEARN Model

L Listen carefully to what the elder is saying. Attend to not just the words but to the nonverbal communication and the meaning behind the stories. Listen to the elder's perception of the situation, the desired goals, and the ideas for treatment.

E Explain your perception of the situation and the problems.

A Acknowledge and discuss both the similarities and the differences between your perceptions and goals and those of the elder.

R Recommend a plan of action that takes both perspectives into account.

N Negotiate a plan that is mutually acceptable.

Source: Berlin EA, Fowkes WC: A teaching framework for cross-cultural health care: application in family practice, *West J Med* 139(6):934-938, 1983.

Box 4-4	The Explanatory Model for Culturally Sensitive Assessment

1. How would you describe the problem that has brought you here? (*What do you call your problem; does it have a name?*)
   a. Who is involved in your decision making about health concerns?
2. How long have you had this problem?
   a. When do you think it started?
   b. What do you think started it?
   c. Do you know anyone else with it?
   d. Tell me what happened to that person when dealing with this problem.
3. What do you think is wrong with you?
   a. How severe is it?
   b. How long do you think it will last?
4. Why do you think this happened to you?
   a. Why has it happened to the involved part?
   b. What do you fear most about your sickness?
5. What are the chief problems your sickness has caused you?
6. What do you think will help clear up this problem? (*What treatment should you receive; what are the most important results you hope to receive?*)
   a. If specific tests and/or medications are listed, ask what they are and do.
7. Apart from me, who else do you think can make you feel better?
   a. Are there therapies that make you feel better that I do not know? (*Maybe in another discipline?*)

Modified from Kleinman A: *Patient and healers in the context of culture: an exploration of the borderland between anthropology, medicine, and psychiatry,* Berkeley, 1980, University of California Press; Pfeifferling JH: A cultural prescription for mediocentrism. In Eisenberg L, Kleinman A, editors: *The relevance of social science for medicine,* Boston, 1981, Reidel.

and other health care providers. Finding out more about the person's beliefs about disease causation and the type of treatments he or she believes are appropriate in the given circumstances will allow the nurse to navigate the cultures of the medical establishment and that of the patient and work to promote better health.

Nurses should not attempt to change the person's beliefs. It is difficult, if not impossible, and usually counterproductive. This is particularly so when working with older adults who carry a lifetime of beliefs and illness experience. However, negotiating health, treatment, or prevention options is helpful. The nurse attempts to preserve helpful beliefs and practices, accommodate beliefs that are neither helpful nor harmful, or help clients to give up beliefs or practices that have been shown to be harmful. For the nurse who has little or no knowledge of a belief or practice, it will be necessary to study and evaluate it to determine its helpfulness or its potential harm. In this way beliefs and practices can be preserved whenever possible. Respectfully explaining concern about potentially harmful practices with the offer of possible alternatives may show the person that the nurse is considering the person's preferences.

When care is provided in the home, nurses must adapt home care strategies to the beliefs and culture of the individual and the family if they hope to promote healthy aging and wellness. Special attention should be given to caregivers who are torn between their acculturated beliefs such as nursing home stays, work:caregiver demands, and expectations of the role of the child. The fictionalized accounts portrayed in Amy Tan's *The Bonesetter's Daughter* and Julia Alvarez' *Yo!* present some of the dilemmas and conflicts between the traditional elder and the acculturated children. Nurses work with the family to attempt to find a solution to potential cross-cultural and intergenerational conflicts in the caregiving and health care settings. The nurse also focuses on the elder's overall health and assists the elder and the family in gaining access to needed services. This is done by ascertaining the following: affordability, efficacy, accessibility, and availability of information; client satisfaction; illness perspective; and informal support systems. Maintaining respect for clients' health beliefs is always paramount.

Cross-Cultural Caring in the Long-Term Care Setting

The term *long-term care* refers to ongoing assistance provided to persons who are physically or mentally fragile and unable to independently meet their basic needs

(see Chapter 26). In many cultures outside the United States and in subcultures in the United States, families are expected to take care of their older members, and thus institutional long-term care is less often used than in families of European descent (see Figure 4-1) (Jett, 2006). Long-term care takes place in family homes, group homes, assisted living, skilled nursing facilities, and hospices. The preference for where care is received is culturally determined but often economically influenced. Senior centers also provide a type of on-going long-term care, most of it social in nature. Many centers attract primarily long-term community members; rarely do they provide service or a setting that is welcoming to other groups, such as new immigrants (Box 4-6).

The On Lok Project in San Francisco is the ultimate model for the provision of long-term care services to diverse elders. Originally designed to meet the home care needs of Chinese and Italian immigrants, it now has the capacity to provide every level of short- and long-term care to the diverse populations of San Francisco. Services are provided in the language of the elder and in the manner that optimizes each person's cultural heritage (Kornblatt et al, 2003). Nurses can learn from the work of On Lok and other programs to enhance the care and encourage the health of ethnically diverse elders.

Box 4-6	Providing Culturally Welcoming Services

Dr. Ruth McCaffrey and colleagues received a grant in 2006 and "integrated" Haitian elders into a senior center in the very diverse community of Belle Glade, Florida. The center's staff and usual participants were introduced to culturally oriented ideas, music, art, and language. They were given an opportunity to ask questions of the local Haitian priest. The Haitian elders were similarly oriented. On a prearranged date, transportation was provided to the Haitian elders and a "welcoming" party was held; the event was facilitated by a bilingual native speaker-advocate-helper. The project was a success; both the long-term participants of the center and the newer participants expressed a new appreciation of each other and of the center.

Summarized from McCaffrey RG: Integrating Haitian older adults into a senior center in Florida: understanding cultural barriers for immigrant older adults, *J Gerontol Nurs* 33(12):13-18, 2007.

Modifications to existing long-term care services that On Lok and others have found to enhance the well-being of ethnically diverse elders includes:

1. Ensuring that the resident has access to professional interpreter services if needed
2. Developing programs that reflect the diversity of the residents and the staff
3. Considering monocultural facilities or units, where population demographics warrant
4. Attempting to employ staff that reflects the diversity of the residents or participants

The study of the uniqueness and individuality of each elder is one of the most complex and intriguing opportunities of our day. Realistically it is almost impossible to become familiar with the whole range of clinically relevant cultural differences of older adults one may encounter. Caring for elders holistically and sensitively is the most challenging and potentially satisfying opportunity.

Culture, Nursing, and Maslow's Hierarchy of Needs

Promoting healthy aging in the care of ethnically diverse elders frequently provides the gerontological nurse with new challenges and necessitates a slightly different conceptualization of Maslow's hierarchy. Unfortunately, poverty is very common in many households of persons of color, and meeting basic needs (level one) may be difficult. The nurse can be sensitive to this possibility without making assumptions. The nurse can assess the components of biological integrity and, if necessary, facilitate the elder or the family in obtaining whatever supports (e.g., food stamps, home-delivered meals) are possible and appropriate.

Although some ethnically diverse elders did not experience trauma during their move to the United States there are many others who have suffered horrifically in their home country prior to the move or during their immigration process and for whom safety and security (level two) may have special meaning. The staff of a nursing home for Jewish residents complained that it was particularly difficult getting some of the residents with dementia to shower. Many of the residents were Holocaust survivors. It was some time before the staff realized that as the residents' dementia progressed, they were no longer able to distinguish the difference between a shower for hygiene and the fear of "going to the showers" (i.e., to the gas chamber) in the concentration camps of their youth (Weissman, 2004) (see Chapter 24).

Cultural identity may be one of the major elements of self-concept and a key to self-esteem—increasingly so as a person becomes more mentally or physically frail. Often elders of a distinct ethnic background are closely tied to family and community. Estrangement from their country of origin may be ameliorated if they live in homogeneous communities and exacerbated if they live in social isolation or away from persons with similar backgrounds (Averill, 2005). The ethnic community (e.g., barrios, Nihonmachi, Chinatown) serves as a buffer and a means of strengthening social cohesiveness for elders and others of various cultural groups (Chiang-Hanisko, 2005). Within the community, members are protected from discrimination and the language and customs of the society outside.

Family, religion, community, and history are important reference points for self-worth and identity for any ethnic group. Familial supports vary among groups, social classes, and subcultures, yet the nuclear or extended family is the chief avenue of transmitting cultural values, beliefs, customs, and practices. In many groups, elders are considered repositories of cultural knowledge. The elder and extended family provides orientation, stability, and often, sanctuary. In gross generalizations, we must consider the possibility of that persons of Asian descent value familial piety; Hispanics, the extended family; African Americans, extended or fictive kin (family "members" due to emotional bond) supports; Native Americans, a system of kinship and line of descent; and persons of northern European descent, the desire for independence and autonomy above all other things (Purnell and Paulanka, 2008).

Changes are threatening the historical role of the older adult in the traditional family (see Chapter 24). Economic independence and mobility of the younger members of the family are chipping away at the insulation afforded by the community (Jett, 2006). Intergenerational discontinuities created by assimilation produce a communication gap between the young and the old. This may cause isolation and estrangement between the oldest and youngest generations. Members of ethnic minorities are extremely vulnerable in old age. They may be devalued by the majority culture because of both age and ethnicity. Nurses can take an active role in facilitating self-actualization by facilitating expression of the uniqueness of the individual, by attending to the elder's spiritual and cultural needs, and by taking the lead in optimizing the abilities of those who seek our care (Box 4-6).

Human Needs and Wellness Diagnoses

Self-Actualization and Transcendence
(Seeking, Expanding, Spirituality, Fulfillment)
Exemplifies beliefs and values of one's culture
Expresses unique cultural perspective in creative ways
Functions to optimal ability within culture

Self-Esteem and Self-Efficacy
(Image, Identity, Control, Capability)
Maintains an ethnic identity
Practices rituals and traditions
Reaffirms values and attitudes
Teaches others

Belonging and Attachment
(Love, Empathy, Affiliation)
Identifies with a cultural group
Participates in cultural activities of his or her group
Maintains role in family
Has ability to perpetuate the culture in family's young

Safety and Security
(Caution, Planning, Protections, Sensory Acuity)
Seeks allies through multicultural agencies
Learns enough of dominant language for elemental communication

Biological and Physiological Integrity
(Air, Fluids, Comfort, Activity, Nutrition, Elimination, Skin Integrity)
Has basic needs met

These are not all the possible wellness diagnoses that may be identified. The above
are examples of nursing diagnoses that should be considered when planning care
for the older adult

▶ **KEY CONCEPTS**

▶ Population diversity will continue to increase rapidly for many years. This suggests that nurses will be caring for a greater number of ethnically diverse elders than in the past.

▶ Recent research has revealed significant and persistent disparities in the outcomes of health for persons from minority groups, with the members of these groups bearing the burden of morbidity and mortality in most areas.

▶ Nurses can contribute to the reduction of health disparities through increasing their own cultural awareness, knowledge, and skills.

▶ Negative stereotyping is never appropriate.

▶ Cultural awareness, knowledge, and skills are necessary to increase cultural competence.

▶ Nurses caring for ethnically diverse elders must let go of their own ethnocentrism before they can give effective care.

▶ Many ethnically diverse elders hold health beliefs that are different from those of the biomedical or Western medicine used by most health care professionals in the United States.

▶ Lack of awareness of the elder's health beliefs has the potential to produce conflict in the nursing situation.

▶ The more complex the communication or decision-making needs in a given situation, the greater the need for skilled interpreter services for persons with limited English proficiency.

▶ Programs staffed by persons who reflect the ethnic background of the participants and speak their language may be preferred by the elderly.

▶ The explanatory model and the LEARN Model provide a useful framework for working with elders of any ethnicity or background.

ACTIVITIES AND DISCUSSION QUESTIONS

1. Discuss your personal beliefs regarding health and illness and how they fit into the three major classifications of health systems. How can this affect culturally competent care for ethnically diverse elders?

2. Explain the types of questions that would be helpful in assessing an elder's health problem or problems in a way that is respectful of the person and his or her cultural background and ethnic identity.

3. Propose strategies that would be helpful in planning care for elders from different ethnic backgrounds.

4. Identify sensitive areas in which discussion is frequently needed with older adults, and suggest how these would be affected by differences in the cultural backgrounds of client and nurse.

5. Discuss your familial and culturally determined views of aging and the elderly after speaking to older family members.

RESOURCES

Organizations
Stanford Geriatric Education Center
http://sgec.stanford.edu
A repository of reputable information related to cultural knowledge, including a core curriculum for ethnogeriatrics, on-line modules, and resources. The center sponsors periodic training in cultural competence.

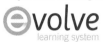

For additional resources, please visit evolve.elsevier.com/Ebersole/gerontological.

REFERENCES

Averill JB: Studies of rural elderly individuals: merging critical ethnography with community-based action research, *J Gerontol Nurs* 31(2):11-18, 2005.

Berlin EA, Fowkes WC: A teaching framework for cross-cultural health care: application in family practice, *West J Med* 139(6):934-938, 1983.

Chiang-Hanisko L: Transnational perspective: ethnic identity and older adult immigrant's health care decision making, *Geriatr Nurs* 26(6):349, 2005.

Caminha-Bacote J: People of African American heritage. In Purnell L, Paulanka BJ, editors: *Transcultural health care: a culturally competent approach*, Philadelphia, 2008, FA Davis.

Cole T: *The journey of life: cultural history of aging in America,* Cambridge, England, 1997, Cambridge University Press.

Enslein J, Tripp-Reimer T, Kelley LS et al: Evidence-based protocol: interpreter facilitation for individuals with limited English proficiency, *J Gerontol Nurs* 28(7):5-13, 2002. Available on-line from http://www.nursing.uiowa.edu/products_services/documents/June07Catalog.pdf. Accessed September 22, 2008.

Gelfand D: *Aging and ethnicity: knowledge and service,* ed 2, New York, 2003, Springer.

Jett K: Mind-loss in the African American community: a normal part of aging, *J Aging Stud* 20(1):1-10, 2006.

Kleinman A, Eisenberg L, Good B: Culture, illness, and care: clinical lessons from anthropologic and cross-cultural research, *Ann Intern Med* 88(2):251-258, 1978.

Kornblatt S, Eng C, Hansen JC: Cultural awareness in health and social services: the experience of On Lok, *Generations* 26(3):46-53, 2003.

McIntosh P: *White privilege: unpacking the invisible knapsack*, 1989. Working paper #189. Wellesley College Center for Research on Women. Accessed September 22, 2008 from http://www.case.edu/president/aaction/UnpackingTheKnapsack.pdf.

Purnell L, Paulanka BJ: *Transcultural health care: a culturally competent approach*, Philadelphia, 2008, FA Davis.

Schim SN, Doorenbos A, Benkert R, Miller J: Culturally congruent care: putting the pieces together, *J Transcult Nurs* 18(2):57-62, 2007.

Shen Z: Cultural competence models in nursing: a selected annotated bibliography, *J Transcult Nurs* 15(4):317-322, 2004.

Smedley B, Stith A, Nelson A, editors: *Unequal treatment: confronting racial and ethnic disparities in health care,* Special report, Institute of Medicine, Washington, DC, 2002, National Academy Press. Available at http://www.nap.edu/catalog.php?record_id=10260. Accessed September 22, 2008.

Spector RE: *Cultural diversity in health and illness*, ed 6, Upper Saddle River, NJ, 2004, Prentice-Hall Health.

Wang Y, Paulanka BJ: People of Chinese culture, pp. 129-144. In Purnell L, Paulanka BJ, editors: *Transcultural health care: a culturally competent approach*, Philadelphia 2008, FA Davis.

Weissman G: Personal communication, April 10, 2004.

Documentation for Optimal Care

5

LEARNING OBJECTIVES

Upon completion of this chapter, the reader will be able to:

- Describe the reasons for accurate and thorough documentation in gerontological nursing.
- Identify potential problems in documentation.
- Identify ways in which errors in documentation and communication are especially dangerous when caring for older adults.
- Compare the major documention methods used in acute, long-term, and home care.
- Describe the responsibilities of the nurse in protecting the privacy of patients.
- Identify ways to reduce the possibility of errors through the use of documentation and the special importance of this when caring for older adults.

GLOSSARY

HIPAA Health Insurance Portability and Accountability Act of 1996, which legislated the handling of confidential patient information.

THE LIVED EXPERIENCE

I was so happy to be able to make a big difference in Mrs. Jones's life. She was 97 and had grown slowly confused over the years. She was also profoundly hard of hearing. She spent the majority of time calling for "Mary," her deceased sister. We really could not communicate effectively with her; we could only show her we cared and keep her safe. Eventually she became acutely ill, and a decision had to be made about CPR (cardiopulmonary resuscitation). When we tried to find out what her wishes were, we could not immediately find any record of them, and she had no living relatives or friends, just an attorney. I searched and searched and finally found documentation about her wishes. We were able to provide her the comfort she wanted because of a nurse's careful documentation years before.

Kathleen, GNP, age 45

DOCUMENTATION

Nursing documentation is an age-old practice of making a permanent record of the conditions of our patients, our actions, and the patients' responses to our actions or those of others. There is probably not a nurse alive who does not know the mantra, "If you didn't document it—you didn't do it!"

Clinical documentation chronicles, supports, and communicates the condition of the patient or resident at all times. Good documentation will help the nurse identify, monitor, and evaluate treatment or interventions. The recorded assessment provides the data needed for the careful development of the individualized plan of care and the evaluation of patient outcomes. Documentation also provides the communication needed to ensure that a person continues to receive the care that is needed from one shift to another, and one caregiver to another. The nurse who provides care to a patient for whom the previous nurse did not document knows well the potential errors that can be made and the added risk to the patient. At the same time, documentation is the major means for the nurse to demonstrate the quality of care he or she provides (Joint Commission, 2008).

Careful and accurate documentation is especially important in gerontological nursing. In the acute care setting the older adult is seriously ill and at special risk for accidents and iatrogenic problems because the normal changes of aging are superimposed on the acute and complex problems. The older adult is at the greatest risk for iatrogenic and adverse reactions to our interventions and medical treatments.

Most older adults require care across all settings at some point in their lives. Since reimbursement for skilled home care has been significantly limited in recent years, continuity from one visit to the next is especially important and made possible only with careful documentation. In skilled nursing facilities the nurse and the nurse's aide provide the majority of the care. Since both long-term care facilities and home health services are nurse-driven, documentation also serves as a basis for the calculation of the amount of reimbursement for the nursing care provided.

Since the Patient Self-Determination Act was passed in 1991, all persons entering a health care facility or who begin to receive skilled home care are asked if they have an advance directive and, if not, are provided information about them (see Chapter 26). The nursing records supplement this documentation with more details regarding a person's wishes and include who they want involved in their care, who they want to have access to their records, and their wishes related to everything from organ donation to the use of cardiopulmonary resuscitation (CPR) and the handling of their bodies after death. Patients often discuss these things with nurses during quiet moments. By recording these conversations in the clinical record we are able to both officially document this important information and share it with other members of the health care team. This will better ensure that the patient's wishes are respected.

DOCUMENTATION ACROSS HEALTH CARE SETTINGS

Documentation begins as soon as the person enters the health care system. Done correctly, ongoing documentation not only provides the basis for care and the evaluation of the interventions and treatments provided, but also forms the basis of providing continuity of care when a patient moves from one setting to another or is discharged home.

This chapter provides an overview of nursing documentation to optimize care of vulnerable elders in acute, long-term, and home health settings.

Acute Care Setting

Documentation in the acute care setting has undergone a significant change in recent years. Computers can be found at the bedside, in nurses' pockets, and in strategic locations around the unit. Nurses are given passwords that may be more important than their name tags. Bar codes are scanned both for access to records and the administration of treatments and medications. The use of checklists, flow sheets, and standardized tools has become the norm (see Chapter 14), as has the use of electronic format for everything from the documentation of vital signs to discharge planning. Care maps are used to predict and document the care provided within a preestablished trajectory and to anticipate the day of discharge. Electronic notations are required when the patient does not follow the anticipated path.

In some settings, "lower-tech" approaches may still used. There, documentation is done in the form of problem-oriented notes made in the clinical record. The patient is assessed (usually with a checklist); nursing diagnoses are identified using the diagnoses of the North American Nursing Diagnosis Association (NANDA); and care plans of interventions using the Nursing Interventions Classification (NIC) are created or selected from preprinted forms. NANDA diagnoses, NIC, and Nursing Outcomes Classification (NOC) are the taxonomies most often used by nurses to categorize their findings, interventions, and outcomes; these sources provide a standardization of language and ease of communication between nurses.

When the nurse needs to document a particular event in the course of the patient stay, a "SOAP" note may be used. SOAP is the acronym for *s*ubjective, *ob*jective, *a*ssessment, and *p*lan. If SOAPE is used, the *e* represents *e*ducation. The subjective section of the note, also called the chief complaint, represents the patient's own words regarding how he or she is feeling. The objective portion includes the data that the nurse can measure, see, feel, touch, or smell related to the chief complaint. The assessment is the result of the nurse's analysis of the patient's condition considering both the subjective and the objective data. The plan includes those nursing interventions that have been done or will be done to address the chief complaint. The education section includes the patient teaching that has been done or is needed (see Box 5-1). This system is very useful for the succinct communication of information related to a specific problem. However, if the patient has multiple problems, as do many older adults, this form of documentation can be complicated and lengthy.

Documentation in Long-Term Care Facilities

The term long-term care facility is applied to a number of settings, including family care homes, assisted living facilities (board and care homes), nursing facilities, skilled nursing facilities (SNFs), and "swing beds" in rural hospitals (beds that serve for either acute or long-term care, depending on the patient's needs).

In family care homes and assisted living facilities, documentation generally occurs only if a nurse has been hired or is under contract with the facility. This service is always optional and is usually limited to administration of medications or the delegation of this act to nurse's aides.

Many persons enter a nursing home at sometime in their lives, either for a short stay for rehabilitation or for a permanent stay. When people enter long-term care

---

Box 5-1	Example of a SOAP Note

S "I have to go to the toilet too much and it burns . . . started last week and getting worse." Denies history of urinary tract infections.

O 72-year-old white female. Temp 99, pulse 94, blood pressure 140/86, respirations 18. Urine is dark yellow with strong, foul odor, skin slightly damp, face flushed, abdomen tender.

A Altered elimination, elevated temp, mild distress, possible infection.

P Call nurse practitioner with report, ask patient to drink extra water every hour, check vital signs every 4 hours until this is resolved.

N, Nurse, RN

---

facilities they are usually functionally impaired because of physical problems, cognitive limitations, the onset or exacerbation of an acute problem, or other related factors. They are dependent on assistance for their activities of daily living (see Chapter 14). The level of documentation required varies by setting and is proscribed by state or jurisdiction statutes.

Documentation in nursing and skilled nursing facilities encompasses the recording of day-to-day care such as eating and bowel movement as well as vital signs, periodic assessment, medication and treatment administration, assessment of any unusual event or change in condition, and periodic mandated comprehensive assessments. Documentation in SNFs includes narrative progress notes, flow sheets, checklists, and mandated standardized and comprehensive instruments (see next section). When a resident's care is no longer covered by Medicare, narrative notes may be reduced to "problem-oriented only" and be completed on an "as-needed" and weekly or monthly basis depending on the facility. Good documentation is an expectation of both trained and licensed staff that provide professional care; the nurse is ultimately responsible for both the quality of the care provided and the completeness and accuracy of the documentation of the care.

Resident Assessment Instrument for Use in Skilled Nursing Facilities

In 1986 the Institute of Medicine (IOM) completed a study indicating that although there was considerable variation, residents in nursing care facilities were receiving an unacceptably low quality of care. As a result, nursing home reform was legislated as part of the Omnibus Budget Reconciliation Act (OBRA) of 1987. The creators of OBRA recognized the challenging work of caring for sicker and sicker persons discharged from acute care settings to nursing homes and, along with this, the need for comprehensive assessment and complex decision making regarding the care that is needed, planned, implemented, and evaluated.

In 1990 a Resident Assessment Instrument (RAI) was created and mandated for use in all long-term care facilities that receive compensation from either Medicare or Medicaid (see Chapter 23) (Dellefield, 2007). The RAI is composed of three parts, the 450-item Minimum Data Set (MDS) with associated Utilization Guidelines, and the Resident Assessment Protocols (RAPs). The RAPs are structured, problem-oriented frameworks for the organization and direction of the care. Finally, the information forms the basis for the Resource Utilization Group data (RUGs), used to determine the reimbursement rate. The exhaustive and thorough assessment and documentation requirement is an attempt to improve and standardize the quality of care provided and help long-term care residents achieve the highest level of functioning and highest quality of life possible (Centers for Medicare and Medicaid Services [CMS], 2008; Dellefield, 2007). The RAPs and the RUGs are quality indicators and quality measures.

Nurses are responsible for the coordination of the RAI shortly after a person's admission, at preset intervals (see current requirements at www.cms.gov), and at any time there is a significant change in the resident's health. The RAI process is dynamic and solution-oriented. It is used to gather definitive information on the resident's functioning. As MDS reassessments are done, the nurse and other members of the care team are able to both document and track the progress toward the resolution of identified problems and make changes to the plan of care as necessary. An identified actual or potential social, medical, or psychological problem that appears in the RAP is known as a trigger. The trigger prompts the nurse to conduct a more detailed assessment, following utilization guidelines (UGs). The care plan is modified as a result of the trigger. The type and level of documentation called for in the RAI facilitates reliable and measurable communication and, when used properly, improves outcomes for residents. The resulting picture of the resident is as clear as possible. For persons who will benefit from active rehabilitation, the outcomes include discharge to a lower level of care, such as returning home. For persons whose condition is one of progressive decline, the RAI process can lead to increased comfort and appropriate care. While the MDS is completed jointly by all members of the interdisciplinary team, the nurse is responsible for verifying the accuracy and completion of the assessment with his or her signature.

The RAI is entered into computer software for ease of analysis and communication of patient profiles to the federal Centers for Medicare and Medicaid (CMS). These data then become part of an aggregate national database used to better respond to the needs of residents in skilled nursing facilities.

Documentation and Reimbursement

In an attempt to control the increasing costs associated with long-term care, the Balanced Budget Act of 1997 set the reimbursement rate for long-term care in an SNF on a PPS. In SNFs, the daily rate is calculated based on the results of the MDS through the use of RUGs. This means that the payment is determined by which RUG the resident falls in and is weighted by the relative amount of staff time that is expected to be needed for the specific person with specific problems, strengths, and weaknesses. Like the diagnostic-related groups (DRGs) used in the acute care setting, the payment is preset and not based on the actual costs. Facilities whose nurses provide high quality, efficient care have the potential to benefit financially, whereas those whose staff is inefficient may incur higher costs than the payment they receive.

Documentation in Home Care

When rehabilitation is needed, it may also be provided in the home setting. While personal care in this setting is provided informally by family and friends (see Chapters 24 and 27), the requisite skilled care is provided through home visits from nurses, occupational therapists, and physical therapists.

Informal caregivers will often develop documentation systems of their own to track appointments, medication administration, and health care provider instruction. This system increases the continuity of care. Nurses may need to assist the family in developing and using effective systems.

Medicare and Medicaid have very strict criteria for documenting skilled home health care. Like the requirements for standardized documentation in the SNF setting above, home care was also affected by the Balanced Budget Act of 1997. The Outcomes and Assessment Information Set (OASIS) was implemented to provide the format for a comprehensive assessment, which forms the basis for planning care and measuring patient outcomes–based quality improvement (OBQI) (CMS, 2007). As with all other documentation systems, OASIS is used both to improve the quality of care and the communication about the individual and, it serves as a guide for reimbursement. OASIS is completed in the person's home, recorded directly on portable or hand-held computers, and later transferred to a central database. Home health agencies are also required to electronically transmit OASIS results to a central, national database. Nurses supplement the data collected in OASIS to include pertinent information personalizing the care provided.

IMPLICATIONS FOR GERONTOLOGICAL NURSING AND HEALTHY AGING

Health care documentation contains highly personal and private information relating to clients, patients, or residents, whether it is written or electronic. For many years the confidentiality of health and medical information was protected through professional codes of ethics. The expectation has always been that the nurse and other health care providers will only access information that relates to a specific individual on a "need to know" basis. Nursing students are taught to avoid talking about patients in hallways, elevators, and lunch rooms or with persons outside their clinical groups, such as friends and family members. The nurse who notes that a neighbor has been admitted to the unit is expected to not review the chart unless he or she is the nurse assigned to provide the care.

However, we have not been as respectful of people's privacy as we should be. This, coupled with the electronic exchange of personal health information, has significantly increased the risk for breaches of confidentiality. In 1996 the Health Insurance Portability and Accountability Act (HIPAA) was passed, legislating the strict protection of the privacy of medical records. The Department of Health and Human Services has the responsibility to ensure this protection. Patients may request that reasonable steps are taken to ensure that their verbal communications are confidential as well and that they have complete control as to who has access to their information. It is expected that nursing actions to protect privacy include closing the patient's or resident's door before having health-related conversations or staff's not discussing patient or residents' needs or condition in a location where it could be overheard, for example in hallways or some nurses' stations.

Communication through documentation has become critical to ensure patients' rights, adequate care, and the economic survival of providers. It is the responsibility of the nurse to make sure that communication and documentation are of the highest quality so as to provide error-free and appropriate care and continuity and to maximize both patient outcomes and accurate reimbursement.

KEY CONCEPTS

▶ Excellence in documentation sets the stage for excellence in patient care.

▶ Standardized instruments for patient evaluation are integral to consistent determination of the needs and health status of patients and appropriate reimbursement for care provided.

▶ Documenting patient status and needs accurately is a key responsibility of the licensed nurse.

▶ Nurses have a responsibility to protect patient confidentiality at all times, both in spoken communication and in the clinical record.

ACTIVITIES AND DISCUSSION QUESTIONS

1. Discuss the origins and purpose of the development of standardized documentation systems.
2. Discuss problems you have experienced with incomplete data or poor documentation in a health facility.
3. Discuss the potential uses of the RAI, MDS, and OASIS.
4. Discuss ways in which patient confidentiality is breached and what the nurse can do about this.
5. Explain the reasons why documentation is critical to patient care.

RESOURCES

Publications
MDS 2.0; The Long Term Care Facility Resident Assessment Instrument (RAI) User's Manual. Obtain copies from Briggs Health Care Products, Customer Service Department, (800) 247-2343. Updated January 2008.

Websites
Center for Medicare and Medicaid Services
www.cms.gov

United States Department of Health and Human Services (USDHHS): *Fact sheet: protecting the privacy of patients' health information,* 2007.
www.hhs.gov/news/facts/privacy.html.

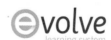

For additional resources, please visit evolve.elsevier.com/Ebersole/gerontological

REFERENCES

Center for Medicare and Medicaid Services (CMS): *CMS's Resident Assessment Instrument (RAI) version 2.0 manual,* Washington, DC, 2007, U.S. Government Printing Office. Available at www.cms.hhs.gov. Updated RAI January 2008.

Center for Medicare and Medicaid Services (CMS): *OASIS: background,* 2007. Accessed March 11, 2008 from www.cms.hhs.gov.

Dellefield ME: Implementation of the Resident Assessment Instrument/Minimum Data Set in the nursing home as organization: implications for quality improvement in RN clinical assessment, *Geriatr Nurs* 28(6):377-386, 2007.

The Joint Commission: Performance measurement systems. Accessed November 21, 2008 from www.jointcommission.org.

Theories and Physical Changes of Aging

6

LEARNING OBJECTIVES

Upon completion of this chapter, the reader will be able to:

- Identify the physical changes that are associated with normal aging.
- Begin to differentiate normal age-related changes from those that are potentially pathological.
- Make a plan of care for the older adult that targets prevention and health promotion.

GLOSSARY

Glomerular filtration rate (GFR) The rate at which the kidneys filter blood.
Kyphosis C-shaped curvature of the cervical vertebrae.
Presbycusis Progressive, bilaterally and symmetrical age-related hearing loss.

Presbyopia Reduced near vision occurring normally with age, usually resulting in improved distance vision.
Xerostomia Excessive mouth dryness.

THE LIVED EXPERIENCE

Strange how these things creep up on you. I really was surprised and upset when I first realized it was not the headlights on my car that were dim but only my aging night vision. Then I remembered other bits of awareness that forced me to recognize that I, that 16-year-old inside me, was experiencing changes that go along with getting older.

Sally, age 60

Later life is a time of challenge and opportunity. Among the challenges are those related to age-related physical changes. Some changes are considered a normal part of aging and others the result of pathological conditions that are mistakenly considered to be an expected part of the aging process.

Aging comprises a series of complex changes and occurs in all living organisms. Most of these changes are intrinsic, coming from within; others are a result of extrinsic, environmental factors, such as exposure to smoke or other pollutants. Just why the changes occur has been of interest to scientists for decades as they have unceasingly searched for the mythical "fountain of youth." It is

known that the triggers of aging are influenced by genetics and by injury to or abuse of the body earlier in life.

In this chapter the prominent biological theories of aging and some of the major physical changes associated with normal aging are discussed. For a more thorough discussion see Toward Healthy Aging (Jett, 2008a, pp. 65-87) . We also discuss some of the changes that indicate pathological conditions commonly seen in older adults. With this knowledge the nurse can begin to differentiate normal aging from health problems that necessitate treatment and help facilitate prompt intervention, which in turn promotes healthy aging. When health is optimized the person can more easily move toward self-actualization (see Chapter 1).

BIOLOGICAL THEORIES OF AGING

A theory is an explanation that makes sense to us of some phenomenon. Theories remain reasonable explanations until someone finds them to be incorrect. Most theories can neither be proved nor disproved, but they are useful as points of reference. Each theory in its own right provides a clue to the aging process. However, many unanswered questions remain.

The biological theories of aging today have evolved from the early study of changes over the life span of the organism. Two related theoretical views form the foundation of biological theories, error (stochastic) theories and predetermined aging (nonstochastic theories). Although they differ, both viewpoints agree that, in the end, the cells in the body become disorganized or chaotic and are no longer able to replicate, and cellular death occurs. When enough cells die, so does the organism. In recent years, research on the biological theories of aging has emphasized the cells and the genes and other components within the cell. A short description of emerging theories can be found in Box 6-1.

Error (Stochastic) Theories

Error theories explain aging as the result of an accumulation of errors in the synthesis of cellular DNA and RNA, the basic building blocks of the cell (Short et al, 2005). With each replication, more errors occur, until the cell is no longer able to function. The visible signs of aging, such as gray hair, are thought to be the result of the accumulation of these cellular errors. Three of the most common theories of error are wear-and-tear, cross-linkage, and free radical.

Wear-and-Tear Theory

One of the earliest theories of aging is known as "wear-and-tear." According to this theory, cell errors are the result of "wearing out" over time because of continued use and trauma. Internal and external stressors increase the numbers of errors and the speed with which they occur (e.g., in shoulder joints of pitchers or knees of

---

Box 6-1   Emerging Biological Theories of Aging

Neuroendocrine Control or Pacemaker Theory
The neuroendocrine system regulates many essential activities related to an organism's growth and development. The neuroendocrine (or pacemaker) theory focuses on the changes in these systems over time. It may be that common neurons in the higher brain centers act as pacemakers that regulate the biological clock during development and aging, and slow down and eventually "shut off" at the predetermined time. Much of the current research in this area is on the examination of the influence of hormones on neuroendocrine functioning over time, especially dehydroepiandrosterone (DHEA) and melatonin.

Caloric Restriction (Metabolic) Theory
Some animal studies since the 1930s have found that reductions in caloric intake by 30% have multiple positive effects, such as increasing the life span, slowing metabolism, lowering body temperature, and delaying the onset of most age-related diseases (NIA, 2003). In particular, caloric restriction has been found to reduce the level of lipid peroxidation and subsequent damage from oxidation. Speculation is that lower body temperature slows body biochemical reactions and lowers levels of pentosidine, a substance found to strongly correlate with onset of age-related diseases (Bokov et al, 2004).

Genetic Research
As the human genome is being mapped, scientists continue to examine the roles that genetics and RNA have in both random and programmed aging and may eventually be able to explain senescence. Among the findings are telomeres, which serve to cap the ends of the chromosomes. With each cellular reproduction, the telomere is shortened, until a time when the telomere disappears and the cell can no longer reproduce and dies. Abnormal cells such as cancer cells produce an enzyme called *telomerase,* which actually lengthens the telomeres, enabling the cells to continue to reproduce. Learning to manipulate telomerase may have significant implications for controlling both cellular reproduction and aging.

Meiner S, Lueckenotte A: *Gerontologic nurisng,* ed 3, St. Louis, 2005, Mosby.

runners). These errors may cause a progressive decline in cellular function.

Cross-Link Theory

Cross-link theory explains aging in terms of the accumulation of errors by cross-linking, or the stiffening of proteins in the cell. Proteins link with glucose and other sugars in the presence of oxygen and become stiff and thick (Marin-Garcia, 2008). Because collagens are the most plentiful proteins in the body, this is where the cross-linking is most easily seen. Skin that was once smooth, silky, firm, and soft becomes drier and less elastic with age. Collagen is also a key component of the lungs, the arteries, and the tendons, and similar changes can be seen there, such as in stiffened joints.

Free Radical Theory

The free radical theory of aging is among those most understood and accepted. Free radicals are natural by-products of cellular activity and are always present to some extent. It is believed that cellular errors are the result of random damage from molecules in the cells called free radicals.

It is known that exposure to environmental pollutants increases the production of free radicals and increases the rate of damage. The best-known pollutants include smog and ozone, pesticides, and radiation (Abdollahi et al, 2004). Other environmental sources thought to cause increases in free radicals are gasoline, by-products from the plastic industry, and drying linseed oil paints. In youth, naturally occurring vitamins, hormones, enzymes, and antioxidants neutralize the free radicals as needed (Valko et al, 2005). However, with aging, the damage caused by free radicals occurs faster than the cells can repair themselves, and cell death occurs (Marin-Garcia, 2008).

Programmed Aging (Nonstochastic Theories)

The nonstochastic theories attribute the changes of aging to a process that is thought to be predetermined or "programmed" at the cellular level. This means that each cell has a natural life expectancy. As more and more cells cease to replicate, the signs of aging appear, and ultimately the person dies at a "predetermined" age (Hayflick, 1983). These theories evolved from the groundbreaking work of Hayflick and Moorehead (1981). They referred to this process as the inner "biological clock." In other words, each cell is "born" with a limited number of replications and then it dies.

Neuroendocrine-Immunological Theory

Closely tied to both programmed and free radical theory is the immunity theory of aging. It is based on changes in the integrated neuorendocrine and immune systems. In this case, the emphasis is on the programmed deaths of the immune cells from damage caused by the increase of free radicals as aging progresses (Effros et al, 2005; Marin-Garcia, 2008). The immune system in the human body is a complex network of cells, tissues, and organs that function separately and together to protect the body from substances from the outside, such as bacteria. It is highly dependent on the release of hormones. In the simplest terms, the specialized B lymphocytes (humoral) and the T lymphocytes (cellular) protect the body against invasion by infection or other matter that is considered foreign, such as tissue or organ transplants. The results of animal studies have demonstrated that the cells of the immune system become progressively more diversified with age and in a somewhat predictable fashion lose some of their ability to self-regulate. The T lymphocytes show more signs of "aging" than do the B lymphocytes. The reduced T cells are thought to be responsible for hastening the age-related changes caused by autoimmune reactions as the body battles itself; healthy cells are mistaken for foreign substances and are attacked.

It is important for the nurse to understand that the exact cause of aging is unknown, that there is considerable variation in the aging process. Not only is there variation between persons but also between the systems of any one person. Aging is a wholly unique and individual experience.

PHYSICAL CHANGES THAT ACCOMPANY AGING

Integument

The skin is composed of the epidermis, the dermis, and the hypodermis. As the largest, most visible organ of the body, the various layers of the skin mold and model the individual to give much of his or her personal and sexual identity; hair provides recognizable characteristics. The skin is important both in health and in illness. It provides clues to hereditary, racial, dietary, physical, and emotional conditions.

Many age-related changes in the skin are functionally inconsequential, but others have implications for organs throughout the body and have more far-reaching impact. Skin changes occur due to both genetic (intrinsic) factors and environmental (extrinsic) factors such as wind, sun, and pollution, to which skin is especially sensitive. Cigarette smoking causes coarse wrinkles, and the photo-damage of the sun is evidenced by rough, leathery texture, itching, and mottled pigmentation, among other signs. Changes that may be genetic, environmental, or both include dryness, thinning, decreased elasticity, and the development of prominent small blood vessels. Skin tears, purpura (large purple spots), and xerosis (excessive dryness) are common but not normal aspects of physical aging. Visible changes of the skin—quality of color, firmness, elasticity, and texture—affirm that one is aging.

Epidermis

The epidermis is the outer layer of skin and is composed primarily of tough keratinocytes and squamous cells. Melanocytes produce melanin, which gives the skin color. With age, the epidermis thins, making blood vessels and bruises much more visible. T-cell function declines, and there may be a reactivation of latent conditions such as herpes zoster (shingles) or herpes simplex.

Cell renewal time increases by up to one third after 50 years of age; 30 or more days may be necessary for new epithelial replacement (Gosain and DiPietro, 2004). This change significantly affects wound healing. In a younger adult, if the skin is injured (e.g., a cut or scrape), the surrounding tissue becomes erythematous almost immediately. This inflammatory response is the first step in the natural healing process. In an older adult, this inflammatory first step may take 48 to 72 hours. A laceration that becomes pink several days after the event may be misinterpreted by the nurse as having become "infected," when in reality, the healing process has only just started. Evidence of true skin infection in older adults is no different than in younger adults, namely, increasing redness and purulent drainage.

The number of melanocytes in the epidermis decreases. Fewer melanocytes means a lightening of the overall skin tone, regardless of original skin color, and a decrease in the amount of protection from ultraviolet rays; the importance of sunscreen is thus significantly increased (see Chapter 12). However, in some body areas, melanin synthesis is increased. Pigment spots (freckles and nevi) enlarge and can become more numerous with increased exposure to natural and artificial light. Lentigines appear, commonly referred to as "age spots" or "liver spots." They are frequently found on the backs of the hands and the wrists, and on the faces of light-skinned persons older than 50 years. Thick, brown, raised lesions with a "stuck on" appearance (seborrheic keratoses) are more common in men and are of no clinical significance but can become cosmetically disfiguring if severe.

Dermis

The dermis, lying beneath the epidermis, is a supportive layer of connective tissue composed of a matrix of yellow elastic fibers that provide stretch and recoil and white fibrous collagen fibers that provide tensile strength. It also supports hair follicles, sweat and sebaceous glands, nerve fibers, muscle cells, and blood vessels, which provide nourishment to the epidermis. Sun exposure accelerates skin tissue changes by hastening collagen fiber alterations.

Many of the visible signs of aging skin are reflections of changes in the dermis. The dermis loses about 20% of its thickness (Friedman, 2006a). The thinness of the dermis is what causes older skin to look more transparent and fragile. Dermal blood vessels are reduced, which accounts for resultant skin pallor and cooler skin temperature. Collagen synthesis decreases, causing the skin to "give" less under stress and tear more easily. Elastin fibers thicken and fragment, leading to loss of stretch and resilience and a "sagging" appearance. Loss of elasticity accentuates jowls and elongated ears and contributes to the formation of a "double" chin. Breasts that were full and firm begin to sag and become pendulous. As will be seen, the impact of the change in elastin has implications for a number of other systems as well.

Hypodermis: Subcutaneous Layer

The hypodermis is the inner-most layer of the skin, and it contains connective tissues, blood vessels, and nerves, but the major component is subcutaneous fat (adipose tissue). The primary purposes of the adipose tissue are to store calories and provide thermal regulation. It also provides shape and form to the body and acts as a shock absorber against trauma (Merck Manual of Geriatrics, 2006). With age, some areas of the hypodermis atrophy. As the natural insulation of fat decreases, a person becomes more sensitive to the cold.

Changes in the hypodermis also increase the chance for hyperthermia as a result of the reduced efficiency of the eccrine (sweat) glands. Sweat glands are located all over the body and respond to thermostimulation and neurostimulation in response to internal changes (e.g. fever, menopausal "hot flashes") or increases in environmental temperatures. The usual body response to heat is to produce moisture or sweat from these glands and thus cool the skin by evaporation. With aging, the glands become fibrotic, and surrounding connective tissue becomes avascular, leading to a decline in the efficiency of the body to cool down. It is not uncommon for persons to complain of being either too hot or too cold in environments that are comfortable to others.

Sebaceous glands which secrete sebum (oil) also atrophy. Sebum protects the skin by preventing the evaporation of water from the epidermis; it possesses bactericidal properties and contains a precursor of vitamin D. When the skin is exposed to sunlight, vitamin D is produced and absorbed into the skin. Continuing to produce Vitamin D is especially important because of the high incidence of osteoporosis (see later section on "Structure, Posture, and Body composition" and Chapters 12 and 27). All people need some sunshine or vitamin D supplementation every day, including those living in residential care facilities who are dependent on others to help them get it.

Older adults are at significant risk for both hyperthermia and hypothermia. When caring for frail older adults, gerontological nurses can assist their patients to avoid extremes of temperature, to prevent drying, and to prevent exposure to toxic products.

Hair and Nails

Hair, as part of the integument, has biological, psychological, and cosmetic value. Hair is composed of tightly fused horny cells that arise from the dermal layer of the skin and obtain coloration from melanocytes. Genetics, race, sex, and testosterone and estrogen hormones influence hair distribution in both men and women.

Race, sex, and hormones also determine the maximum amount of body and scalp hair and the changes that will occur throughout life. Men and women in all racial groups have less hair as they grow older. Hair on the head thins. Scalp hair loss is prominent in men, beginning as early as the twenties. The hair in the ears, the nose, and the eyebrows of older men increases and stiffens. Women have less pronounced scalp hair loss (Luggen, 2005). For some, the accustomed hair color remains, but for most, there is a gradual loss of pigmentation (melanin) and it becomes dryer and coarser. Older women develop chin and facial hair because of the decreased estrogen to testosterone ratio. Leg, axillary, and pubic hair lessens and in some instances disappears in postmenopausal women. The absence of leg hair can be misinterpreted as a sign of peripheral vascular disease in the older adult, whereas it is a normal change of aging.

The various races have distinctive hair characteristics, which should be kept in mind when caring for or assessing the person. Almost all Asians have sparse facial and body hair that is dark, straight, and silky. Blacks have slightly more head and body hair than Asians; however, the hair texture varies widely. It is always fragile, and it ranges from straight to spiraled, and thin to thick. Whites have the most head and body hair, with an intermediate texture and form ranging from straight to curly, fine to coarse, and thick to thin.

The nail becomes harder and thicker, and more brittle, dull, and opaque. It changes shape, becoming at times flat or concave instead of convex. Vertical ridges appear because of decreasing water, calcium, and lipid content. The blood supply, as well as the rate of nail growth, decreases. The half moon (lunule) of the fingernail may entirely disappear, and the color of the nails may vary from yellow to gray. The development of a fungal infection of the nails (onychomycosis) is not the result of aging but is quite common. Fungus invades the space between the layers of the nails, leaving a thick and unsightly appearance. The slowness of growth and the reduced circulation in the older nail make treatment very difficult.

For suggestions of nursing interventions that promote healthy skin during aging see Box 6-2.

Musculoskeletal

A functioning musculoskeletal system is necessary for the body's movement in space, for gross responses to environmental forces, and for the maintenance of posture. This complex system comprises bones, joints, tendons, ligaments, and muscles.

Although none of the age-related changes to the musculoskeletal system are life-threatening, any of them could affect one's ability to function and therefore one's quality of life. Some of the changes are visible to others and have the potential to affect the individual's self-esteem. As seen with the skin, changes in the musculoskeletal system are influenced by many factors, such as age, sex, race, and environment; signs begin to become obvious in the forties.

Box 6-2	Promoting Healthy Skin While Aging

- Avoid excessive exposure to ultraviolet light.
- Keep skin moisturized.
- Avoid use of drying soaps.
- Always use sunscreens.
- Keep well hydrated.

The musculoskeletal changes that have the most effect on function are related to the ligaments, tendons, and joints; over time these become dry, hardened, more rigid, and less flexible. In joints that had been subjected to trauma earlier in life (injuries or repetitive movement), these changes can be seen earlier and in more severe form. If joint space is reduced, arthritis is diagnosed.

Muscle mass can continue to build until the person is in his or her 50s. However, between 30% and 40% of the skeletal muscle mass of a 30-year-old may be lost by the time the person is in his or her 90s (Crowther, 2006). Disuse of the muscles accelerates the loss of strength. Age-related changes to muscles are known as *sarcopenia* and are seen almost exclusively in the skeletal muscle. Muscle tissue mass decreases (atrophies), whereas adipose tissue increases in key areas. The replacement of lean muscle by adipose tissue is most noticeable in men in the area of the waist and in women between the umbilicus and the symphysis pubis. The nurse can encourage older adults to exercise, especially through weight-bearing exercises, to help maintain healthy bones and muscles and flexibility (Box 6-3). See Chapter 10 for discussion on exercise.

Structure, Posture, and Body Composition

Changes in stature and posture are two of the more obvious signs of aging and are associated with multiple factors involving skeletal, muscular, subcutaneous, and fat tissue. Vertebral disks become thin as a result of dehydration, causing a shortening of the trunk. These changes may begin to be seen as early as the fifties (Manolagas, 2000). The trunk shortens as a result of gravity and dehydration of the vertebral disks. The person may have a stooped appearance from kyphosis, a curvature of the cervical vertebrae arising from reduced bone mineral density (BMD). Some loss of BMD in women is associated with the reduction of estrogen levels after menopause. With the shortened appearance, the bones of the arms and the legs may appear disproportionate in size. If a person's bone mineral density is very low, it is diagnosed as osteoporosis and a loss of 2 to 3 inches in height is not uncommon (see Chapter 18).

Alteration in body shape and weight occurs as lean body mass declines and body water is lost: 54% to 60% in men; 46% to 52% in women (Kee and Paulanka, 2000). Fat tissue increases until 60 years of age; therefore body density is higher in youth because of the density of muscle compared to the lightness of fat. From 25 to 75 years of age, fat content of the body increases by 16%. Cellular solids and bone mass decline; extracellular water, however, remains relatively constant. The water loss has significant implications for the dramatically increased risk for dehydration (see Figure 6-1).

Cardiovascular

The cardiovascular system is responsible for the transport of oxygen and nutrient-rich blood to the organs and the transport of metabolic waste products to the kidneys and the bowels. The most relevant age-related changes in this system are myocardial and blood vessel stiffening and decreased responsiveness to sudden changes in demand (McCance, 2006). Changes in the cardiovascular (CV) system are progressive and cumulative.

Cardiac

The age-related changes of the heart (presbycardia) are structural, electrical, and functional. The size of the heart remains relatively unchanged in healthy adults. However, the left ventricle wall thickens by as much as 50% by 80 years of age, and the left atrium increases in size slightly—an adaptation that enhances ventricular filling (Taffet and Lakatta, 2003). Maximum coronary artery blood flow, stroke volumes, and cardiac output are decreased. In health, the changes have little or no effect on the heart's ability to function in day-to-day life. The changes only become significant when there are environmental, physical, or psychological stresses. With sudden demands for more oxygen the heart may not be able to respond adequately (Marin-Garcia, 2008). It takes longer for the heart to accelerate and then return to a resting state.

For the gerontological nurse, this means that the increased heart rate one might expect to see when the person is in pain, anxious, febrile, or hemorrhaging may not be present or will be delayed. Similarly, the older heart may not be able to respond to other calls for

Box 6-3	Promoting Healthy Bones and Muscles

- Ensure regular intake of vitamin D and calcium.
- Engage in regular weight-bearing exercise, for example, tai chi.
- Engage in regular flexibility and balance exercises, for example, yoga.
- For women: consider preventive pharmacotherapeutics.

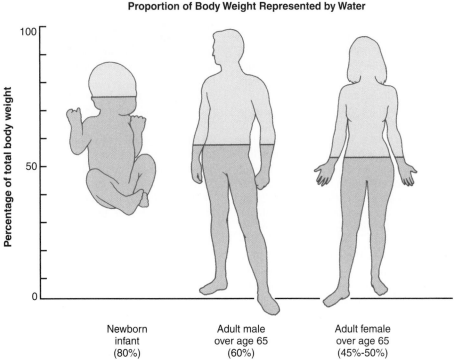

Proportion of Body Weight Represented by Water

Percentage of total body weight

Newborn infant (80%)	Adult male over age 65 (60%)
	Adult female over age 65 (45%-50%)

Fig. 6-1   Changes in body water distribution. *(From Thibodeau GA, Patton KT:* Structure and function of the body, *ed 12, St Louis, 2004, Mosby.)*

increased cardiac demand such as infection, anemia, pneumonia, cardiac dysrhythmias, surgery, diarrhea, hypoglycemia, malnutrition, and drug-induced and noncardiac illnesses such as renal disease and prostatic obstruction. Instead, the nurse must depend on other signs of distress in the older patient and be diligently alert to signs of rapid decompensation of both the previously well elder and one who is already medically fragile, such as those in nursing homes.

Heart disease is the number one cause of nonaccidental death world-wide. Often the changes associated with disease are thought to be "normal," but they are not. The nurse promotes healthy aging with recommendations for heart-healthy life choices and obtaining excellent health care.

Blood Vessels

Several of the same age-related changes seen in the skin and muscles affect the lining (intima) of the blood vessels, especially the arteries. Like in the skin, the most significant change is decreased elasticity and recoil. The blood supply to various organs deceases, and peripheral resistance increases. Change in flow to the coronary ar-

teries and the brain is minimal, but decreased perfusion of other organs, especially the liver and kidneys, has potentially serious implications for medication use (see Chapter 15). When a person already has or develops arteriosclerosis or hypertension, the age-related changes can have serious consequences.

Less dramatic changes are found in the veins, although they do become somewhat stretched and the valves less efficient. This means that lower extremity edema develops more quickly and that the older adult is more at risk for deep vein thrombosis because of the increased sluggishness of the venous circulation. The normal changes, when combined with long-standing but unknown weakness of the vessels, may become visible in marked varicosities and explain the increased rate of stroke and aneurysms in older adults. However, the promotion of a healthier heart is possible (see Box 6-4).

Respiratory

The respiratory system is the vehicle for ventilation and gas exchange, particularly the transfer of oxygen into and the release of carbon dioxide from the blood. The

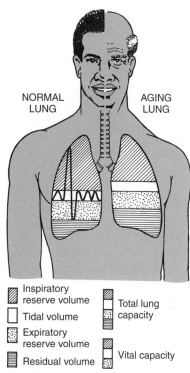

Fig. 6-2 Changes in lung volumes with aging. *(From McCance KL, Huether SE, editors:* Pathophysiology: the biologic basis for disease in adults and children, *ed 5, St Louis, 2006, Mosby.)*

respiratory structures depend on the musculoskeletal and nervous systems to function fully. The respiratory system matures by the age of 20 and then begins to decline even in healthy individuals. Although subtle changes occur in the lungs, the thoracic cage, the respiratory muscles, and the respiratory centers in the central nervous system, the changes are small and, for the most part, insignificant. The specific changes include loss of elastic recoil, stiffening of the chest wall, inefficiency in gas exchange, and increased resistance to air flow (Figure 6-2). Respiratory problems are common but almost always the result of exposure to environmental toxins (e.g., pollution, cigarette smoke) rather than the aging process (Sheahan and Musialowski, 2001).

Like the cardiovascular system, the biggest change is in the efficiency, in this case, of gas exchange. Under usual conditions, this has little or no effect on the performance of customary life activities. However, when an individual is confronted with a sudden demand for increased oxygen, a respiratory deficit may become evident. Chemoreceptor function is altered or blunted at the peripheral and central chemoreceptor sites in the central nervous system, with reduced ability to respond to hypoxia or hypercapnia.

The changes that occur in the anatomical structures of the chest and the altered muscle strength can significantly affect one's ability to cough forcefully enough to quickly expel materials that accumulate in or obstruct airways. In addition, the respiratory cilia are less effective. The reduced effectiveness of the cough response and cough reflex places the person at high risk of potentially life-threatening infections and aspiration. With impairments such as dysphagia or decreased esophageal motility, the risk is significantly increased. The lack of basilar inflation, an ineffective cough response, and a less efficient immune system pose potential problems for older adults who are sedentary, bedridden, or limited in activity. All of these

make the administration of annual influenza immunizations of the highest importance. In promoting the appropriate use of immunizations the nurse is promoting healthy aging (see Box 6-5).

Renal

The renal system is responsible for regulating water and salts in the body and maintaining the acid/base balance in the blood. With each beat of the heart the blood passes through the nephrons in the kidneys for filtering. The glomerulus is the key structure that controls the rate of filtering (glomerular filtration rate, GFR). Kidney function is measured indirectly by means of the plasma creatinine through the calculation of the creatinine clearance rate (CrCl) (see Chapter 15).

Among the many changes to the kidneys are those of blood flow and the ability to regulate body fluids. Blood flow through the kidneys decreases by about 10% per

Box 6-5	Promoting Healthy Lungs

- Obtain pneumonia immunization.
- Obtain annual influenza immunization.
- Avoid exposure to smoke and pollutants.
- Do not smoke.
- Avoid persons with respiratory illnesses.
- Seek prompt treatment of respiratory infections.
- Wash hands frequently.
- Eat meals in relaxed atmosphere.
- Practice thorough regular oral hygiene

decade, from about 1200 ml/min in young adults to about 600 ml/min by the age of 80, as a result of vascular and fixed anatomical and structural changes (Wiggins, 2003; MacAas-Naaez and Cameron, 2005). The kidneys lose as many as 50% of the nephrons with little change in the body's ability to regulate body fluids and maintain adequate day-to-day fluid homeostasis. There is no significant variation by sex or race (MacAas-Naaez and Cameron, 2005). The age-related decrease in size and function occurs primarily in the kidney cortex, begins in the thirties, and becomes significant by the seventies (MacAas-Naaez and Cameron, 2005). However, renal reserve is lost and the ability to respond to either a salt or water load or deficit is compromised.

Whereas plasma creatinine is constant throughout life, urine creatinine shows a decline even in healthy aging because of the reduced lean muscle mass. The creatinine clearance, a measurement of GFR, is decreased to 100 ml/min by the age of 80. The urine creatinine clearance is an important indicator for appropriate drug therapy, reflecting the ability to handle medications passing through and metabolized by the kidneys (see Chapter 14). Persons with a reduced creatinine clearance usually need a reduction in the dosages of their medications to prevent potential toxicity, and caution must be used in the administration of fluids (see Chapter 19).

Age-related changes in the renal system are significant due to resultant heightened susceptibility to fluid and electrolyte imbalance and structural damage from medications and contrast media of diagnostic tests. Under normal circumstances, renal function is sufficient to meet the regulation and excretion demands of the body (MacAas-Naaez and Cameron, 2005). However, with the stress of disease, surgery, or fever, the kidneys have reduced capacity to respond and are therefore at greater risk for renal insufficiency and failure.

Endocrine

The endocrine system, working in tandem with the neurological system, provides regulation and control of the integration of body activities through the secretion of hormones from glands throughout the body. As the body ages, most glands atrophy and decrease their rate of secretion. However, other than the decrease in estrogen, which causes menopause, the impact of the changes is not clear.

Pancreas

The endocrine pancreas secretes insulin, glucagon, somatostatin, and pancreatic polypeptides. The secretion of these substances does not appear to decrease to any level of clinical significance. However, for reasons unknown, the tissues of the body often develop decreased sensitivity to insulin. When combined with increased needs for insulin in the presence of obesity, the result is often the development of type two diabetes. Older adults have the highest rate of type two diabetes of any other age group, with significant variation by ethnicity and region (see Chapter 18). When the pancreas is stressed with sudden concentrations of glucose, blood levels are higher for longer. These temporary levels of increased blood glucose make the diagnosis of diabetes or glucose intolerance difficult.

Thyroid

Slight changes occur in the structure and function of the thyroid gland, which may explain the increased incidence of hypothyroidism in older adults (Huether, 2006b). Some atrophy, fibrosis, and inflammation occurs. Although other evidence of change is inconclusive at this time, diminished secretion of thyroid-stimulating hormone (TSH) and thyroxine (T_4) and decreased plasma triiodothyronine (T_3) appear to be age-related. Serum T_3 decreases with age (Jett, 2008b, pp. 88-103), perhaps as a result of decreased secretion of TSH by the pituitary gland. When thyroid replacement is needed, lower doses are necessary and higher doses contraindicated. The required dose of thyroxin may change over time.

Collective signs, such as a slowed basal metabolic rate, thinning of the hair, and dry skin, are characteristic of hypothyroidism in the young but are normal manifestations in the aged who have no history of thyroid deficiencies, also making the recognition of thyroid disturbances difficult.

Reproductive

The reproductive systems in men and women serve the same physiological purpose—human procreation. Although both aging men and women undergo age-related changes, the changes affect women significantly more than men. Women lose the ability to procreate after the cessation of ovulation (menopause), whereas men remain fertile their entire lives. Regardless of the physical changes, sexual needs remain (see Chapter 24).

Female Reproductive System

As menopause signals the end of the reproductive phase in a woman's life, several other age-related changes occur, particularly in breast tissue and urogenital structures. Older breasts are smaller, pendulous, and less firm. Outwardly, the labia majora and minora become less prominent and pubic hair thins. The ovaries, cervix, and uterus slowly atrophy. The vagina shortens, narrows, and loses some of its elasticity, typical of aging muscle and skin. Vaginal walls also lose their ability to lubricate quickly, especially if the woman is not sexually active. More stimulation is needed to achieve orgasm. The vaginal epithelium changes considerably; the pH rises from 4.0 to 6.0 before menopause to 6.5 to 8.0 afterward (Deneris and Huether, 2006). The vaginal changes result in the potential for dyspareunia (painful intercourse), trauma during intercourse, and more susceptibility to infection.

Male Reproductive System

Although men have the ability to produce sperm beginning at puberty, they also experience changes in the functioning of the reproductive and the urogenital organs in late life. The changes are usually more subtle and noticed only as they accumulate, beginning when men are in their 50s. The testes atrophy and soften. The seminiferous tubules thicken, and obstruction caused by sclerosis and fibrosis can occur. Although sperm count does not decrease, fertility may be reduced because of the higher number of sperm lacking motility or because of structural abnormalities. Erectile changes are also seen: more stimulation is needed to achieve a full erection, ejaculation is slower and less forceful, and refractory periods are longer (Deneris and Huether, 2006). As with women, alterations in hormone balances may play a part in the age-related changes in

men. Testosterone level is reduced in all men but only rarely to the level at which it would be considered a true deficiency.

By the age of 80 years, up to 80% of men have some degree of prostatic enlargement (Kamel and Dornbrand, 2004). The condition known as *benign prostatic hypertrophy* (BPH) is so common that some are beginning to call it a normal part of aging. The only time it is considered a problem is when the enlargement is such that it causes compression of the urethra. As a result, the man may experience urinary retention leading to repeated urinary tract infections and overflow incontinence. Intervention is pursued only when the symptoms of BPH interfere with the man's quality of life (Kamel and Dornbrand, 2004).

Gastrointestinal

The digestive system includes the gastrointestinal (GI) tract and the accessory organs that aid in digestion. Like the endocrine system, few true age-related changes affect function. However, a number of common health problems can have a great effect on the digestive system. Changes in other systems can also affect GI structure and function; changes can be seen as early as the fifties (Huether, 2006b).

Mouth

Age-related changes affect both the teeth and the mouth. With the wear and tear of years of use, the teeth eventually lose enamel and dentin and then become more vulnerable to decay (caries). The roots become more brittle and break more easily. For unknown reasons, the gums are also more susceptible to periodontal disease. Without care, teeth may be lost. Taste buds decline in number, and salivary secretion lessens. A very dry mouth (xerostomia) is common. It is still common to care for persons over 70 or 80 who have had all of their teeth removed (edentulous) and who may or may not wear dentures. It is important that the nurse ensure the fit and cleanliness of the dentures or the appropriate choice of diet. Even in health, these changes when combined have the potential to decrease the pleasure and comfort of eating, which can lead to anorexia and weight loss. A number of medications taken for common health problems can quickly exacerbate potential problems, especially xerostomia. When the gerontological nurse administers medications to an older adult or conducts medication education, he or she should warn persons about this potential (see Chapter 18).

Esophagus

In youth, food passes quickly through the esophagus to the stomach because of the strong and coordinated contractions of associated muscle and peristalsis. In aging, the contractions increase in frequency but are more disordered, and therefore propulsion is less effective. This is called presbyesophagus. The sluggish emptying of the esophagus forces the lower end to dilate, creating greater stress in this area and possibly causing digestive discomfort. Pathological processes that are increasingly seen as adults become older include gastroesophageal reflux disease (GERD) and hiatal hernias.

Stomach

Decreased gastric motility and volume and reductions in the secretion of bicarbonate and gastric mucus are also associated with aging (Huether, 2006b). The reductions are caused by gastric atrophy and result in hypochlorhydria (insufficient hydrochloric acid). Decreased production of intrinsic factor can lead to pernicious anemia if the stomach is not able to utilize ingested B_{12} vitamins. The protective alkaline viscous mucus of the stomach is lost because of the increase in stomach pH. This makes the stomach more susceptible to peptic ulcer disease, particularly with the use of nonsteroidal antiinflammatory drugs such as aspirin and ibuprofen. Loss of smooth muscle in the stomach delays emptying time, which may lead to anorexia or weight loss as a result of distention, meal-induced fullness, and the feeling of satiety (Price and Wilson, 2002).

Intestines

The age-related changes of the small intestine include those noted earlier that involve smooth muscles and those related to the villi, the anatomical structures in the intestinal walls that are essential for absorption of nutrients. The villi become broader and shorter and less functional. Nutrient absorption is affected; proteins, fats, minerals (including calcium), vitamins (especially B_{12}), and carbohydrates (especially lactose) are absorbed more slowly and in lesser amounts (Huether, 2006b). Changes in motility, epithelial membranes, vascular perfusion, and gastrointestinal membrane transport may affect absorption of lipids, amino acids, glucose, calcium, and iron.

Peristalsis is slowed with aging and there is blunted response to rectal filling; the extent of the change should not be such to cause problems with defecation. In other words, constipation, which is often thought of as a normal part of aging, is not. Instead, constipation is more often a side effect of medications, life habits, immobility, inadequate fluid intake, and lack of attention to the gastrocolic reflex, the postprandial urge to defecate. The role of the gerontological nurse and elimination needs are presented in Chapter 8 and suggestions on promoting healthy digestion are found in Box 6-6.

Accessory Organs

The accessory organs of the digestive system are the liver and the gall bladder. The liver continues to function throughout life despite a decrease in volume and weight (mass) and a concomitant decrease in liver blood flow of 30% to 40% by the late nineties (Hall, 2003); this carries implications for impaired drug metabolism and is associated with an increased half-life of fat-soluble medications (see Chapter 15). While slow, liver regeneration is not greatly impaired and liver function tests remain unaltered with age.

There does not seem to be a specific change in the gallbladder; however, the incidence of gallstones increases (Huether, 2006b). This is possibly caused by the increased lipogenic composition of bile from biliary cholesterol. The decrease in bile salt synthesis increases the incidence of cholelithiasis and cholecystitis (Hall, 2003). In addition, the decrease in bile acid synthesis causes a reduction in hydroxylation of cholesterol. This, in conjunction with a decrease in hepatic extraction of low-density lipoprotein (LDL) cholesterol from the blood, increases the level of serum cholesterol in the older adult. For women, the increase in cholesterol begins to be seen following menopause.

Box 6-6   Promoting Healthy Digestion

- Practice good oral hygiene.
- Wear properly fitting dentures.
- Seek prompt treatment of dental caries and periodontal disease.
- Eat meals in relaxed atmosphere.
- Maintain adequate intake of fluids.
- Provide time for response to gastrocolic reflex.
- Respond promptly to urge to defecate.
- Eat a balanced diet.
- Avoid prolonged periods of immobility.
- Avoid tobacco products.

Neurological

Contrary to popular belief, the older nervous system, including the brain, is remarkably resilient and changes in cognitive functioning are not a normal part of aging. Neither the patient nor the nurse should accept an assessment of "confusion" without making sure the cause is identified and treated if at all possible. Although many neurophysiological changes occur with aging, they do not occur in all older persons and do not affect everyone the same way. For example, the presence of neurofibrillary tangles is a classic sign of dementia and is found in the brains of all persons with Alzheimer's disease, but they are found also in the brains of persons without dementia. Although it is very difficult to show a true cause-and-effect of age-related changes in the nervous system, some changes appear to be consistent.

Central Nervous System (CNS)

The major changes in the aging nervous system are found in the CNS. With aging, the dendrites appear to be "wearing out," and the number of neurons found decreases with the correlating decrease in brain weight and size (see Figure 6-3). This change in size is seen primarily in the frontal lobe and appears as "atrophy" on computed tomography (CT) scans or magnetic resonance imaging (MRI), considered clinically insignificant. Decreased adherence of the dura mater to the skull, fibrosis, thickening of the meninges, narrowing of the gyri, widening of the sulcus, and increase in the subarachnoid space also occur (Sugarman, 2006).

Sleep disturbances may also be a normal part of aging as a result of changes in the reticular formation (RF). The RF is a set of neurons that extend from the spinal cord through the brainstem and into the cerebral cortex. With aging, a loss of deep sleep (stages 3 and 4) may be seen. Elders spend more time in bed to get the same amount of "sleep" since the time in light sleep increases in proportion to that spent in deep sleep (Friedman, 2006b). However, excessive daytime somnolence is not expected and, if it occurs, should lead to a thorough assessment of causative factors aside from aging, especially side effects of medication and depression.

Subtle changes in cognitive and motor functioning occur in the very old. Mild memory impairments and difficulties with balance may be seen as normal age-related changes in neurodegeneration and neurochemistry (see Chapters 7 and 21). Intellectual performance of the older adult without brain dysfunction remains constant; however, the performance of tasks may take longer, which is an indication that central processing is slowed. There are also decreasing levels of the neurotransmitters

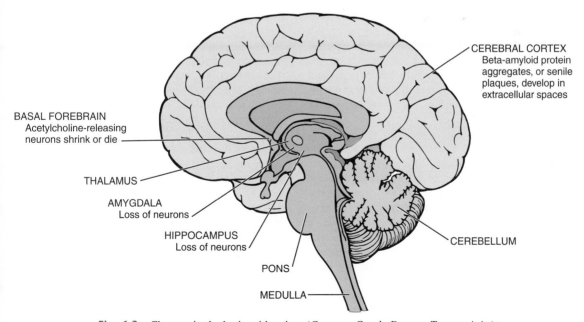

CEREBRAL CORTEX
Beta-amyloid protein aggregates, or senile plaques, develop in extracellular spaces

BASAL FOREBRAIN
Acetylcholine-releasing neurons shrink or die

THALAMUS

AMYGDALA
Loss of neurons

HIPPOCAMPUS
Loss of neurons

PONS

MEDULLA

CEREBELLUM

Fig. 6-3   Changes in the brain with aging. *(Courtesy Carole Donner, Tucson, Ariz.)*

choline acetylase, serotonin, and catecholamines. Other enzymes such as monoamine oxidase (MAO) increase. Redundancy of brain cells may forestall the effects of these changes, but the exact number of cells required for certain functions is unknown.

Peripheral Nervous System

The most important effect of the normal changes in the aging peripheral nervous system is the increased risk for injury. Vibratory sense in the lower extremities may be nonexistent. Somesthetics, or tactile sensitivity, decreases in connection with the loss of nerve endings in the skin. This is most notable in the fingertips, the palms of the hands, and the lower extremities. This decreased sensitivity is translated into delayed reactions to things such as hot surfaces, significantly increasing the risk for burns and the extent of burns should they occur. The presence of a functioning smoke detector is particularly important for healthy and safer aging.

Kinesthetic sense, or proprioception (one's position in space), is altered because of changes in both the peripheral and central nervous systems. If one is less aware of body position and has less tactile awareness, the risk for falling is dramatically increased. The person may be walking on a flat surface when it suddenly becomes uneven. With reduced proprioception, it takes a little longer to realize the surface is uneven and a little longer still to realize that one has tripped (changed position in space). Where a younger person would be able to immediately right herself or himself and prevent a fall, this slight delay may result in a fall in an older adult. Conditions such as arthritis, stroke, some cardiac disorders, or damage to the structures of the inner ear may also affect peripheral and central mechanisms of mobility and exacerbate. Further discussion of sensory alterations appears in Chapter 13.

Sensory Changes

A number of changes occur in the sensory organs as a result of a combination of intrinsic and extrinsic factors. As we age, we cannot totally escape some loss of smell, sight, sound, and touch. The creative gerontological nurses can make a big difference in the quality of life for the person with sensory changes (see Boxes 6-7 and 6-8). See Chapter 3 for discussion of communicating with elders with vision and hearing impairments.

Eye and Vision. Changes in vision and eyes begin very early and are both functional and structural. All the changes affect visual acuity and accommodation, or

Box 6-7	Promoting Healthy Eyes

- Protect eyes from ultraviolet light.
- Avoid eye strain; use a bright light when needed.
- See health care provider promptly if there are changes in vision.
- Have yearly dilated eye examination.

Box 6-8	Promoting Healthy Ears

- Avoid exposure to excessively loud noises.
- Avoid injury with cotton-tipped applicators and other cleaning materials.
- Use assistive devices as appropriate, for example, hearing aids.
- See health care provider promptly if there are sudden changes in hearing.

the ability for the vision to adjust to changes in the environment.

Presbyopia is an age-related decrease in near vision that begins to become noticeable in midlife. Nearly 95% of adults older than 65 years wear glasses for close vision (Burke and Laramie, 2000), and 18% also use a magnifying glass for reading and close work. Although presbyopia is first seen between 45 and 55 years of age, 80% of those older than 65 years have fair to adequate far vision past 90 years of age.

Extraocular. Like the skin elsewhere age-related changes affect both form and function of the eye. The eyelids lose elasticity, and drooping (senile ptosis) results. In most cases, this only affects appearance. In extreme cases the lids sag far enough to block vision. Spasms of the orbicular muscle may cause the lower lid to turn inward. If it stays this way, it is called *entropion.* The lower lashes that curl inward irritate and scratch the cornea. Surgery may be needed to prevent permanent injury. Decreases in the orbicular muscle strength may result in *ectropion,* or an out-turning of the lower lid. Without the integrity of the trough of the lower lid, tears run down the cheek instead of bathing the cornea. This and an inability to close the lid completely lead to excessively dry eyes and the need for artificial tears. The person may need to tape the eyes shut during sleep. Exacerbating this problem, the number of goblet cells that provide mucin, essential for eye lubrication and movement, decreases. A severe deficiency of lubrication is known as "dry eye syndrome."

Ocular. The cornea is the avascular transparent outer surface of the eye globe that refracts (bends) light rays entering the eye through the pupil. With aging, the cornea becomes flatter, less smooth, thicker, and duller in appearance. The result is increased far-sightedness (hyperopia). For the person who was myopic (near-sighted) earlier in life, this change may actually improve vision. Arcus senilis, a gray-white to silver ring or partial ring, may be observed 1 to 2 mm inside the limbus at the juncture of the iris and cornea; it is composed of deposits of calcium and cholesterol salts. It does not appear to have any clinical significance.

The anterior chamber is the space between the cornea and the lens. The edges of the chamber include canals that control the volume and movement of aqueous fluid within the space. With aging, the chamber decreases slightly in size and capacity because of thickening of the lens. Resorption of the intraocular fluid becomes less efficient with age. If the decrease is significant, it can lead to increased intraocular pressure and glaucoma (Huether and DeFriez, 2006). Any acute changes in vision or eye pain should be considered medical emergencies and responded to accordingly. The ability to adjust to changes in light and the need for greater levels of lighting are the result of reduced responsiveness of the pupils and changes in the lens. The lens, a small, flexible, biconvex, crystal-like structure just behind the iris, is most responsible for visual acuity; it adjusts the light entering the pupil and focuses it on the retina. Age-related changes in the lens are probably universal and begin in the forties. The origins of these changes are not fully understood, although ultraviolet rays of the sun contribute to the problem, with cross-linkage of collagen creating a more rigid and thickened lens structure.

Light scattering increases, and color perception decreases. As a result, glare is a problem, not only that created by sunlight outdoors, but also the reflection of light on any shiny object, such as light striking polished floors and surfaces (Meisami et al, 2003). Eventually people require 3 times as much light to see things as they did when they were in their twenties. It is more effective to place high-intensity light on the object or surface to be observed rather than increasing the intensity of the light in the entire room. For example, it would be more effective to focus a light directly on the newspaper a person was reading.

Intraocular. The retina, which lines the inside of the eye, has less distinct margins and is duller in appearance than in younger adults. Color clarity diminishes by 25% in the sixth decade and by 59% in the eighth decade, especially that of the blues, the violets, and the greens of the spectrum; light colors such as reds, oranges, and yellows are more easily seen. Some of this difficulty is linked to the yellowing of the lens and impaired transmission of light to the retina. Finally, the number of rods and associated nerves at the periphery of the retina is reduced, resulting in peripheral vision that is not as clear or is absent (Tumosa, 2000). Arteries in back of the eye may show atherosclerosis and slight narrowing. Veins may show indentations (nicking) as they pass over the arteries if the person has a long history of hypertension. As long as these changes are not accompanied by distortion of objects or a significant decrease in vision, they are not clinically significant.

Ear and Hearing. Like the eye, age-related changes affect both the structure and the function of the ear. Some hearing loss affects about one third of all adults between 65 and 74 years of age and about one half of those aged 75 to 79 years. This is a high-frequency, sensorineural loss is known as presbycusis, which affects more than 10 million people (Williams, 2000).

There are several age-related changes to the appearance of the ear, especially in men. The auricle loses flexibility and becomes longer and wider as a result of diminished elasticity. The lobe sags, elongates, and wrinkles. Together, these changes make the ear appear larger. Coarse, wiry, stiff hairs grow at the periphery of the auricle, and the tragus enlarges in men.

The auditory canal narrows through inward collapse. Stiffer and coarser hairs line the canal. Cerumen glands atrophy, causing thicker and dryer wax, which is more difficult to remove. This is a substantial cause for temporary, reversible obstructive hearing loss. The gerontological nurse should be sensitive to this possibility and be skilled at safe cerumen removal.

On otoscopic examination the tympanic membrane appears dull and gray. Structurally, the ossicle joints between the malleus and the stapes become calcified, causing reduced vibration of these bones and a mechanical reduction in the amount of sound transmitted to the auditory nerve.

In sensorineural hearing loss (presbycusis) there is a decrease in vestibular sensitivity as a result of degeneration of the organ of Corti in the cochlea and otic nerve loss, and transmission of sound waves to the brain is therefore impaired. Genetically influenced changes in electrophysiological function of the organ of Corti are the basis of metabolic hearing loss. Hearing loss develops slowly. Whereas obstructive causes are reversible, sensorineural ones are not. Presbycusis is primarily the loss of the ability to hear high frequency sounds such as consonants, the chirping of birds, and the rustling of leaves. The phrase "The Cat in the Hat" may be heard as "e at in e at." Although the person may be able to decipher what is said if it is within context, this processing takes longer than usual or language is processed incorrectly. It is important to note that with normal age-related hearing loss the person can still hear but may not be able to make sense of the partially heard words. Inaccurate responses too often lead to the incorrect suspicion of dementia or confusion when in fact it is a hearing loss.

Immune

The immune system functions to protect the host from invasions from foreign substances and organisms. To do so, it must be able to differentiate the self from the non-self (Kishiyama, 2006). The immune system includes elements of many of the systems already discussed, including white blood cells, bone marrow, thymus, lymph nodes, and spleen.

A number of age-related changes have been implicated in the increased risk for infection in the older adult. For example, the skin is thinner and therefore less resistant to bacterial invasion. The reduced number of cilia in the lungs leads to the increased risk for pneumonia. The friability of the urethra increases the risk for urinary tract infections, especially in women. But perhaps the most important of all is the reduced immunity at the cellular level, which is now understood to have a significant genetic underpinning.

Late life brings a decrease in T-cell function that results from a decrease in innate immunity, adaptive immunity, and self-tolerance (see p. 78). The response to foreign antigens decreases, but immunoglobulins increase, creating an autoimmune response not associated with autoimmune diseases that may have developed earlier (Michel, 2000; Proust, 2000). Being alert for signs and symptoms of autoimmune changes is especially important to gerontological nursing, as is the responsibility to promote disease prevention and protection from infection for the older adult (Box 6-9).

The changes in immune function affect the older person's response to illness. Early studies by Stengel (1983) found oral temperature norms in well elders significantly lower. In women older than 80 years, the temperature was lower than in younger women; older men consistently had an even lower temperature than women of comparable age. This means that a febrile response suggestive of infection is no longer restricted to a temperature above 98.6° or 99° F. Instead, an older adult may have a core temperature elevation at much lower numbers. The old-old may have an average normal temperature of 96° F, with an average range of 95° to 97° F. (Hogstel, 1994). These findings emphasize the need to carefully evaluate the basal temperature of older adults and recognize that even low-grade fevers (98.6° F) in the elderly may signify serious illness. When this is combined with the age-related delay in the increases in the white blood cell count compared to younger adults, early detection of serious illness is difficult in many cases. *A lack of fever (temperature greater than 98.6° F) or a normal white blood count cannot be used to rule out an infection.*

Box 6-9   *Healthy People 2010* Immunization Rates and Infections

Objective 1-9c: Reduce hospitalizations for preventable pneumonia or influenza—persons 65 years and older
Baseline: 10.6 persons per 10,000 (1996)
2010 Target: 8.0 persons per 10,000
Objective 14-5: Reduce invasive pneumococcal infections
Baseline and 2010 Target:

| | | RATE PER 100, | |
OBJECTIVE		1997 Baseline	2010 Target
14-5b	New invasive pneumococcal infections Adults 65 years and older	62	42
14-5d	Invasive penicillin-resistant pneumococcal infections Adults 65 years and older	9	7

From U.S. Department of Health and Human Services: *Healthy People 2010: national health promotion and disease prevention objectives,* Washington, DC, 2000, The Department.

Based on the current biological theories of aging, with support of clinical evidence, it can be concluded that complex functions of the body decline more than simple body processes; that coordinated activity, which relies on interacting systems such as nerves, muscles, and glands, has a greater decremental loss than single-system activity; and that a uniform and predictable loss of cell function occurs in all vital organs. Yet older adults are able to function effectively within the physical dictates of their body and continue to live to a healthy old age, capable of wisdom, judgment, and satisfaction.

Human Needs and Wellness Diagnoses

Self-Actualization and Transcendence
(Seeking, Expanding, Spirituality, Fulfillment)
Is able to cope with adverse physical conditions
Expresses self appropriately
Overcomes physical adversity with spirituality

Self-Esteem and Self-Efficacy
(Image, Identity, Control, Capability)
Has a strong self-esteem
Has multiple hobbies
Solves problems effectively
Is well groomed

Belonging and Attachment
(Love, Empathy, Affiliation)
Expresses an adequate sense of belonging
Participates in group activities
Appropriately expresses affection toward others

Safety and Security
(Caution, Planning, Protections, Sensory Acuity)
Adapts to changes in sensory acuity
Problem solves satisfactorily
Has adequate mobility
Travels alone

Biological and Physiological Integrity
(Air, Fluids, Comfort, Activity, Nutrition, Elimination, Skin Integrity)
Has adequate cardiac output
Has intact skin
Maintains adequate nutrition
Maintains adequate fluid intake
Has sufficient range of motion

These are not all the possible wellness diagnoses that may be identified. The above are examples of nursing diagnoses that should be considered when planning care for the older adult.

APPLICATION OF MASLOW'S HIERARCHY

The normal physical changes with aging have the potential to affect the person at all levels of Maslow's Hierarchy. For example, the most basic need for air can be compromised by the combination of decreased pulmonary cilliary movement, cough reflex, and immunity. The need for safety may be compromised by reduced sensory function, such as the slightly reduced ability to smell and escape a fire emergency in time. Meeting belonging needs can be compromised when decreased response time restricts the ability to drive safely and social opportunities are missed. Self-esteem may be threatened by changes in appearance, especially in skin and hair color. Finally, the overall changes with aging require a readjustment in how one looks at transcendence—what is most important in later life will probably be very different from what was most important in earlier periods of life.

The physical changes that accompany aging affect every body system, and the theories of why they occur are many. Although there are numerous ways nurses can promote healthy aging in the presence of these changes, when nurses are able to begin to differentiate these normal changes from signs and symptoms of potential health problems, the positive effect of the nurse's interventions is multiplied.

KEY CONCEPTS

▶ There are many physical changes that accompany aging; however, a number of these are relatively insignificant in the absence of disease or unusual stress.

▶ Physiological aging begins at birth and is universal, progressive, and intrinsic.

▶ There are enormous individual variations in the rate of aging of body systems and functions.

▶ Many of the normal changes with aging may be misinterpreted as being pathological, and some pathological conditions may be mistaken for normal changes of aging.

▶ Careful assessment of individual aging changes, lifestyle, and desires is fundamental to caring and quality nursing care of persons in later life.

ACTIVITIES AND DISCUSSION QUESTIONS

1. Identify at least two normal changes that accompany aging and two abnormal physical and/or physiological changes that are commonly seen in older adults, for each body system.
2. Discuss the changes of aging you would find most difficult to accept.

3. Develop a nursing care plan using wellness and NANDA diagnoses.

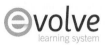

For additional resources, please visit evolve.elsevier.com/Ebersole/gerontological

REFERENCES

Abdollahi M, Ranjbar A, Shadnia S et al: Pesticides and oxidative stress: a review, *Med Sci Monit* 10(6):RA141-147, 2004.

Burke M, Laramie JA: *Primary care of the older adult: a multidisciplinary approach,* ed 2, St. Louis, 2003, Mosby.

Crowther CL: Structure and function of the musculoskeletal system. In McCance KL, Huether SE, editors: *Pathophysiology: the biologic basis for disease in adults and children,* ed 5, St Louis, 2006, Mosby.

Deneris A, Huether SE: Structure and function of the reproductive systems. In McCance KL, Huether SE, editors: *Pathophysiology: the biologic basis for disease in adults and children,* ed 5, St Louis, 2006, Mosby.

Effros RB, Dagarag M, Spaulding C, Man J: The role of CD8+ T-cell replicative senescence in human aging. *Immunol Rev* 205:147-157, 2005.

Friedman S: Integumentary function. In Meiner SE, Lueckenotte AG, editors: *Gerontologic nursing,* ed 3, St. Louis, 2006a, Mosby.

Friedman S: Pain, temperature regulation, sleep, and sensory function. In McCance KL, Huether SE, editors: *Pathophysiology: the biologic basis for disease in adults and children,* ed 5, St Louis, 2006b, Mosby.

Gosain A, DiPietro LA: Aging and wound healing, *World J Surg* 28(3):321-326, 2004.

Hall KE: Effect of aging on gastrointestinal function. In Hazzard WR, Blass J, Halter B et al, editors: *Principles of geriatric medicine and gerontology,* ed 5, New York, 2003, McGraw-Hill.

Hayflick L: Theories of aging. In Cape R, Coe R, Rossman I, editors: *Fundamentals of geriatric medicine,* New York, 1983, Raven Press.

Hayflick L, Moorehead PS: The serial cultivation of human diploid cell strains, *Exp Cell Res* 25:585, 1981.

Hogstel MO: Vital signs are really vital in the old-old, *Geriatr Nurs* 15(5):253, 1994.

Huether SE: Structure and function of the digestive system. In McCance KL, Huether SE, editors: *Pathophysiology: the biologic basis for disease in adults and children,* ed 5, St Louis, 2006b, Mosby.

Huether SE, DeFriez CB: Pain, temperature regulation, sleep, and sensory function. In McCance KL, Huether SE, editors: *Pathophysiology: the biologic basis for disease in adults and children,* ed 5, St Louis, 2006, Mosby.

Jett K: Physiological changes with aging. In Ebersole P, Touhy T, Hess P et al, editors: *Toward healthy aging,* 2008a, St. Louis, Mosby.

Jett K: Laboratory values and diagnostics. In Ebersole P, Touhy T, Hess P et al, editors: *Toward healthy aging,* 2008b, St. Louis, Mosby.

Kamel H, Dornbrand L: Health issues of the aging male. In Landefeld CS, Palmer R, Johnson MA et al, editors: *Current geriatric diagnosis and treatment,* New York, 2004, McGraw-Hill.

Kee JL, Paulanka BJ: Fluids and their influence on the body. In Kee JL, Paulanka BJ: *Handbook of fluids, electrolytes and acid-base imbalances,* Albany, NY, 2000, Delmar.

Kishiyama JL: Disorders of the immune system. In McPhee SJ, Ganong WF, editors: *Pathophysiology of disease: an introduction to clinical medicine,* ed 5, Lange, 2006, McGraw-Hill.

Luggen AS: Rapunzel no more: hair loss in older women, *Adv Nurse Pract* 13(10):28-33, 2005.

MacAas-Naaez JF, Cameron JS: the ageing kidney. In Davison AM et al, editors: *Oxford textbook of clinical nephrology,* ed 3, 2005, Oxford University Press.

Manolagas S: Aging musculoskeletal system. In Beers MH, Berkow R, editors: *The Merck manual of geriatrics,* ed 3, Whitehouse Station, NJ, 2000, Merck Research Laboratories.

Marin-Garcia J: *Aging and the heart: a post genomic view,* New York, 2008, Springer.

McCance KL: Structure and function of the cardiovascular systems. In McCance KL, Huether SE, editors: *Pathophysiology: the biologic basis for disease in adults and children,* ed 5, St Louis, 2006, Mosby.

Meisami E, Brown CM, Emerle HF: Sensory systems: normal aging, disorders, and treatments of vision and hearing in humans. In Timiras PS, editor: *Physiological basis of aging and geriatrics,* ed 3, New York City, 2002, CRC Press.

Merck Manual of Geriatrics (online): Age-related changes in skin structure and function, 2006 (website): www.merck.com/mrkshared/mmg/sec15/ch122/ch122b.jsp. Accessed July 1, 2006.

Michel J: Aging and the immune system. In Beers MH, Berkow R, editors: *The Merck manual of geriatrics,* ed 3, Whitehouse Station, NJ, 2000, Merck Research Laboratories.

Price S, Wilson L: *Pathophysiology: clinical concepts of disease processes,* ed 6, St Louis, 2002, Mosby.

Proust J: Aging and the immune system. In Beers MH, Berkow R, editors: *The Merck manual of geriatrics,* ed 3, Whitehouse Station, NJ, 2000, Merck Research Laboratories.

Sheahan SL, Musialowski R: Clinical implications of respiratory system changes in aging, *J Gerontolog Nurs* 27(5):26, 2001.

Short KR, Bigelow ML, Kahl J et al: Decline in skeletal muscle mitochondrial function with aging in humans, *Proc Natl Acad Sci USA* 102(15):5618, 2005.

Stengel GB: Oral temperature in the elderly, *Gerontologist* 23(special issue):306, 1983.

Sugarman RA: Structure and function of the neurologic system. In McCance KL, Huether SE, editors: *Pathophysiology: the biologic basis for disease in adults and children,* ed 5, St Louis, 2006, Mosby.

Taffet GE, Lakatta EG: Aging of the cardiovascular system. In Hazzard WR, Blass J, Halter B et al, editors: *Principles of geriatric medicine and gerontology,* ed 5, New York, 2003, McGraw-Hill.

Tumosa N: Aging and the eye. In Beers MH, Berkow R, editors: *The Merck manual of geriatrics,* ed 3, Whitehouse Station, NJ, 2000, Merck Research Laboratories.

Wiggins J: Changes in renal function. In Hazzard WR, Blass J, Halter B et al, editors: *Principles of geriatric medicine and gerontology,* ed 5, New York, 2003, McGraw-Hill.

Williams TF: History and physical examination. In Beers MH, Berkow R, editors: *The Merck manual of geriatrics,* ed 3, Whitehouse Station, NJ, 2000, Merck Research Laboratories.

Valko M, Morris H, Cronin M et al: Metals, toxicity and oxidative stress, *Curr Med Chem* 12(10):1161-1208, 2005.

Social, Psychological, Spiritual, and Cognitive Aspects of Aging

▶ LEARNING OBJECTIVES

Upon completion of this chapter, the reader will be able to:

- Explain the major cognitive, psychological, and sociological theories of aging.
- Discuss the influence of culture and cohort on psychological and social adaptation.
- Discuss the importance of spirituality to healthy aging.
- Explain several normal cognitive changes of aging.
- Discuss factors influencing learning in late life and appropriate teaching and learning strategies.

▶ GLOSSARY

Cognition The mental process characterized by knowing, thinking, learning, and judging.

Cross-sectional A study design in which data are collected at one point in time on several variables such as gender, income, educatiion, and health status.

Eurocentric The practice of viewing the world from a European perspective, with an implied belief, either consciously or subconsciously, in the preeminence of European (and more generally, of Western) culture, concerns and values at the expense of non-Europeans.

Face validity "The extent to which a measuring instrument looks as though it is measuring what it purports to measure." (Polit and Beck, 2006, p. 500).

Geragogy The application of the principles of adult learning theory to teaching for older adults.

Health literacy The degree to which individuals have the ability to obtain, process, and understand basic health information and services needed to make appropriate health decisions.

Longitudinal research A study design that studies a group of subjects over time, assessing their experiences at predetermined stages. The Harvard Nurses' Study is an example of this in that a large group of nurses have been assessed every few years for more than 20 years.

▶ THE LIVED EXPERIENCE

If I Had My Life to Live Over

I'd dare to make more mistakes next time, I'd relax, I would limber up. I would be sillier than I've been this trip. I would take fewer things seriously. I would take more chances. I would climb more mountains and swim more rivers. I would eat more ice cream and less beans. I would perhaps have more actual troubles, but I'd have fewer imaginary ones.

You see, I'm one of those people who live sensibly and sanely hour after hour, day after day. Oh, I've had my moments, and if I had to do it over again, I'd have more of them. In fact, I'd try to have nothing else. Just moments, one after another, instead of living so many years ahead of each day. I've been one of those persons who never goes anywhere without a thermostat, a hot water bottle, a raincoat, and a parachute. If I had it to do again, I would travel lighter than I have.

If I had my life to live over, I would start barefoot earlier in the spring and stay that way later in the fall. I would go to more dances. I would ride more merry-go-rounds. I would pick more daisies.

Nadine Stair

SOCIAL, PSYCHOLOGICAL, SPIRITUAL, AND COGNITIVE ASPECTS OF AGING

There are normal biological, psychological, social, and cognitive changes in the process of aging. The biological changes are discussed in Chapter 6. This chapter is meant to provide the reader with information on the psychological, social, cognitive, and spiritual aspects of aging. Factors influencing learning in late life and appropriate teaching and learning strategies for older adults are also discussed.

Each individual has unique life experiences and because of this must be seen holistically, through the lens of his or her time, place, culture, gender, and personal history. The close relationship among biological, social, and psychological development that exists through childhood and adolescence varies more in adulthood because of the greater variations in life experiences and demands as one matures.

LIFE SPAN DEVELOPMENT APPROACH

Human development goes on throughout life and is a lifelong process of adaptation. Life span development refers to an individual's progress through time and an expected pattern of change: biological, sociological, and psychological. A summary of the key principles of the life span developmental approach, provided by Papalia et al (2002), is based on the work of Paul Baltes and colleagues (Baltes, 1987; Baltes et al, 1998). Principles include the following:

▶ Development is lifelong. Each part of the life span is influenced by the past and will affect the future. Each period of the life span has unique characteristics and value; none is more important than any other.
▶ Development depends on history and context. Each person develops within a certain set of circumstances or conditions defined by time and place. Humans are influenced by historical, social, and cultural context.

▶ Development is multidimensional and multidirectional and involves a balance of growth and decline. Whereas children usually grow consistently in size and abilities, in adulthood, the balance gradually shifts. Some abilities, such as vocabulary, continue to increase, whereas others, such as speed of information retrieval, may decrease. New abilities, such as wisdom and expertise, may emerge as one ages.
▶ Development is plastic rather than rigid. Function and performance can improve throughout the life span with training and practice. However, there are limits on how much a person can improve at any age.

TYPES OF AGING

People age in a number of ways. Aging can be viewed in terms of *chronological age, biological age, psychological age*, and *social age*. These ages may or may not be the same. Chronological age is measured by the number of years lived. Biological age is predicted by the person's physical condition and how well vital organ systems are functioning. Psychological age is expressed through a person's ability and control of memory, learning capacity, skills, emotions, and judgment. Maturity and capacity will direct the manner in which one is able to adapt psychologically over time to the requirements of the physical and social environment. Social age may be quite different from chronological age and is measured by age-graded behaviors that conform to an expected status and role within a particular culture or society. A person may be chronologically aged 80 but biologically aged 60 because he or she has remained fit with a healthy lifestyle. Or, a person with a chronic illness may be biologically aged 70 but psychologically is much younger because he or she has remained active and involved in life.

There are several psychological and sociological theories of aging. In contrast to biological theories of aging (see Chapter 6), the psychological and sociological theories are not always based on empirical evidence because of methodological and measurement-related problems. The majority of these theories were developed from a Eurocentric perspective and may be less useful to describe aging within other cultures, especially those that are collective rather than individualistic (see Chapter 4). The importance of opportunity, ethnicity, gender, and social status is largely ignored. In addition, they have little to do with personal meaning and motivation; however, they may be useful as a guide in helping us understand the world around us and move toward and into healthy aging. As current generations of elders move through this period of life development, many of the ideas we have about this period of life are being, and will continue to be, redefined.

SOCIOLOGICAL THEORIES OF AGING

Sociological theories of aging attempt to explain and predict the changes in roles and relationships in middle and late life, with an emphasis on adjustment. The basic theories were developed in the 1960s and 1970s and must be viewed within the context of the historical period from which they emerged. Some of the theories continue to generate interest and thought, such as modernization and social exchange theories, and others, such as disengagement theory, are no longer considered relevant.

Disengagement Theory

The disengagement theory states that "aging is an inevitable, mutual withdrawal or disengagement, resulting in decreased interaction between the aging person and others in the social system he belongs to" (Cumming and Henry, 1961, p. 2). This means that withdrawal from one's society and community is natural and acceptable for the older adult and his or her society. The measures of disengagement are based on age, work, and decreased interest or investment in societal concerns. The theory is seen as universal and applicable to older people in all cultures, although there are expected variations in timing and style.

Activity Theory

The activity theory is based on the belief that remaining as active as possible in the pursuits of middle age is the ideal in later life. Because of improved general health and wealth, this is more possible than it was 40 years ago when Maddox (1963) proposed this theory. The activity theory may make sense when individuals live in a stable society, have access to positive influences and significant others, and have opportunities to participate meaningfully in the broader society if they continue to desire to do so. Attempts at clarifying activity theory as a general concept of satisfactory aging have not been supported.

Continuity Theory

The continuity theory, proposed by Havighurst and co-workers (1968), explains that life satisfaction with engagement or disengagement depends on personality traits. Three ideas about personality (Neugarten et al, 1968) are important to understanding continuity theory:

▶ In the normal progression of aging, personality traits remain quite stable.
▶ Personality influences role activity and one's level of interest in particular roles.
▶ Personality influences life satisfaction regardless of role activity.

Age-Stratification Theory

Age-stratification theory is a newer approach to understanding the role, the reactions, and the adaptations of older adults. Like continuity theory, it specifically challenges activity theory and disengagement theory. Age-stratification theory goes beyond the individual to the age structure of society (Marshall, 1996). The structuring of different ages can take a number of different forms, including the conceptualization of "young," "middle-aged," and "old" or Thomas's (2004) proposal of the state of "elderhood" following "childhood" and "adolescence."

Historical context is a key component of age-stratification theory. Elders can be understood as members of cohorts along with others who have shared similar historical periods in their lives, with age-graded systems of expectations and rewards. They have been exposed to similar events and conditions and common global, environmental, and political circumstances (Riley et al, 1972). Hooks (2000) reminds us that race must be considered when understanding cohort effects.

This theory may be particularly useful to examine aging within a global context. The definitions of age strata usually encompass social and cultural expressions of aging as well as who is placed in a given stratum and when. The cohort effect can be used as a powerful tool for understanding the potential life experiences of people from not only different cultures, but also different parts of the world.

Social Exchange Theory

Challenging both activity theory and disengagement theory, social exchange theory is based on the consideration of the cost-benefit model of social participation (Dowd, 1980). It explains that withdrawal or social isolation is the result of an imbalance in the exchanges between older persons and younger members of society and that the balance is what determines one's personal satisfaction and social support at any point in time.

Older adults are often viewed as unequal partners in the exchange and may need to depend on metaphorical reserves of contributions to the pool of reciprocity. This may be seen in the expectation of elderly African Americans for care as "pay-back" for their providing care to others earlier in their lives (Jett, 2006). Other elders care for younger grandchildren so that their adult children can work. For this they may receive total support (i.e., room, board, income). Although this exchange may appear uneven, it can also be viewed from the more holistic perspective of a lifetime of exchanges and contributions. Hooyman and Kiyak (2008) noted that "although older individuals may have fewer economic and material resources, they often have nonmaterial resources such as respect, approval, love, wisdom, and time for civic engagement and giving back to society" (p. 317). Intergenerational programs are an example of the value of social exchange between generations.

Modernization Theory

Modernization theory attempts to explain the social changes that have resulted in the devaluing of both the contributions of elders and the elders themselves. Historically (before about 1900 in the United States), materials and political resources were controlled by the older members of society (Achenbaum, 1978). The resources included not only their time, as shown in the examples just described, but also their knowledge, traditional skills, and experience. According to this theory, the status, and therefore the value, of elders is lost when their labors are no longer considered useful. Kinship networks are dispersed, the information they hold is no longer useful to the society in which they live, and the culture in which they live no longer reveres them. It is proposed that these changes are the result of advancing technology, urbanization, and mass education.

Treatment of the elderly in modern Japan was long considered evidence of the inaccuracy of the theory. Historically, Japanese elders were given the highest status and held the greatest power. This did not seem to change with the industrialized advances after World War II. However, today Japan not only is a highly modern country from an industrial point but also is showing signs of "modernization" in social relations with elders. Other researchers have also found support of the modernization theory in other societies such as India and Taiwan (Dandekar, 1996; Silverman et al, 2000).

Symbolic Interaction Theories

Symbolic interaction theories propose that the kind of aging process people experience is a result of interactions between the environment, the individual, and the meaning the person attributes to his or her activities (Gubrium, 1973; Hooyman and Kiyak, 2008). "Whether a new activity increases or decreases life satisfaction depends on an elder's resources (health, socioeconomic status, and social support), along with the environmental norms for interpreting activities" (Hooyman and Kiyak, 2008, p. 313). With this perspective, one has to examine how the individual's resources and activities, as well as the environmental demands, can be altered to enhance satisfaction and self concept. For example, if an elder needs to move to a nursing home, a useful line of thinking involves looking at how the new environment can be structured to support the individual's resources and lifestyle so that he or she can continue to maintain a positive self-concept and experience life satisfaction

IMPLICATIONS FOR GERONTOLOGICAL NURSING AND HEALTHY AGING

The sociological theories of aging provide the gerontological nurse with useful information and a background for enhancing healthy aging and adaptation (Box 7-1). Although these theories have neither been proved nor disproved, many of the ideas they discuss have withstood the test of time. The theories have been adapted and applied to contemporary approaches to aging in many ways, from the concept of senior centers (activity theory) to nursing assessments of social support (social exchange theory). And, unfortunately, the disengagement theory is still applied any time one incorrectly assumes depression and isolation to be a "normal" part of aging. Further research is needed to explore how culture, ethnicity, and gender influence

Box 7-1	Areas of Potential Nursing Assessment and Education Consistent with the Sociological Theories of Aging

- Currently held roles, role satisfaction, and emerging roles (*Role*)
- Individual's and family's expectations of age norms and effect on self-esteem (*Role*)
- Current level of activity and satisfaction with such (*Activity*)
- Effect of changes in health on usual roles and activities (*Role, Activity*)
- Cultural beliefs and expectations related to roles, activity, and both engagement and disengagement related to these (*Role, Activity, Disengagement*)
- Usual life patterns and personality and attention to any change in these as an indication of a potential problem (*Continuity*)
- Knowledge of the historical context of the individual and its potential influence on perception and responses (*Age-Stratification*)
- Complexity of social support and network (*Social/Exchange*)
- Opportunities for contributions of knowledge to society (*Modernization*)
- Sense of self and self-worth (*Modernization*)

aging and adaptation. This is particularly important in light of the expected growth of a very diverse aging population.

PSYCHOLOGICAL THEORIES OF AGING

Psychological theories presuppose that aging is one of many developmental processes experienced between birth and death. Life, then, is a dynamic process. Although these are widely accepted because of their face validity, like the sociological theories, they are not well suited to testing or measurement and do not address the influence of culture, gender, and ethnicity.

Jung's Theories of Personality

Psychologist Carl Jung (1971), a contemporary of Freud, proposed a theory of the development of a personality throughout life, from childhood to old age. He was one of the first psychologists to define the last half of life as having a purpose of its own, quite apart from species survival. The last half of life is often a time of inner discovery, quite different from the biological and social issues that demand a great deal of outward attention during the first half of life. The last half of life, ideally, is less intensely demanding and allows more time for inner growth, self-awareness, and reflective activity.

According to this theory, a personality is either extroverted and oriented toward the external world or introverted and oriented toward the subjective inner world of the individual. Jung suggested that aging results

in the movement from extraversion to introversion. Beginning perhaps at midlife, individuals begin to question their own dreams, values, and priorities. The potentially resulting crisis or emotional upheaval is a step in the process of personality development. With chronological age and personality development, Jung proposed that the person is able to move from a focus on outward achievement to one of acceptance of the self and to the awareness that both the accomplishments and challenges of a lifetime can be found within oneself. The development of the psyche and the inner person is accomplished by a search for personal meaning and the spiritual self. This personality of late life can easily be compared to Erikson's ego integrity and Maslow's self-actualization (see Chapter 1).

Developmental Theories

Psychologist Eric Erikson is well known for articulating the developmental stages and tasks of life, from early childhood to later "elderhood." Most students have studied Erikson's eight-stage or task model. Erikson (1963) theorized a predetermined order of development and specific tasks that were associated with specific periods in one's life course. He proposed that one needed to successfully accomplish one task before complete mastery of the next was possible and originally articulated these in "either/or" language. He proposed that all persons would return again and again to a task that had been poorly resolved in the past.

Erikson's task of middle age is generativity. If successful in this task, one establishes oneself and contributes in meaningful ways for the future and future generations. Failure to accomplish this task results in stagnation. Erikson saw the last stage of life as a vantage point from which one could look back with ego integrity or despair on one's life. Ego integrity implies a sense of completeness and cohesion of the self. In achieving this final task, individuals can look back over their lives, at the joys and the sorrows, the mistakes and the successes, and feel satisfied with the way they lived.

In later years, as octogenarians, Erikson and his wife, Joan, reconsidered his earlier work from the perspective of their own aging. They modified their "either/or" stance of the developmental tasks to the recognition of the balance of each of the tasks. Thus ego integrity is tinged with some regrets, wisdom is balanced with frivolity, and letting go is balanced with hanging on (Erikson et al, 1986).

Peck (1968) expanded on the original work of Erikson with the identification of specific tasks of old age that must be addressed to establish ego integrity. Peck's tasks represent the process or movement toward Erikson's final stage.

▶ *Ego differentiation* versus *work role preoccupation.* The individual is no longer defined by his or her work.

▶ *Body transcendence* versus *body preoccupation.* The body is cared for but does not consume the interest and attention of the individual.

▶ *Ego transcendence* versus *ego preoccupation.* The self becomes less central, and one feels a part of the mass of humanity, sharing their struggles and their destiny.

To achieve ego integrity, according to Peck's theoretical model, one must develop the ability to redefine the self, to let go of occupational identity, to rise above bodily discomforts, and to establish meanings that go beyond the scope of self-centeredness. Although these are admirable and idealistic goals, they place a considerable burden on the older person. Not everyone may have the courage or the energy to laugh in the face of adversity or surmount all of the assaults of old age. The wisdom of old age involves a crisis of understanding in which the ordinary structures are shaken and the meaning of life is reexamined. It may or may not include the wisdom of questioning assumptions in the search for meaning in the last stage of life.

Robert Havighurst (1971) is another developmental theorist who has proposed specific tasks to be accomplished in middle age and later maturity. Havighurst's developmental tasks are presented in Box 7-2.

Box 7-2   Havighurst's Developmental Tasks

Middle Age
- Assisting teenage children to become responsible and happy adults
- Achieving adult social and civic responsibility
- Reaching and maintaining satisfactory performance in one's occupational career
- Developing adult leisure-time activities
- Relating to one's spouse as a person
- Accepting and adjusting to the physiological changes of middle age
- Adjusting to aging parents

Later Maturity
- Adjusting to decreasing physical strength and health
- Adjusting to retirement and reduced income
- Adjusting to death of a spouse
- Establishing an explicit affiliation with one's age group
- Adopting and adapting social roles in a flexible way
- Establishing satisfactory living arrangements

From: Havighurst R: *Developmental tasks and education,* ed 3, New York, 1971, Longman.

Theory of Gerotranscendence

Tornstam (1994, 1996, 2005) theorizes that human aging brings about a general potential for what he terms *gerotranscendence*, a shift in perspective from the material world to the cosmic and, concurrent with that, an increasing life satisfaction. Gerotranscendence is thought to be a gradual and ongoing shift that is generated by the normal processes of living, sometimes hastened by serious personal disruptions. It is associated with wisdom and spiritual growth, similar to Erikson's concept of integrity and Maslow's self-actualization. Characteristics of gerotranscendence include the following:

▶ A high degree of life satisfaction
▶ Midlife patterns and ideals are no longer prime motivators
▶ Complex and active coping patterns
▶ A greater need for solitary philosophizing, meditation, and solitude
▶ Social activities are not essential to well-being
▶ Satisfaction with self-selected social activities
▶ Less concern with body image and material possessions

▶ Decreased fear of death
▶ Affinity with past and future generations
▶ Decreased self-centeredness and increased altruism

SPIRITUALITY AND AGING

Spirituality has been defined as a "quality of a person derived from the social and cultural environment that involves faith, a search for meaning, a sense of connection with others, and a transcendence of self, resulting in a sense of inner peace and well-being" (Delgado, 2007, p. 230). The spiritual aspect of people's lives transcends the physical and psychosocial to reach the deepest individual capacity for love, hope, and meaning. Erickson's concept of ego integrity and Maslow's concept of self-actualization seem closely related to development of a spiritual self.

Although religious needs are important for many older people, spiritual needs are much broader and more personal than adherence to any religious persuasion would normally comprise. However, nurses must be knowledgeable and respectful of the rites and rituals of varying religions, cultural beliefs, and values. Religious and spiritual resources such as pastoral visits should be available in all settings where older people reside. It is important to avoid imposing one's own beliefs and to respect the person's privacy on matters of spirituality and religion (Touhy and Zerwekh, 2006).

Spirituality must be considered a significant factor in understanding healthy aging. Rowe and Kahn's (1998) model of successful aging includes active engagement in life, minimal risk and disability, and high cognitive and physical function. Crowther and colleagues (2002) maintain that spirituality must be the fourth element of the model and is interrelated with all of the others. Spirituality and religiosity may be particularly important to healthy aging in "historically disadvantaged populations who display remarkable strengths despite adversities in their lives" (Hooyman and Kiyak, 2005, p. 213).

Aging as a biological process has been studied extensively. Less attention has been paid to the study of aging as a spiritual process. As people age and move closer to death, spirituality may become more important. Declining physical health, loss of loved ones, and a realization that life's end may be near often challenge older people to reflect on the meaning of their lives (Touhy, 2001a).

Nursing research on spirituality and aging indicates that spirituality is a source of hope (Touhy, 2001b); aids in adaptation to illnesses (Potter and Zausniewski, 2000); and has a positive influence on quality of life in chronically ill older adults (O'Brien, 2003; Delgado, 2007). Spirituality is an important component of healthy aging, and gerontological nurses have many opportunities to assist elders in reflecting on the meaning and purpose of life and achieving spiritual well-being (Box 7-3). Spiritual well-being can be considered the ability to experience and integrate meaning and purpose in life through connectedness with self others, art, music, literature, nature, or a power greater than oneself (NANDA International, 2004; Gaskamp et al, 2006).

A comprehensive, evidence-based guideline for promoting spirituality in the older adult (Gaskamp et al, 2006) provides a framework for spiritual assessment and interventions. Suggestions for assessment of spiritual resources, identification of older adults who may be at risk for spiritual distress, and spiritual nursing responses are presented in Boxes 7-4 and 7-5.

IMPLICATIONS FOR GERONTOLOGICAL NURSING AND HEALTHY AGING

Knowledge about the process of life span development and the various ways people experience growing older assists gerontological nurses in understanding the

---

Box 7-3	Spiritual Nursing Responses

- Relief of physical discomfort, which permits focus on the spiritual
- Comforting touch, which fosters nurse-patient connection
- Authentic presence
- Attentive listening
- Knowing the patient as a person
- Listening to life stories
- Sharing fears and listening to self-doubts or guilt
- Fostering forgiveness and reconciliation
- Sharing caring words and love
- Fostering connections to that which is held sacred by the person
- Respecting religious traditions and providing for access to religious objects and rituals
- Referring the person to a spiritual counselor

Sources: Gaskamp C, Sutter R, Meraviglia M et al: Evidence-based practice guideline: promoting spirituality in the older adult, *J Gerontol Nurs* 32(11):8-11, 2006; Touhy T, Brown C, Smith C: Spiritual caring: end of life in a nursing home, *J Gerontol Nurs* 31(9):27-35, 2004; Touhy T, Zerwekh H: Spiritual caring. In Zerwekh J: *Nursing care at the end of life: palliative care for patients and families*, Philadelphia, 2006, FA Davis.

Box 7-4	Brief Assessment of Spiritual Resources and Concerns

Instructions: Use the following questions as a guide to interview the older adult (or caregiver if the older adult is unable to communicate).
- Does your religion or spirituality provide comfort or serve as a cause of stress? (*Ask to explain in what ways spirituality is a comfort or stressor.*)
- Do you have any religious or spiritual beliefs that might conflict with health care or affect health care decisions? (*Ask to identify any conflicts.*)
- Do you belong to a supportive church, congregation, or faith community? (*Ask how the faith community is supportive.*)
- Do you have any practices or rituals that help you express your spiritual or religious beliefs? (*Ask to identify or describe practices.*)
- Do you have any spiritual needs you would like someone to address? (*Ask what those needs are and if referral to spiritual professional is desired.*)
- How can we (health care providers) help you with your spiritual needs or concerns?

From Gaskamp C, Sutter R, Meraviglia M et al: Evidence-based guideline: promoting spirituality in the older adult, *J Gerontol Nurs* 32(11):8-11, 2006, p. 10; Adapted from Meyer CL. Dissertation Abst Int 55(6):2158B, UMI No 9428614, 2003; Koenig HG, Brooks RG: Religion, health, and aging: implications for practice and public policy, *Public Policy Aging Rep* 12(4):13, 2002.

Box 7-5	Identifying Elders at Risk for Spiritual Distress

- Individuals experiencing events or conditions that affect the ability to participate in spiritual rituals
- Diagnosis and treatment of a life-threatening, chronic, or terminal illness
- Expressions of interpersonal or emotional suffering, loss of hope, lack of meaning, need to find meaning in suffering
- Evidence of depression
- Cognitive impairment
- Verbalized questioning or loss of faith
- Loss of interpersonal support

Data from Gaskamp C, Sutter R, Meraviglia M et al: Evidence-based guideline: promoting spirituality in the older adult, *J Gerontol Nurs* 32(11): 8-11, 2006.

meaning of healthy aging for each individual. Future generations of older adults will redefine what we now consider the "norms" for aging. People can expect to spend 30 or more years in "late life," and there are still many important tasks to be accomplished during this period. Concerns of the young are to become established as adults; middle-aged persons are overwhelmed with the requirements of success and survival. Focusing on the reason for being and the meaning of life is the concern of elders.

COGNITION AND AGING

Cognition is both a biological and a psychological factor that must be considered in caring for the older adult. Processes of normal cognition and learning in late life are discussed in this chapter. Care of older adults with impairment of cognition is discussed in Chapter 21.

Cognition is the process of acquiring, storing, sharing, and using information. Cognitive function includes the following 12 categories: attention span, concentration, intelligence, judgment, learning ability, memory, orientation, perception, problem-solving, psychomotor ability, reaction time, and social intactness (McDougall et al, 2003).

It has been generally believed that cognitive function declines in old age because of a decreased number of neurons, decreased brain size, and diminished brain weight. Although these losses are features of aging, they are not consistent with deteriorating mental function (Sugarman, 2006), nor do they interfere with everyday routines. Neuron loss occurs mainly in the brain and spinal cord and is most pronounced in the cerebral cortex. The neuronal dendrites atrophy with aging, resulting in impairment of the synapses and changes in the transmission of the chemical neurotransmitters dopamine, serotonin, and acetylcholine. This causes a slowing of many neural processes. However, overall cognitive abilities remain intact. There are many myths about aging and the brain that may be believed by both health professionals and older adults. It is important to understand cognition, memory and learning in late life and dispel the myths that can have a negative effect on wellness and may, in fact, contribute to unnecessary cognitive decline (Box 7-6).

The determination of intellectual capacity and performance has been the focus of a major portion of gerontological research. In general, cognitive functions may remain stable or decline with increasing age. The cognitive functions that remain stable include attention span, language skills, communication skills, comprehension and discourse, and visual perception. The cognitive skills that decline are verbal fluency, logical analysis, selective attention, object naming, and complex visuospatial skills (Hooyman and Kiyak, 2008).

Early studies about cognition and aging were cross-sectional rather than longitudinal and were often conducted with older adults who were institutionalized or had coexisting illnesses. The cognitive development of older people is often measured against the norms of young or middle-aged people, which may not be appropriate to the distinctive characteristics of older adults. In addition, most tests of cognitive ability were designed to test young children, and most do not address cultural or ethnic differences. Other reasons have been advanced for the variations of intellectual performance of the older adult being tested (Box 7-7).

Therefore, these tests may have little relevance for the daily function of older people. Intelligence in old age is dynamic, and certain abilities change and even improve with age (Figure 7-1).

More recent research, conducted longitudinally, is investigating the influence of various factors such as health, personality, life experiences, activity, emotion, socialization patterns, education, and culture on cognition in late life. More recent research, conducted longitudinally, is investigating the influence of various factors such as health, personality, life experiences, activity, emotion, socialization patterns, education, and culture on cognition in late life. Rates of cognitive impairment among older Americans have dropped from 12.2% in 1993 to 8.7% in 2002 among people age 70 and older. Education and financial status appeared overall to protect against the development of cognitive impairment, and improved treatment for stroke, heart disease, and vascular conditions may also have contributed to the decline (Lang et al, 2008).

Strategies to maintain and even improve cognitive function are being researched, and many older adults are taking proactive steps to keep both their bodies and their brains fit. The phrase "use it or lose it" applies to cognitive function as well as physical. *The Healthy Brain Initiative: A National Public Health Road Map*

Box 7-6   Myths About Aging and the Brain

MYTH: People lose brain cells every day and eventually just run out.
FACT: Most areas of the brain do not lose brain cells. Although you may lose some nerve connections, it can be part of the reshaping of the brain that comes with experience.
MYTH: You can't change your brain.
FACT: The brain is constantly changing in response to experiences and learning, and it retains this "plasticity" well into aging. Changing our way or thinking causes corresponding changes in the brain systems involved, that is, your brain believes what you tell it.
MYTH: The brain doesn't make new brain cells.
FACT: Certain areas of the brain including the hippocampus (where new memories are created) and the olfactory bulb (scent-processing center) regularly generate new brain cells.
MYTH: Memory decline is inevitable as we age.
FACT: Many people reach old age and have no memory problems. Participation in physical exercise, stimulating mental activity, socialization, healthy diet, and stress management helps maintain brain health. The incidence of dementia does increase with age, but when there are changes in memory, older people need to be evaluated for possible causes and receive treatment.
MYTH: There is no point in trying to teach older adults anything since "you can't teach an old dog new tricks."
FACT: Basic intelligence remains unchanged with age, and older adults should be provided with opportunities for continued learning. Minimizing barriers to learning such as hearing and vision loss and applying principles of geragogy enhance learning abilities.

Modified from: American Association of Retired Persons: *Myths about aging and the brain,* 2007. Accessed July 8, 2008 from www.aarp.org/health/brain/aging/myths_about_aging_and_the_brain.html.

Box 7-7	Complexities of Accurately Assessing Intellect in Old Age

- Older adults are most frequently compared with college students, whose chief occupation is proving their intellectual capacity.
- Young adults today are in the habit of being tested and have developed test wisdom, a skill never developed by some older adults or one that in others has grown rusty with disuse.
- Test material may not be relevant to the world of older adults, especially those of different cultures.
- Older people often perform poorly on test items because they are less likely to guess and more likely not to answer any items that seem ambiguous to them.
- Older people may have difficulty ignoring irrelevant stimuli.
- Intellectual performance relying on verbal functions shows little or no decline with age, but speed tests making use of nonverbal psychomotor functions show a decline.
- Social cognition and social context are related in terms of functioning in older adults. The older adults who maintain the best cognitive function are also those with a high social interactional level.

to Maintaining Cognitive Health (Centers for Disease Control and Prevention and The Alzheimer's Association, 2007) (www.cdc.gov/aging/roadmap/) and the *Cognitive and Emotional Health Project: The Healthy Brain* (http://trans.nih.gov/cehp/index.htm) are examples of national efforts to promote cognitive health.

Fluid and Crystallized Intelligence

Fluid intelligence (often called *native intelligence*) consists of skills that are biologically determined, independent of experience or learning. It is associated with flexibility in thinking, inductive reasoning, abstract thinking, and integration. Fluid intelligence "enables people to identify and draw conclusions about complex relationships" (Miller, 2008, p. 187). *Crystallized intelligence* is comprised of knowledge and abilities that the person acquires through education and life. Measures of crystallized intelligence include verbal meaning, word association, social judgment, and number skills. Older people perform more poorly on performance scales (fluid intelligence), but scores on verbal scales (crystallized intelligence) remain stable. This is known as the *classic aging pattern* (Hooyman and Kiyak, 2008). The tendency to do poorly on performance tasks may be related to age-related changes in sensory and perceptual abilities as well as psychomotor skills. Speed of cognitive processing and slower reaction time also affect performance.

Late adulthood is no longer seen as a period when growth has ceased and cognitive development halted; rather it is seen as a life stage programmed for plasticity and the development of unique capacities. Older people

do maintain their ability to understand situations and learn from new experiences. These findings are significant to satisfaction in late life, because the capacity for effective lifestyle management and one's cognitive resources contribute to adaptation and enjoyment. If brain function becomes impaired in old age, it is a result of disease, not aging.

Memory

Memory is defined as the ability to retain or store information and retrieve it when needed. Memory is a complex set of processes and storage systems. Three components characterize memory: immediate recall; short-term memory (which may range from minutes to days); and remote or long-term memory (Gallo et al, 2003). Biological, functional, environmental, and psychosocial influences affect memory development throughout adulthood. Recall of newly encountered information seems to decrease with age, and memory declines are noted in connection with complex tasks and strategies. Even though some older adults show decrements in the ability to process information, reaction time, perception, and capacity for attentional tasks, the majority of functioning remains intact and sufficient. Familiarity, previous learning, and life experience compensate for the minor loss of efficiency in the basic neurological processes. In unfamiliar, stressful, or demanding situations, however, these changes may be more marked.

Age-associated decline in memory is a major focus of research in aging and dementia. Normal older adults may complain of memory problems, but their symptoms do not meet the criteria for dementia. The term *age-associated memory impairment* (AAMI) has been

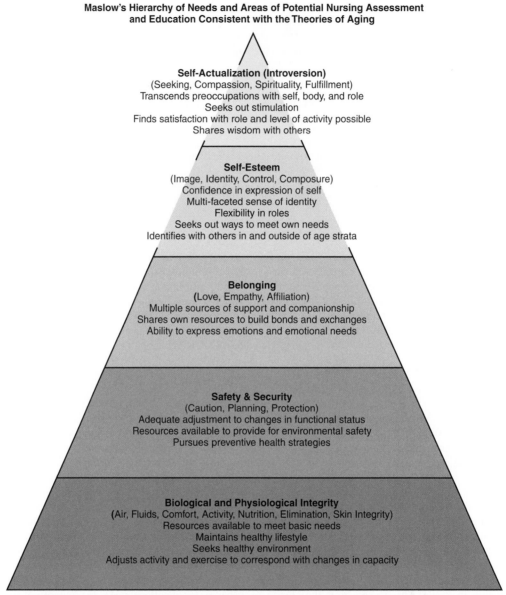

Maslow's Hierarchy of Needs and Areas of Potential Nursing Assessment and Education Consistent with the Theories of Aging

Self-Actualization (Introversion)
(Seeking, Compassion, Spirituality, Fulfillment)
Transcends preoccupations with self, body, and role
Seeks out stimulation
Finds satisfaction with role and level of activity possible
Shares wisdom with others

Self-Esteem
(Image, Identity, Control, Composure)
Confidence in expression of self
Multi-faceted sense of identity
Flexibility in roles
Seeks out ways to meet own needs
Identifies with others in and outside of age strata

Belonging
(Love, Empathy, Affiliation)
Multiple sources of support and companionship
Shares own resources to build bonds and exchanges
Ability to express emotions and emotional needs

Safety & Security
(Caution, Planning, Protection)
Adequate adjustment to changes in functional status
Resources available to provide for environmental safety
Pursues preventive health strategies

Biological and Physiological Integrity
(Air, Fluids, Comfort, Activity, Nutrition, Elimination, Skin Integrity)
Resources available to meet basic needs
Maintains healthy lifestyle
Seeks healthy environment
Adjusts activity and exercise to correspond with changes in capacity

Fig. 7-1   Life span cognitive developmental strengths. *(Developed by Priscilla Ebersole.)*

used to describe memory loss that is considered normal in light of the person's age and educational level. *Mild cognitive impairment* (MCI) (Petersen, 2004) is used when memory impairment is present beyond that which is felt to constitute normal aging, but other aspects of cognitive functioning remain intact. Some research indicates that about 50% of people with MCI will develop dementia within 3 years of diagnosis, but it is unclear

whether MCI is a "transitional state to dementia or a separate condition entirely" (Butler et al, 2004, p. 119). AAMI and MCI refer only to memory loss, whereas dementia is defined as cognitive impairment severe enough to affect daily functioning.

Many medical or psychiatric difficulties (depression, anxiety) also influence memory abilities, and it is important for older adults with memory complaints to have a comprehensive evaluation. In many cases, memory impairment is related to reversible and treatable conditions. Assessment of cognitive function is discussed in Chapter 21. If an irreversible dementia is detected, it is important to accurately diagnose the type of dementia and provide appropriate treatment. Clearly, the knowledge about memory and memory changes related to aging is still developing.

Scientists are finding that nerve cell regeneration does occur in the hippocampus of the brain, where memory function occurs (National Institutes on Aging, 2007). They have found that stress decreases the capacity for generation of new nerve cells, and current research focuses on the factors linking stress and nerve cell regeneration. Still other research on the "plasticity" of the brain is based on physical changes that occur in the brain that result from new memories and the addition of new neurons. Nurses need to educate people of all ages on effective strategies to enhance cognitive health and vitality and to promote cognitive reserve and brain plasticity. Suggested strategies include prevention and management of chronic conditions, maintaining a healthy weight, avoiding excess caloric intake, limiting sodium and fat intake, increasing antioxidant defense by consuming fresh fruits and vegetables, physical activity, participation in mentally stimulating activity, and social engagement (Yevchak, Loeb, Fick, 2008).

Cognitive stimulation and memory training may be helpful for cognitively intact older adults, as well as for those with cognitive impairment (Camp and Skrajner, 2004; Knapp et al, 2006; Unverzagt et al, 2007; Yevchak et al, 2008). Cognitive stimulation and memory training techniques include mnemonics (strategies to enhance coding, storage, and recall), internal and external aids, reasoning and speed-of-processing training, cognitive games (e.g., Scrabble, chess, crossword puzzles), and spaced retrieval techniques. Many games and aids are available that may be useful to enhance memory and stimulate cognitive function. One of the health maintenance organizations (HMOs) (Humana) in Florida offers a free brain fitness computer CD to its members (www.positscience.com). All older adults should remain active and engaged in activities that are stimulating for the mind as well as for the body.

LEARNING IN LATE LIFE

Basic intelligence remains unchanged with increasing years, and older adults should be provided with opportunities for continued learning. Geragogy is the application of the principles of adult learning theory to teaching interventions for older adults (Hayes, 2005). The older adult demands that teaching situations be relevant; new learning must relate to what the elder already knows and should emphasize concrete and practical information. Box 7-8 presents additional strategies to enhance the learning of older adults.

Opportunities for elders to learn are available in many formal and informal modes: self-teaching, college attendance, participation in seminars and conferences, public television programs, CDs, Internet courses, and countless others. In most universities, older people are taking classes of all types. Fees are usually lower for individuals older than 60 years, and elders may choose to work toward a degree or audit classes for enrichment and enjoyment. The Elderhostel program is an example of a program designed for elders to participate in that combines continued learning with travel (www.elderhostel.org).

The Internet has become one of the major vehicles of learning for older adults. Increasingly, elders are taking charge of their own learning and scanning the Internet for information about health and lifestyles. Many reliable Internet resources related to health and aging are available. The National Institute on Aging (NIA) website (www.nia.nih.gov/health/) provides excellent resources for health-related topics as well as training materials to help older adults find reliable online health information. The NIA "Age-Page" series is especially helpful and includes a variety of one-page informational sheets for consumers and health professionals.

Barriers to Learning

Aging may also present barriers to learning such as hearing and vision losses and cognitive impairment; moreover, the process of aging may accentuate other challenges that had already been factors in a person's life, such as cultural and cohort variations, education, and low literacy levels. Many elders may have special learning needs based on educational deprivation in their early years and consequent anxiety about formalized learning. Nurses must discover the preferred learning mode and setting appropriate to the needs and desires of the older adult (Figure 7-2).

Vision and hearing deficits interfere with learning, and teaching methods must be designed to enhance both the written and spoken word (see Chapters 3 and 19). Attention to literacy level and cultural variations is important to enhance learning and the usefulness of what is learned. Mood is extremely important in terms of what individuals (young and old) will recall. In other

Box 7-8	Guiding Older Adult Learners

- Make sure the client is ready to learn before trying to teach. Watch for cues that would indicate that the client is preoccupied or too anxious to comprehend the material.
- Be sensitive to cultural, language, and other differences among the older adults you serve. Some suggestions may not be appropriate for everyone.
- Provide adequate time for learning, and use self-pacing techniques
- Create a shame-free environment where older adults feel free to ask questions and stay informed.
- Provide regular positive feedback.
- Avoid distractions, and present one idea at a time.
- Present pertinent, specific, practical and individualized information. Emphasize concrete rather than abstract material.
- Use past experience; connect new learning to what has already been learned.
- Use written material to supplement verbal instruction. Use a list format, a low-literacy level, and large readable font (e.g., Arial, 14 to 16 points).
- Use high contrast on visuals and handout materials (e.g., black print on white paper).
- Consider using Braille and audio-taped information whenever necessary.
- Pay attention to reading ability; use tools other than printed material such as drawings, pictures, and discussion.
- Use bullets or lists to highlight pertinent information.
- Sit facing the client so he or she can watch your lip movements and facial expressions.
- Speak slowly.
- Keep the pitch of your voice low; older people can hear low sounds better than high-frequency sounds.
- Encourage the learner to develop various mediators or mnemonic devices (e.g., visual images, rhymes, acronyms, self designed coding schemes).
- Use shorter, more frequent sessions with appropriate breaks; pay attention to fatigue and physical discomfort.

Modified from: *Bridging principles of older adult learning: reconnaissance phase final report,* Washington, DC, 1999, SPRY Foundation; and Hayes K: Designing written medication instructions: effective ways to help older adults self-medicate, *J Gerontol Nurs 32*(5):5-10, 2005.

words, when we attempt to measure recall of events that may have occurred in a crisis situation or an anxiety state, recall will be impaired. This is significant for health care professionals who give information to elders who are ill or upset. They are very likely not to remember the information provided.

Health Literacy

Health literacy has been defined as "the degree to which individuals have the ability to obtain, process, and understand basic health information and services needed to make appropriate health decisions" (Quick Guide to Health Literacy in Older Adults, 2008). Health literacy is more than the ability to read and write and includes the ability to listen, follow directions, complete forms, perform basic math calculations, and interact with health professionals and health care settings. Factors influencing health literacy include the person's basic literacy skills, culture, and the situations encountered in the health care system as well as the cultural competence and communication skills of health professionals.

Nearly nine out of ten adults do not have proficient health literacy. Individuals residing in urban settings, those with poor education or low income, members of racial and ethnic minorities, older people, people for whom English is a second language, and those with compromised health status are more likely to perform at lower levels of literacy (Wilson et al, 2003). According to the 2003 National Assessment of Adult Literacy, older adults have lower health literacy scores than all other age groups with only 3% measured as proficient (Kutner et al, 2007). Chronic health conditions and vision and hearing impairments may further limit health literacy.

Limited literacy skills influence learning, as well as understanding, of health-related information such as prescription directions, consent documents, and health education materials. Consequences of limited literacy include poorer health, less importance assigned to health-related information and poorer adherence to instructions, increased hospitalizations, and increased health care costs (Cho et al, 2008; Hayes, 2000). "Limited literacy is, in fact, an occult, silent disability and a secret that

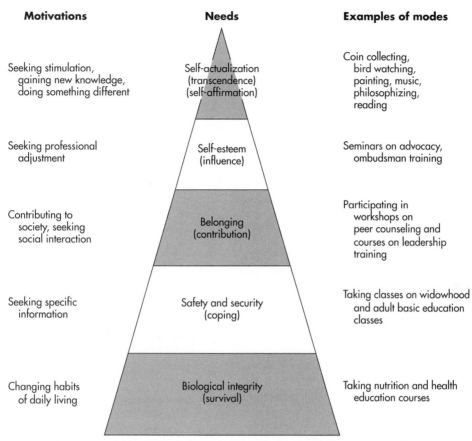

| Motivations | Needs | Examples of modes |

Fig. 7-2   Learning and growing in later life. *(Developed by Priscilla Ebersole.)*

most people do not share even with members of their own family" (Dreger and Tremback, 2002, p. 282).

Educational level cannot be relied upon as an indicator of literacy skills for medical information. Health literacy level is "approximately five grade levels lower than the last school year completed" (Hayes, 2000, p. 7). Many health education materials, as well as information on the World Wide Web, are written at reading levels above the recommended fifth-grade reading level. Innovations such as a user-friendly talking computer touchscreen are being used with good outcomes to assist low-literacy elders in health and disease prevention initiatives (Hahn et al, 2004). *The Quick Guide to Health Literacy in Older Adults* (2008) provides information for health care professionals related to health literacy and strategies for communicating effectively. Resources for assisting health care professionals in constructing low-literacy materials for use with the elderly are presented in Box 7-9.

IMPLICATIONS FOR GERONTOLOGICAL NURSING AND HEALTHY AGING

Caring for older adults means caring for body, mind, and spirit—holistic nursing at its finest. Understanding and appreciating the social, psychological, spiritual, and cognitive aspects of aging provides a foundation for nursing interventions that enhance lifelong growth, development, health, and well-being. A rich and stimulating environment should be available to all older adults in all settings so that they can thrive, not merely survive, in old age.

APPLICATION OF MASLOW'S HIERARCHY

Nurses can provide the opening for elders to discuss the process of aging and its psychological and social effects. In our highly biomedicalized approach to

| Box 7-9 | Resources for Constructing Low-Literacy Teaching Materials |

- Fleish-Kincaid Reading Level: Available in Microsoft Word tool setting.
- Rapid Estimate of Adult Literacy in Medicine (REALM) (Hayes, 2000) is a reading recognition test that estimates a reading grade level. A short (7-item) version of this instrument is now available (REALM-SF) (Arozullah A et al, 2007).
- Clinical Teacher's PET developed by LOGICARE Corporation (www.logicare.com) provides patient teaching materials at the fourth- through sixth-grade reading levels with free-text options.
- On-line Reference Point software (www.charm.net/%Erps/medsheet/index.htm) provides medication instruction sheets that are data-based and can be printed in large font, and also allows for free text information. The program can also be used to store and recall information about the patient and medications used.
- *Quick Guide to Health Literacy, Fact Sheet.* Available at www.health.gov/communication/literacy/quickguide/factsliteracy.htm.

From: Arozullah A, Yarnold P, Bennett C et al: Development and validation of a short-form rapid estimate of adult literacy in medicine, *Med Care* 45(11):1026-1033, 2007; Hayes K: Designing written medication instructions: effective ways to help older adults self-medicate, *J Gerontol Nurs* 31(5):5-10, 2005; Hayes K: Literacy for health information of adult patients and caregivers in the rural emergency department, *Clinical Excellence for Nurse Practitioners,* 4(1):35-40, 2000. *Quick guide to health literacy, fact sheet.* Accessed July 8, 2008 from www.health.gov/communication/literacy/quickguide/factsliteracy.htm.

aging, it is imperative that we seek to know individuals beyond the problem that brings them to the attention of the health care team. Care addressing only of the body and biological needs robs older people of the opportunity to grow toward self-actualization—a major task of late life. Ask elders, "How has aging affected your inner life and outlook?" "What gives your life meaning and purpose?" Listen to the answers, and learn. We are all aging, and those we serve are our best teachers.

KEY CONCEPTS

▶ Normal aging involves a gradual process of biopsychosocial change over the course of time.
▶ Life span development theorists tend to study the total life course of cohort groups to determine the influence of major historical events on their development.
▶ The impact of gender, culture, and cohort must always be considered when discussing the validity of biopsychosocial theories.
▶ Spirituality must be considered a significant factor in understanding healthy aging.
▶ Late adulthood is no longer seen as a period of when growth ceases and cognitive development halts; rather it is seen as a life stage programmed for plasticity and the development of unique capacities.
▶ Cognitive stimulation and attention to brain health is just as important as attention to physical health.

▶ Learning in late life can be enhanced by utilizing principles of geragogy and adapting teaching strategies to minimize barriers such as hearing and vision impairment and low literacy.

ACTIVITIES AND DISCUSSION QUESTIONS

1. Identify and discuss the major flaws in the sociological theories of aging.
2. How well do the psychological and sociological theories of aging "fit" within your own cultural perspective?
3. Discuss the variables that must constantly be considered when assessing the psychosocial aspects of the aging experience. Identify and discuss those that seem most significant.
4. Discuss some of the problems of adequately testing the cognitive function of elders.
5. How would you respond to the following myth of aging: "You can't teach an old dog new tricks"?
6. Discuss some ways that nurses can respond to the spiritual needs and concerns of older adults.

RESOURCES

Publications

Quick Guide to Health Literacy. Fact Sheet. Available at www.health.gov/communication/literacy/quickguide/factsliteracy.htm.
The Healthy Brain Initiative: A National Public Health Road Map to Maintaining Cognitive Health (Centers for Disease

Control and Prevention and The Alzheimer's Association, 2007). Available at www.cdc.gov/aging/roadmap/.

Organizations

National Institute on Aging, Senior Health. Age Pages, convenient one-page information sheets on health and aging www.nihseniorhealth.gov

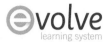

For additional resources, please visit evolve.elsevier.com/Ebersole/gerontological

REFERENCES

Achenbaum WA: *Old age in a new land,* Baltimore, 1978, Johns Hopkins Press.

Arozullah A, Yarnold P, Bennett C et al: Development and validation of a short-form rapid estimate of adult literacy in medicine, *Med Care* 45(11):1026-1033, 2007

Baltes PB: Theoretical propositions on life-span developmental theory: on the dynamics between growth and decline, *Dev Psychol* 23(5):611-626, 1987.

Baltes PB, Lindenberger U, Staudinger U: Life-span theory in developmental psychology. In Lerner R, editor: *Handbook of child psychology,* vol 1. *Theoretical models of human development,* New York, 1998, Wiley.

Butler R, Forette F, Greengrass B: Maintaining cognitive health in an ageing society, *J Royal Soc Prom Health* 124(3):119-121, 2004.

Camp C, Skrajner J: Resident-assisted Montessori programming (RAMP): training persons with dementia to serve as activity group leaders, *Gerontologist* 44(3):426-431, 2004.

Cho Y, Lee S, Arozullah A, Crittenden K: Effects of health literacy on health status and health service utilization amongst the elderly, *Social Sci and Medicine* 66:1809-1816, 2008.

Crowther M, Parker M, Achenbaum W et al: Rowe and Kahn's model of successful aging revisited: positive spirituality— the forgotten factor, *Gerontologist* 42(5):613, 2002.

Cumming E, Henry W: *Growing old,* New York, 1961, Basic Books.

Dandekar K: *The elderly in India,* Thousand Oaks, CA, 1996, Sage.

Delgado C: Sense of coherence, spirituality, stress and quality of life in chronic illness, *J Nurs Scholarsh* 39(3):229-234, 2007.

Dowd JJ: *Stratification among the aged,* Monterey, CA, 1980, Brooks Cole.

Dreger V, Tremback T: Optimize patient health by treating health literacy and language barriers, *AORN J* 75(2):278, 280-283, 285, 289-293, 297-300, 303-304, 2002.

Erikson EH: *Childhood and society,* ed 2, New York, 1963, WW Norton.

Erikson EH, Erikson JM, Kivnick HQ: *Vital involvement in old age: the experience of old age in our time,* New York, 1986, WW Norton.

Gallo JJ, Fulmer T, Paveza G: *Handbook of geriatric assessment,* ed 3, Boston, 2003, Jones & Bartlett.

Gaskamp C, Sutter R, Meraviglia M et al: Evidence-based guideline: promoting spirituality in the older adult, *J Gerontol Nurs* 32(11):8-11, 2006.

Gubrium JF: *The myth of the golden years,* Springfield, IL, Charles C. Thomas, 1973.

Hahn EA, Cella D, Dobrez D et al: The talking touch screen: a new approach to outcomes assessment in low literacy, *Psychooncology* 13(2):86-95, 2004.

Hayes K: Literacy for health information of adult patients and caregivers in the rural emergency department, *Clinical Excellence for Nurse Practitioners,* 4(1):35-40, 2000.

Hayes K: Designing written medication instructions: effective ways to help older adults self-medicate, *J Gerontol Nurs* 32(5):5-10, 2005.

Havighurst R, Neugarten B, Tobin S: Disengagement and patterns of aging. In Neugarten BL, editor: *Middle age and aging,* Chicago, 1968, University of Chicago Press.

Havighurst R: *Developmental tasks and education,* ed 3, New York, 1971, Longman.

Hooks B: *Feminist theory: from margin to center,* Cambridge, MA, 2000, South End Press.

Hooyman N, Kiyak H: *Social gerontology,* ed 8, Boston, 2008, Pearson.

Jett KR: Mind loss in the African-American community: a normal part of aging, *J Aging Stud* 20(1):1, 2006.

Jung C: The stages of life. In Campbell J, editor: *The portable Jung,* New York, 1971, Viking Press (translated by RFC Hull).

Knapp M, Thorgrimsen L, Patel A et al: Cognitive stimulation therapy for people with dementia: cost-effectiveness analysis, *Br J Psychiatr* 188:574-580, 2006.

Kutner M, Greenberg E, Jen Y, Paulsen C: The health literacy of America's adults: results from the 2003 National Assessment of Adult Literacy, 2007. Accessed July 8, 2008 from http://nces.ed.gov/Pubsearch/pubsinfo.asp?pubid=2006483.

Langa K, Larson E, Karlawish J et al: Trends in the prevention and mortality of cognitive impairment in the US: is there evidence of a compression of morbidity?, *Alzheimer's and Dementia: J Alzheimer's Assoc,* 4(2):134-144, 2008.

Maddox G: Activity and morale: a longitudinal study of selected older adult subjects, *Soc Forces* 42(2):195, 1963.

Marshall V: The state of theory in aging and the social sciences. In Binstock RH, Geroge LK, editors: *Handbook of aging and the social sciences,* ed 4, San Diego, 1996, Academic Press.

Maslow A: *Motivation and personality,* New York, 1954, Harper and Row.

McDougall G, Montgomery K, Eddy N et al: Aging memory self-efficacy: elders share their thoughts and experience, *Geriatr Nurs* 24(3):162-168, 2003.

Miller C: *Nursing for wellness in older adults,* Philadelphia, 2008, Wolters Kluwer–Lippincott Williams & Wilkins.

NANDA International: *Nursing diagnoses: definitions and classification 2003-2004,* Philadelphia, 2004, Author.

National Institute on Aging: *Inside the Human Brain,* 2007. Accessed July 7, 2008 from www.nia.nih.gov/Alzheimers/Publications/UnravelingTheMystery/Part1/InsideBrain.htm.

Neugarten BL, Havighurst R, Tobin SS: Personality and patterns of aging. In Neugarten B, editor: *Middle age and aging,* Chicago, 1968, University of Chicago Press.

Neugarten BL, Tobin SS: Disengagement and patterns of aging. In Neugarten BL, editor: *Middle age and aging,* Chicago, 1968, University of Chicago Press.

O'Brien ME: *Spirituality in nursing: standing on holy ground,* Boston, 2003, Jones & Bartlett.

Papalia D, Sterns H, Feldman R, Camp C: *Adult development and aging,* Boston, 2002, McGraw-Hill.

Peck R: Psychological developments in the second half of life. In Neugarten B, editor: *Middle age and aging,* Chicago, 1968, University of Chicago Press.

Petersen R: MCI as a useful clinical concept, *Geriatric Times* 5(1), 2004. Accessed July 8, 2008 from www.geriatrictimes.com/g040215.html.

Polit D, Beck C: *Essentials of nursing research: methods, appraisal and utilization,* ed 6, Philadelphia, 2006, Lippincott Williams & Wilkins.

Potter ML, Zausniewski J: Spirituality, resourcefulness, and arthritis impact on health perceptions of elders with rheumatoid arthritis, *J Holist Nurs* 18(4):311-331, 2000.

Quick Guide to Health Literacy in Older Adults. U.S .Department of Health and Human Services, 2007, Accessed 4/16/08 from www.health.gov/communication/literacy/olderadults/literacy.htm.

Riley M, Johnson M, Forner A: *Aging and society: a sociological of age stratification,* vol 3, New York, 1972, Russell Sage Foundation.

Rowe JW, Kahn RL: *Successful aging,* New York, 1998, Pantheon-Random House.

Satir N: *If I had my life to live over,* In Martz S, editor: *If I had my life to live over I would pick more daisies,* Watsonville, CA, 1992, Papier Mache Press.

Silverman P, Hecht L, McMillin J: Modeling life satisfaction among the aged: a comparison of Chinese and Americans, *J Cross Cult Gerontol* 15(4):289, 2000.

Sugarman RA: Structure and function of the nervous system. In McCance KL, Huether SE, editors: *Pathophysiology: the biologic basis for disease in adults and children,* ed 5, St Louis, 2006, Mosby.

Thomas W: *What are old people for: how elders will save the world,* New York, 2004, VanderWyk & Burnham.

Tornstam L: Gerotranscendence: a theoretical and empirical exploration. In Thomas LE, Eisenhandler SA, editors, *Aging and the religious dimension,* Westport, CT, 1994, Greenwood Publishing Group.

Tornstam L: Gerotranscendence: a theory about maturing into old age, *J Aging Identity* 1(1):37, 1996.

Tornstam L: *Gerotranscendence: a developmental theory of positive aging,* New York, 2005, Springer.

Touhy T: Nurturing hope and spirituality in the nursing home, *Holist Nurs Pract* 15(4):45-56, 2001a.

Touhy T: Touching the spirit of elders in nursing homes: ordinary yet extraordinary care, *Int J Human Caring* 6(1):12-17, 2001b.

Touhy T and Zerwekh J: Spiritual caring. In Zerwekh J: *Nursing care at the end of life: palliative care for patients and families,* Philadelphia, 2006, FA Davis.

Unverzagt FW, Kasten L, Johnson KE et al: Effect of memory impairment in training outcomes in ACTIVE, *J Int Neuropsycholog Soc* 13(6): 953-960, 2007.

Wilson F, Racine E, Tekieli V, Williams B: Literacy, readability and cultural barriers: critical factors to consider when educating older African Americans about anticoagulant therapy, *J Clin Nurs* 12(2):275-282, 2003.

Yevchak A, Loeb S, Fick D: Promoting cognitive health and vitality: a review of clinical implications, *Ger Nurs,* 29(5): 302-330, 2008.

Nutritional Needs

LEARNING OBJECTIVES

Upon completion of this chapter, the reader will be able to:

- Discuss nutritional requirements for older adults.
- Identify factors affecting the nutrition of older adults.
- Discuss interventions to promote improved nutrition for older adults.
- Discuss assessment and interventions for older adults with dysphagia.
- Identify strategies to ensure adequate nutrition for older adults experiencing hospitalization, institutionalization, and physical and cognitive impairments.
- Discuss interventions that promote healthy bowel function and good oral hygiene for older people.

GLOSSARY

Chemosenses The senses of taste and smell.
Dysphagia Sensation of impaired passage of food from the mouth to the esophagus and stomach; difficulty swallowing.
Gastroesophageal reflux disease (GERD) Backward flow of stomach contents into the esophagus.

Presbyesophagus Age-related change in the esophagus affecting motility.
Soul food Food possessing emotional significance and providing personal satisfaction; often has some cultural or traditional origins.
Xerostomia Dry mouth.

THE LIVED EXPERIENCE

If I do reach the point when I can no longer feed myself, I hope that the hands holding my fork belong to someone who has a feeling for who I am. I hope my helper will remember what she learns about me and that her awareness of me will grow from one encounter to another. Why should this make a difference? Yet, I am certain that my experience of needing to be fed will be altered if it occurs in the context of my being known... I will want to know about the lives of the people I rely on, especially the one who holds my fork for me. If she would talk to me, if we could laugh together, I might even forget the chagrin of my useless hands. We could have a conversation rather than a feeding."

From Lustbader W: Thoughts on the meaning of frailty, Generations 13(4):21-22, 1999.

NUTRITION AND AGING

Adequate nutrition is critical to preserving the health of older people and an integral part of health, happiness, independence, quality of life, and physical and mental functioning. Proper nutrition means that all of the essential nutrients (carbohydrates, fat, protein, vitamins, minerals, water) are adequately supplied and used to maintain optimal health and well-being. Increased amounts of calcium and vitamins D and B_{12} are needed in late life. Total caloric intake should decline in response to corresponding changes in metabolic rate and a general decrease in physical activity.

Nutrition is a leading indicator in *Healthy People 2010* and will be used over the next 10 years to measure the health of the nation (U.S. Department of Health and Human Services [USDHHS], 2002) (Box 8-1).

The Modified MyPyramid for adults older than 70 years has been adapted from the United States Department of Agriculture's (USDA) MyPyramid. The Modified MyPyramid provides the types and amounts of food that should be eaten to optimize nutrient intake. Figure 8-1 illustrates the Modified MyPyramid. The pyramid emphasizes a higher ratio of nutrients to calories. Fluid is emphasized because thirst mechanisms may be less responsive in older people. With proper instruction, the Modified MyPyramid is an easy and systematic way for a person to evaluate his or her own nutritional intake and independently make corrective adjustments. Pictures can be used to transcend cultural and speech barriers and educational limitations. The USDA also provides ethnic-cultural and vegetarian food pyramids (www.fda.gov).

The major nutrition-related concerns in older adults include obesity and malnutrition. Approximately 71% of women and 76% of men aged 65 to 74 and 69% of women and 67% of men aged 75 and older have a body mass index (BMI) greater than or equal to 25 and are considered overweight (DiMaria-Ghalili, 2008). "The growing prevalence of obesity (OB) in late life could further exacerbate the seriousness of a number of age-related health concerns, depending on the body weight gain patterns and the health history of the obese individuals. Studies of the mortality/body weight relationship favor maintaining weight in older persons who become OB after age 65, while intervention trials show clinically significant benefits of weight reduction with regard to osteoarthritis, physical function, and possible

---

Box 8-1 — Healthy People 2010 and Nutritional Goals: Key Recommendations for Older Adults

- Consume adequate nutrients within calorie needs.
- Consume a variant of nutrient-dense foods and drinks among the basic food groups, eliminating intake of saturated and trans fats, cholesterol, added sugar, salt, and alcohol.
- Meet energy needs by adopting a balanced eating pattern such as the United States Department of Agriculture (USDA) food guide (www.usda.gov/wps/portal/usdahome) or the Dietary Approaches to Stop Hypertension (DASH) eating plan.
- Consume vitamin B_{12} in crystalline form (fortified foods or supplements).
- Consume extra vitamin D from fortified foods and/or supplements, especially older adults with dark skin or those exposed to insufficient ultraviolet-band radiation.
- Maintain body weight in a healthy range, balancing calories from foods and beverages with calories expended. At a minimum, do moderately intense cardio or aerobic activity 30 minutes/day most days of the week.
- Prevent or delay onset of hypertension. Increase potassium intake; reduce salt intake; eat a healthful diet; and engage in regular physical activity to achieve a healthy weight.
- If hypertensive or African American, aim to consume no more than 1500 mg/day of sodium and meet the potassium recommendation of 4700 mg/day with food.
- To prevent or delay onset of heart disease, eat less fat. Fats that are solid at room temperature are the saturated and trans fats that increase risk of heart disease. Eat fewer than 10% of calories from saturated fats. Wise fat choices include fish, nuts, and vegetable oils.
- If the level of low-density lipoproteins (LDLs), the dangerous lipids, is elevated, decrease saturated fat calories to fewer than 7% of total calories.
- If alcoholic beverages are consumed, take no more than two drinks/day for men and one drink/day for women. Avoid activities that require attention, skill, or coordination such as driving. Note than many medications interact with alcohol.
- Older adults are compromised immunologically. Do not eat or drink raw, unpasteurized milk or any products made from raw milk. Do not eat raw or partially cooked eggs or foods containing raw eggs or raw or undercooked meat and poultry, raw or undercooked fish or shellfish, unpasteurized juices, or raw sprouts.
- Increase or maintain fiber-rich foods to 14 g/1000 calories consumed.

(See also the American Public Health Association [APHA] *Fact Sheet: Healthy lifestyle for older adults:* Washington, DC, 2005, The Association.)

From U.S. Department of Health and Human Services: *Healthy People 2010: national health promotion and disease prevention objectives,* Washington, DC, 2000, The Department.

Modified MyPyramid for Older Adults

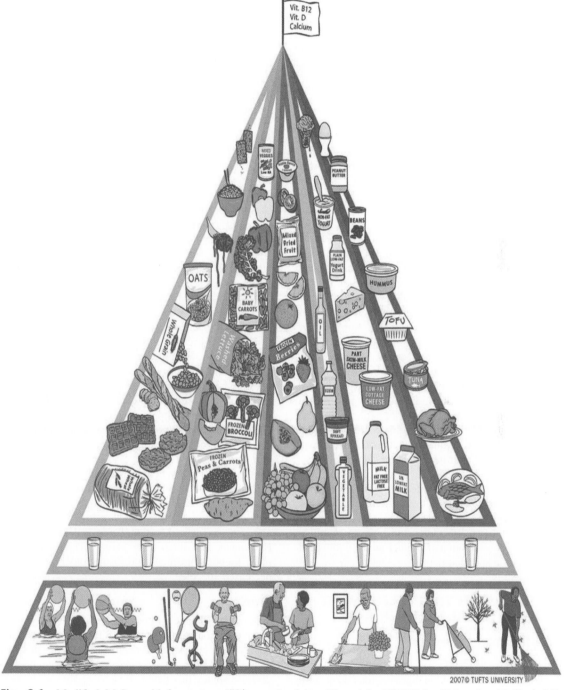

Fig. 8-1 Modified MyPyramid for mature (70$^+$ years) adults. *(Copyright 2007 Tufts University, Medford, MA. See http://nutrition.tufts.edu/docs/pdf/releases/ModifiedMyPyramid.pdf.)*

diabetes mellitus type 2 and coronary heart disease. Given these findings, decisions about whether or not to institute a weight loss intervention for OB older persons must be carefully considered on an individualized basis, with special attention to the weight history and the medical conditions of each individual" (Bales and Buhr, 2008, p. 311). Maintaining a healthy weight throughout life is one of the most important goals for people of all ages.

Malnutrition is a major concern because it is often "unrecognized and impacts morbidity, mortality, and quality of life. Malnutrition is a precursor to frailty in older adults" (DiMaria-Ghalili, 2008, p. 354). It is important to note that obese elders are also at risk for malnutrition, particularly if they lose weight because of the onset of acute or chronic illness (Locher, 2008). Malnutrition is discussed in more depth later in this chapter.

Although some age-related changes in the gastrointestinal system do occur, these changes are rarely the primary factors in inadequate nutrition. Fulfillment of an older person's nutritional needs is more often affected by numerous other factors, including lifelong eating habits, ethnicity, socialization, income, transportation, housing, food knowledge, health, and dentition.

Data from the National Health and Nutrition Examination Survey (NHANES) showed that only 17% of older adults consumed a "good" quality diet, with non-Hispanic white persons having the highest scores on the Healthy Eating Index (HEI) and non-Hispanic black persons the lowest scores. Edentulous persons and those who rated their health as fair or poor generally ate fewer servings of fruit and vegetables, ate a less varied diet, and had a poorer quality diet than persons with teeth or who rated their health higher (Ervin, 2008).

This chapter discusses the dietary needs of older adults, age-related changes affecting nutrition, risk factors contributing to inadequate nutrition, bowel function in aging, dental health concerns, the effect of diseases and functional impairments on nutrition, malnutrition, and special considerations for older adults with cognitive and physical impairments.

FACTORS AFFECTING FULFILLMENT OF NUTRITONAL NEEDS IN AGING

Age-Related Changes

Some age-related changes in the senses of taste and smell (chemosenses) and the digestive tract do occur as an individual ages and may affect nutrition. For most older people, these changes do not seriously interfere with eating, digestion, and the enjoyment of food. However, combined with other factors affecting fulfillment of nutritional needs, they may contribute to inadequate nutrition and decreased eating pleasure.

Taste

The sense of taste has many components and primarily depends on receptor cells in the taste buds. Taste buds are scattered on the surface of the tongue, the cheek, the soft palate, the upper tip of the esophagus, and other parts of the mouth and throat. Components in food stimulate taste buds during chewing and swallowing, and tongue movements enhance flavor sensation. Fine, subtle taste to discriminate between flavors is an olfactory function, whereas crude taste (e.g., sweet and sour) depends on the taste buds. Individuals have varied levels of taste sensitivity that seem predetermined by genetics and constitution, as well as age variations. Early studies suggested that a decline in the number of taste cells occurs with aging, but more recent studies suggest that "taste cells can regenerate but that the lag time of this turnover may account for the diminished taste response in older adults" (Miller, 2008, p. 363).

Age-related changes do not affect all taste sensations equally, and with age, the ability to detect sweet taste seems to remain intact whereas the ability to detect sour, salty, and bitter tastes declines. Many denture wearers say they lose some of their satisfaction in food, possibly because dentures cover the palate and because texture is a very important element in food enjoyment. Difficulty in flavor appreciation comes from individual variables, such as smoking, olfactory sensitivity, attitude toward food and eating, and the presence of moistening secretions. There are also aberrations in flavor sensation caused by certain medications and medical conditions. The addition of flavor enhancers (bouillon cubes) and concentrated flavors (jellies or sauces) can amplify both taste and smell. Fresh herbs and spices also give an extra boost to flavor and may increase enjoyment and interest in eating. The bland diets often found in hospitals and institutions contribute to decreased appetite.

Smell

Age-related changes in the sense of smell and consequent effect on nutrition call for further research. In the past, studies have shown a decline in the sense of smell as the individual ages. Recent research (Markovic et al, 2007) disputes this belief. Results of this study suggested that for perceived odors, olfactory pleasure increases at later stages in the life span and the perceived intensity of odors remains stable. Decrease in the sense of smell may be related to many factors, including the following: nasal sinus disease, repeated injury to olfactory receptors through viral infections, age-related changes in central nervous system functioning, cigarette smoking, medications, and periodontal disease and other dentition problems. Changes in the sense of smell are also associated with Parkinson's disease and Alzheimer's (Cacchione, 2008).

Smell occurs when nerve receptors in the nose send messages to the brain. The oral and nasal senses interact to give us the impression of a certain food, combining to heighten the sensory perceptions we receive. Smells also create emotional responses (positive or negative) to food because emotions and smell sensations overlap in the brain. Think how the smell of freshly baked chocolate chip cookies makes you feel compared with the smell of burned popcorn. Many older people, particularly those in institutions, no longer cook and never have the experience of smelling food as it is cooking, an important appetite stimulant. Many long-term care institutions have adapted kitchens and dining rooms so that the residents can smell the food cooking and even participate in the preparation of food as a way of increasing interest and enjoyment in food.

Digestive System

Age-related changes in the oral cavity, the esophagus, the stomach, the liver, the pancreas, the gallbladder, and the small and large intestines may influence nutritional status in concert with other factors. However, normal age-related changes do not significantly affect function, and the digestive system remains adequate throughout life. Presbyesophagus, a decrease in the intensity of propulsive waves, may be an age-related change in the esophagus. Some of these changes may be more attributable to pathological conditions rather than to age alone. The functional impact of presbyesophagus seems to be minimal, but combined with other conditions, may contribute to dysphagia. Chapter 6 discusses age-related changes in the digestive system.

Regulation of Appetite

Appetite in persons of all ages is influenced by factors such as physical activity, functional limitations, smell, taste, mood, socialization, and comfort. Appetite is regulated by a combination of a peripheral satiation system and a central feeding drive. Gastrointestinal hormones, such as cholecystokinin, also regulate satiety to varying degrees. However, the physiological basis to appetite regulation differs in older adults

compared with younger adults. Although the specifics await further research, changes in neurotransmitter regulators of appetite have been implicated in impaired appetite and decreased intake associated with aging.

Disease states also increase cytokine levels as a result of its release by diseased tissues. Increase in cholecystokinin levels also occurs in malnourished individuals, which may further decrease appetite. There is also some suggestion that alterations in the endogenous opioid feeding and drinking drive may decline in aging, further contributing to decreased appetite and the risk for dehydration (Morley, 2003).

Lifelong Eating Habits

The nutritional state of a person reflects the individual's dietary history and present food practices. Lifelong eating habits are also developed out of tradition, ethnicity, and religion, all of which collectively can be called culture. Food habits established since childhood may influence the intake of older adults.

Eating habits do not always coincide with fulfillment of nutritional needs. Rigidity of food habits may increase with age as familiar food patterns are sought. Ethnicity determines if traditional foods are preserved, whereas religion affects the choice of foods possible. Throughout life, then, preferences for particular foods bring deep satisfaction and possess emotional significance. Such foods are called soul food or comfort food. Preferences for soul food influence food choices and affect nutrient intake. Foods prepared or served in a special way provide "soul" and are not unique to any one group but, rather, are found all over the world. Rice with every meal and homemade chicken soup given to the individual when ill are examples of what people consider their soul food.

Members of a particular ethnic or religious group will have unique eating patterns, so individual assessment is important. Cultural preferences affect nutrition and culturally and religiously appropriate diets should be available in any institution or congregate dining program.

Lifelong habits of dieting or eating fad foods also echo through the later years. Older people may fall prey to advertisements that claim specific foods maintain youth and vitality or rid one of chronic conditions. Recent studies are showing that diet can affect longevity and, combined with lifestyle changes, can reduce disease risk. Everyone can benefit from improved eating habits, and it's never too late to change dietary habits. Consuming more nutrient- and fiber-rich fruits—brightly colored vegetables (fresh or packaged without extra salt or sugar), whole grains, legumes, lean proteins, and healthy types of fats—and less fatty meat, high-fat dairy, and refined, processed foods is beneficial (Aronson, 2008). Following the Modified MyPyramid guidelines (see Figure 8-1) will help lower the risk of chronic disease and provide health-protective nutrition.

Older adults should be counseled to base their dietary decisions on valid research and consultation with their primary care provider. For the healthy older adults, essential nutrients should be obtained from food sources rather relying on dietary supplements.

Socialization

The fundamentally social aspect of eating has to do with sharing and the feeling of belonging that it provides. All of us use food as a means of giving and receiving love, friendship, or belonging. Often, older adults may be isolated from the mainstream of life because of chronic illness, depression, and other functional limitations. When one eats alone, the outcome is often either overindulgence or disinterest in food. The presence of others during meals is a significant predictor of caloric intake (Locher et al, 2008).

Disinterest in food may also result from the effects of medication or disease processes. Misuse and abuse of alcohol are prevalent among older adults and are growing public health concerns. Excessive drinking interferes with nutrition. Drinking alcohol depletes the body of necessary nutrients and often replaces meals, thus making an individual susceptible to malnutrition. Chapter 24 discusses alcohol use.

The elderly nutrition program, authorized under Title III of the Older Americans Act, provides grants to state agencies on aging to support congregate and home-delivered meals to persons age 60 years and older. Most cities and rural areas throughout the United States have such programs. Congregate nutrition programs and home-delivered nutrition services enable older adults to avoid or delay costly institutionalization and allow them to stay in their homes and communities.

Income

There is a strong relationship between poor nutrition and low income. According to the federal government, fewer than 1 in 10 adults age 65 and older is living in poverty. However, elderly poverty rates among blacks are nearly triple, and among Hispanics more than double, those of whites (Burticka, 2008). Older single women are also at

high risk for poverty. Older adults with low incomes may need to choose among fulfilling needs such as food, heat, telephone bills, medications, and health care visits. Some older people eat only once per day in an attempt to make their income last through the month.

Programs such as the food stamp program have the potential for increasing the purchasing power of older adults who qualify, but older adults are less likely than any other age group to use the food stamp program. Of all older Americans living in poverty, approximately one in five receives food stamps (Fuller-Thomson and Redmond, 2008). Many older people may find that the amount of money required to purchase the food stamps is greater than they think they can afford, or they do not see the benefit to them. Transportation may be limited and the distance too great for an older person to travel to grocery stores or to acquire food stamps, which are sold only at designated locations in cities. In addition, many older people, especially those who lived through the depression, are very reluctant to accept "welfare."

Fuller-Thomson and Redmond (2008) suggest the use of focused outreach programs and public education to destigmatize the food stamp program and encourage greater use by older adults in need. Suggestions to improve use of the food stamp program include creating mobile and satellite food stamp offices separate from welfare offices; increasing availability of online application forms; creating more user-friendly applications; home visits by food stamp workers; more extensive multilingual services; and targeting information to older adults receiving Supplemental Security Income (SSI), Medicaid, those who live in public housing, and those whose Social Security payments are below the poverty line.

Free food programs, such as donated commodities, are also available at distribution centers (food banks) for those with limited incomes. Although this is another valuable option for older people, use of such programs is not always feasible. One takes a chance on the types of food available any particular day or week; quantities distributed are frequently too large for the single older person or the older couple to use or even carry from the distribution site; the site may be too far away or difficult to reach; and the time of distribution of the food may be inconvenient.

Cafeterias and restaurants that provide special meal prices for older people have had to increase their prices as food costs have risen. Thus the previous advantages of eating out have diminished. Yet, many single elders eat out for most meals. More and more are eating fast food.

Transportation

Available and easily accessible transportation may be limited for older people. Many small, long-standing neighborhood food stores have been closed in the wake of the expansion of larger supermarkets, which are located in areas that serve a greater segment of the population. It may become difficult to walk to the market, to reach it by public transportation, or to carry a bag of groceries while using a cane or walker. Fear is apparent in elders' consideration of transportation. They may fear walking in the street and being mugged, not being able to cross the street in the time it takes the traffic light to change, or being knocked down or falling as they walk in crowded streets. Despite reduced senior citizen bus fares, many older people remain very fearful of attack when using public transportation. Functional impairments also make the use of public transportation difficult for some older people.

Transportation by taxicab for an individual on a limited income is unrealistic, but sharing a taxicab with others who also need to shop may enable the older person to go where food prices are cheaper and to take advantage of sale items. Senior citizen organizations in many parts of the United States have been helpful in providing older adults with van service to shopping areas. In housing complexes, it may be possible to schedule group trips to the supermarket. Most communities have multiple sources of transportation available, but the older adult may be unaware of them. It is important for nurses to be knowledgeable about resources in the community that are available to older people.

In addition, many older adults, particularly widowed men, may have never learned to shop and prepare food. Often, older adults have to rely on others to shop for them, and this may be a cause of concern depending on availability of support and the reluctance to be dependent on someone else, particularly family. For older adults who own a computer, shopping over the Internet and having groceries delivered offers advantages, although prices may be higher than in the stores. A new option is easy nutritious meals delivered to the home by Fresh From The Kitchen, a company that prepares and delivers meals without additives or preservatives that can be used immediately or stored for future use (www. freshfromthekitchen.net).

Housing

Poor and near-poor older people are likely to reside in substandard housing. Some who live in single rooms lack storage space for food, a means of refrigeration, and a stove for cooking. At certain times of the year, some single-room dwellers use the window ledges and fire escapes to keep perishables cool for several days' use.

Dentition

Dental health of older adults is a basic need that is increasingly neglected with advanced age, debilitation, and limited mobility. Orodental health is integral to general health. Oral health is a leading indicator in *Healthy People 2010* (USDHHS, 2002). Goals related to the oral health of older adults are presented in Box 8-2.

Poor oral health is recognized as a risk factor for dehydration and malnutrition as well as a number of systemic diseases including, aspiration pneumonia, joint infections, cardiovascular disease, and poor glycemic control in type 1 and type 2 diabetes (O'Connor, 2008; Sarin et al, 2008). Poor oral health, which leads to difficulty chewing, missing teeth, teeth in ill repair, and oral pain, contributes to chewing and swallowing problems that affect adequate nutritional intake (Locher et al, 2008).

The percentage of older people without natural teeth is more than 30%, primarily as a result of periodontitis, which occurs in about 95% of those older than 65 years (American Geriatrics Society [AGS], 2006a). Prevalence of this disease is decreasing as

Box 8-2	*Healthy People 2010* Dental Health Goals for Older Adults

- Reduce the proportion of adults with untreated dental decay.
- Increase the proportion of adults who never had a permanent tooth extracted because of dental caries or periodontal disease.
- Reduce the proportion of adults who have had all of their natural teeth extracted.
- Increase the proportion of oral and pharyngeal cancers detected at the earliest stage.
- Increase the proportion of long-term care residents who use the oral health care system each year.

From U.S. Department of Health and Human Services: *Healthy People 2010: national health promotion and disease prevention objectives,* Washington, DC, 2000, The Department.

knowledge increases and more people use fluorides, improve nutrition, engage in new oral hygiene practices, and take advantage of improved dental health care. However, older people may not have had the advantages of new preventive treatment and those with functional and cognitive limitations may be unable to perform oral hygiene. Oral care is often lacking in institutions (Miller, 2008). Decades ago, dental care was extremely painful, and fear of the dentist still exists (Momeyer and Luggen, 2005). Access to dental care for older people may be limited as well as cost-prohibitive.

In the existing health care system, dental care is a low priority, reflected by the absence or inadequacy of third-party reimbursement for the type of dental care needed by older adults. Medicare does not provide any coverage for oral health care services and only 1 in 5 Americans aged 75 years or older has any type of private dental insurance (Editorial, 2006). Elders have fewer dentist visits than any other age group. Older Americans with the poorest oral health are those who are economically disadvantaged, lack insurance, and are members of racial and ethnic minorities. Being disabled, homebound, or institutionalized increases the risk of poor oral health (Centers for Disease Control [CDC], 2006).

Age-related changes in the buccal cavity also predispose older people to orodental problems (Box 8-3). Aging teeth become worn and darker in color and tend to develop longitudinal cracks. The dentin, or the layer beneath the enamel, becomes brittle and thickens so that pulp space decreases (AGS, 2006a). In addition to years of exposure of the teeth and related structures to microbial assault, the oral cavity shows evidence of wear and tear as a result of normal use (chewing and talking) and destructive oral habits such as bruxism (habitual grinding of the teeth). People who are edentulous and are using complete dentures continue to have oral health care needs. Ill-fitting dentures affect chewing and hence nutritional intake. People without teeth remain susceptible to oral cancer and other oral diseases.

Another common oral problem among older adults is dry mouth (xerostomia). Approximately 25% to 40% of older adults experience xerostomia. More than 500 medications have the side effect of reducing salivary flow. A reduction in saliva and a dry mouth make eating, swallowing, and speaking difficult. It can also lead to significant problems of the teeth and their supporting structure (Editorial, 2006). Artificial saliva preparations are available (avoid those containing sorbitol), and adequate fluid intake is also important when xerostomia occurs. Chewing on xylitol-flavored fluoride tablets, sugar-free candies, or sugar-free gum with xylitol 15 minutes after meals may stimulate saliva flow and promote oral hygiene (Miller, 2008). Medication review is also indicated to eliminate, if possible, medications contributing to xerostomia.

Oral cancers occur more frequently in late life; men are affected twice as often as women. Oral cancers occur more frequently in black men, and the incidence of oral cancer varies in different countries. It is much more common in Hungary and France than in the United States and much less common in Mexico and Japan (AGS, 2006b). For all stages combined, the 5-year survival rate is 59% and the 10-year survival rate is 48%. This has not changed significantly in the past 20 years. Oral examinations are important and can assist in early detection and treatment of oral cancers and other orodental problems. Box 8-4 presents common signs and symptoms of oral cancer.

Risk factors for oral cancer are tobacco use, alcohol use, and exposure to ultraviolet light, especially for cancer of the lips. Pipe, cigar, and cigarette smoking are all implicated. Other risk factors are age, sex, local irritation of the tissues, poor nutrition, mouthwash with high alcohol content, human papillomavirus (HPV) infection, and immune suppression from immunosuppressant drugs. Therapy options are based on diagnosis and staging and include surgery, radiation, and chemotherapy.

Box 8-3   Age-Related Changes of the Buccal Cavity

- Decrease in the cellular compartment
- Loss of submucosal elastin in oral mucosa
- Loss of connective tissue (collagen)
- Increase in thickness of collagen fibers
- Decrease in function of minor salivary glands
- Decrease in number and quality of blood vessels and nerves
- Attrition on occlusive contact surfaces
- Enamel less permeable—teeth more brittle
- Tooth color change
- Excessive secondary dentin formation
- Decrease in rate of cementin deposition
- Decrease in size of pulp chamber and root canals
- Decrease in size and volume of the tooth pulp
- Increase in pulp stones and dystrophic mineralization

Box 8-4	Signs and Symptoms of Oral and Throat Cancer

- Swelling or thickening, lumps or bumps, or rough spots or eroded areas on the lips, gums, or other areas inside the mouth
- Velvety white, red, or speckled patches in the mouth
- Persistent sores on the face, neck, or mouth that bleed easily
- Unexplained bleeding in the mouth
- Unexplained numbness or pain or tenderness in any area of the face, mouth, neck, or tongue
- Soreness in the back of the throat; a persistent feeling that something is caught in the throat
- Difficulty chewing or swallowing, speaking, or moving the jaw or tongue
- Hoarseness, chronic sore throat, or changes in the voice
- Dramatic weight loss
- Lump or swelling in the neck
- Severe pain in one ear—with a normal eardrum
- Pain around the teeth; loosening of the teeth
- Swelling or pain in the jaw; difficulty moving the jaw

If detected early, these cancers can almost always be treated successfully.

Hospitalization and Institutional Living

Older adults in hospitals and long-term care settings are more likely to experience a number of the problems that contribute to inadequate nutrition. In the United States, 40% to 60% of hospitalized older adults are malnourished or at risk for malnutrition (DiMaria-Ghalili, 2008). In addition to the risk factors above, severely restricted diets, long periods of nothing-by-mouth (NPO) status, and insufficient time and staff for feeding assistance contribute to inadequate nutrition. Malnutrition is related to prolonged hospital stay, increased risk for poor health status, institutionalization, and mortality (DiMaria-Ghalili, 2008). Assessment of nutritional status to identify malnutrition and the risk factors for malnutrition is important and required by the Joint Commission. Sufficient time, care, and attention should be given to feeding dependent older people. Malnutrition and strategies for increasing intake are discussed later in the chapter.

The incidence of eating disability in long-term care is high with estimates that 50% of all residents cannot eat independently (Burger et al, 2000). Inadequate staffing in long-term care facilities is associated with poor nutrition and hydration, and as Kayser-Jones (1997, p. 19) states: "Certified nursing assistants (CNAs) have an impossible task trying to feed the number of people who need assistance." Having one staff person for every two or three residents who need feeding assistance would allow the resident 20 to 30 minutes with the CNA (Burger et al, 2000). Reports of a research study (Simmons et al, 2001) supported these recommendations. In this study, 50% of residents significantly increased their oral food and fluid intake during mealtime when they received one-on-one feeding assistance. The time required to implement the feeding assistance (38 minutes) greatly exceeded the time nursing staff spent assisting residents in usual mealtime conditions (9 minutes).

In response to concerns about the lack of adequate assistance during mealtime in long-term care facilities, the Centers for Medicare and Medicaid Services (CMS) implemented a rule that allows feeding assistants with 8 hours of approved training to help residents with eating. Feeding assistants must be supervised by a registered nurse (RN) or licensed practical–vocational nurse (LPN-LVN). Family members may also be willing and able to assist at mealtimes and also provide a familiar social context for the patient. Nurses need to provide guidance and support on feeding techniques, supervise eating, and evaluate outcomes.

The use of restrictive therapeutic diets for frail elders in long-term care (low cholesterol, low salt, no concentrated sweets) often reduces food intake without significantly helping the clinical status of the resident (Morley, 2003). If caloric supplements are used, they should be administered at least 1 hour before meals or they interfere with meal intake. These products are widely used and can be costly. Often, they are not dispensed or consumed as ordered. There is a need for research related to their effectiveness (Kayser-Jones, 2006).

Dispensing a small amount of calorically dense oral nutritional supplement (2 calories/ml) during the routine medication pass may have a greater effect on weight gain than a traditional supplement (1.06 calories/ml) with or between meals. Small volumes of nutrient-dense supplement may have less of an effect on appetite and will enhance food intake during meals and snacks. This delivery method allows nurses to observe and document consumption. Results of a recent pilot study investigating the effect of a nutrient-dense supplement given to residents at high nutritional risk during the medication pass reported maintenance or improvement of weight, improved skin integrity, and improved visceral protein status. Further studies and randomized clinical trials are needed to evaluate the effectiveness of nutritional supplementation (Doll-Shankaruk et al, 2008).

Attention to the environment in which meals are served is important. It is not uncommon to hear over the public address system at mealtimes: "Feeder trays are ready." This reference to the need to feed those unable to feed themselves is, in itself, degrading and erases any trace of dignity the older person is trying to maintain in a controlled environment. It is not malicious intent by nurses or other caregivers but rather a habit of convenience. Feeding older people who have difficulty eating can become mechanical and devoid of feeling. The feeding process becomes rapid, and if it bogs down and becomes too slow, the meal may be ended abruptly, depending on the time the caregiver has allotted for feeding the person. Any pleasure derived through socialization and eating and any dignity that could be maintained is often absent (see "An Elder Speaks" at the beginning of this chapter). Older adults accustomed to certain table manners may feel ashamed at their inability to behave in what they feel is an appropriate manner.

In addition to adequate staff, many innovative and evidence-based ideas can improve nutritional intake in institutions. Many suggestions are found in the literature including the following: restorative dining programs, homelike dining rooms, individualized menu choices including ethnic foods, cafeteria style service, kitchens on the nursing units, availability of food around the clock, choice of mealtimes, liberal diets, finger foods, visually appealing pureed foods with texture and shape, music, touch, verbal cueing, hand-over-hand feeding, and sitting while assisting the person to eat. Other suggestions can be found in Box 8-5.

IMPLICATIONS FOR GERONTOLOGICAL NURSING AND HEALTHY AGING

Assessment

Good oral hygiene and assessment of oral health are essentials of nursing care. In addition to identifying oral health problems, examination of the mouth can serve as an early warning system for some diseases and lead to early diagnosis and treatment. All persons, especially those over 50 years of age, with or without dentures, should have oral examinations on a regular basis. Federal regulations mandate an annual

Box 8-5	Suggestions to Improve Intake

- Serve meals with the person in a chair rather than in bed when possible.
- Provide analgesics and antiemetics on a schedule that provides comfort at mealtime.
- Determine food preferences; include culturally appropriate food.
- Make food available 24 hours/day—provide snacks between meals and at night.
- Do not interrupt meals to administer medication if possible.
- Walk around the dining area or the rooms at mealtime to determine if food is being eaten or if assistance is needed.
- Encourage family members to share the mealtimes for a heightened social situation.
- If caloric supplements are used, offer between meals or with the medication pass.
- Recommend an exercise program that may increase appetite.
- Ensure proper fit of dentures and denture use.
- Provide oral hygiene and allow the person to wash his or her hands.
- Have the person wear his or her glasses during meals.
- Sit while feeding the person who needs assistance, use touch, and carry on a social conversation.
- Provide soft music during the meal.
- Use small, round tables seating six to eight people. Consider using tablecloths and centerpieces.
- Seat people with like interests and abilities together and encourage socialization.
- Use restorative dining programs and the use of adaptive equipment.
- Make diets as liberal as possible depending on health status, especially for frail elders who are not consuming adequate amounts.
- Consider a referral to a speech-language pathologist for persons experiencing difficulties with eating and/or an occupational therapist for adaptive equipment.

examination for residents of long-term care facilities. Although the oral examination is best performed by a dentist, nurses can provide basic screening examinations to persons using an instrument such as The Kayser-Jones Brief Oral Health Status Examination (BOHSE) (Figure 8-2), available at www.hartfordign. org. Gil-Montoya et al (2006) developed an oral clinical history appropriate for residents of long-term care institutions (Figure 8-3).

Interventions

Prescribed oral hygiene for the individual with some or all teeth is to brush, floss, and use a fluoride dentifrice and mouthwash daily. It is best if individuals can brush their teeth after each meal. There is evidence that cleaning the person's teeth with a toothbrush after meals

lowers the risk of developing aspiration pneumonia (Metheny, 2007).

Impaired manual dexterity may make it difficult for elders to adequately maintain their dental routine and remove plaque adequately. The hand grip of manual toothbrushes is too small to grasp and manipulate easily. Using a child's toothbrush or enlarging the handle of an adult-sized toothbrush by adding a foam grip or wrapping it with gauze to increase handle size has been effective in facilitating grasp. The ultrasonic toothbrush is an effective tool for elders or for those who must brush the teeth of elders to use. The base is large enough for easy grasp, and the ultrasonic movement of the bristles in concert with the usual brushing movement is very effective in plaque removal. Use of a commercial floss handle may provide the leverage and ease necessary for the person to continue flossing. Occupational therapists can be helpful

KAYSER-JONES BRIEF ORAL HEALTH STATUS EXAMINATION

Resident's Name _____

Examiner's Name _____

Date _____

TOTAL SCORE _____

CATEGORY	MEASUREMENT	0	1	2
LYMPH NODES	Observe and feel nodes	No enlargement	Enlarged, not tender	Enlarged and tender*
LIPS	Observe, feel tissue, and ask resident, family or staff (e.g., primary caregiver)	Smooth, pink, moist	Dry, chapped, or red at corners*	White or red patch, bleeding or ulcer for 2 weeks*
TONGUE	Observe, feel tissue, and ask resident, family, or staff (e.g., primary caregiver)	Normal roughness, pink and moist	Coated, smooth, patchy, severely fissured or some redness	Red, smooth, white or red patch; ulcer for 2 weeks*
TISSUE INSIDE CHEEK, FLOOR, AND ROOF OF MOUTH	Observe, feel tissue, and ask resident, family, or staff (e.g., primary caregiver)	Pink and moist	Dry, shiny, rough, red, or swollen*	White or red patch, bleeding, hardness; ulcer for 2 weeks*
GUMS BETWEEN TEETH AND/OR UNDER ARTIFICIAL TEETH	Gently press gums with tip of tongue blade	Pink, small indentations; firm, smooth, and pink under artificial teeth	Redness at border around 1-6 teeth; one red area or sore spot under artificial teeth*	Swollen or bleeding gums, redness at border around 7 or more teeth, loose teeth; generalized redness or sores under artificial teeth*
SALIVA (EFFECT ON TISSUE)	Touch tongue blade to center of tongue and floor of mouth	Tissues moist, saliva free flowing and watery	Tissues dry and sticky	Tissues parched and red, no saliva*
CONDITION OF NATURAL TEETH	Observe and count number of decayed or broken teeth	No decayed or broken teeth/roots	1-3 decayed or broken teeth/roots*	4 or more decayed or broken teeth/roots; fewer than 4 teeth in either jaw*
CONDITION OF ARTIFICIAL TEETH	Observe and ask patient, family, or staff (e.g., primary caregiver)	Unbroken teeth, worn most of the time	1 broken/missing tooth, or worn for eating or cosmetics only	More than 1 broken or missing tooth, or either denture missing or never worn*
PAIRS OF TEETH IN CHEWING POSITION (NATURAL OR ARTIFICIAL)	Observe and count pairs of teeth in chewing position	12 or more pairs of teeth in chewing position	8-11 pairs of teeth in chewing position	0-7 pairs of teeth in chewing position*
ORAL CLEANLINESS	Observe appearance of teeth or dentures	Clean, no food particles/tartar in the mouth or on artificial teeth	Food particles/tartar in one or two places in the mouth or on artificial teeth	Food particles/tartar in most places in the mouth or on artificial teeth

Upper dentures labeled: Yes_____ No _____ None _____ Lower dentures labeled: Yes_____ No _____ None _____   Italic*—refer to dentist immediately

Is your mouth comfortable? Yes_____ No _____ If no, explain: _____

Additional comments:_____

Fig. 8-2 Kayser-Jones Brief Oral Health Status Examination. *(With permission of Jeanie Kayser-Jones, RN, PhD, School of Nursing, University of California, San Francisco.)*

Oral Clinical History	
Date of examination:	
Name:	
Room No:	
1. Does he/she have any natural teeth? ( ) No ( ) Yes, Upper ( ) Yes, Lower	
2. Does he/she use removable dental prosthesis? ( ) No ( ) Yes, Upper ( ) Yes, Lower	
3. Are his/her gums inflamed (reddened or bleeding)? ( ) No ( ) Yes	
4. Does he/she have bacterial plaque or tartar on teeth or prosthesis? ( ) No ( ) Medium amount ( ) A lot	
5. Does his/her mouth slow signs of dryness? ( ) No ( ) Yes	
6. He/she carries out hygiene ( ) on his/her own ( ) with some help ( ) someone has to do it for him/her	
7. ( ) Immediate dental care by the dental service is required.	Reason

Recommendations for care of teeth and prostheses

	Encourage/supervise tooth and/or prosthesis brushing
	Remove prostheses at bedtime
	Clean teeth with electric toothbrush
	Clean prostheses with electric toothbrush
	Clean oral mucosa with gauze - 0.12% CLX
	Rinse with 0.12% Chlorhexidine solution
	Moisten/coat lips with vaseline or lip balm
	Transfer for immediate dental care

Dates	Incidences

Fig. 8-3   Oral history. *(From Gil-Montoya JA, de Mello AL, Cardenas CB, Lopez IG: Oral health protocol for the dependent institutionalized elderly,* Geriatr Nurs, *27(2):95-101,2006, p. 98.)*

in assessment of functional impairments and provision of adaptive equipment for oral care.

Foam swabs are available to provide oral hygiene but do not remove plaque as well as toothbrushes. Foam swabs may be used to clean the oral mucosa of an edentulous older adult. Lemon glycerin swabs should never be used for older people. In combination with decreased salivary flow and xerostomia, they dry the oral mucosa and erode the tooth enamel (O'Connor, 2008).

Therapeutic rinses contain an agent that is beneficial to the surface of the teeth and the oral environment. Some therapeutic rinses require a prescription, such as Peridex (chlorhexidine), which contains alcohol but is also a broad-spectrum antimicrobial agent that helps control plaque. The commercial product, Listerine, is an over-the-counter product that carries the American Dental Association approval, but it should not be used by persons taking Antabuse, or who have severe oral mucositis, because it contains a high quantity by volume of alcohol (26.9%). Listerine and generic equivalents that contain alcohol may be mixed with water but should always be used in conjunction with, not instead of brushing.

Infected teeth and poor oral hygiene are associated with pneumonia following aspiration of contaminated oral secretions. Research results indicate that tube feeding in older adults is associated with significant pathologic colonization of the mouth, greater than that observed in people who received oral feeding. Oral care should be provided every 4 hours for patients with gastrostomy tubes, and teeth should be brushed with a toothbrush after each meal to decrease the risk of aspiration pneumonia (Metheny et al, 2008; O'Connor, 2008). The oral mucosa of unconscious or severely cognitively impaired patients should be hydrated using gauze soaked in physiological saline, and lips should be coated with petroleum jelly or lip balm (Gil-Montoya et al, 2006).

When the person is unable to carry out his or her dental/oral regimen, it is the responsibility of the caregiver to provide oral care (Box 8-6). Oral care is an often neglected part of daily nursing care. Poor oral health and lack of attention to oral hygiene are major concerns in institutional settings and contribute significantly to poor nutrition and other negative outcomes such as aspiration pneumonia. Many reasons exist for this deficit including inadequate knowledge of how to assess and provide care, difficulty providing oral care to dependent and cognitively impaired elders, inadequate training and staffing, and lack of appropriate supplies.

Many long-term care institutions have implemented programs such as special training of aides for dental care teams, providing visits from mobile dentistry units on a routine basis, or using dental students to perform oral screening and cleaning of teeth. "Implementation of evidence-based protocols combined with educational training sessions have been shown to have a positive impact on oral care being provided and on the oral health status of older adults" (O'Connor, 2008, p. 394). The use of electric toothbrushes and products such as chlorhexidine, fluoride toothpaste, and rinses or gels for dry mouth are most effective. An oral hygiene protocol can be found at www.consultgerirn.org. Gil-Montoya et al (2006) also provide an oral health protocol for institutionalized elders.

Many elders believe that once they have dentures, there is no longer a need for oral care. Older adults with dentures should be taught the proper home care of their dentures and oral tissue to prevent odor, stain, plaque buildup, and oral infections. Care should include removal of debris under dentures to prevent pressure on and shrinkage of underlying support structures. Dentures and other dental appliances, such as bridges, should be rinsed after each meal and brushed thoroughly once a day, preferably at night (Box 8-7). Dentures should be worn constantly except at night (to allow relief of the compression on the gums) and replaced in the mouth in the morning.

Dentures are very personal and expensive possessions. In communal living situations of nursing homes, hospitals, and other care centers, dentures have often been misplaced or mixed up with those of others. The utmost care should be taken when handling, cleaning, and storing dentures. Dentures should be marked, and many states require all newly made dentures to contain the client's identification. A commercial denture marking system called Identure, produced by the 3M Company, provides a simple, efficient, and permanent means of marking dentures.

Box 8-6   Dental Care: Instructions for Caregivers

1. If the patient is in bed, elevate his or her head by raising the bed or propping it with pillows, and have the patient turn his or her head to face you. Place a clean towel across the chest and under the chin, and place a basin under the chin.
2. If the patient is sitting in a stationary chair or wheelchair, stand behind the patient and stabilize his or her head by placing one hand under the chin and resting the head against your body. Place a towel across the chest and over the shoulders. (It may be helpful to secure it with a safety pin.) The basin can be kept handy in the patient's lap or on a table placed in front of or at the side of the patient. A wheelchair may be positioned in front of the sink.
3. If the patient's lips are dry or cracked, apply a light coating of petroleum jelly or use lip balm.
4. Brush and floss the patient's teeth as you have been instructed (use an electric toothbrush if possible, with sulcular brushing). It may be helpful to retract the patient's lips and cheek with a tongue blade or fingers in order to see the area that is being cleaned. Use a mouth prop as needed if the patient cannot hold his or her mouth open. If manual flossing is too difficult, use a floss holder or interproximal brush to clean the proximal surfaces between the teeth. Use a dentifrice-containing fluoride.
5. Provide the conscious patient with fluoride rinses or other rinses as indicated by the dentist or hygienist.

Box 8-7   **Instructions for Denture Cleaning**

1. Rinse your denture or dentures after each meal to remove soft debris.
2. Once each day, preferably before retiring, remove your denture and brush it thoroughly.
   a. Although an ordinary soft toothbrush is adequate, a specially designed denture brush may clean more effectively. (CAUTION: Acrylic denture material is softer than natural teeth and may be damaged by being brushed with very firm bristles.)
   b. Brush your denture over a sink lined with a facecloth and half-filled with water. This will prevent breakage if the denture is dropped.
   c. Hold the denture securely in one hand, but do not squeeze. Hold the brush in the other hand. It is not essential to use a denture paste, particularly if dentures are soaked before being brushed to soften debris. Never use a commercial tooth powder, because it is abrasive and may damage the denture materials. Plain water, mild soap, or sodium bicarbonate may be used.
   d. When cleaning a removable partial denture, great care must be taken to remove plaque from the curved metal clasps that hook around the teeth. This can be done with a regular toothbrush or with a specially designed clasp brush.
3. After brushing, rinse your denture thoroughly; then place it in a denture-cleaning solution and allow it to soak overnight or for at least a few hours. (NOTE: Acrylic denture material must be kept wet at all times to prevent cracking or warping.) In the morning, remove your denture from the cleaning solution, rinse it thoroughly, and then insert it into your mouth. Use denture paste if necessary to secure dentures.

Broken or damaged dentures and dentures that no longer fit because of weight loss are a common problem for older adults. Rebasing of dentures is a technique to improve the fit of dentures. Ill-fitting dentures or dentures that are not cleaned contribute to oral problems as well as to poor nutrition and reduced enjoyment of food. Daily removal and cleaning of dentures and brushing of teeth should be a part of the care routines in institutions.

Both nursing students and nursing staff need to be knowledgeable about oral hygiene and techniques to care for teeth and dentures. Oral hygiene protocols and appropriate oral care equipment should be available in institutions. Patients and families also need education on the importance of good oral health in older adults and techniques for providing adequate oral care.

HEALTH CONDITIONS AFFECTING NUTRITION

Chronic Diseases and Conditions

Many chronic diseases and their sequelae pose nutritional challenges to older adults including osteoporosis, gastrointestinal disorders, obesity, diabetes, cardiovascular and respiratory diseases, cancer, dysphagia, and dementia. Functional impairments associated with chronic disease interfere with the person's ability to shop, cook, and eat independently.

For example, heart failure and chronic obstructive pulmonary disease (COPD) are associated with fatigue,

increased energy expenditure, and decreased appetite. Alzheimer's disease and other dementias affect adequate nutritional intake, and in late dementia, weight loss becomes a considerable concern. Depression can cause changes in appetite (weight loss or weight gain) and the side effects of antidepressant medications affect appetite and nutrition (see Chapters 14 and 24). Dysphagia, often a result of stroke and dementia, significantly affects nutrition. A number of prevalent disorders of the gastrointestinal (GI) tract are associated with nutritional concerns including gastroesophageal reflux disease (GERD), ulcers, constipation, diverticulosis, and colon cancer.

The following section discusses nutritional concerns and nursing interventions related to dementia, dysphagia, constipation, and fecal impaction. For more detailed information on health conditions and chronic diseases in older persons, see Chapters 15, 17, 18, 20 and 21, as well as a comprehensive geriatric medicine text. More detailed information on chronic illness and nutrition can be found in a nutrition text.

Dementia

Dementia affects adequate nutritional intake, and in late dementia, weight loss becomes a considerable concern. The loss of weight may be the result of physiological changes, cognitive deficits, lack of awareness of the need to eat, depression, increased energy output caused by pacing or wandering, increased incidence of infections, and/or loss of independence for self-feeding (McCance and Huether, 2006).

One of the best strategies for managing poor intake is establishing a routine so the elder does not have to remember times and places for eating. Caregivers should continue to serve well-balanced foods and fluids that the person likes and has always eaten (Kempler, 2005). Nutrient-dense foods are preferred. Attention to mealtime ambience is important, and the person should be able to take as much time as needed to eat the food. Food should be available 24 hours a day and the person should be allowed to follow his or her accustomed eating schedule (e.g., late breakfast, early dinner). Remove any items that should not be eaten and hot items that might be spilled. Finger foods may be a good choice because utensils may be too difficult to manage. Serving one dish and using only one utensil at a time may assist in promoting adequate intake. Demonstrate eating motions that the person can imitate; use hand-over-hand feeding technique to guide self-feeding, use verbal cueing and prompting (e.g., take a bite, chew, swallow). Offer small amounts of fluid between bites of food and throughout the day. Refreshment stations with easy access to juices, water, and healthy snacks also promote adequate intake. Amella and Lawrence (2007) provide a protocol: *Eating and Feeding Issues in Older Adults with Dementia.* Chapter 21 provides more discussion of dementia.

Dysphagia

Dysphagia may occur as a result of neurologic diseases such as stroke, Parkinson's disease, multiple sclerosis, and dementia. Dysphagia is a serious problem and has negative consequences including weight loss, malnutrition, dehydration, and aspiration (Leibovitz et al, 2007). Dysphagia carries a sevenfold increased risk of aspiration pneumonia and is an independent predictor of mortality (Metheny et al, 2008). In the older adult, dysphagia is superimposed on the slowed swallowing rate associated with normal aging, creating an even greater risk of complications.

The exact prevalence of dysphagia is unknown, but studies indicate that it may be present in approximately 14% of individuals over 60 years of age. In patients who have experienced a stroke, the prevalence of dysphagia ranges from 25% to 70%. Dysphagia is present in 25% to 30% of adults admitted to acute trauma centers; 41% of individuals admitted to rehabilitation centers, and 30% to 75% of patients in nursing homes (American Speech and Hearing Association, 2008).

Dysphagia can be classified as oropharyngeal or esophageal. Oropharyngeal dysphagia refers to difficulty in the passage from the mouth to the esophagus.

In esophageal dysphagia, there is disordered passage of food through the esophagus. The two types can be distinguished based on medical history, specific signs and symptoms during a physical examination, and diagnostic tests. Oropharyngeal dysphagia is the more common type, and stroke is its most common cause. Esophageal dysphagia is most often due to actual blockages within the esophagus that are referred to as structural disorders (e.g., esophageal cancer, strictures) (American Speech and Hearing Association, 2008).

IMPLICATIONS FOR GERONTOLOGICAL NURSING AND HEALTHY AGING

Assessment

It is important to obtain a careful history of the elder's response to dysphagia and to observe the person during mealtime. Symptoms that alert the nurse to possible swallowing problems and aspiration are presented in Box 8-8.

Interventions

Aspiration is the most profound and dangerous problem for older adults experiencing dysphagia. Aspiration during swallowing is best detected by procedures such

---

Box 8-8   Symptoms of Dysphagia or Possible Aspiration

- Difficult, labored swallowing
- Drooling
- Copious oral secretions
- Coughing, choking at meals
- Holding or pocketing of food in the mouth
- Difficulty moving food or liquid from mouth to throat
- Difficulty chewing
- Nasal voice or hoarseness
- Wet or gurgling voice
- Excessive throat clearing
- Sensation of something stuck in the throat during swallowing; sensation of a lump in the throat
- Reflux of food or liquid into the throat, mouth, or nose
- Heartburn
- Chest pain
- Hiccups
- Weight loss
- Frequent respiratory infections, pneumonia

as video-fluoroscopy or fiberoptic endoscopy, but clinical observations and evaluation by a speech-language pathologist are important as well. Aspiration pneumonia is under-diagnosed in older adults, and signs and symptoms manifest themselves differently in this age group. Small-volume aspirations that produce few overt symptoms are common and often not discovered until the condition progresses to aspiration pneumonia (Metheny et al, 2008). An elevated respiratory rate and alterations in mental status may be early symptoms of aspiration pneumonia.

It is important to have suctioning equipment available at bedside or in the dining room in institutional settings. In the home setting, if the person is having trouble breathing, is choking, or has stopped breathing, it is important to call for emergency help immediately. Perform first-aid and cardiopulmonary resuscitation (CPR) if necessary. People with dysphagia should have supervision at mealtimes, and observation for aspiration pneumonia should be on-going in high-risk persons.

The gerontological nurse must work closely with other members of the interdisciplinary team, such as speech-language pathologists, in implementing suggested interventions to prevent aspiration. Research on the appropriate management of swallowing disorders in older people, particularly during acute illness and in long-term care facilities, is very limited, and additional study is essential. A comprehensive protocol for preventing aspiration in older adults with dysphagia is available from www.hartfordign.org (Metheny, 2007). A video presentation of assessment of dysphagia can be found at www.nursingcenter.com/prodev/ce_article. asp?tid=771463. Suggested interventions helpful in preventing aspiration during hand feeding are presented in Box 8-9.

Constipation

Bowel function of the older adult, although normally only slightly altered by physiological changes of age, can be a source of concern and a potentially serious problem, especially for the older person who is functionally impaired. Normal elimination should be an easy passage of feces, without undue straining or a feeling of incomplete evacuation or defecation. The urge to defecate occurs when the distended walls of the sigmoid and the rectum, which are filled with feces, stimulate pressure receptors to relax the sphincters for the expulsion of feces through the anus. Evacuation of feces is accomplished by relaxation of the sphincters and contraction of the diaphragm and abdominal muscles, which raises the intraabdominal pressure.

Box 8-9 | **Interventions to Prevent Aspiration in Patients with Dysphagia: Hand Feeding**

- Provide a 30-minute rest period before feeding; a rested person will likely have less difficulty swallowing.
- The person should sit at 90 degrees during all oral (PO) intake.
- Maintain 90-degree positioning for at least 1 hour after PO intake.
- Adjust rate of feeding and size of bites to the person's tolerance; avoid rushed or forced feeding.
- Alternate solid and liquid boluses.
- Follow speech therapist's recommendation for safe swallowing techniques and modified food consistency (may need thickened liquids, puree foods).
- If facial weakness is present, place food on the nonimpaired side of the mouth.
- Avoid sedatives and hypnotics that may impair cough reflex and swallowing ability.
- Keep suction equipment ready at all times.
- Supervise all meals.
- Monitor temperature.
- Observe color of phlegm.
- Visually check the mouth for pocketing of food in cheeks.
- Provide mouth care every 4 hours.

Adapted from: Metheny N, Boltz M, Greenberg S: Preventing aspiration in older adults with dysphagia, *Am J Nurs* 108(2):45-46, 2008.

Constipation is the most common GI complaint made to the health care provider, with about 60% of community-based elders and 74% of older adults in long-term care reporting daily laxative use (Beers and Berkow, 2000). The annual estimated expenditure for laxatives in the general population of the United States is $800 million annually. This figure is probably low since many people use over-the-counter medications before they seek out prescription medications. Annual direct costs attributable to chronic constipation is estimated in the billions of dollars (Cash, 2005). The extensive use of laxatives among older adults in the United States can be considered a cultural habit. During earlier times, weekly doses of rhubarb, cascara, castor oil, and other types of laxatives were consumed and believed by many to promote health. The belief that cleaning out the colon and having a daily bowel movement is paramount to maintaining good health still persists in some groups.

Constipation is a symptom. It is a reflection of poor habits, postponed passage of stool, and many chronic illnesses—both physical and psychological—as well as a common side effect of medication. Constipation can also signal more serious underlying problems such as colonic dysmotility or mass lesions. Diet and activity level play a significant role in constipation. Numerous precipitating factors or condition can cause or worsen constipation (Box 8-10).

Fecal Impaction. Fecal impaction is a major complication of constipation. It is especially common in incapacitated and institutionalized older people. Symptoms of fecal impaction include malaise, urinary retention, elevated temperature, incontinence of bladder or bowel, alterations in cognitive status, fissures, hemorrhoids, and intestinal obstruction. Unrecognized, unattended, or neglected constipation eventually leads to fecal impaction. Leakage of liquid stool from around the impaction is frequently seen, and if there is oozing liquid stool, the person should have a rectal examination to assess for impaction. Continued obstruction by a fecal mass may eventually impair sensation, leading

to the need for larger stool volume to stimulate the urge to defecate, which contributes to megacolon (Edwards, 2002). Valsalva's maneuvers done during straining at stool defecation can cause transient ischemic attacks and syncope, especially in the frail elderly.

Removal of a fecal impaction is at times worse than the misery of the condition. Management of fecal impaction requires the digital removal of the hard, compacted stool from the rectum with use of lubrication containing lidocaine jelly. Generally this is preceded by an oil-retention enema to soften the feces in preparation for manual removal. Use of suppositories is not effective, because their action is blocked by the amount and size of the stool in the rectum. Suppositories do not facilitate the removal of stool in the sigmoid, which may continue to ooze once the rectum is emptied.

Several sessions or days may be necessary to totally cleanse the sigmoid colon and rectum of impacted feces. Once this is achieved, attention should be directed to planning a regimen that includes adequate fluid intake, increased dietary fiber, administration of stool softeners if needed, and many of the suggestions presented for

---

Box 8-10   Precipitating Factors for Constipation

Physiological
Dehydration
Insufficient fiber intake
Poor dietary habits

Functional
Decreased physical activity
Inadequate toileting
Irregular defecation habits
Irritable bowel disease
Weakness

Mechanical
Abscess or ulcer
Fissures
Hemorrhoids
Megacolon
Pelvic floor dysfunction
Postsurgical obstruction
Prostate enlargement
Rectal prolapse
Rectocele
Spinal cord injury

Strictures
Tumors

Other
Lack of abdominal muscle tone
Obesity
Recent environmental changes
Poor dentition

Psychological
Avoidance of urge to defecate
Confusion
Depression
Emotional stress

Systemic
Diabetic neuropathy
Hypercalcemia
Hyperparathyroidism
Hypothyroidism
Hypokalemia
Porphyria
Uremia

Parkinson's disease
Cerebrovascular disease
Defective electrolyte transfer

Pharmacological
ACE-inhibitors
Antacids: calcium carbonate, aluminum hydroxide
Antiarrhythmics
Anticholinergics
Anticonvulsants
Antidepressants
Anti-Parkinson's medications
Calcium channel blockers
Calcium supplements
Diuretics
Iron supplements
Laxative overuse
Nonsteroidal antiinflammatories
Opiates
Phenothiazines
Sedatives
Sympathomimetics

ACE, Angiotensin-converting enzyme.

Adapted from Allison OC, Porter ME, Briggs GC: Chronic constipation: assessment and management in the elderly, *J Am Acad Nurse Pract* 6(7):311, 1994; Tabloski PA: *Gerontological nursing,* Upper Saddle River, NJ, 2006, Pearson/Prentice Hall.

prevention of constipation. For patients who are hospitalized or residing in long-term care settings, accurate bowel records are essential; unfortunately, they are often overlooked or inaccurately completed. Education about the importance of bowel function and the accurate reporting of size, consistency, and frequency of bowel movements, should be provided to all direct care providers. This is especially important for frail or cognitively impaired elders to prevent fecal impaction, a serious and often dangerous condition for older people.

IMPLICATIONS FOR GERONTOLOGICAL NURSING AND HEALTHY AGING

Assessment

The precipitants and causes of constipation must be included in the evaluation of the patient. A review of these factors will also determine if the patient is at risk for altered bowel function. Older people at high risk for constipation and subsequent fecal impaction are those who have hypotonic colon function, who are immobilized and debilitated, or who have central nervous system lesions. It is important to note that alterations in cognitive status, incontinence, increased temperature, poor appetite, or unexplained falls may be the only clinical symptoms of constipation in the cognitively impaired or frail older person.

Recognizing constipation can be a challenge because there may be a significant disconnect between patient definitions of constipation and those of clinicians. Constipation has different meanings to different people. Assessment begins with clarification of what the patient means by constipation. A bowel history is also important to obtain, including usual patterns, frequency of bowel movements, size, consistency, and any changes. Many clinicians think of constipation as bowel movement infrequency but according to several large epidemiological studies, patients with chronic constipation are more likely to report straining, a sense of incomplete or ineffective defecation, and hard or lumpy stools as the most bothersome symptoms of constipation (Cash, 2005).

The Rome III criteria for defining chronic functional constipation in adults can be used to guide the evaluation and treatment of constipation (Box 8-11). The Bristol Stool Form Scale can also be used to provide a visual depiction of stool appearance (Lewis and Heaton, 1997).

A physical examination is needed to rule out systemic causes of constipation such as neurological, endocrine, or metabolic disorders. Symptoms that may suggest the presence of an underlying GI disorder are abdominal pain, nausea, cramping, vomiting, weight loss, melena, rectal bleeding, rectal pain, and fever. A review of food and fluid intake may be necessary to determine the amount of fiber and fluid ingested. Questions should be asked about the level of physical activity and the use of medications. A psychosocial history with attention to depression, anxiety, and stress management is also indicated.

The abdomen is examined for masses, distention, tenderness, and high-pitched or absent bowel sounds. A rectal examination is important to reveal painful anal

---

Box 8-11	Rome III Criteria for Defining Chronic Functional Constipation in Adults

Chronic constipation is defined by symptoms that have persisted for the last 3 months with an onset at least 6 months before diagnosis. All three of the following criteria must be met:
- At least two of the following:
  –Hard or lumpy stool in ≥25% of defecations
  –Straining during ≥25% of defecations
  –Sensation of incomplete evacuation in ≥25% of defecations
  –Sensation of anorectal obstruction or blockage for ≥ of defecations
  –Manual maneuvers (e.g. digital evacuation or pelvic floor support to facilitate ≥25% of defecations
  –Fewer than three defecations per week
- Loose stools rarely present without the use of laxatives. However, it is important to check for impaction if loose stools are present.
- Insufficient criteria for irritable bowel syndrome (IBS)

Adapted from: Cash B: Chronic constipation—defining the problem and clinical impact, *Medscape Gerontol* 7(1), 2005, Available at www.medscape.com/viewarticle/501467_print; Longstreth GF, Thompson WG, Chey WD et al: Functional bowel disorders, *Gastroenterology* 130(5):1480-1491, 2006.

disorders, such as hemorrhoids or fissures, that will impede the evacuation of stool and to evaluate sphincter tone, rectal prolapse, stool presence in the vault, strictures, masses, anal reflex, and enlarged prostate. Biochemical tests should include a complete blood count, fasting glucose, chemistry panel, and thyroid studies. Other diagnostic studies such as flexible sigmoidoscopy, colonoscopy, computed tomography (CT) scan of the abdomen or abdominal x-ray study may also be indicated. Colonic transit and anorectal function can be evaluated. Other tests are available for chronic constipation including the use of radiopaque markers, defecating proctography, and anorectal manometry (Beers and Berkow, 2000).

Interventions

The first intervention is to examine the medications the person is taking and eliminate those that are constipation-producing, preferably changing to medications that do not carry that side effect. Medications are the leading cause of constipation, and almost any drug can cause it. Drugs that affect the central nervous system, nerve conduction, and smooth muscle function are associated with the highest frequency of constipation. Anticholinergics, pain opiates, and many psychoactive medications can be especially problematic.

Nonpharmacological interventions for constipation that have been implemented and evaluated can be grouped into four areas: (1) fluid- and fiber-related, (2) exercise, (3) environmental manipulation, and (4) a combination of these. Adequate hydration is the cornerstone of constipation therapy with fluids coming mainly from water (Beers and Berkow, 2000).

A low-fiber diet and insufficient fluid intake contribute to constipation. Fiber is an important dietary component that many older people do not consume in sufficient quantities. Fiber, the indigestible material that gives plants their structure, is abundant in raw fruits and vegetables and unrefined grains and cereals. Fiber facilitates the absorption of water, increases bulk, and improves intestinal motility. Fiber helps to prevent or reduce the incidence of constipation by increasing the weight of the stool and shortening the transit time.

Individuals who can chew foods well could benefit from eating increased amounts of fresh fruits and vegetables daily or combining unsweetened bran with other types of food. Those who have difficulty chewing can sprinkle bran on cereals or in soups, meat loaf, or casseroles. The quantity of bran depends on the individual, but generally 1 to 2 tablespoons daily

is sufficient. Individuals who have not used bran should begin with 1 teaspoon and progressively increase until the quantity of fiber intake is enough to accomplish its purpose. If bran is used in larger amounts to start, bloating, gas, diarrhea, and other colon discomforts will initially occur and discourage further use of this important dietary ingredient. Adequate fluid intake is also important. If megacolon or colonic dilation from bowel obstruction is suspected, fiber supplements are not advised; most of these patients are placed on fiber-restricted diets.

Exercise

Exercise is important as an intervention to stimulate colon motility and bowel evacuation. Daily walking for 20 to 30 minutes is helpful, especially after a meal. Pelvic tilt exercises, and range of motion (passive or active) exercises are beneficial for those who are less mobile or who are bedridden.

Positioning

The squatting or sitting position, if the patient is able to assume it, facilitates bowel function. A similar position may be obtained by leaning forward and applying firm pressure to the lower abdomen or placing the feet on a stool. Massaging the abdomen may help stimulate the bowel.

Regularity

Establishing a routine for toileting promotes or normalizes bowel function (bowel retraining). The gastrocolic reflex occurs after breakfast or supper and may be enhanced by a warm drink. Given privacy and ample time (a minimum of 10 minutes), many will have a daily bowel movement. However, any urge to defecate should be followed by a trip to the bathroom. Older people dependent on others to meet toileting needs should be assisted to maintain normal routines and provided opportunities for routine toilet use. Additional information on bowel management programs can be found in Chapter 9.

Laxatives

When changes in diet and lifestyle are not effective, the use of laxatives is considered. Older persons receiving opiates need to have a constipation-prevention program in place, because these drugs delay gastric emptying and decrease peristalsis. Correction of constipation associated with opiate use calls for a senna or osmotic laxative to overcome the strong opioid effect. Stool softeners and bulking agents alone are inadequate.

Commonly used laxatives used in chronic constipation include the following:

▶ Bulking agents (e.g., psyllium, methylcellulose)
▶ Stool softeners (e.g., docusate sodium)
▶ Osmotic laxatives (e.g., lactulose, sorbitol)
▶ Stimulant laxatives (e.g., senna, bisacodyl)
▶ Saline laxatives (e.g., Milk of Magnesia)

Bulk laxatives are often the first prescribed because of their safety. Bulk laxatives absorb water from the intestinal lumen and increase stool mass. Adequate fluid intake is essential, and use of these laxatives is contraindicated in the presence of obstruction or compromised peristaltic activity. A saline or osmotic laxative can be added if the bulk laxative is not effective. Use of saline laxatives should be avoided in patients with poor renal function or congestive heart failure because they may cause electrolyte imbalances. Stimulant laxatives should be used when other laxatives are ineffective. The emollient laxative, mineral oil, should be avoided because of the risk of lipoid aspiration pneumonia. Stool softeners have shown little effect when given to older adults with limited mobility, and use should be limited to patients in whom excessive straining or painful defecation occurs or for individuals at high risk for developing constipation (Hall et al, 2007; Thomas et al, 2003).

Combinations of natural fiber, fruit juices, and natural laxative mixtures are often recommended in clinical practice, and some studies have found an increase in bowel frequency and a decrease in laxative use when these mixtures are used. A recent study (Hale et al, 2007) showed that older long-term care residents receiving the Beverley-Travis natural laxative mixture (Beverley and Travis, 1992) at a dosage of 2 tablespoons twice a day had a significant increase in number of bowel movements compared with residents receiving daily prescribed laxatives (Box 8-12). Box 8-13 presents the

---

Box 8-12   Evidence-Based Practice: Pilot Study of the Feasibility and Effectiveness of a Natural Laxative Mixture

Purpose
To determine the effect of the Beverley-Travis natural laxative mixture given in a dosage of 2 tablespoons (tbs) twice daily compared with daily prescribed laxatives on bowel movement frequency in elderly long-term care (LTC) residents

Sample and Setting
Participants included 34 residents (control group:18; treatment group: 16) of a 200-bed Midwestern hospital-affiliated skilled long-term care facility. Inclusion criteria consisted of age 65 to 100 years, admission to the study site, ability to ingest soft foods actively and fluids orally, positive history of constipation, and current treatment with a prescription laxative.

Method
The study was conducted over 8 weeks, with the first 4-week period constituting baseline data collection without any changes in current bowel management. During the second 4-week period, control subjects continued with their currently prescribed once-daily laxative regime and treatment group subjects had their prescribed laxatives discontinued and received 2 tbs of the Beverley-Travis natural laxative mixture (see Box 8-13) twice a day. No dietary changes were made for either group, and fluid intake of 1500 ml per day was ordered for both groups.
    Daily bowel movement records were kept by registered nursing staff according to established criteria. A modified version of the Beverley-Travis Ease of Administration of Natural Laxative Mixture tool was used to measure subject resistance, ease of swallowing mixture, and overall ease of administration.

Results
Elderly LTC residents receiving the Beverley-Travis natural laxative mixture had a significant increase in number of bowel movements compared with residents receiving daily prescribed laxatives. Ninety percent of the staff rated the natural laxative mixture as easy to administer. Total retail cost of the natural laxative mixture was estimated at $0.30 /day compared with $0.52/day for prescribed laxatives.

Implications
Even with a small sample size and lack of a double-blind design, a natural laxative recipe may provide an alternative to commonly prescribed pharmaceutical laxatives in the prevention and treatment of constipation. Further study with a larger number of subjects across a variety of patient populations and health care settings is necessary.

Box 8-13 | Natural Laxative Recipes

1. Beverley-Travis Natural Laxative Mixture
Ingredients
1 cup raisins
1 cup pitted prunes
1 cup figs
1 cup dates
1 cup currants
1 cup prune concentrate

Directions
Combine contents together in grinder or blender to a thickened consistency. Store in refrigerator between uses

Dosage
Administer 2 tablespoons (tbs) twice a day (once in the morning and once in the evening). May increase or decrease according to the frequency of bowel movements.

Nutritional Composition
Each 2-tbs dose contains the following:
61 calories
137 mg potassium
8 mg sodium
11.9 g sugar
0.5 g protein
1.4 g fiber

2. Power Pudding
Ingredients
1 cup wheat bran
1 cup applesauce
1 cup prune juice

Directions
Mix and store in refrigerator. Start with administration of 1 tbs/day. Increase *slowly* until desired effect is achieved and no disagreeable symptoms occur.

Beverley-Travis Natural Laxative Mixture from: Hale E, Smith E, St. James J et al: Pilot study of the feasibility and effectiveness of a natural laxative mixture, *Geriatr Nurs* 28(2):104-111, 2007.

Beverley-Travis natural laxative recipe and an additional recipe for an alternative natural laxative mixture.

Enemas

Enemas of any type should be reserved for situations in which other methods produce no response or when it is known that there is an impaction. Enemas should not be used on a regular basis. A normal saline or tap water enema (500 to 1000 ml) at a temperature of 105° F is the best choice. Soapsuds and phosphate enemas irritate the rectal mucosa and should not be used. Oil retention enemas are used for refractory constipation and in the treatment of fecal impaction (Reuben et al, 2006).

A program to prevent as well as treat constipation that incorporates a high-fiber diet, liberal fluid intake, daily exercise, and environmental modifications that promote a regular pattern of bowel elimination must be developed for each client. Interventions in any setting are based on a thorough assessment. Assessment and management of bowel function is an important nursing responsibility.

MALNUTRITION

The occurrence of malnutrition among the elderly has been documented in elders in acute care, long-term care, and the community. Protein-calorie malnutrition (PCM) is the most common form of malnutrition in older adults. PCM is characterized by the presence of clinical signs (muscle wasting, low BMI) and biochemical indicators (decreased albumin or other serum protein) indicative of insufficient intake. Many of the factors discussed previously contribute to the occurrence of malnutrition in older adults (Box 8-14).

The prevalence of PCM varies with the population observed and the definition of malnutrition. In the United States, estimates indicate that 50% of nursing home patients, 50% of hospitalized patients, and 44% of home health patients over the age of 65 are malnourished (Crogan and Pasvogel, 2003). Thomas and colleagues (2002) reported that more than 91% of patients admitted to a subacute facility are either malnourished or at risk of malnutrition. The high prevalence of malnutrition in nursing homes and subacute facilities may in part reflect transfer of malnourished patients from acute care to long-term care following an acute illness.

Malnutrition has serious consequences, including infections, pressure ulcers, anemia, hypotension, impaired cognition, hip fractures, and increased mortality and morbidity. The majority of pathological causes of weight loss are considered reversible.

Depression, frequent in older adults, is a common and reversible cause of weight loss. Screening for depression using validated tools, such as the Geriatric Depression Scale or the Cornell Scale for Depression in Dementia, should be included in assessment of older people with weight loss (see Chapter 25). A thorough medication review is important when assessing nutritional concerns since many medications affect appetite and can affect nutritional status. Medications most frequently associated with malnutrition include digoxin, theophylline, nonsteroidal antiinflammatory drugs (NSAIDs), iron supplements, and psychoactive drugs.

Box 8-14	Factors Potentiating Malnutrition in Older Adults

Psychosocial Risk Factors
Limited income
Abuse of alcohol and other central nervous system depressants
Bereavement, loneliness, or living alone
Removal from usual cultural patterns
Memory loss
Depression

Mechanical Risk Factors
Decreased or limited strength and mobility
Neurological deficits, arthritis, impairment of hand-arm coordination, loss of tongue strength, dysphagia
Decreased or diminished vision or blindness
Inability to shop, prepare food, and/or feed self and lack of adequate assistance
Pressure ulcers
Loss of teeth, poor-fitting dentures, or chewing problems
Difficult breathing
Polypharmacy
Surgery, nothing by mouth (NPO) orders for extended periods of time, and patients being maintained on intravenous therapy only

In light of current population projections, the number of older adults requiring hospitalization, subacute care, and nursing home care will dramatically increase, leading to increased hospital stays, increased costs, and considerable mortality (Crogan and Pasvogel, 2003). Since the risk of malnutrition rises as soon as a person joins one of these groups, malnutrition is clearly a serious challenge for health professionals in all settings.

IMPLICATIONS FOR GERONTOLOGICAL NURSING AND HEALTHY AGING

Assessment

Older people are less likely than younger people to show signs of malnutrition and nutrient malabsorption. Evaluation of nutritional health can be difficult in the absence of severe malnutrition, but a comprehensive assessment and physical examination can reveal deficits (Baker, 2007).

A nutritional assessment that provides the most conclusive data about a person's actual nutritional state consists of the following steps: interview, physical examination, anthropometrical measurements, and biochemical analysis. The collective results can provide the nurse with the data needed to identify the immediate and the potential nutritional problems of the client. The nurse can then begin to establish plans for supervision, assistance, and education in the attainment of adequate nutrition for the older person.

A Nutrition Screening Initiative (1991) checklist (Figure 8-4) can be used by older people to identify risk factors for poor nutrition. The Mini Nutritional Assessment (MNA), developed by Nestle of Geneva, Switzerland, is intended for use by professionals to screen for malnutrition (www.hartfordign.org). A video demonstration of the MNA can be found at www.nursingcenter.com/prodev/ce_article.asp?tid=771461.

The Minimum Data Set (MDS) includes assessment information that can be used to identify potential nutritional problems, risk factors, and the potential for improved function. The nutrition and dehydration Resident Assessment Protocols (RAPs) guide staff in assessment of nutritionally related problems. Triggers for more thorough investigation of problems include weight loss, alterations in taste, medical therapies, prescription medications, hunger, parenteral or intravenous feedings, mechanically altered or therapeutic diets, percentage of food left uneaten, pressure ulcers, and edema. See Chapter 13 for further information on MDA and RAPs. An evidence-based guideline, *Nutritional management in long-term care: development of a clinical guideline,* is available at www.guideline.gov/summary/summary.aspx?ss=15&doc_id=5235&nbr=3577.

Interview

The interview provides background information and clues to the nutritional state and actual and potential problems of the older adult. Questions about the individual's state of health, social activities, normal patterns, and changes that have occurred should be asked. The nurse must explore the individual's needs, the manner in which food is obtained, and the client's ability to prepare food.

Information concerning the relationship of food to daily events will provide clues to the meaning and significance of food to that person. The older person who eats alone is considered a candidate for malnutrition. Information about occupation and daily activities will suggest the degree of energy expenditure and caloric intake most appropriate for the overall activity. One's economic status will have a direct bearing on nutrition.

Read the statements below. Circle the number in the Yes column for those that apply to you or someone you know. For each "yes" answer, score the number listed. Total your nutritional score.

	YES
I have an illness or condition that made me change the kind or amount of food I eat.	2
I eat fewer than two meals per day.	3
I eat few fruits, vegetables or milk products.	2
I have three or more drinks of beer, liquor, or wine almost every day.	2
I have tooth or mouth problems that make it hard for me to eat.	2
I don't always have enough money to buy the food I need.	4
I eat alone most of the time.	1
I take three or more different prescriptions or over-the-counter drugs each day.	1
Without wanting to, I have lost or gained 10 pounds in the past 6 months.	2
I am not always physically able to shop, cook, and/or feed myself.	2

Total Nutritional Score _____

0-2 indicates good nutrition
3-5 moderate risk
6+ high nutritional risk

Fig. 8-4 Nutrition Screening Initiative checklist to determine nutritional health. *(From the Nutrition Screening Initiative, 1010 Wisconsin Avenue NW, Suite 800, Washington, DC 2000. The Nutrition Screening Initiative is funded in part by a grant from Ross Products Division of Abbott Laboratories.)*

It is therefore important to explore the client's financial resources to establish the income available for food.

Medications being taken should be included in the nutrition history. Additional medical information should include the presence or absence of mouth pain or discomfort, visual difficulty, bowel and bladder function, and history of illness. As noted earlier, depression is a major cause of weight loss in long-term care settings, accounting for up to 36% of residents who lose weight. An evaluation for depression should be obtained for residents with anorexia (Thomas, 2000).

Diet Histories. Frequently a 24-hour diet recall compared with MyPyramid can provide an estimate of nutritional adequacy. When the older person cannot supply all of the information requested, it may be possible to obtain data from a family member or another source. There will be times, however, when information will not be as complete as one would like, or the older person, too proud to admit that he or she is not eating, will furnish erroneous information. Even so, the nurse will be able to obtain additional data from the other three areas of the nutritional assessment.

Keeping a dietary record for 3 days is another assessment tool. What one ate, when food was eaten, and the amounts eaten must be carefully recorded. Computer analysis of the dietary records provides information on energy and vitamin and mineral intake. Printouts can provide the older person and the health care provider with a visual graph of the intake. Accurate completion of 3-day dietary records in hospitals and nursing homes can be problematic, and intake may be either underestimated or overestimated. Standardized observational protocols should be developed to ensure accuracy of oral intake documentation as well as the adequacy and quality of feeding assistance during mealtimes. Nurses should ensure that direct caregivers are educated on the proper observation and documentation of intake and should closely monitor performance in this area.

Physical Examination

The physical examination furnishes clinically observable evidence of the existing state of nutrition. Data such as height and weight; vital signs; condition of the tongue, lips, and gums; skin turgor, texture, and color; and functional ability are assessed, and the overall general appearance is scrutinized for evidence of wasting. Height should always be measured and never estimated or given by self-report. If the person cannot stand, an alternative way of measuring standing height is knee-height using knee-height calipers (DiMaria-Ghalili, 2008). BMI should be calculated to determine if weight for height is within the normal range of 22-27. A BMI below 22 is a sign of undernutrition (DiMaria-Ghialli, 2008).

A detailed weight history should be obtained along with current weight. History should include a history of weight loss, whether the weight loss was intentional or unintentional, and during what period it occurred. Debate continues in the quest to determine the appropriate weight charts for an older adult. Although weight alone does not indicate the adequacy of diet, unplanned fluctuations in weight are significant and should be evaluated.

Accurate weight patterns are sometimes difficult to obtain. Procedures for weighing people should be established and followed consistently to obtain an accurate picture of weight changes. Weighing procedure should be supervised by licensed personnel and changes reported immediately to the provider. One might meet correct weight values for height, but weight changes may be the results of fluid retention, edema, or ascites and merit investigation. An unintentional weight loss of more than 5% of body weight in 1 month, more than 7.5% in 3 months, or more than 10% in 6 months is considered a significant indicator of poor nutrition as well as an MDS trigger.

Anthropometrical Measurements

Anthropometrical measurements include height, weight, midarm circumference, and triceps skinfold thickness. These are obtained by simple body measurement procedures, which take less than 5 minutes to perform. These measurements offer information about the status of the older person's muscle mass and body fat in relation to height and weight. Muscle mass measurements are obtained by measuring the arm circumference of the nondominant upper arm. The arm hangs freely at the side, and a measuring tape is placed around the midpoint of the upper arm, between the acromion of the scapula and the olecranon of the ulna. The centimeter circumference is recorded and compared with standard values.

Body fat and lean muscle mass are assessed by measuring specific skinfolds with Lange or Harpenden calipers. Two areas are accessible for measurement. One area is the midpoint of the upper arm, the triceps area, which is also used to obtain arm circumference. The nondominant arm is again used. The nurse lifts the skin with the thumb and forefinger so that it parallels the humerus. The calipers are placed around the skinfold, 1 cm below where the fingers are grasping the skin. Two readings are averaged to the nearest half centimeter. If there is a neuropathological condition or hemiplegia following a stroke, the unaffected arm should be used for obtaining measurements.

Biochemical Examination

The final step in a nutritional assessment is the biochemical examination. Suggested biochemical parameters include serum albumin, cholesterol, hemoglobin, and serum transferrin. Although these parameters may also be abnormal in several conditions unassociated with malnutrition, they are useful as guides to interventions (Thomas, 2000). Serum albumin of more than 4 g/dl is desired; less than 3.5 g/dl is an indicator of poor nutritional state. Prealbumin level may be a better indicator of protein loss because it changes rapidly in the presence of malnutrition. Transferrin, an iron transport protein, is diminished in protein malnutrition. However, it increases in iron deficiency anemia, which is common in older adults, so it is not a sensitive indicator of PCM. Laboratory test results, although not definitive for malnutrition, provide important clues to nutritional status but should be evaluated in relation to the person's overall health status. Unintentional weight loss remains the most important indicator of potential nutritional deficits.

Interventions

Interventions are formulated around the identified nutritional problem or problems. Nursing interventions are centered on techniques to increase food intake and enhance and manage the environment to promote increased food intake (DiMaria-Ghialli, 2008). Collaboration with the interdisciplinary team (dietitian, pharmacist, social worker, occupational or speech therapist) is important in planning interventions. For the community-dwelling elder, nutrition education and problem solving with the elder and family members on how to best resolve the potential or actual nutritional deficit is important.

Causes of poor nutrition are complex, and all of the factors emphasized in this chapter are important to assess when planning individualized interventions to insure adequate nutrition for older people. Box 8-15 presents a list of protocols and practice guidelines that may be used to guide assessment and nursing interventions.

Pharmacological Therapy

Drugs that stimulate appetite (orexigenic drugs) should be considered to reverse resistant anorexia after all other interventions have been tried. They must be monitored closely for side effects and have had little evaluation in frail older people. Benefits are restricted to small weight gains without indication of decreased morbidity or mortality or improved quality of life or functional ability.

Megestrol (Megace) may be effective at a dosage of 800 mg daily for 3 months. Patients should be

Box 8-15	Protocols and Guidelines: Resources for Assessment and Management of Nutritional Concerns in Older Adults

Unintentional weight loss in the elderly (www.guideline.gov)
Mealtime difficulties for older persons: assessment and management (www.guideline.gov)
Preventing aspiration in older adults with dysphagia (www.hartfordign.org)
Assessing nutrition in older adults (www.hartfordign.org)
Eating and feeding issues in older adults with dementia. Part I: Assessment (www.hartfordign.org)
Eating and feeding issues in older adults with dementia. Part II: Interventions (www.hartfordign.org)
Nutrition in the elderly: Nursing Standard of Practice Protocol: Nutrition in Aging (www.consultgerirn.org)

monitored closely for adrenocortical insufficiency, and it should not be used with bedridden patients because of the risk for deep venous thrombosis. Dronabinol (Marinol), although not adequately tested in older people, has shown some potential benefits and may be an appropriate drug for end-of-life and palliative care because it stimulates appetite, has antinausea properties, decreases pain, and enhances general well-being. Weight gain from the use of these two drugs is primarily adipose tissue as opposed to lean body mass (University of Texas, 2006).

Oxandrolone (Osandrin), an exogenous anabolic hormone, is used to increase net protein synthesis and is the only oral anabolic steroid that is safe for weight loss and protein energy malnutrition (PEM). Studies have not shown that it leads to weight gain. For older adults who are depressed and have a poor appetite or weight loss, mitrazapine (Remeron), an antidepressant, has been shown to increase appetite and weight gain as well as improve depressed mood (University of Texas, 2006).

Patient Education

Education in the area of reading nutritional information on labels is needed. Since 1994, the U.S. Food and Drug Administration (FDA) has required producers of processed foods to list nutrition information on the amounts of nutrients and fiber that are desirable in daily diets of 2000 to 2500 calories. These nutrients were chosen based on evidence suggesting that eating too much or too little of these substances has the greatest impact of one's health. The FDA defines a "good source" as a food that contains 10% to 19% of the daily value per serving. The daily totals for fat, cholesterol, and sodium should be less than 100%. Medicare covers nutrition therapy for select diseases, such as diabetes and kidney disease, which creates unprecedented opportunities for older

Americans to access information. Balance should be emphasized as the key to a healthful diet.

Feeding Tubes

A common approach to problems with nutritional intake in older people has been the insertion of a feeding tube. Comprehensive assessment of swallowing problems and other factors that influence intake must be conducted before initiating severely restricted diet modifications or considering the use of feeding tubes, particularly for older people with advanced dementia. Use of feeding tubes for patients with advanced dementia to prevent aspiration, pneumonia, malnutrition, and infections provides few long-term benefits and may, in fact, contribute to further decline. Tube feeding has never been shown to reduce the risk of regurgitating gastric contents and cannot be expected to prevent aspiration of oral secretions (Finucane et al, 1999, 2001; Teno et al, 2002; Metheny et al, 2008).

The use of percutaneous endoscopic gastrostomy (PEG) feeding tubes has increased at an astonishing rate in older adults over recent years. Few complications occur with the insertion of a PEG tube; however, numerous complications occur from having one (AGS, 2006b). Aspiration pneumonia, diarrhea, metabolic problems, and cellulitis are just a few of these complications. Persons who aspirate oral feedings are also likely to aspirate tube feedings, either via nasogastric tubes or gastrostomy tubes (Metheny et al, 2008).

As discussed earlier, food and eating are closely tied to socialization, comfort, pleasure, love, and the meeting of basic biological needs. Decisions about artificial feeding are some of the most challenging of the many decisions that face families, health care providers, and the institutions that care for older adults with dementia. Decisions to use or not to use a feeding tube must be made carefully. Health care providers must take the time to listen to the wishes and concerns of the patient and the family. Individuals have the right to use or not to use a feeding tube but should be given accurate information about both the risks and benefits of enteral feeding in late-stage dementia (AGS, 2005).

Discussion about advance directives and feeding support should begin early in the course of the illness rather than waiting until a crisis develops. The best advice is for individuals to state preferences for the use of a feeding tube in a written advance directive. Surrogate decision makers should use advance directives and previously expressed wishes to decide what the patient with advanced dementia who is not eating would want under the present circumstances.

Hospitals, nursing homes, and other care settings must promote choice and honor patient preferences about enteral feeding and should not exert pressure on patients or medical providers to institute artificial feeding (Finucane et al, 2001). Nursing homes should have policies to ensure that patients with remediable causes of weight loss are appropriately evaluated and treated and that enteral feeding is not regarded as the only treatment of choice (Mitchell et al, 2003; AGS, 2005).

It is important that everyone involved in the care of the patient be informed about the benefits and risks of tube feeding for patients with dementia and the uncertainty of whether enteral feeding provides any benefit to the patient. The decision should never be understood as a question of tube feeding versus no feeding. No family should be made to feel that they are starving their loved one to death if the decision is made not to institute enteral feeding. Comprehensive attempts to continue to provide nutrition should always continue. Patients should be able to take any type of nutrition they desire, any time they desire.

Strict dietary restrictions such as low salt or no concentrated sweets should be replaced with liberalized diet choices. Attention to all factors contributing to inadequate intake should be investigated, including attention to mealtime ambience, feeding techniques, food preferences, medication side effects, and treatment of depression if present (Finucane et al, 2001). Excellent information for patients and families about enteral feeding can be found at www.chcr.brown.edu/dying/consumerfeedingtube.htm. The Northern California chapter of the National Gerontological Nurse Practitioners has produced a brochure about nutrition and hydration for caregivers, families of persons with dementia, and the health care team (available at www.ncgnp.org) (Hess, 2008).

Short-term enteral feeding may be indicated for some conditions (e.g., after a hip fracture when serum albumin is low), but the evidence to support the effectiveness of feeding tubes for older people with dementia is scant. When tube feeding is indicated, the nurse and dietician must work closely together to determine the appropriate formula and rate of administration, as well as observation of tolerance, weight, and hydration status. Keep the head of the bed elevated at least 30 degrees for patients receiving continuous tube feedings. When feeding by bolus, keep the head of the bed elevated at least 30 degrees during feeding and for 1 hour after feeding. Gavi et al (2008) provide a guide to management of feeding tube complications in the long-term care resident.

IMPLICATIONS FOR GERONTOLOGICAL NURSING AND HEALTHY AGING

Maintenance of adequate nutritional health as a person ages is extremely complex. Knowledge of normal nutrition in later years and the many factors contributing to inadequate nutrition is essential for the gerontological nurse and should be a part of every assessment of an older person. Working with members of the interdisciplinary team in appropriate assessment and development of therapeutic interventions is a major role in community, hospital, and long-term care settings. Use of evidence-based practice protocols is important in determining nursing interventions to support and enhance nutritional status and promote adequate bowel function. Prevention of undernutrition and malnutrition and the maintenance of dietary needs and food enjoyment until the end of life are also ethical responsibilities. No older person should be hungry or thirsty because he or she cannot shop, cook, or buy food. Nor should any older persons have to suffer because of a lack of assistance with these activities in whatever setting in which they may reside.

APPLICATION OF MASLOW'S HIERARCHY

Food is a basic human need for people of all ages. Attention must be paid to more than just adequate caloric intake to sustain life. Not only does adequate nutrition satisfy biological needs, but also the experience of eating provides opportunities for belonging. Being able to eat independently and enjoy meals or being provided with kind and competent assistance if unable to be independent promotes self-esteem and a feeling of worth.

KEY CONCEPTS

▶ Recommended dietary patterns for the older adult are similar to those of younger persons, with some reduction in the caloric intake based on decreased caloric requirements.

▶ Many factors affect adequate nutrition in late life, including lifelong eating habits, income, chronic illness, dentition, mood disorders, capacity for food preparation, and functional limitations.

▶ Protein-caloric malnutrition (PCM) is the most common form of malnutrition in older adults. Estimates indicate that 50% of nursing home patients, 50% of hospitalized patients, and 44% of home health patients over the age of 65 are malnourished.

▶ A comprehensive nutritional assessment is an essential component of the assessment of older adults.

▶ Making mealtime pleasant and attractive for the older adult who is unable to eat unassisted is a nursing challenge; mealtime must be made enjoyable, and adequate assistance must be provided.

▶ Dental health of older adults is a basic need that is increasingly neglected. Poor oral health is a risk factor for dehydration, malnutrition, and aspiration pneumonia.

▶ Bowel function in older adults is minimally affected by physiological changes of aging. Constipation is a common complaint and nonpharmacological interventions such as exercise and increased fluid and fiber intake are important to maintain normal bowel function.

ACTIVITIES AND DISCUSSION QUESTIONS

1. What are the factors affecting the nutrition of the older adult?
2. How can the nurse intervene to provide better nutrition for elders in the community, in acute care, and in long-term care settings?
3. What are the causes of malnutrition?
4. What is included in the nutritional assessment of an older person?
5. What are the factors contributing to alterations in bowel function as one ages?
6. What proactive measures can the nurse take to promote adequate bowel function for older adults in the community, in acute care, and in long-term care settings?
7. How is dysphagia assessed, and what interventions may be helpful in preventing aspiration?
8. Develop a nursing care plan for an older adult at risk for malnutrition using wellness and North American Nursing Diagnosis Association (NANDA) diagnoses.

RESOURCES

Publications

Healthy eating index scores among adults, 60 years of age and over, by sociodemographic and health characteristics: United States, 1999–2002, by R. Bethene Ervin, PhD, RD, Division of Health and Nutrition Examination Surveys. Available at www.cdc.gov/nchs/data/ad/ad395.pdf.

Websites

Oral Health: Preventing Cavities, Gum Disease, and Tooth Loss, 2008
www.cdc.gov/nccdphp/publications/aag/pdf/doh.pdf

U.S. Department of Agriculture and Health and Human Services
www.mypyramid.gov

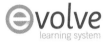

For additional resources, please visit evolve.elsevier. com/Ebersole/gerontological

REFERENCES

Amella E, Lawrence J: Eating and feeding issues in older adults with dementia. Accessed June 30, 2008 from www.hartfordign.org.

American Geriatrics Society: Feeding tube placement in elderly patients with advanced dementia, 2005. Accessed June 30, 2008 from www.americangeriatrics.org/products/positionpapers/feeding_tube_placement.pdf.

American Geriatrics Society (AGS): *Geriatrics at your fingertips,* New York, 2006a, The Society.

American Geriatrics Society (AGS): *Geriatric review syllabus,* New York, 2006b, The Society.

American Speech and Hearing Association: Communication facts: special populations: Dysphagia, 2008 edition. Accessed May 8, 2008 from www.asha.org/members/research/reports/dysphagia.html.

Arce D, Ermocilla C, Costa H: Evaluation of constipation, *Am Fam Physician,* June 1, 2002. Accessed June 30, 2008 from www.aafp.org/afp/20020601/2283.html.

Aronson D: Nutrition for health and longevity, *Aging Well* 1(2):20-24, 2008.

Baker H: Nutrition in the elderly: diet pitfalls and nutrition advice, *Geriatrics* 62(10):24-26, 2007.

Bales C, Buhr G: Is obesity bad for older persons? A systematic review of the pros and cons of weight reduction in later life, *JAMDA* 9(2):302-312, 2008.

Beers M, Berkow R: *Merck manual of geriatrics,* ed 3, Whitehouse Station, NJ, 2000, Merck Research Laboratories.

Beverley L, Travis I: Constipation: proposed natural laxative mixtures, *J Gerontol Nurs* 18(10):5-12, 1992.

Burger S, Kayser-Jones J, Bell J: Malnutrition and dehydration in nursing homes: key issues in prevention and treatment,

2000. Accessed July 23, 2004 from http:www.cmwf.org/programs/elders/burger_mal_386.asp.

Burticka B: Do assets change the racial profile of poverty among older adults, *The Urban Institute* 8, 2008. Accessed June 30, 2008 from www.urban.org/UploadedPDF/411620_racial_poverty.pdf.

Cacchione PZ: Sensory changes, In Capezuti E, Zwicker D, Mezey M, Fulmer T, editors: *Evidence-based geriatric nursing protocols for best practice*, ed 3, New York, 2008, Springer.

Cash B: Chronic constipation—defining the problem and clinical impact, *Medscape Gastroenterology* 7(1), 2005. Accessed September 15, 2008 from www.medscape.com/viewarticle/501467_print.

Centers for Disease Control and Prevention: Oral health for older Americans, 2006. Accessed June 2, 2008 from www.cdc.gov/Oralhealth/publications/factsheets/adult_older.htm.

Crogan NL, Pasvogel A: The influence of protein-calorie malnutrition on quality of life in nursing homes, *J Gerontol* 58:M159-164, 2003.

DiMaria-Ghalili R: Nutrition. In Capezuti E, Zwicker D, Mezey M, Fulmer T, editors: *Evidence-based geriatric nursing protocols for best practice,* ed 3, New York, 2008, Springer.

Doll-Shankaruk M, Yau W, Oekle C: Implementation and effects of a medication pass nutritional supplement program in a long-term care facility, *J Gerontol Nurs* 34(5):45-50, 2008.

Editorial: Oral health care services for older adults : a looming crisis, *Am J Pub Health* 94(5):699-702, 2004.

Edwards W: Gastrointestinal problems. In Cotter UT, Strumpf NE, editors: *Advanced practice nursing with older adults,* New York, 2002, McGraw Hill.

Ervin B: *Healthy eating index scores among adults, 60 years of age and over, by sociodemographic and health characteristics: United States, 1999-2002.* Advance data from vital and health statistics; no. 395. Hyattsville, MD: National Center for Health Statistics, 2008. Accessed June 30, 2008 from www.cdc.gov/nchs/data/ad/ad395.pdf.

Finucane TE, Mitchell SL, Christmas C, McCann R: Tube feeding for elderly patients. Caring for the older adult: innovations in research and practice. Presented at the American Geriatrics Society Annual Scientific Meeting, May 12, 2001, Chicago, Illinois, Symposium. Accessed June 30, 2008 from www.medscape.com/viewarticle/420780.

Fuller-Thomson E, Redmond M: Falling through the social safety net: food stamp use and nonuse among older impoverished Americans, *Gerontologist* 48(2):235-244, 2008.

Gavi S, Hensley J, Cervo F et al: Management of feeding tube complications in the long-term care resident, *Ann Long-Term Care* 16(4):28-32, 2008.

Gil-Montoya J, Ferreira A, Lopez I: Oral health protocol for the dependent institutionalized elderly, *Geriatric Nurs* 27(2):95-101, 2006.

Hale E, Smith E, St. James J et al: Pilot study of the feasibility and effectiveness of a natural laxative mixture, *Geriatr Nurs* 28(2):104-111, 2007.

Hall K, Karstens M, Rakel B et al: Managing constipation in the elderly, *Geriatrics* A CME-Accredited Supplement, August: 2007.

Hess P: Artificial nutrition and hydration for the person with dementia: creation of a brochure, *Geriatr Nurs* 29(3):172-3, 2008.

Kayser-Jones J: Inadequate staffing at mealtime: implications for nursing and health policy, *J Gerontol Nurs* 23(8):14-21, 1997.

Kayser-Jones J: Use of oral supplements in nursing homes: remaining questions, *J Am Geriatr Soc* 54(9):1463, 2006.

Kempler D: *Neurodegenerative disorders in aging,* Thousand Oaks, California, 2005, Sage.

Leibovitz A, Baumoehl E, Lubart A et al: Dehydration among long-term care elderly patients with oropharyngeal dysphagia, *Gerontology* 53(4):179-183, 2007.

Lewis SJ, Heaton KW: Stool form scale as a useful guide to intestinal transit time, *Scand J Gastroenterol* 32(9):920-924, 1997.

Locher J, Ritchie C, Robinson C et al: A multidimensional approach to understanding under-eating in homebound older adults: the importance of social factors, *Gerontologist* 48(2):223-234, 2008.

Lustbader W: Thoughts on the meaning of frailty, *Generations* 13(4):21-22, 1999.

Markovic K et al: Good news for elderly persons: olfactory pleasure increases at later stages of the life span, *Jour Gerontology: Medical Sci* 62A(11):1287-1293, 2007.

McCance K, Huether S: *Pathophysiology: the biologic basis for disease in adults and children*, ed 5, St. Louis, 2006, Mosby.

Metheny M: Preventing aspiration in older adults with dysphagia, *Try This: Best practices in nursing care to older adults,* Issue 20, revised 2007. Accessed June 30, 2008 from www.hartfordign.org/publications/trythis/issue_20.pdfwww.hartfordign.org.

Metheny M, Boltz M, Greenberg S: Preventing aspiration in older adults with dysphagia, *Am J Nurs* 108(2):45-46, 2008.

Miller C: *Nursing for wellness in older adults*, ed 5, Philadelphia, 2008, Wolters Kluwer–Lippincott Williams & Wilkins.

Mitchell SL, Kiely, DK, Hamel MB et al: Clinical and organizational factors associated with feeding tube use among nursing home residents with advanced cognitive impairment, *JAMA* 290(1):73-80, 2003.

Momeyer A, Luggen AS: Periodontal disease in older adults, *Geriatr Nurs* 26(3):197-200, 2005.

Morley JE: Why do physicians fail to recognize and treat malnutrition in older persons? *J Am Geriatr Soc* 39(11):1139-1140, 1991.

Morley JE: Anorexia and weight loss in older persons, *J Gerontol A Biol Sci Med Sci* 58(2):131-137, 2003.

Morley JE, Silver AJ: Nutritional issues in nursing home care, *Ann Intern Med* 123(11):850-859, 1995.

Nutrition Screening Initiative, project of American Academy of Family Physicians, American Dietetic Association, and

National Council on Aging. Grant from Ross-Abbott Laboratories, Inc, 1991.

O'Connor L: Oral health care. In Capezuti E, Zwicker D, Mezey M, Fulmer T, editors: *Evidence based geriatric nursing protocols for best practice,* ed 3, New York, 2008, Springer.

Reuben D, Herr K, Pacala J et al: *Geriatrics at your fingertips 2006-7,* ed 8, New York, 2006, American Geriatrics Society.

Sarin J, Balasubramanian R, Colcoran A: Reducing the risk of aspiration pneumonia among elderly patients in long-term care facilities through oral health interventions, *JAMDA* 9(2):128-135, 2008.

Simmons S, Osterweil D, Schnelle J: Improving food intake in nursing home residents with feeding assistance, *J Gerontol A Biol Sci Med Sci* 56A(12):M790-M794, 2001.

Teno J, Mor V, DeSilva D et al: Use of feeding tubes in nursing home residents with severe cognitive impairment, *JAMA* 287(24):3211-3212, 2002.

Thomas D: Nutritional management in long-term care: development of a clinical guideline, *J Gerontol A Biol Sci Med Sci* 55(12):M725, 2000.

Thomas D, Zdrowski C, Wilson M et al: Malnutrition in sub-acute care, *Am J Clin Nutr* 75(2):308-313, 2002.

Thomas D, Forrester L, Gloth F et al: Clinical consensus: the constipation crisis in long-term care, *Ann Long-Term Care Suppl* (October):1-16, 2003. Accessed June 30, 2008 from www.aafp.org/afp/20020601/2283.html

University of Texas: *Unintentional weight loss in the elderly,* Austin, TX, University of Texas School of Nursing, 2006. Accessed June 15, 2008 from www.guideline.gov.

U.S. Department of Health and Human Services (USDHHS): *Healthy people 2010,* Hyattsville, MD, 2002, Public Health Service. Accessed June 30, 2008 from www.healthypeople.gov.

Fluids and Continence

9

▶ LEARNING OBJECTIVES

Upon completion of this chapter, the reader will be able to:

- Identify risk factors for dehydration.
- Discuss interventions to prevent or treat dehydration.
- Define urinary and fecal incontinence.
- List factors contributing to urinary and fecal incontinence.
- Explain the types of urinary incontinence and their causes.
- Discuss nursing interventions for urinary and fecal incontinence.

▶ GLOSSARY

Detrusor A body part that pushes down, such as the bladder muscle.

Incontinence The inability to control excretory function.

Micturition Urination.

Transient Temporary.

▶ THE LIVED EXPERIENCE

"UI (urinary incontinence) is like being a bad kid or a big baby."

"There's nothing that can be done. Well, I don't think there is anything else but a diaper."

"It is very, very embarrassing being incontinent and it affects your self-esteem."

"Sometimes I have to wet my bed before they get here, you know, and they are all busy and I have to wait for somebody, then I can't control it."

"I do something that is very wrong. I try not to drink too much but that's so wrong. So how can you drink a lot, you would be soaked all the time."

Comments from participants in a study of living with urinary incontinence in long-term care (MacDonald and Butler, 2007).

UI is a preventable and treatable condition and yet, "continence remains undervalued and UI remains underassessed. Even though UI is a basic nursing issue, nurses are not claiming it as one."

Comment from nurses in expert continence care (Mason et al, 2003, p. 3).

FLUIDS

Hydration Management

Hydration management is the promotion of an adequate fluid balance, which prevents complications resulting from abnormal or undesirable fluid levels (www. consultgerirn.org). Water, an accessible and available commodity to almost all people, is often overlooked as an essential part of nutritional requirements. Water's function in the body includes thermoregulation, dilution of water-soluble medications, facilitation of renal and bowel function, and creation of requisite conditions for and maintenance of metabolic processes.

Daily needs for water can usually be met by functionally independent older adults through intake of fluids with meals and social drinks. However, a significant number of older adults (up to 85% of those 85 years of age and over) drink less than 1 liter of fluid per day. Older adults, with the exception of those requiring fluid restrictions, should consume at least 1500 ml of fluid per day (Mentes, 2006).

Maintenance of fluid balance (fluid intake equals fluid output) is essential to health, regardless of a person's age (Mentes, 2006). Age-related changes, medication use, functional impairments, and comorbid medical and emotional illnesses, place some older adults at risk for changes in fluid balance, especially dehydration (Mentes, 2008). A comprehensive hydration management guideline (Mentes, 2004) can be found at www. guideline.gov/summary/summary.aspx?ss=15&doc_ id=4832&nbr=3479.

Dehydration

Dehydration is defined clinically as "a complex condition resulting in a reduction in total body water. This can be due primarily to a water deficit (water loss dehydration) (hyperosmolar) or both a salt and water deficit (salt loss dehydration) (hypoosmolar). In older people, dehydration most often develops as a result of disease, age-related changes, and/or the effects of medication and NOT primarily due to lack of access to water" (Thomas et al, 2008, p. 293). Dehydration is considered a geriatric syndrome frequently associated with common diseases (e.g. diabetes, respiratory illness, heart failure) and declining stages of the frail elderly (Crecelius, 2008).

Dehydration is a problem prevalent among older adults in all settings. If not treated adequately,

mortality from dehydration can be as high as 50% (Faes et al, 2007). Dehydration is a significant risk factor for delirium, thromboembolic complications, infections, kidney stones, constipation and obstipation, falls, medication toxicity, renal failure, seizure, electrolyte imbalance, hyperthermia, and delayed wound healing (Mentes, 2006; Faes et al, 2007). Thomas et al (2008) comment that there are few diagnoses that generate as much concern about causes and consequences as does dehydration. A recent study reported that physicians misdiagnose dehydration in at least a third of patients admitted to the hospital. Due to a lack of understanding of the pathogenesis and consequences of dehydration in older adults, the condition is often attributed to poor care by nursing home staff and/or physicians. However, the majority of older people develop dehydration as a result of increased fluid losses combined with decreased fluid intake, related to decreased thirst. The condition is rarely due to neglect.

Risk Factors for Dehydration

Most healthy older adults maintain adequate hydration, but the presence of physical or emotional illness, surgery, or trauma or conditions of higher physiologic demands increase the risk of dehydration. "The limited capacity of homeostatic mechanisms to maintain fluid balance only becomes important when fluid balance is at risk" (Faes et al, 2007).

Age-related changes in the thirst mechanism, decrease in total body water (TBW), and decreased kidney function increase the risk for dehydration. TBW decreases with age. In young adults, TBW is about 60% of body weight in men and 52% in women. In older people, TBW decreases to about 52% of body weight in men and 46% in women. The loss of muscle mass with age increases the proportion of fat cells. This loss is greater in women because they have a higher percentage of body fat and less muscle mass than men. Because fat cells contain less water than muscle cells, older people have a decreased intracellular fluid volume (Mentes, 2006).

Thirst sensation diminishes, resulting in the loss of an important defense against dehydration (American Geriatrics Society, 2006). In a mechanism that is not well understood, thirst in older adults is not "proportional to metabolic needs in response to dehydrating conditions" (Mentes, 2008, p. 371). Creatinine clearance also declines with age, and the kidneys are less able to concentrate urine. These changes are more pronounced in older people with illnesses affecting kidney function. (See Chapter 6.)

Old age and black race have both been associated with an increased risk of dehydration. Other risk factors for dehydration include medications, particularly those that directly affect renal function and fluid balance (diuretics, laxatives, angiotensin-converting enzyme [ACE] inhibitors) and psychotropic medications that have anticholinergic effects (dry mouth, urinary retention, constipation). The use of four or more medications is also a risk factor (Mentes, 2006; Faes et al, 2007).

Functional deficits, communication and comprehension problems, oral problems, dysphagia, depression, dementia, hospitalization, low body weight, diagnostic procedures necessitating fasting, inadequate assistance with fluid intake, diarrhea, fever, vomiting, infections, bleeding, draining wounds, artificial ventilation, fluid restrictions, high environmental temperature, and multiple comorbidities have all been noted as risk factors for dehydration in older people (Mentes, 2006; Faes et al, 2007). Nothing by mouth (NPO) requirements for diagnostic tests and surgical procedures should be as short as possible for older adults and adequate fluids given once tests and procedures are completed. A 2-hour suspension of fluid intake is recommended for many procedures (www.asahq.org/publicationsAndServices/NPO.pdf). Box 9-1 presents a simple screen for dehydration.

Hyponatremia is defined as a decrease in sodium plasma concentration (<136 mEq/L) and is caused by an excess of water relative to solute. When a person is hyponatremic, the differential diagnosis includes the syndrome of inappropriate antidiuretic hormone (SIADH) (Thomas et al, 2008). Selective serotonin reuptake inhibitors (SSRIs) increase the risk of hyponatremia with the risk being greatest in the first 2 weeks of treatment. Monitoring of sodium level and fluid intake in patients recently prescribed SSRIs is important. Changes in mental status, including lethargy or acute confusion, should be investigated immediately. Other risk factors include age, renal insufficiency, postsurgical status, presence of malignancy, and use of diuretics (Mentes, 2006; Craig, 2008). Hyponatremia has been observed in approximately 30% of patients in the intensive care unit (Craig, 2008).

IMPLICATIONS FOR GERONTOLOGICAL NURSING AND HEALTHY AGING

Assessment

Prevention of dehydration is essential, but assessment is complex in older people. Clinical signs may not appear until dehydration is advanced. Attention to risk factors for dehydration in older adults using a screen (Box 9-1) is very important. In addition, the MDS has 12 triggers for dehydration/fluid maintenance and 7 additional risk factors. Education should be provided to older people and their caregivers on the need for fluids and the signs and symptoms of dehydration. Acute situations such as vomiting, diarrhea, or febrile episodes should be identified quickly and treated. Older adults over the age of 85 years who have experienced volume deficits, weight loss, malnutrition, or infections, and those with dementia, delirium, and functional impairments are at high risk for dehydration.

Typical signs of dehydration may not always be present in older people. "The large variability in the way different organs are affected by dehydration will cause symptoms to remain atypical in older adults" (Faes et al, 2007, p. 3). Skin turgor, assessed at the sternum and commonly included in the assessment of dehydration, is an unreliable marker in older adults because of the loss of subcutaneous tissue with aging. Dry mucous membranes in the mouth and nose, longitudinal furrows on the tongue, orthostasis, speech incoherence, extremity weakness, dry axilla, and sunken eye may indicate dehydration. However, the diagnosis of dehydration is biochemical (Thomas et al, 2008).

If dehydration is suspected, laboratory tests include blood urea nitrogen (BUN), sodium, creatinine, glucose, and bicarbonate. Osmolarity should be either directly

Box 9-1	Simple Screen for Dehydration

Drugs, e.g., diuretics
End of life
High fever
Yellow urine turns dark
Dizziness (orthostasis)
Reduced oral intake
Axilla dry
Tachycardia
Incontinence (fear of)
Oral problems/sippers
Neurological impairment (confusion)
Sunken eyes

From: Thomas D, Cote T, Lawhorne L et al: Understanding clinical dehydration and its treatment, *Journal of the American Medical Directors Association* 9(5):292-301, 2008.

measured or calculated. While most cases of dehydration have an elevated BUN, there are many other causes of an elevated BUN/creatinine ratio and this test cannot be used alone to diagnose dehydration in older adults (Thomas et al, 2008). Mentes (2006) notes that "as is true with other standard tests, serum markers confirm a diagnosis of dehydration once it is too late to prevent it from occurring" (Mentes, 2006, p. 5). Attention to risk factors is important to identify possible dehydration and to intervene early. Body weight changes should also be assessed as indicators of changes in hydration (Faes et al, 2007).

Urine color, measured using a urine color chart, has been suggested as helpful in assessing hydration status (not dehydration) in older individuals in nursing homes with adequate renal function (Mentes, 2008). The urine color chart has eight standardized colors, ranging from pale straw (number 1) to greenish brown (number 8) approximating urine specific gravities of 1.003 to 1.029 (Mentes, 2006, 2008). Urine color should be assessed and charted over several days. Pale straw–colored urine usually indicates normal hydration status, and as urine darkens, poor hydration may be indicated (after taking into account discoloration by food or medications). For older adults, a reading of 4 or less is preferred (Mentes, 2006). If a person's urine becomes darker than his or her usual color, fluid intake assessment is indicated and fluids can be increased before dehydration occurs (Mentes, 2008).

Interventions

Interventions are derived from a comprehensive assessment and consist of risk identification and hydration management (Mentes, 2008). Hydration management involves both acute and ongoing management of oral intake. Oral hydration is the first treatment approach for dehydration. Individuals with mild to moderate dehydration who can drink and do not have significant mental or physical compromise due to fluid loss may be able to replenish fluids orally (Thomas et al, 2008). Water is considered the best fluid to offer, but other clear fluids may also be useful depending on the person's preference. One study found a significant reduction in lab values indicative of dehydration among nursing home residents who received verbal prompting and were given the type of beverage they requested (Simmons et al, 2001).

Rehydration methods depend on the severity and the type of dehydration and may include intravenous or hypodermoclysis. A general rule is to replace 50% of the loss within the first 12 hours (or 1 L/day in afebrile

elders) or sufficient quantity to relieve tachycardia and hypotension. Further fluid replacement can be administered more slowly over a longer period of time.

Hypodermoclysis is safe, easy to administer, and a useful alternative to intravenous administration for persons with mild to moderate dehydration, particularly those patients with altered mental status. Normal saline (0.9%), half-normal saline (0.45%), 5% glucose in water infusion (D5W), or Ringer's solution can be used (Thomas et al, 2008). Hypodermoclysis can be administered in almost any setting so hospital admissions may be avoided. Hypodermoclysis is "an evidence-based low-cost therapy in geriatrics" (Faes et al, 2007).

Ongoing management of oral intake includes the following five components: (1) calculate a daily fluid goal; (2) compare individual's current intake to the amount calculated from applying the standard, to evaluate the individual's hydration status; (3) provide fluids consistently throughout the day; (4) plan for at-risk individuals; and (5) perform fluid regulation and documentation (Mentes, 2008; www.consultgeririn.org) (Box 9-2).

CONTINENCE

Bladder Function

Normal bladder function requires an intact brain and spinal cord, competent lower urinary tract function, the motivation to maintain continence, functional ability to recognize voiding signals and use a toilet, and an environment that facilitates the process (Dowling-Castronovo and Bradway, 2008). A full bladder increases pressure and signals the spinal cord and the brainstem center of the desire to micturate. Social training then dictates whether micturition should be attended to or should be postponed until there is an appropriate opportunity to seek out toilet facilities. However, when the bladder contents reach 500 ml or more, the pressure is such that it becomes more difficult to control the urge to void. As volume increases, emptying the bladder becomes an uncontrollable act.

Age-Related Changes in Bladder Function

Bladder changes with aging include a decreased capacity, increased irritability, contractions during filling, and incomplete emptying. These changes may lead to frequency, nocturia, urgency, and vulnerability to infection. The warning period between the desire to void and actual micturition is shortened. This, in combination with age-related changes, illness, cognitive impairments, difficulty in walking to the toilet, or handling a bedpan

Box 9-2	Ongoing Management of Oral Intake

1. Calculate a daily fluid goal
   - All older adults should have an individualized fluid goal determined by a documented standard for daily fluid intake. At least 1500 ml of fluid/day should be provided.
2. Compare current intake to fluid goal to evaluate hydration status
3. Provide fluids consistently throughout the day
   - 75% to 80% of fluids delivered at meals and the remainder offered during nonmeal times such as medication times
   - Offer a variety of fluids and fluids that the person prefers
   - Standardize the amount of fluid that is offered with medication administration—for example, at least 6 oz
4. Plan for at-risk individuals
   - Fluid rounds midmorning and midafternoon
   - Provide 2 8-oz glasses of fluid in the morning and evening
   - "Happy hour" or "tea time," when residents can gather for additional fluids and socialization
   - Modified fluid containers based on resident's abilities—for example, lighter cups and glasses, weighted cups and glasses, plastic water bottles with straws (attach to wheel chairs, deliver with meals)
   - Make fluids accessible at all times and be sure residents can access them—for example, filled water pitchers, fluid stations, or beverage carts in congregate areas
   - Allow adequate time and staff for eating or feeding. Meals can provide two thirds of daily fluids
   - Encourage family members to participate in feeding and offering fluids
5. Perform fluid regulation and documentation
   - Teach individuals, if they are able, to use a urine color chart to monitor hydration status
   - Document complete intake including hydration habits
   - Know volumes of fluid containers to accurately calculate fluid consumption
   - Frequency of documentation of fluid intake will vary among settings and is dependent on the individual's condition. In most settings, at least one accurate intake and output recording should be documented, including amount of fluid consumed, difficulties with consumption, and urine specific gravity and color. For individuals who are not continent, teach caregivers to observe incontinent pads or briefs for amount and frequency of urine, color changes, and odor and report variations from individual's normal pattern

Adapted from: Mentes JC: Managing oral hydration. In Capezuti E, Zwicker D, Mezey M, Fulmer T, editors: *Evidence-based geriatric nursing protocols for best practice*, ed 3, New York, 2008, Springer; www.consultgerirn.org.

or urinal, and problems manipulating clothing, can affect an older person's ability to maintain continence. Drugs that increase urinary output and sedatives, tranquilizers, and hypnotics, which produce drowsiness, confusion, or limited mobility, promote incontinence by dulling the transmission of the desire to urinate.

Urinary Incontinence

Urinary incontinence (UI) is the involuntary loss of urine sufficient to be a problem (Dowling-Castronovo and Bradway, 2008). UI is a stigmatized, underreported, underdiagnosed, undertreated condition that is erroneously thought to be part of normal aging (Levy and Muller, 2006). About half of persons with UI have never discussed the concern with their primary care provider, and only 1 in 8 who have experienced bladder control problems have been diagnosed. On average, women wait 6.5 years from the first time they experience symptoms

until they obtain a diagnosis for their bladder control problems (Muller, 2005).

Individuals may not seek treatment for UI because of embarrassment in talking about the problem or because they do not know that successful treatments are available. Men may be unlikely to report UI to their primary care provider because they feel it is a woman's disease. A Swedish study reported that 24% of the sample of men aged 40 to 80 years reported at least one symptom of UI but the majority had not reported the symptoms to their health care provider (Engstrom et al, 2003). Further research is necessary to explore the prevalence and experience of UI in men. Older people want more information about bladder control, and nurses must take the lead in implementing approaches to continence promotion and public health education about UI (Palmer and Newman, 2006).

Without an adequate knowledge base of continence care and use of evidence-based practice guidelines, nursing care will continue to consist of containment strategies, such as the use of pads and briefs, to manage UI (Dowling-Castronova and Bradway, 2008). UI tends to be viewed as an inconvenience rather than a condition requiring assessment and treatment (MacDonald and Butler, 2007). Nurses in all practice settings with older adults should be prepared to assess data that relate to urine control and implement nursing interventions that promote continence (Dowling-Castronova and Bradway, 2008) Resources for evidence-based practice in continence care are presented in Box 9-3.

Prevalence of UI

UI affects an estimated 200 million adults worldwide (Sampselle et al, 2004). Of those who experience UI, 75% to 80% are female; the prevalence of UI increases with age and functional dependency. Estimates are that 39% of community-living older women and 30% to 70% of nursing home residents are incontinent, More than half of nursing home residents are incontinent upon admission (Shamliyan et al, 2007).

Box 9-3	Evidence-Based Resources for Continence Care

- Nursing Standard of Practice Protocol: Urinary Incontinence (UI) in Older Adults Admitted to Acute Care (Dowling-Castronova and Bradway, 2008)
- The American Geriatrics Society provides a comprehensive toolkit for management of urinary incontinence in older adults in primary care: (www.americangeriatrics.org/education/urinary_incontinence.shtml).
- The Center for Medicare and Medicaid Services (CMS) has published new interpretive guidelines for incontinence in long-term care settings (Johnson and Ouslander, 2006).
- The Borun Center provides training modules in incontinence management useful to nurses in the long-term care setting: (www.geronet.ucla.edu/centers/borun/modules/Incontinence_management/default.htm).
- Urinary Incontinence Assessment in Older Adults: Part I: Transient Urinary Incontinence (Dowling-Castronova, 2007) and Part II: Established Urinary Incontinence (Dowling-Castronova, 2008) (www.hartfordign.org)
- Prevention of Urinary and Fecal Incontinence in Adults (AHRQ) (www.ahrq.gov/downloads/pub/evidence/pdf/fuiad/fuiad.pdf)

UI is more prevalent than diabetes, Alzheimer's disease, and many other chronic conditions that have prompted more attention and treatment. Incontinence is also costly; the indirect costs are estimated at more than $16 billion annually. UI costs exceed those of coronary artery bypass surgery and renal dialysis combined (Weiss, 2005; Dowling-Castronova and Bradway, 2008).

UI is an important yet neglected geriatric syndrome (Lawhorne et al, 2008). A recent study on UI in nursing facilities (Lawhorne et al, 2008) reported that physicians, geriatric nurse practitioners, and directors of nursing evaluated and managed UI significantly less often than five other geriatric syndromes (falls, dementia, unintended weight loss, pain, and delirium). Nursing assistants were more likely to be involved in care provision for UI than any other syndrome and rated UI second only to pain with respect to its effect on quality of life. Reasons for less then optimal care for UI are multifactorial and include inadequate knowledge and skills about UI, inability to implement specific guidelines for UI care in nursing facilities, insufficient staffing, and poor communication among professionals and nursing assistants. "Because of its high prevalence and chronic but preventable nature, UI is most appropriately considered a public health problem. Nursing research is needed to test prevention programs for UI using a population-based public health focus" (Sampselle et al, 2004, p. S61).

Consequences of UI

UI affects quality of life and has physical, psychosocial, and economic consequences. UI is associated with falls, skin irritations and infections, urinary tract infections (UTIs), and pressure ulcers. UI affects self-esteem and increases the risk for depression, anxiety, social isolation, and avoidance of sexual activity. Older adults with UI experience a loss of dignity, independence, and self-confidence, as well as feelings of shame and embarrassment (MacDonald and Butler, 2007; Dowling-Castronova and Bradway, 2008). The psychosocial impact of UI affects the individual as well as the family caregivers. Two instruments are available to assess the psychological effects of UI, the Incontinence Impact Questionnaire (Uebersax et al, 1995) and the Male Urinary Symptom Impact Questionnaire (MUSIQ) (Robinson and Shea, 2002).

Risk Factors for UI

Cognitive impairment, limitations in daily activities and institutionalization are associated with higher risks of UI. Stroke, diabetes, obesity, poor general health, and comorbidities are also associated with UI (Shamliyan et al, 2007). Older people with dementia are at high risk for UI. Hospital patients with dementia are more likely than other older people to develop new incontinence. One study reported that those with dementia are 5 times more likely to develop new urinary incontinence when hospitalized (Mecocci et al, 2005).

In a study of nursing home residents with dementia, 48% were incontinent of urine upon admission, and that number increased to 81% 6 months following admission. Dementia does not cause urinary incontinence but affects the ability of the person to find a bathroom and recognize the urge to void. Mobility problems and dependency in transfers are better predictors of continence status than dementia, suggesting that persons with dementia may have the potential to remain continent as long as they are mobile. Making toilets easily visible, providing assistance to the bathroom at regular intervals, and implementing prompted voiding protocols can assist in continence promotion for people with dementia. Box 9-4 presents risk factors for UI.

Types of UI

Incontinence is classified as either transient (acute) or established (chronic). Transient incontinence has a sudden onset, is present for 6 months or less, and is usually caused by treatable factors such as UTIs, delirium, constipation and stool impaction, and increased urine production caused by metabolic conditions such as hyperglycemia and hypercalcemia. Iatrogenic (or treatment-induced) incontinence is a type of transient UI that results from the use of restraints, limited fluid intake, bed rest, or intravenous (IV) fluid administration. Use of medications such as diuretics, anticholinergic agents, antidepressants, sedatives, hypnotics, calcium channel blockers, and alpha-adrenergic agonists and blockers can also lead to transient UI (Specht, 2005).

Established UI may have either a sudden or gradual onset and is categorized into the following types: urge, stress, overflow, functional, mixed, reflex, and total incontinence.

▶ *Urge incontinence* (overactive bladder) is defined as involuntary urine loss that occurs soon after feeling an urgent need to void. The bladder muscles are overactive and cause a sudden urge to void—the "Gotta Go Right Now" syndrome (Bucci, 2007). Defining characteristics include loss of urine in moderate to large amounts before getting to the toilet and an inability to suppress the need to urinate. Frequency and nocturia may also be present. Postvoid residual urine reveals a low volume. Bladder changes in aging predispose

Box 9-4	Risk Factors for Urinary Incontinence

- Age
- Immobility, functional limitations
- Diminished cognitive capacity (dementia, delirium)
- Medications (those with anticholinergic properties, sedatives, diuretics)
- Smoking
- High caffeine intake
- Obesity
- Constipation, fecal impaction
- Pregnancy, vaginal delivery, episiotomy
- Low fluid intake
- Environmental barriers
- High-impact physical exercise
- Diabetes
- Stroke
- Parkinson's disease
- Hysterectomy
- Pelvic muscle weakness
- Childhood nocturnal enuresis
- Prostate surgery
- Estrogen deficiency
- Arthritis
- Hearing and vision impairments

Adapted from DeMaagd G: Urinary incontinence: treatment update with a focus on pharmacological management, *US Pharmacist* 32(6):34-44, 2007. Available from: www.uspharmacist.com/index.asp?show=article&page=8_2047.htm; Dowling-Castronova A, Bradway C: Urinary incontinence. In Capezuti E, Zwicker D, Mezey M, Fulmer T, editors: *Evidence-based nursing protocols for best practice*, ed 3, New York, Springer, 2008.

older adults to urge incontinence. Urge UI is the most common type of urinary incontinence in older adults (Bucci, 2007; Specht, 2005; Dowling-Castronova and Bradway, 2008).

▶ *Stress incontinence* (outlet incompetence) is defined as an involuntary loss of less than 50 ml of urine associated with activities that increase intraabdominal pressure (e.g., coughing, sneezing, exercise, lifting, bending). Stress UI is more common in women because of short urethras and poor pelvic muscle tone. Stress UI occurs in men who have experienced prostatectomy and radiation. Postvoid residual urine is low (Bucci, 2007; Specht, 2005; Dowling-Castronova and Bradway, 2008).

▶ *Overflow incontinence* is defined as the involuntary loss of urine associated with overdistention of the bladder. Causes include obstruction of the urethra by fecal impaction or an enlarged prostate, smooth muscle relaxants that relax the bladder muscle and increase bladder capacity, tumors, strictures, or an impaired ability to contract the bladder (e.g., peripheral neuropathy secondary to diabetes, neurological disorder such as multiple sclerosis). The bladder becomes overdistended, leading to frequent or constant loss of urine (dribbling). Other symptoms include hesitancy, slow urine stream, passage of infrequent or small volumes of urine, a feeling of incomplete bladder emptying, and large postvoid residuals (Bucci, 2007; Specht, 2005; Dowling-Castronova and Bradway, 2008).

▶ *Functional incontinence* refers to a situation in which the lower urinary tract is intact but the individual is unable to reach the toilet because of environmental barriers, physical limitations, or severe cognitive impairment. Individuals may be dependent on others for assistance to the toilet but have no genitourinary problems other than incontinence. Older adults who are institutionalized have higher rates of functional incontinence (Bucci, 2007; Specht, 2005; Dowling-Castronova and Bradway, 2008). Functional UI may also occur in the presence of other types of UI.

▶ *Mixed incontinence* is a combination of more than one urinary incontinence problem, usually stress and urge. Mixed UI is the most prevalent type of incontinence in older women (Shamliyan et al, 2007). With increasing age, older women with stress UI begin to experience urge UI (Specht, 2005).

▶ *Reflex incontinence* occurs when the bladder empties autonomically without the sensation to void. Reflex UI occurs with spinal cord injuries.

▶ *Total incontinence* is the continuous and unpredictable loss of urine as a result of anatomical abnormalities. It usually results from surgery, trauma, or malformation (Specht, 2005).

IMPLICATIONS FOR GERONTOLOGICAL NURSING AND HEALTHY AGING

Assessment

Continence must be routinely addressed in the initial assessment of every older person, yet many older people do not bring up their concerns about incontinence, and many health professionals do not ask.

Health care personnel must begin to change their thinking about incontinence and acknowledge that incontinence can be cured. If it cannot be cured, it can be treated to minimize its detrimental effects. Nurses are often the ones to identify urinary incontinence, but neither nurses nor physicians have been particularly aggressive in its management.

Assessment is multidimensional. It includes a health history, targeted physical examination, urinalysis, and determination of postvoid residual urine. More extensive examinations are considered after the initial findings are assessed. A thorough health history should focus on the medical, neurological, and genitourinary history; functional assessment; cognitive assessment; psychosocial effects; strategies currently used to control UI; medication review of both prescribed and over-the-counter drugs; a detailed exploration of the symptoms of the urinary incontinence; and associated symptoms and other factors. In care facilities, an environmental assessment including the accessibility of bathrooms, room lighting, and the use of aids such as raised toilet seats or commodes is also important.

In the nursing home, the completed Minimum Data Set (MDS) may trigger the Resident Assessment Protocol (RAP) for incontinence. New Center for Medicare and Medicaid Services (CMS) guidelines (F-Tag 315) requires comprehensive continence assessment, treatment, and evaluation for nursing home residents. The CHAMMP (Continence, History, Assessment, Medications, Mobility, and Plan) tool (Bucci, 2007) was developed by a certified wound, ostomy, and continence nurse to guide comprehensive continence assessment and implementation of individualized plans of care in nursing homes (Figure 9-1). The Rapid Assessment of Urinary Incontinence (Penn et al, 1996) is another instrument that can be used in all settings.

One of the best ways to establish the presence of and describe incontinence problems is with a voiding diary. The is considered the "gold standard" for obtaining objective information about the person's voiding patterns and the UI episodes and their severity (Dowling-Castronova and Bradway, 2008, p. 314) (Figure 9-2). The voiding diary can be used by both community-dwelling and institutionalized elders. Older adults in the community can usually keep a bladder diary without much difficulty. Bladder diaries for those in long-term care are usually maintained by the staff. The character of the urine (color, odor, sediment, or clear) and difficulty starting or stopping the urinary stream should be recorded. Activities of daily living (ADLs) such as ability to reach a toilet and use

CHAMP TOOL

(<u>C</u>ontinence, <u>H</u>istory, <u>A</u>ssessment, <u>M</u>edications, <u>M</u>obility, <u>P</u>lan)

C Resident is continent? Yes ___ No ___

H Medical / Surgical History:
    a. Diagnosis often associated with continence? Yes ___ No ___
        ___ BPH (prostate) ___ Diabetes ___ MS
        ___ CHF ___ Fracture ___ Osteoporosis
        ___ Constipation ___ Heart Disease ___ Pain
        ___ Contractures ___ HTN ___ Parkinson's
        ___ CVA ___ Immobility ___ Spinal Cord Injury
        ___ Dementia ___ Kidney Stones ___ UTI (last 90 days)
        ___ Depression
    b. Recent Acute Medical Condition (last 30 days)? Yes ___ No ___
        If yes, date and type:
    c. Recent Surgery (last 30 days)? Yes ___ No ___
        If yes, date and type:
    d. Surgical History: Hysterectomy ___ Bladder Repair ___ Prostate (TURP) ___ Other ___
    e. Lab Data ___ Urodynamic Studies ___ Imaging Studies ___
        Date and type:

A Assessment of Urinary Incontinence:
    Trigger Event (surgery, accident, other)? Yes ___ No ___
    Leak urine when cough, sneeze, laugh, stand up, change position? Yes ___ No ___
    Urge to go (Need to be there NOW)? Yes ___ No ___
    Wet without feeling the need to go? Yes ___ No ___
    Number of night time voids? ___
    Leak only at night? Yes ___ No ___
    Difficult to start or stop stream? Yes ___ No ___
    Weak stream? Yes ___ No ___
    Dribbling? Yes ___ No ___
    Products used? _____

M1 Medications.
    a. Current Medication:

___ Anticholinergic	___ Diuretic	___ Narcotic
___ Antidepressant	___ Hypnotic	___ OTC Cold Remedies
___ Antihypertensive	___ Laxative	___ Sedative
___ Other:		

    b. Medications to treat Incontinence:

___ Antibiotic	___ Estrogen	___ Proscar
___ Detrol	___ Flomax	___ Sanctura
___ Ditropan	___ Imipramine	___ VESIcare
___ Enablex	___ Other:	

M2 Mobility Status: I Independent, A Assist, D Dependent

___ Ambulation	___ Dressing	___ Toileting
___ Transfer		

    Can access bedpan, BSC, urinal, toilet independently (Circle):___ Yes ___ No

P Plan of care:
    a. Resident is motivated to toilet: ___ Yes ___ No ___ not oriented
    b. Resident is candidate for treatment program? Yes ___ No ___
    If no, reason:
    c. Care Plan interventions: (Circle Suggestions)
        ○ Incontinence, functional–Prompted voiding, behavioral modification (i.e., timed voiding), restorative toileting, physical and/or occupational therapy, environmental modifications
        ○ Incontinence, overflow–clean intermittent catheterization
        ○ Incontinence, stress–pelvic muscle exercises, behavior modification, medications
        ○ Incontinence, urge–pelvic muscle exercises, behavior modification, medication Incontinence, mixed (stress and urge)–pelvic muscle exercises, behavior modification, medications
        ○ Incontinence, total–check and change
    d. Bladder treatment initiated (date):
    Nurse Signature: _____ Date: _____

Fig. 9-1 *CHAMMP tool. (From Bucci A: Be a continence champion: use the CHAMMP tool to individualize the plan of care,* Geriatr Nurs *28(2):123, 2007.)*

Time Interval	Urinated in Toilet	Incontinent Episode[1]	Reason for Episode[1]	liquid Intake[3]	Bowel Movement	Product Use[3]
A.M. HOURS 12:00–01:00 AM						
01:00–02:00 AM						
02:00–03:00 AM						
03:00–04:00 AM						
04:00–05:00 AM						
05:00–06:00 AM						
06:00–07:00 AM						
07:00–08:00 AM						
08:00–09:00 AM						
09:00–10:00 AM						
10:00–11:00 AM						
11:00–12:00 PM						
P.M. HOURS 12:00–01:00 PM						
01:00–02:00 PM						
02:00–03:00 PM						
03:00–04:00 PM						
04:00–05:00 PM						
05:00–06:00 PM						
06:00–07:00 PM						
07:00–08:00 PM						
08:00–09:00 PM						
09:00–10:00 PM						
10:00–11:00 PM						
11:00–12:00 AM						

[1] **Incontinent episodes:** (++) = SMALL: did not have to change pad/ clothing; (+++) = LARGE: needed to change pad/clothing
[2] **Examples of reasons for incontinent episodes:** leaked while sneezing; leaked while running to the bathroom
[3] **Examples of type and amount of liquid intake:** 12 oz can of cola, 2 cups regular coffee
[4] **Examples of product use:** pad, undergarment; track times you changed

Fig. 9-2 Sample voiding or bladder diary. *(Adapted from Fantl C, Newman, DK, Colling J et al: Urinary incontinence in adults: acute and chronic management. Clinical Practice Guideline No. 2. AHCPR Publication No. 96-0682. Rockville, MD, 1996, Agency for Health Care Policy and Research, U.S. Department of Health and Human Services.)*

it and finger dexterity for clothing manipulation should be documented.

Interventions

Behavioral

Urinary incontinence can be improved when appropriate care is provided. A number of behavioral interventions have a good basis in research and can be implemented by nurses without extensive and expensive evaluation. These treatments are viewed as healthy bladder behavior skills (HBBSs) (Dowling-Castronova and Bradway, 2008). These interventions will do no harm and if there is no improvement, further evaluation can be sought. Behavioral techniques such as scheduled voiding, prompted voiding, bladder training, biofeedback, and pelvic floor muscle exercises (PFMEs) are recommended as first-line treatment of UI.

Selection of a modality and interventions will depend on a comprehensive assessment, the type of incontinence and its underlying cause, and whether the outcome is to cure or to minimize the extent of the incontinence. Interventions for UI should be multidisciplinary and everyone involved with the person's care should be involved in the treatment plan. If the person has mobility impairments, physical and occupational therapy and/or restorative nursing programs should be implemented as part of the treatment plan for UI. Box 9-5 lists the numerous modalities available in the treatment of incontinence. Nursing interventions focus primarily on the therapeutic modality of supportive measures and designing restorative therapeutic modalities.

▶ *Scheduled (timed) voiding* is used to treat urge and functional UI in both cognitively intact and cognitively impaired older adults. The schedule or timing of voiding is based on the person's bladder diary patterns or common voiding patterns (voiding upon arising, before and after meals, midmorning, midafternoon, and bedtime). Generally, toileting is scheduled at 2- to 4-hour intervals. People can be taught to do this

---

| **Box 9-5** | **Therapeutic Modalities in the Treatment of Incontinence** |

Support Measures
  Appropriate attitude
  Accessible toilet substitutes (bedpan, urinal, commode)
  Avoidance of iatrogenic conditions (urinary tract infections, constipation/impaction, excessive sedation, inaccessible toilets, drugs adversely affecting the bladder or urethral function)
  Protective undergarments
  Absorbent bed pads
  Behavioral techniques: bladder training, scheduled (timed) voiding, prompted voiding, biofeedback, pelvic floor muscle exercises (PFMEs)
  Good skin care

Drugs
  Bladder relaxants
  Bladder outlet stimulants

Surgery
  Suspension of bladder neck
  Prostatectomy
  Prosthetic sphincter implants
  Urethral sling
  Bladder augmentation

Mechanical and Electrical Devices Catheters
  External (condom or "Texas" catheter)
  Intermittent
  Suprapubic
  Indwelling

---

routinely or they can be assisted to the bathroom according to the scheduled intervals (Specht, 2005).

▶ *Prompted voiding* combines scheduled voiding with monitoring, prompting, and verbal reinforcement. For cognitively intact people, the objective is to increase self-initiated voiding and decrease the number of episodes of UI. For people with cognitive impairment, caregivers regularly ask whether or not they need toileting assistance. The person is assisted to the toilet if he or she requests it and receives positive feedback if he or she voids successfully. Prompted voiding may improve incontinence in 25% to 50% of residents in long-term care who are incontinent, and can also be successful in homebound older adults (Specht, 2005).

Research results indicate that prompted voiding programs are successful in long-term care but are hard to sustain. "*Targeting residents* who are likely to be successful may be of benefit in establishment of prompted voiding programs and direct scarce staff resources to residents most likely to benefit" (Lekan-Rutledge, 2006, p. 508). Barriers to implementation include inadequate staffing, lack of knowledge about UI and existing protocols, and insufficient professional staff.

Continence programs in nursing homes are both needed and required by new CMS regulations. Monitoring and documentation of continence status in relation to implemented continence care should be a *quality of care indicator* for nursing homes (Shamliyan et al, 2007). "The success of any intervention to improve continence care will need to address individual, group, organizational, and environmental level factors" (Holroyd-Leduc et al, 2006, p. 31). McConnell and colleagues (2004) reported on the success of a comprehensive continence program in a long-term care facility involving geriatric nurse practitioner students that addressed all of these factors.

▶ *Bladder training* aims to increase the time interval between the urge to void and voiding. This method is appropriate for people with urge UI who are cognitively intact and independent in toileting. Improvements in UI ranging from 44% to 100% have been reported (Specht, 2005). The person follows an established voiding schedule until UI episodes cease. Once this is achieved, the interval between voidings is extended and techniques for overcoming the urge and postponing urination are taught (pelric floor muscle exercises).

▶ *Pelvic Floor Muscle Exercises* (PFMEs), also called Kegel exercises, involve repeated voluntary pelvic floor muscle contraction. The targeted muscle is the pubococcygeal muscle, which forms the support for the pelvis and surrounds the vagina, the urethra, and the rectum. The goal of the repetitive contractions is to strengthen the muscle and decrease UI episodes. PFMEs are recommended for stress, urge, and mixed UI in older women. PFMEs have also been shown to be helpful for men who have undergone prostatectomy. Contractions should be repeated 30 to 100 times a day; the contraction is held for 10 seconds and followed by 10 seconds of relaxation.

Correct identification of the pelvic floor muscles and adherence to the exercise regimen are key to success. Improvement may not be noted until 2 to 4 weeks of exercises have been successfully completed. To help identify the correct muscle groups, it may be helpful to tell the person to try to tighten the anal sphincter (as if to control the passage of flatus or feces) and then tighten the urethral and/or vaginal muscles (as if to stop the flow of urine). The stomach, thigh, or buttocks muscles should not be contracted since this increases intraabdominal pressure. PFMEs may be taught during a vaginal or rectal examination when the clinician manually assists the person to identify the pelvic muscles by instructing the patient to squeeze around a gloved examination finger (Dowling-Castronova and Bradway, 2008). Biofeedback may be helpful in identifying the correct muscle and visualizing the strength and time of the contraction (Specht, 2005; Holroyd-Leduc et al, 2006).

▶ Vaginal weight training was introduced in Europe as an alternative for women who have difficulty identifying the pelvic floor muscles. Graded-weight vaginal balls or cones are worn during two 15-minute periods each day or are used in addition to PFMEs. When the weighted cone is placed in the vagina, the pelvic floor muscle contractions keep it from slipping out. Although this technique involves less time and is more easily taught than PFMEs, difficulty inserting the cones and discomfort have been noted as deterrents to use (Wyman, 2003).

Lifestyle Modifications

Several lifestyle factors are associated with either the development or exacerbation of UI. These include dietary factors (increased fluid, avoidance of caffeine), weight reduction, smoking cessation, bowel management, and physical activity. Box 9-6 presents other interventions helpful to noninstitutionalized elders to control or eliminate incontinence.

Box 9-6	Helpful Interventions for Noninstitutionalized Elders to Control or Eliminate Incontinence

- Empty bladder completely before and after meals and at bedtime.
- Urinate whenever the urge arises; never ignore it.
- A schedule of urinating every 2 hours during the day and every 4 hours at night is often helpful in retraining the bladder. Use of an alarm clock may be necessary.
- Drink 1½ to 2 quarts of fluid a day before 8 pm. This helps the kidneys to function properly. Limit fluids after supper to ½ to 1 cup (except in very hot weather).
- Eliminate or reduce the use of coffee, tea, brown cola, and alcohol, since they have a diuretic effect.
- Take prescription diuretics in the morning upon rising.
- Limit the use of sleeping pills, sedatives, and alcohol because they decrease sensation to urinate and can increase incontinence, especially at night.
- If overweight, lose weight.
- Exercises to strengthen pelvic muscles that help support the bladder (PFMEs) are often helpful for women with stress, urge, and mixed UI. May also be helpful for men after prostatectomy
- Make sure the toilet is nearby with a clear path to it and good lighting, especially at night. Grab bars or a raised toilet seat may be needed.
- Dress protectively with cotton underwear and protective pants or incontinent pads if necessary.

Urinary Catheters

Intermittent catheterization may be used in people with urinary retention related to a weak detrusor muscle (e.g., diabetic neuropathy), those with a blockage of the urethra (e.g., benign prostatic hypertrophy), or those with reflux incontinence related to a spinal cord injury. The goal is to maintain 300 ml or less of urine in the bladder. Most of the research on intermittent catheterization has been conducted with children or young adults with spinal cord injuries but may be useful for older adults who are able to self-catheterize. It provides an important alternative to indwelling catheterization (Specht, 2005).

Clinical guidelines indicate that indwelling catheter use is not appropriate for long-term (more than 30 days) management. Continuous indwelling catheter use is indicated for urethral obstruction or urinary retention or in patients with the following conditions:

▶ When surgical or pharmacological interventions are inappropriate or unsuccessful
▶ If contraindications are present to intermittent catheterization to treat retention
▶ When changes of bedding, clothing, and absorbent products may be painful or disruptive for a patient with an irreversible medical condition, such as metastatic terminal disease, coma, or end-stage congestive heart failure
▶ For patients with severely impaired skin integrity
▶ For patients who live alone without a caregiver or with a caregiver who is unable to routinely change the person (Newman and Palmer, 2003)

Regulatory standards in nursing homes follow these same guidelines, and the use of indwelling catheters must be justified based on medical conditions and failure of other efforts to maintain continence. The use of indwelling catheters in hospitals is often unjustified, and they are used inappropriately (convenience for staff) or left in place too long. Misuse of catheterization should be considered a medical error. About 1 in 4 indwelling catheters in hospitalized patients aged 70 and older and 1 in 3 in patients aged 85 and older turn out to be unnecessary (Inelman et al, 2007). Urinary catheterization without a specific medical indication is associated with greater risk of death and longer hospital stay (Holroyd-Leduc et al, 2007). Cognitive impairment and the presence of pressure ulcers almost doubles the risk of receiving a catheter and severe functional decline is associated with a 4-fold risk of catheter placement (Inelmen et al, 2007).

Long-term catheter use increases the risk of recurrent urinary tract infections leading to urosepsis, urethral damage in men secondary to urethral erosion, urethritis or fistula formation, and bladder stones or cancer. UTIs are the most common infections in residents in long-term care. Asymptomatic bacteria in the urine are considered benign in older people and should not be treated with antibiotics. Screening urine cultures should also not be performed in patients who are asymptomatic (Midthun et al, 2004). Symptomatic UTIs necessitate antibiotic treatment, but it is important to pay attention to the range of symptoms older patients may present. Fever, dysuria, and flank pain may not be present. Changes in mental status, decreased appetite, abdominal pain, new onset of incontinence, or even respiratory distress may signal a possible UTI in older people. Catheter care should consist of washing the meatal area with soap and water daily.

External catheters (condom catheters) are used in male patients who are incontinent and cannot be toileted. Long-term use of external catheters can lead to fungal skin infections, penile skin maceration, edema, fissures, contact burns from urea, phimosis, UTIs, and septicemia. The catheter should be removed and replaced daily and the penis cleaned, dried, and aired to prevent irritation, maceration, and the development of pressure ulcers and skin breakdown. If the catheter is not sized appropriately and applied and monitored correctly, strangulation of the penile shaft can occur.

Absorbent Products

A variety of protective undergarments or adult briefs are available for the older adult who is incontinent. Disposable types come in several sizes determined by hip and waist measurements, or one size may fit all. Many of these undergarments look like regular underwear and contribute more to dignity than the standard "diaper." Referring to protective undergarments as diapers is demeaning and infantilizing to older people and should be avoided. Some individuals may prefer to use absorbent products in addition to toileting interventions to maintain "social continence," and there is a wide variety of products available.

Pharmacological

Pharmacological treatment may be indicated for urge UI and overactive bladder (OAB). OAB symptoms include urgency, frequency, and nocturia. Drugs for urge UI and OAB include anticholinergic (antimuscarinic) agents. Commonly prescribed medications include oxybutynin (Ditropan), tolterodine (Detrol), and trospium chloride, darifenacin, and solifenacin as well as a transdermal formulation of oxybutynin. Dosages should be started very low in older adults and titrated slowly with careful attention to side effects and drug interactions. A trial of 4 to 8 weeks is adequate and recommended; there is no clear advantage in terms of efficacy between the different medications (DeMaagd, 2007). Undesirable side effects of anticholinergic medications such as dry mouth and eyes, constipation, confusion, or the precipitation of glaucoma are problematic in older people. These medications can be especially problematic for older adults with cognitive impairment (Barton et al, 2008). Medications are not considered first-line treatment; behavioral therapies are more effective and should be implemented first (Weiss, 2005).

Medications for the treatment of benign prostatic hypertrophy include the alpha-adrenergic blockers and the 5-alpha-reductase inhibitors. Alpha-adrenergic blockers are usually the therapy of choice in early, mild disease. Careful monitoring of side effects and drug interactions is necessary. The herbal saw palmetto, reported to have 5-alpha-reductase inhibitor activity, may also be used, but reports about its effectiveness are mixed (DeMaagd, 2007).

Surgical

Surgical intervention is appropriate for some conditions of incontinence. Surgical suspension of the bladder neck (sling procedure) in women has proved effective in 80% to 95% of persons electing to have this surgical corrective procedure. Outflow obstruction incontinence secondary to prostatic hypertrophy is generally corrected by prostatectomy. Sphincter dysfunction resulting from nerve damage following surgical trauma or radical perineal procedures is 70% to 90% repairable through sphincter implantation. Periurethral bulking has been added to the number of surgical procedures that address urinary incontinence. Collagen or polytetrafluoroethylene (PTFE) is injected into the periurethral area to increase pressure on the urethra. This adds bulk to the internal sphincter and closes the gap that allowed leakage to occur.

Nonsurgical Devices

Stress UI can be treated with intravaginal support devices, pessaries, and urethral plugs. An extracorporeal magnetic innervation chair (ExMI) may also be of benefit in stress UI. The ExMI strengthens pelvic floor muscles through application of a low-intensity magnetic field (Weiss, 2005). Another option is the pessary, which is primarily used to prevent uterine prolapse. The pessary is a device that is fitted into the vagina and exerts pressure to elevate the urethrovesical junction of the pelvic floor. The patient is taught to insert and remove the pessary, much like inserting and removing a diaphragm used for contraception. The pessary is removed weekly or monthly for cleaning with soap and water and then reinserted. Adverse effects include vaginal infection, low back pain, and vaginal mucosal erosion. Another concern is the danger of forgetting to remove the pessary.

Fecal or Bowel Incontinence

Fecal incontinence (FI) is defined as "continuous or recurrent uncontrolled passage of fecal material for at least 1 month in a mature person" (Stevens and Palmer, 2007, p. 35). Estimates are that more than 6.5 million Americans have fecal incontinence. Accurate estimates are hard to obtain since many people are reluctant to discuss this disorder and many primary care providers do not ask about it. Prevalence varies with the study population: 2% to 17% in community-dwelling older people, 50% to 65% in older adults in nursing homes, and 33% in hospitalized older adults. Higher prevalence rates are found among patients with diabetes, irritable bowel syndrome, stroke (new onset 30%; 15% at 3 years post-stroke), multiple sclerosis, and spinal cord injury (Roach and Christie, 2008).

Often FI is associated with urinary incontinence and as many as 50% to 70% of patients with UI also carry the diagnosis of FI. FI can be transient (episodes of diarrhea, acute illness, fecal impaction) or persistent. Fecal incontinence, like urinary incontinence, has devastating social ramifications for the individuals and families who experience it. UI and FI share similar contributing factors including damage to the pelvic floor as a result of surgery or trauma, neurologic disorders, functional impairment, immobility, and dementia. Bowel continence and defecation depend on coordination of sensory and motor innervation of the rectum and anal sphincters. Impairment of the anorectal unit, such as weakness from prolonged straining secondary to constipation or overt anal tears seen after vaginal delivery in women (35%) are common causes of FI. Injury from obstetric trauma is often delayed in onset and many women do not manifest symptoms until after the age of 50 years (Roach and Christie, 2008).

IMPLICATIONS FOR GERONTOLOGICAL NURSING AND HEALTHY AGING

Assessment

Assessment should include a complete client history as in urinary incontinence (described earlier in this chapter) and investigation into stool consistency and frequency, use of laxatives or enemas, surgical and obstetrical history, medications, effect of FI on quality of life, focused physical exam with attention to the gastrointestinal system, and a bowel record. A digital rectal examination should be performed to identify any presence of a mass, impaction, or occult blood.

Fecal impaction (Chapter 8) can be quite common in older adults. Fecal impaction is reported to occur in more than 40% of older adults admitted to the hospital (Roach and Christie, 2008). Paradoxical diarrhea, caused by the leakage of fecal material around the impacted mass, may occur. Reports of diarrhea in older adults must be thoroughly assessed before the use of anti-diarrheal medications which further complicate the problem of fecal impaction. Digital rectal examination for impacted stool and an abdominal plain film will confirm the presence of impacted stool. Stool analysis for *clostridium difficile* toxin should be ordered in patients who develop new onset diarrhea with incontinence (Bharucha et al, 2005). Other tests may be indicated based on assessment findings. Comprehensive assessment is needed to search for causes of FI that are amenable to therapeutic interventions. Maintenance of healthy bowel function and prevention of constipation are discussed in Chapter 8.

Interventions

Nursing interventions are aimed at managing and/or restoring bowel continence. Therapies similar to those used to treat urinary incontinence such as environmental manipulation (access to toilet), diet alterations, habit-training schedules, improving transfer and ambulation ability, sphincter training exercises, biofeedback, medications, and/or surgery to correct underlying defects are effective.

Keeping accurate bowel records and identifying triggers that initiate incontinence is important. For example, eating a meal stimulates defecation 30 minutes following the completion of the meal, or defecation occurs following the morning cup of coffee. If the fecal incontinence is only once or twice each day, it can be controlled by being prepared. Placing the individual on the toilet, commode, or bedpan at a given time following the trigger event facilitates defecation in the appropriate place at the appropriate time. The judicious use of nonirritant laxatives can help to maintain bowel function and prevent constipation. Suggestions for a bowel training program are presented in Box 9-7.

The effectiveness of interventions in fecal incontinence will be self-evident but will take time. As in treatment of urinary incontinence, goals must be realistic. It cannot be stated too often or too strongly that the nurse must always provide immaculate skin care to persons with incontinence because self-esteem and skin integrity depend on it.

"Caring for persons with elimination problems has been integral to basic nursing care since Florence Nightingale's time" (Wells, 1994). Gerontological nurses have a pivotal role in continence care. "In all clinical settings, people have the right to be continent" (Mason et al, 2003, p. 3). It is important that nurses and other health care providers understand the causes of UI, risk factors, and evidence-based protocols for interventions. Health promotion education, comprehensive assessments of UI, education of informal and formal caregivers, and use of evidence-based interventions should be part of individualized care for all older people experiencing UI symptoms. Gerontological nurses also need to be knowledgeable about appropriate products and devices as management options.

Resources listed at the end of this chapter and at evolve.elsevier.com/Ebersole/gerontological will be valuable to the gerontological nurse as he or she prepares for practice. Gerontological nurses may wish to pursue advanced training and certification through specialty organizations such as The Society of Urologic Nurses and Associates (www.suna.org) and the Wound, Ostomy, and Continence Nurses Society (www.wocncb.org).

APPLICATION OF MASLOW'S HIERARCHY

Meeting elimination needs is basic to the maintenance of biological and physiological integrity, but its importance reaches far higher on the hierarchy. Inadequate attention to this basic need can cause excess disability, cause insecurity, affect safety, cause social isolation and curtailment of meaningful activities and relationships, and interfere with the ability of the older person to achieve a meaningful and fulfilling life.

Box 9-7	Bowel Training Program

1. Obtain bowel history, complete a bowel record, and establish a schedule for the bowel training program that is normal and comfortable for the patient and conforms to his or her lifestyle.
2. Ensure adequate fiber and fluid intake (normalize stool consistency).
   a. Fiber
      (1) Add high-fiber foods to diet (dried fruit, dried beans, vegetables, and wheat products).
      (2) Suggest adding 1 to 3 tablespoons (tbs) bran to diet 1 or 2 times/day or use a bulk laxative (Metamucil, Citrocel, FiberCon). Titrate dosage based on response.
      (3) Use a natural laxative recipe: 1 cup wheat bran, 1 cup applesauce, 1 cup prune juice. Mix and store in re-frigerator. Start with 1 tbs/day and increase slowly until desired effect is achieved. (See Chapter 8.)
   b. Fluid
      (1) Two to three liters daily (unless contraindicated).
      (2) Four ounces of prune, fig, or pear juice (or a warm fluid) may be given daily as a stimulus (e.g., 30 to 60 minutes before the established time for defecation).
3. Encourage exercise program.
   a. Pelvic tilt, modified sit-ups for abdominal strength
   b. Walking for general muscle tone and cardiovascular system
   c. More vigorous program if appropriate
4. Establish a regular time for the bowel movement.
   a. Established time depends on the patient's schedule.
   b. Best times are 20 to 40 minutes after regularly scheduled meals, when gastrocolic reflex is active.
   c. Attempts at evacuation should be made daily within 15 minutes of the established time and whenever the pa-tient senses rectal distention.
   d. Instruct patient in normal posture for defecation. (The patient normally sits on the toilet or bedside commode; for the patient who is unable to get out of bed, the left side–lying position is best.)
   e. Instruct the patient to contract the abdominal muscles and "bear down."
   f. Have patient lean forward to increase the intraabdominal pressure by use of compression against the thighs.
   g. Stimulate anorectal reflex and rectal emptying if necessary, with one of the following alternatives:
      (1) Insert a rectal suppository or minienema into the rectum 15 to 30 minutes before the scheduled bowel movement, placing the suppository against the bowel wall
      (2) Insert a gloved, lubricated finger into the anal canal and gently dilate the anal sphincter.

KEY CONCEPTS

▶ Age-related changes in the thirst mechanism, de-crease in TBW, and decreased kidney function increase the risk for dehydration in older adults.

▶ Most healthy older adults maintain adequate hydra-tion, but the presence of physical or emotional ill-ness, surgery, trauma, or conditions of higher physi-ologic demands increase the risk of dehydration.

▶ Urinary incontinence is not a part of normal aging. UI is a symptom of an underlying problem and calls for thorough assessment.

▶ Urinary incontinence can be minimized or cured, and there are many therapeutic modalities available for treatment of UI that nurses can implement.

▶ Health promotion teaching, identification of risk fac-tors, comprehensive assessments of UI, education of informal and formal caregivers, and use of evidence-based interventions are basic continence competen-cies for nurses.

▶ A number of interventions for urinary incontinence are applicable to the management of bowel incontinence.

ACTIVITIES AND DISCUSSION QUESTIONS

1. Explain the problems associated with dehydration in the older adult.
2. Identify the signs and symptoms of dehydration in the elderly.
3. Discuss interventions to prevent and treat dehy-dration.
4. Discuss risk factors for UI in older adults.
5. Conduct a UI history with a partner or with an older adult.

6. What measures can be taken to cure or decrease urinary incontinence in the community and long-term care settings?

7. Devise a nursing care plan for an elder with urinary incontinence or fecal incontinence.

RESOURCES

Websites

National Association for Continence (*lay and professional education, UI products*)
website: www.nafc.org

Wound, Ostomy and Continence Nurses Society
website: www.wocn.org

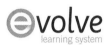

For additional resources, please visit evolve.elsevier. com/Ebersole/gerontological.

REFERENCES

American Geriatrics Society (AGS): *Geriatric review syllabus,* ed 6, New York, 2006, The Society.

Barton C, Sklenicka J, Sayegh P, Yaffe K: Contraindicated medication use among patients in a memory disorders clinic, *Am J Geriatr Pharmacother* 6(3):147-152, 2008.

Bharucha AE, Zinmeister A, Locke G et al: Prevalence and burden of fecal incontinence: population based study in women, *Gastroenterology* 129(1):42-49, 2005.

Bucci A: Be a continence champion: use the CHAMMP tool to individualize the plan of care, *Geriatr Nurs* 28(2): 120-124, 2007.

Craig S: Hyponatremia. Accessed May 7, 2008 from www.emedicine.com/emerg/topic275.htm.

Crecelius C: Dehydration: myth and reality, *J Am Med Dir Assoc* 9(5):287-288, 2008.

DeMaagd G: Urinary incontinence: treatment update with a focus on pharmacological management, *US Pharmacist* 32(6):34-44, 2007. Accessed May 10, 2008 from www.uspharmacist.com/index.asp?show=article&page= 8_2047.htm.

Donnelly G: Chronicity: concepts and reality, *Holis Nurs Prac* 8(1):1-7, 2003.

Dowling-Castronovo A: Urinary incontinence assessment in older adults: Part I—Transient urinary incontinence, 2007. Accessed December 23, 2008 from http://consultgerirn.org/uploads/File/trythis/issue11-1.pdf.

Dowling-Castronova A, Bradway C: Urinary incontinence. In Capezuti E, Zwicker D, Mezey M, Fulmer T, editors: *Evidence-based geriatric nursing protocols for best practice,* ed 3, New York, Springer, 2008.

Dowling-Castronovo A, Spiro E: Urinary incontinence assessment in older adults: Part II—Established urinary incontinence. Accessed December 23, 2008 from http://consultgerirn.org/uploads/File/trythis/issue11-2.pdf.

Engstrom G, Walker-Engstrom ML, Loof L, Leppert J: Prevalence of three lower urinary tract symptons in men—a population-based study, *Fam Pract* 20(1):7-10, 2003.

Faes MC, Spift MG, Olde Rikkert MGM: Dehydration in geriatrics, *Geriatr Aging* 10(9):590-596, 2007.

Holroyd-Leduc JM, Lyder C, Tannebaum C: Practical management of urinary incontinence in the long-term care setting, *Ann Long-Term Care* 14(2):30-37, 2006.

Holroyd-Leduc J, Sen S, Bertenthal D et al: The relationship of indwelling catheters to death, length of hospital stay, functional decline, and nursing home admission in hospitalized older medical patients, *J Am Geriatr Soc* 55(2): 227-233, 2007.

Inelmen E, Giuseppe S, Giuliano E: When are indwelling catheters appropriate in elderly patients? *Geriatrics* 62(10):18-22, 2007.

Jirovec MM, Wyman J, Wells T: Addressing urinary incontinence with educational continence—care competencies, *Image J Nurs Sch* 30(4):375-378, 1998.

Johnson T, Ouslander J: The newly revised F-Tag 315 and surveyor guidance for urinary incontinence in long-term care, *JAMDA* 7(9):594-600,2006.

Lawhorne L, Ouslander J, Parmelee P et al: Urinary incontinence: a neglected geriatric syndrome in nursing facilities, *J Am Med Dir Assoc* 9(1):9-35, 2008.

Lekan-Rutledge D: The new F-tag 315, *J Am Med Dir Assoc* 7(9):607-610, 2006.

Levy R, Muller N: Urinary incontinence: economic burden and new choices in pharmacological treatment, *Adv Ther* 23(4):556-573, 2006.

MacDonald C, Butler L: Silent no more: elderly women's stories of living with urinary incontinence in long-term care, *J Gerontol Nurs* 33(1):14-20, 2007.

Mason DJ, Newman DK, Palmer MH: Changing UI practice, *Am J Nurs* 3(Suppl):2-3, 2003.

McConnell E, Lekan-Rutledge D, Nevidjon B, Anderson R: Complexity theory: a long-term care specialty practice exemplar for the education of advanced practice nurses, *J Nurs Educ* 43(2):84-87, 2004.

Mecocci P, von Strauss E, Cherubini A et al: Cognitive impairment is the major risk factor for development of geriatric syndromes during hospitalization: results from the GIFA study, *Dement Geriatr Cogn Disord* 20(4):262-269, 2005.

Mentes JC: *Hydration management,* University of Iowa Gerontological Nursing Interventions Research Center, Research Dissemination Core, 2004. Accessed July 6, 2008 from www.guideline.gov.

Mentes JC: Managing oral hydration. In Capezuti E, Zwicker D, Mezey M, Fulmer T, editors: *Evidence-based geriatric nursing protocols for best practice,* ed 3, New York, 2008, Springer.

Mentes JC: Oral hydration in older adults: greater awareness is needed in preventing, recognizing and treating dehydration, *Am J Nurs* 106(6):40-49, 2006.

Midthun S, Paur R, Lindseth G: Urinary tract infections, *J Gerontol Nurs* 30(6):4-9, 2004.

Muller N: What Americans understand and how they are affected by bladder control problems: highlights of recent nationwide consumer research, *Urol Nurs* 25(2):109-115, 2005.

Newman DK, Palmer MH, editors: The state of the science on urinary incontinence, *Am J Nurs* 3(Suppl):1-58, 2003.

Palmer MH, Newman D: Bladder control educational needs of older adults, *J Gerontol Nurs* 32(10):28-32, 2006.

Penn C, Lekan-Rutledge D, Joers A et al: Assessment of urinary incontinence, *J Gerontol Nurs* 22(1):8-19, 1996.

Robinson JP, Shea JA: Development and testing of a measure of health-related quality of life for men with urinary incontinence, *J Am Geriatr Soc* 50(5):935–945, 2002.

Roach M, Christie J: Fecal incontinence in the elderly, *Geriatrics* 63(2):13-22, 2008.

Sampselle CM, Palmer M, Boyington A et al: Prevention of urinary incontinence in adults: population-based strategies. *Nurs Res* 53(6 Suppl):S61-S67, 2004. Review.

Shamliyan T, Wyman J, Bliss DZ et al: *Prevention of fecal and urinary incontinence in adults.* Evidence Report/Technology Assessment No. 161 (Prepared by the Minnesota Evidence-based Practice Center under Contract No. 290-02-0009) AHRQ Publication No 08-E003. Rockville, MD. Agency for Healthcare Research and Quality, 2007. Accessed July 6, 2008 from www.ahrq.gov/downloads/pub/evidence/pdf/fuiad/fuiad.pdf.

Simmons SF, Alessi C, Schnelle JF: An intervention to increase fluid intake in nursing home residents: prompting and preference compliance, *J Am Geriatr Soc* 49(7):926-933, 2001.

Specht J: 9 myths of incontinence in older adults: both clinicians and the over-65 set need to know more, *Am J Nurs* 105(6):58-68, 2005.

Stevens T, Palmer R: Fecal incontinence in LTC patients, *LTC Clin Interface* 8(4):35-39, 2007.

Thomas D, Cote T, Lawthorne L et al: Understanding clinical dehydration and its treatment, *Journal of the American Medical Directors Association* 9(5):292-301, 2008.

Uebersax JS, Wyman JF, Shumaker SA, McClish DK, Fantl JA: Short forms to assess life quality and symptom distress for urinary incontinence in women: the Incontinence Impact Questionnaire and the Urogenital Distress Inventory. Continence Program for Women Research Group. *Neurourol Urodyn* 14(2):131-9, 1995.

Weiss B: Selecting medications for the treatment of urinary incontinence, *Am Fam Physician* 71(2):315, 2005.

Wells TJ: Nursing research on urinary incontinence, *Urol Nurs* 14(3):109-112, 1994.

Wyman J: Treatment of urinary incontinence in men and older women, *Am J Nurs* 3(Suppl):38-45, 2003.

Xiao H, Barber J, Campbell E: Economic burden of dehydration among hospitalized elderly patients, *Am J Health Syst Pharm* 61(23):2534-2540, 2004.

Rest, Sleep, and Activity

10

LEARNING OBJECTIVES

Upon completion of this chapter, the reader will be able to:

- Identify age-related changes that affect rest, sleep, and activity.
- Discuss the importance of sleep and activity to the health and well-being of older adults.
- Describe nursing assessment relevant to rest, sleep, and activity.
- Explain nursing interventions useful in the promotion of rest, sleep, and activity.

GLOSSARY

Circadian rhythm Regular recurrence of certain phenomena in cycles of approximately 24 hours.
Insomnia Subjective perception of insufficient or nonrestorative sleep.
Non–rapid eye movement (NREM) sleep First four stages of sleep.

Obstructive sleep apnea Repetitive cessation (>10 seconds) of respiration during sleep.
Rapid eye movement (REM) sleep Wakeful and active form of sleep during which dreaming occurs or tension is discharged.

THE LIVED EXPERIENCE

You know, I never get a decent night's sleep. I wake up at least 4 times every night, and I just know I won't get back to sleep. I really don't want to keep taking pills for sleep, but when I lie there awake, I just think of all the difficult times and situations I can't manage. After a while, I'm really in a stew about everything.

Richard, a 67-year-old recent retiree

This is really beginning to tire me out. Richard keeps waking me at night because he can't sleep. I try to tell him to get up and read or something. I really need my sleep if I'm going to get to work on time. I wonder if Richard needs to see a doctor. Maybe he is depressed about being retired and alone while I'm at work. I'll talk to him about it.

Clara, Richard's wife

Rest, sleep, and activity depend on one another. Inadequacy of rest and sleep affects any activity, whether it is considered strenuous exertion or falls under the heading of the activities of daily living. Activity, in turn, is necessary to maintain physical and physiological integrity, such as cardiopulmonary endurance and function, musculoskeletal strength, agility, and structure, and it helps a person obtain adequate sleep. Rest, sleep, and activity contribute greatly to overall physical and mental well-being.

REST AND SLEEP

The human organism needs rest and sleep to conserve energy, prevent fatigue, provide organ respite, and relieve tension. Sleep is an extension of rest, and both are physiological and mental necessities for survival. Sleep is a basic need. Rest occurs with sleep in sustained unbroken periods. Sleep is restorative and recuperative and is necessary for the preservation of life. Nearly one-third of our lives are spent in rest and sleep.

In older adults, sleep is a barometer of health. Sleep assessment and interventions for sleep concerns should receive as much attention as other vital signs (Zee and Bloom, 2006). Complaints of sleep difficulty are common among older adults. Aging is associated with changes in the amount of sleep, sleep quality, and specific sleep pathologies and disorders such as insomnia, sleep apnea, restless legs syndrome, and circadian rhythm disturbances (Zee and Bloom, 2006; Subramanian and Surani, 2007).

Biorhythm and Sleep

Our lives proceed in a series of rhythms that influence and regulate physiological function, chemical concentrations, performance, behavioral responses, moods, and the ability to adapt. Gerontologists are beginning to seriously study the relevance of age-related changes in circadian rhythms to health and the process of aging. It is clear that body temperature, pulse, blood pressure, neurotransmitter excretion, and hormonal levels change significantly and predictably in a circadian rhythm.

With aging, there is a reduction in the amplitude of all of these circadian endogenous responses. The most important and obvious biorhythm is the circadian sleep-wake rhythm. Abnormalities of this endogenous cycle may be responsible for some of the difficulties of old age.

Sleep and Aging

The predictable pattern of normal sleep is called sleep architecture (Subramanian and Surani, 2007). The body progresses through the five stages of the normal sleep pattern consisting of rapid eye movement (REM) sleep and non–rapid eye movement (NREM) sleep. Sleep structure is shown in Box 10-1.

Sleep architecture changes in aging, and the older the individual, the more changes that will be experienced. Less time is spent in stages 3 and 4 sleep and more time spent awake or in stage 1 sleep. Declines in stages 3 and 4 sleep begin between 20 and 30 years of age and are nearly complete by the age of 50 to 60 years. The amount of deep sleep in stages 3 and 4 contributes to

---

Box 10-1   Sleep Structure

Four Stages of Non–Rapid Eye Movement (NREM) Sleep
Stage 1
  Lightest level
  Easy to awaken
  Comprises 5% of sleep in young
Stage 2
  Decreases with age
  Low-voltage activity on electroencephalogram (EEG)
  May cease in old age
Stage 3
  Decreases with age
  High-voltage activity on EEG
  May cease in old age
Stage 4
  Decreases with age
  High-voltage activity on EEG
  Comprises 15% of sleep in elders

Rapid Eye Movement (REM) Sleep
  Alternates with NREM sleep throughout the night
  Rapid eye movements are the key feature
  Breathing increases in rate and depth
  Muscle tone relaxed
  85% of dreaming occurs in REM sleep

Adapted from Beers MH, Berkow R: *The Merck manual of geriatrics,* ed 3, Whitehouse Station, NJ, 2000, Merck Research Laboratories.

---

how rested and refreshed a person feels the next day. Time spent in REM sleep also declines with age, and transitions between stages 1 and 2 are more common.

Among older adults, sleep is lighter, more fragmented, and characterized by frequent awakenings (Subramanian and Surani, 2007). Older people report more time in bed, reduced total sleep time, prolonged sleep latency (time it takes to fall asleep), more frequent awakenings, increased wakefulness after sleep onset, and increased frequency of daytime naps (Cefalu, 2004). Sleep deprivation and fragmentation of sleep in older adults may adversely affect cognitive functioning, pain, respiratory function, and general health status. (Missildine, 2008).

In the National Sleep Foundation (NSF) 2006 survey of sleep patterns and complaints of people aged 55 to 84 years (www.sleepfoundation.org), approximately two thirds of the 1506 respondents complained of a sleep problem at least a few nights a week (Zee and Bloom, 2006). Sleep deprivation and fragmentation of sleep may be greater when older adults are hospitalized or in a nursing home (Chaperon et al, 2007). The changes that occur in sleep with aging are summarized in Box 10-2.

"Age-related diminishment of circadian regulation and synchrony of body temperature, rest/activity, and melatonin rhythms with the environment are known to disrupt sleep" (Chaperon et al, 2007, p. 22). Older people may not be exposed to adequate amounts of bright outdoor light, particularly in certain climates or when residing in nursing homes. Bright-light therapy (exposure to bright outdoor light or the use of an indoor light box later in the afternoon) may assist in resetting the circadian rhythm (Chaperon et al, 2007; La Reau et al, 2008).

Older adults with good general health, positive moods, and engagement in more active lifestyles and meaningful activities report better sleep and fewer sleep complaints. "Poor sleep is not an inevitable consequence of aging. Also, contrary to popular opinion, healthy elderly persons do not need less sleep than do younger ones" (Zee and Bloom, 2006). Poor

sleep is an indicator of health status and calls for investigation.

Sleep Disorders

Insomnia

Insomnia is a "subjective perception of insufficient or nonrestorative sleep (Subramanian and Surani, 2007). Insomnia can be classified as sleep-onset insomnia, sleep-maintenance insomnia, or nonrestorative sleep (awakening without feeling refreshed or rested). Insomnia has a higher prevalence in older adults and is the result of numerous factors (Box 10-3).

Comorbid medical and psychiatric conditions contribute to insomnia in older adults. Nocturia was the most common reason for interrupted sleep in the NSF

Box 10-2	Age-Related Sleep Changes

- More time spent in bed awake before falling asleep
- Total sleep time and sleep efficiency are reduced
- Awakenings are frequent, increasing after age 50 (>30 minutes of wakefulness after sleep onset in >50% of older subjects).
- Daytime napping
- Changes in circadian rhythm (early to bed, early to rise)
- Sleep is subjectively and objectively lighter (more stage 1, little stage 4, more disruptions)
- Rapid eye movement (REM) sleep is short, less intense, and more evenly distributed.
- Frequency of abnormal breathing events is increased
- Frequency of leg movements during sleep is increased

Adapted from: Subramanian S, Surani S: Sleep disorders in the elderly, *Geriatrics* 62(12):10-32, 2007, Accessed 12/17/07 from http://geri.com/geriatrics/content/printContentPopup.jsp?id=477152.

Box 10-3	Factors Contributing to Sleep Problems in Older Adults

- Age-related changes in sleep architecture
- Comorbidities (cardiovascular disease, diabetes, pulmonary disease, musculoskeletal disorders), CNS disorders (Parkinson's disease, seizure disorder, dementia), GI disorders (hiatal hernia, GERD, PUD), urinary disorders (incontinence, BPH)
- Depression, anxiety, delirium, psychosis
- Polypharmacy
- Life stressors
- Limited exposure to sunlight
- Environmental noises, institutional routines
- Poor sleep hygiene
- Lack of exercise
- Excessive napping
- Caregiving for a dependent elder
- Sleep apnea
- Restless legs syndrome
- Periodic leg movement
- Rapid eye movement behavior disorder
- Alcohol
- Smoking

BPH, Benign prostatic hyperplasia; *CNS*, central nervous system; *GI*, gastrointestinal; *GERD*, gastroesophageal reflux disease; *PUD*, peptic ulcer disease.
Adapted from: Subramanian S, Surani S: Sleep disorders in the elderly, *Geriatrics* 62(12):10-32, 2007, Accessed 12/17/07 from: http://geri.com/geriatrics/content/printContentPopup.jsp?id=477152.

study. Gastroesophageal reflux disease (GERD) is a common cause of sleeplessness. More than 20% more acid is produced during REM sleep. Because the esophageal sphincter at the gastric inlet is more relaxed in elders, acid refluxes into the esophagus, which does not have the same protective lining as the stomach. Over time, the lining of the esophagus becomes scarred and protective secretions emerge into the back of the throat, resulting in frequent coughing during sleep. Treatment includes elevating the head of the bed (not just the mattress) 7 to 8 inches so gravity keeps the secretions in the lower part of the esophagus. Other treatments include avoidance of caffeine and alcohol and the use of proton pump inhibitor medications.

Sleep problems among older adults with dementia can include sleeping too much or too little, wandering during the night, or early rising (Voelker, 2007). "Disturbances in rest-activity rhythm where nighttime sleep is severely fragmented and daytime activity is disrupted by multiple napping episodes are prominent and disabling symptoms in Alzheimer's disease" (Subramanian and Surani, 2007). A high incidence of sleep-disordered breathing (SDB) has been reported in patients with Alzheimer's disease and has been shown to be related to agitation.

Anxiety and depression also contribute to insomnia. A recent study reported that female caregivers with high depressive symptoms were twice as likely to report sleep problems than noncaregivers (Kochar et al, 2007). Prescription and nonprescription medications contribute to insomnia in older people. The side effects of many common medications used by older people include sleep disturbances (Box 10-4). A medication review is always indicated when investigating sleep complaints.

Sleep Apnea

Obstructive sleep apnea (OSA) is a disorder characterized by repetitive cessation (>10 seconds) of respiration during sleep (Reuben et al, 2006). It may be further characterized by hypopnea—a transient reduction in airflow during sleep with diminished oxygen saturation for longer then 10 seconds. When breathing is inadequate, a "fire alarm" goes off and the person is aroused from slumber, normal ventilation then occurs, and the person tries to go back to sleep.

Symptoms of OSA include daytime fatigue, loud periodic snoring, broken sleep with frequent awakenings, gasping and choking on awakenings, unusual nighttime activity such as sitting upright or falling out of bed, morning headache, poor memory and intellectual functioning, and irritability and personality change.

Box 10-4   Medications That Can Cause Insomnia

Antidepressants
- Selective serotonin reuptake inhibitors (SSRIs)
- Monoamine oxidase inhibitors (MAOIs)
- Bupropion
- Venlafaxine

Antihypertensives
Clonidine
β-blockers (Propranolol, Atenolol)
Methyldopa
Reserpine

Anticholinergics
- Ipratropium (Atrovent)

Antineoplastics
- Medroxyprogesterone
- Pentostatin
- Interferon
- Leuprolide

Sympathomimetic Amines
- Bronchodilators
- Xanthine derivatives (theophylline)
- Decongestants (pseudoephedrine, phenylpropanolamine)

Hormones
- Thyroid preparations
- Cortisone
- Progesterone

Neurologic Agents
- Phenytoin
- Topiramate
- Levodopa

Miscellaneous
- Alcohol
- Nicotine
- Opiates
- Quinadine
- Excedrin
- Cough and cold medications
- Anacin
- Diuretics (if used late in the day, they produce nocturia, waking the person)

Adapted from Zee P, Bloom H: Understanding and resolving insomnia in the elderly, *Geriatrics (Suppl* May):1-12, 006.

Sleep is very fragmented and not restorative or refreshing. Older adults with sleep apnea demonstrate significant cognitive decline compared to younger people with the same disease severity. The diagnosis of sleep apnea is often delayed in older adults and symptoms blamed on age (Subramanian and Surani, 2007).

Age-related decline in the activity of the upper airway muscles, which results in compromised pharyngeal patency, predisposes older adults to OSA. Identification, evaluation, and appropriate treatment of OSA are included in the goals of *Healthy People 2010* (U.S. Department of Health and Human Services, 2002). Risk factors for sleep apnea are listed in Box 10-5.

Assessment. Assessment includes information from the sleeping partner, and a sleep study is usually considered. Recognition of OSA in older adults may be more difficult since many are widowed and may not have a sleeping partner to report symptoms (Subramanian and Surani, 2007). If there is a sleeping partner, he or she may move to another room to sleep because of the disturbance to his or her own rest. Physical assessment often reveals that the individual is obese. The neck is often short and thick. The uvula is large, and the soft palate hangs low. Tonsils may be enlarged; adenoids are enlarged; and there may be a small or receded chin. It is important to observe for upper airway tumors or cysts.

Interventions. Therapy will depend on the severity of the sleep apnea. Specific treatment of sleep apnea may involve weight loss, avoidance of alcohol and sedatives, cessation of smoking, and avoiding supine sleep positions. There should be risk counseling about impaired judgment from sleeplessness and the possibility of accidents when driving. Continuous positive airway pressure (CPAP) is the most effective treatment and the treatment of choice for older adults.

Restless Leg Syndrome

Restless legs syndrome (RLS) is a sensorimotor neurologic disorder characterized by the uncontrollable need to move the legs, often accompanied by discomfort in the legs. Other symptoms include paresthesias; creeping sensations; crawling sensations; tingling, cramping, burning sensations; pain; or even indescribable sensations. RLS occurs at rest or during inactivity and may be temporarily relieved by movement. The estimated prevalence of RLS among people over 65 years of age is 10% to 20%. RLS disrupts sleep, and sleep complaints are the primary reason patients seek treatment (Winkelman et al, 2007).

Secondary RLS occurs with Parkinson's disease, iron-deficiency anemia, uremia, and polyneuropathies. Antidepressants and neuroleptic medications can aggravate RLS symptoms. Diagnosis of RLS includes ruling out and/or treating as indicated any medical condition. Oral iron supplements should be prescribed for patients with serum iron levels lower than 45 mcg/L (Winkelman et al, 2007). Nonpharmacological therapy includes mild to moderate physical activity, hot baths, and engrossing mental activity before bedtime, avoidance of alcohol, and antidepressants and dopamine antagonist medications. Dopamine-receptor agonists (pramipexole, ropinirole) are the drugs of choice for RLS. Gabapentin may also be effective for individuals with comorbid RLS and peripheral neuropathy (Winkelman et al, 2007).

Rapid Eye Movement Sleep Behavior Disorder

Rapid eye movement sleep behavior disorder (RBSD) is a sleep disorder common in older adults. The mean age at emergence is 60 years, and RBSD is more common in males. "RBSD is characterized by loss of normal voluntary muscle atonia during REM sleep associated with complex behavior while dreaming" (Subramanian and Surani, 2007). Patients report elaborate enactment of their dreams, often with violent content, during sleep. This may include violent behaviors such as punching

---

Box 10-5	**Risk Factors for Sleep Apnea**

- Increasing age
- Increased neck circumference
- Male sex
- Anatomical abnormalities of the upper airway
- Upper airway resistance and/or obstruction
- Family history
- Excess weight
- Use of alcohol, sedatives, or tranquilizers
- Smoking
- Hypertension

Data from: McCance KL, Huether SE, *Pathophysiology: the biologic basis for disease in adults and children,* ed 5, St. Louis, 2006, Mosby; Phillips B: Sleep apnea, periodic leg movement, restless legs syndrome and cardiovascular complications. In Sleep disorders in the geriatric population: implications for health, *Clin Geriatrics* (Suppl Dec):2005, American Geriatrics Society.

and kicking, with the potential for injury of both the patient and the bed partner.

RBSD may be primary or secondary to neurodegenerative diseases such as Parkinson's disease, diffuse Lewy body disease, Alzheimer's disease, and progressive supranuclear palsy. RBSD may be an early sign of Parkinson's disease. Within 5 to 8 years of being diagnosed with RBSD, 60% to 80% of individuals develop Parkinson's disease (Brooks and Peever, 2008). Caffeine and some medications (selective serotonin reuptake inhibitors [SSRIs], tricyclic antidepressants [TCAs]) may also contribute to RBSD. Interventions include neurological examination, removal of aggravating medications, and counseling related to safety measures in the sleep environment. Clonazepam and/or melatonin may be effective in treating RBSD (Boeve et al, 2004).

IMPLICATIONS FOR GERONTOLOGICAL NURSING AND HEALTHY AGING

Assessment

Sleep habits should be reviewed with older adults in all settings. Many people do not seek treatment for insomnia and may blame poor sleep on the aging process. Nurses are in an excellent position to assess sleep, to improve the quality of the older person's sleep, and to study sleep or assist in sleep research by being available at customary sleep times.

The nurse should learn how well the person sleeps at home, how many times the person is awakened at night, what time the person retires, and what rituals occur at bedtime. Rituals include bedtime snacks, watching television, listening to music, or reading—activities whose execution is crucial to the individual's ability to fall asleep. Other assessment data should include the amount and type of daily exercise; favorite position when in bed; room environment, including temperature, ventilation, and illumination; activities engaged in several hours before bedtime; medications taken for sleep as well as information about all medications taken. Additional assessment data includes information about the individual's involvement in hobbies, life satisfaction, perception of health status, and assessment for depression. The patient's bed partner, caregivers, and/or family members can also provide valuable information about the person's sleep habits and lifestyle.

Subjective and objective measures included in sleep assessment that are available to nurses include visual analog scales, subjective rating scales (e.g., 0 to 10 or 0 to 100), questionnaires that determine if one's sleep is disturbed, interviews, and daily sleep charts. A self-rating scale, the Pittsburgh Sleep Quality Index (PSQI), can be used to measure the quality and patterns of sleep in the older adult (www.hartfordign.org). An on-line video demonstrating assessment of sleep using the PSQI can be found at http://links.lww.com/A262. Objective measures include polysomnography conducted in sleep laboratories, including electroencephalograms (EEGs), electromyograms (EMGs), and direct observations.

The sleep diary or log is noted as an important part of assessment. This information will provide an accurate account of the person's sleep problem and help identify the sleep disturbance. Usually a family member, or the caregiver if the older person is institutionalized, records specific behaviors on a flow sheet. A period of 2 to 4 weeks is needed to obtain a clear picture of the sleep problem (Box 10-6).

Interventions

Interventions begin after a thorough sleep history has been recorded and, if possible, a sleep log obtained. Management is directed at identifiable causes. Pharmacological treatment should be considered an adjuvant treatment to nonpharmacological interventions. Attention to sleep hygiene principles is important to promote good sleep habits (Box 10-7). Cognitive behavioral therapy (CBT) using stimulus control, sleep restriction

Box 10-6	Sleep Diary

Instructions: Record the following for 2 to 4 weeks. To be completed by the person or caregiver if the person is unable.
1. The number of times a call for assistance to the bathroom or for pain medication or subjective symptoms of inability to sleep (e.g., anxiety) occur
2. Whether the person appears to be asleep or awake when checked during the night
3. If sleep medication was given and if repeated
4. The time the person awakens in the morning (approximation)
5. Where the person falls asleep in the evening
6. Daytime naps

Box 10-7	Sleep Hygiene Rules

1. Make sure the bedroom is restful and comfortable.
2. Use the bedroom only for sleep and sex; do not watch television from bed or work in bed.
3. Have a regular bedtime and wake-up time even on weekends.
4. Avoid naps. If you must nap, sleep no longer than 30 minutes in early afternoon (before 3 PM).
5. Get regular exercise, but avoid exercising within 4 hours of bedtime.
6. Get regular exposure to natural light.
7. Wind down during the evening; have a bedtime routine, such as *brush teeth, set alarm clock, and read.*
8. Limit caffeine (tea, cola, coffee, chocolate), nicotine, and diuretics, especially late in the day.
9. Avoid alcohol for at least 2 hours before bedtime, and don't use alcohol to promote sleep.
10. If you have reflux, eat the evening meal at least 3 to 4 hours before bedtime; have a light snack if needed before bedtime. Avoid being too hungry or too full at bedtime.
11. Give attention to the bed environment (comfortable bed, pillows between the knees, quiet, darkness, comfortable temperature).
12. Do not watch the clock, which increases anxiety and pressure to sleep; if anxious, take a warm bath.
13. Avoid working on the computer before bedtime.
14. If you cannot fall asleep, get up and go to another room. Stay up as long as needed to feel sleepy. Return to bed when sleepy. If unable to sleep again after 10 minutes, repeat and get up as long as needed.

Adapted from Beers MH, Berkow R: *Merck manual of geriatrics,* ed 3, Whitehouse Station, NJ, 2000; Zee P, Bloom H: Understanding and resolving insomnia in the elderly, *Geriatrics* (Suppl May):1-12, 2006.

therapy, and relaxation therapy are effective and produce sustained positive effects. Box 10-8 presents other nonpharmacologic therapies for sleep disorders.

McCurry and colleagues (2005) conducted a treatment program using behavioral strategies with persons with dementia and their caregivers living in the community. Results indicate that persons with AD benefit from behavioral techniques (sleep hygiene education, daily walking, increased light exposure). In institutional settings, promotion of a good sleep environment

is important. A sleep improvement protocol, including do-not-disturb periods; provision of usual bedtime routines; and use of soft music, relaxation techniques, massage, and aromatherapy might improve sleep in hospital and nursing home settings. A multidisciplinary approach to identify sources of noise and light, such as equipment and staff interactions, could result in modification without compromising safety and quality of patient care (Missildine, 2008). Alessi and colleagues (2005) reported a significant reduction in daytime sleeping and an increased participation in social and physical activity and social conversations among nursing home residents with the following interventions:

▶ Encouraging residents to stay out of bed between 8:00 AM and 8:00 PM
▶ Providing 30 minutes or more of sunlight exposure in a comfortable outdoor location
▶ Providing low-level physical activity 3 times a day
▶ Keeping noise down, reducing light in hallways and resident rooms, and performing necessary care (e.g. turning, changing) when the individual is awake rather than waking the individual up between the hours of 10:00 PM and 6:00 AM

Further research is needed, and gerontological nurses should take an active role in design of such studies. Box 10-9 provides additional suggestions to promote sleep in nursing homes.

Aromatherapy has also been mentioned as beneficial in sleep promotion. Common essential oils to try for insomnia include *Lavandula angustifolia* (true lavender), *Chamaemelum nobile* (Roman chamomile), *Salvia sclarea* (Clary sage), *Santalum album* (sandalwood), and *Rosa damascene* (rose). Ethnicity and learned memory of smell influence the choice of essential oil. Hispanics and Latinos tend to prefer *Origanum majorana* (sweet marjoram) to lavender, African Americans often prefer *Elettaria cardamomum* (cardamom) to lavender, and Asians prefer *Cananga odorata* (ylang-ylang). Assessment for allergies as well as individual taste is important. The person can place a cotton ball with a few drops of oil under the pillowcase when going to bed, pin a handkerchief with oil to the pajamas, drop oil in a diffuser, or add a few drops to a before-bedtime bath (Buckle, 2002).

Medications may be used in combination with behavioral interventions but must be chosen carefully, started at the lowest possible dosage, and monitored closely to avoid untoward effects in older adults. Patients should be educated on the proper use of medications and their side effects. Sedatives and hypnotics, including benzodiazepines and barbiturates, should be

Box 10-8	Nonpharmacological Therapies for Sleep Disorders

Behavioral Therapy
Stimulus control therapy: The bedroom is to be used for sleep and sexual activity only. Goal is to strengthen the emotional association of the bedroom with sleeping instead of insomnia.

Relaxation Techniques
Progressive relaxation exercises, guided imagery, meditation, and electromyographic biofeedback techniques. Goal is to minimize physical and emotional stressors that affect sleep.

Temporal Control Therapy
Goal is to promote the consistency of the sleep-wake cycle by maintaining a set time to go to bed and get up, regardless of the quality and quantity of sleep. Daytime napping is to be avoided.

Sleep Restriction Therapy
Time spent in bed is limited to actual sleeping. Mild sleep deprivation is allowed to develop, which is expected to enhance ability to sleep.

Exercise
Regular exercise during the day enhances sleep ability. Exercise is to be avoided within 4 hours of bedtime

Light Therapy
Exposure to natural light, use of a light box, eliminating nighttime light (especially in institutions). "Light is the main external stimulus responsible for setting the body's internal clock to time of day. Lack of natural light or artificial day-night light cycles may distort the natural day-night light cycle and disturb natural cures for external rhythms. The amount of light needed for synchrony of rhythms to time of day is assumed to be approximately 3 hours of 1000 lux during the active phase" (Chaperon et al, 2007, p. 23).

Data from Chaperon C, Farr L, LoChiano E: Sleep disturbance of residents in a continuing care retirement community, *J Gerontol Nurs* 33(10):21-28, 2007; Zee P, Bloom H: Understanding and resolving insomnia in the elderly, *Geriatrics (Suppl* May):1-12, 2006.

Box 10-9	Suggestions to Promote Sleep in Nursing Homes

- Limit intake of caffeine and other fluids in excess before bedtime.
- Provide a light snack or warm beverage before bedtime.
- Maintain a quiet environment: soft lights, quiet music, and limited noise and staff intrusions when possible.
- Reduce nursing interruptions for resident medication administration by modifying dose schedule if possible.
- Discontinue invasive treatments when possible (Foley catheters, percutaneous gastrostomy tubes [PEG] tubes, intravenous lines).
- Encourage and assist to the bathroom before bed and as needed.
- Give pain medication before bedtime for patients with pain.
- Provide regular exercise or walking programs.
- Allow resident to stay out of bed and out of the room for as long as possible before bed if possible.
- Institute same time for resident to arise and get out of bed every morning.
- Maintain comfortable temperature in room; provide blankets as needed.
- Provide meaningful activities during the daytime.

Adapted from Cefalu C: Evaluation and management of insomnia in the institutionalized elderly, *Ann Long-Term Care* 12(6):25, 2004.

avoided. Over-the-counter (OTC) drugs such as diphen-hydramine, often thought to be relatively harmless, should be avoided because of antihistaminic and anti-cholinergic side effects. The benzodiazepine receptor agonists such as zolpidem, eszopiclone, and zaleplon have shorter half-lives and more favorable safety profiles for older adults. A new medication, ramelteon, a melatonin receptor agonist that promotes sleep via action on the circadian system, may cause less psychomotor and cognitive impairment in older people (Zee and Bloom, 2006; Subramanian and Surani, 2007).

ACTIVITY

Activity is a direct use of energy in voluntary and involuntary physical and mental ways that alters the microenvironment and the macroenvironment of the individual. Few factors contribute as much to health in aging as being physically active. Improving participation for people of all ages in regular physical activity to improve functional fitness and overall physical and mental health is one of the goals of *Healthy People 2010* (Box 10-10) (U.S. Department of Health and Human Services, 2002). Regular physical activity throughout life is likely to enhance health and functional status as people age while also decreasing the number of chronic illnesses and mobility and functional limitations often assumed to be part of growing older.

Physical activity is important for all older people, not just active healthy elders. Studies have found that increasing physical activity improves health outcomes in persons with chronic illnesses (regardless of severity) and in those with functional impairment (Fahlman et al, 2007; Ferrucci and Simonsick, 2006). The benefit of exercise (improvement in walking speed, strength, functional abilities) of frail nursing home residents with

diagnoses ranging from arthritis to lung disease and dementia has also been shown (Fiatarone et al, 1994; Hughes et al, 2005b). Regardless of age or situation, the older person can find some activity suitable for his or her condition. It is important to keep older people moving any way possible for as long as possible.

Despite a large body of evidence about the benefits of physical activity to maintain and improve function, 33% of men and 50% of women older than 75 years engage in no physical activity (CDC, 2007). Only 4% of sedentary older adults have met the *Healthy People 2010* (USDHHS, 2000) physical activity and strength training objectives (Struck and Ross, 2006). Older people are less likely to receive exercise counseling from primary care providers than younger individuals (Centers for Disease Control [CDC], 2007).

The prevalence of inactivity varies by race, sex, and ethnic group, with older women and black elders having higher rates of inactivity (Hughes et al, 2005a). The levels of physical activity among older adults have not improved over the past decade in the United States. Inactivity poses serious health hazards to young and old alike. It can lead to hypertension, coronary artery disease, osteoporosis, obesity, tension, chronic fatigue, premature aging, depression, poor musculature, inadequate flexibility, and decreased cognitive function (Colcombe et al, 2006).

Many older people mistakenly believe that they are too old to begin an active fitness program. Even a small amount of time (at least 30 minutes of moderate activity several days a week) can improve health. Ferrucci and Simonsick comment that the "health benefits of exercise also result in considerable improvements in health and quality of life and a sizeable reduction in health care costs" (2006, p. 1155). These authors call for a new "societal and cultural appreciation of exercise

---

Box 10-10	*Healthy People 2010* **Physical Activity and Fitness Goals and Objectives (Adults)**

- Reduce the proportion of adults who engage in no leisure-time physical activity.
- Increase the proportion of adults who engage regularly, preferably daily, in moderate physical activity for at least 30 minutes per day.
- Increase the proportion of adults who engage in vigorous physical activity that promotes the development and maintenance of cardiorespiratory fitness 3 or more days per week for 20 or more minutes per occasion.
- Increase the proportion of adults who perform physical activities that enhance and maintain muscular strength and endurance.
- Increase the proportion of adults who perform physical activities that enhance and maintain flexibility.

U.S. Department of Health and Human Services: *Healthy people 2010*, Hyattsville, MD, 2002, Public Health Service.

in old age . . . and the development of new and creative ways of making exercise a joyful and rewarding experience, particularly for the lifelong sedentary"(p. 1155).

IMPLICATIONS FOR GERONTOLOGICAL NURSING AND HEALTHY AGING

Assessment

Assessment of functional abilities and exercise counseling should be included as part of the health assessment of all older adults. "Appropriate screening prior to beginning a physical activity/exercise program is recommended to insure that older adults engage in safe physical activity programs that optimize function and overall health status and prevent injuries" (Resnick et al, 2006, p. 2). Two tools, both available in web format, the Exercise and Screening for You (EASY) tool (www.easyforyou.info/), and the Physical Activity Readiness Questionnaire (PAR-Q) (www.stanford.edu/dept/pe/fitness/parq.pdf), can be used to screen older adults before initiating a moderate level of physical activity. Based on the results of the initial screening, older adults may need to be evaluated by their primary care provider. Frail or vulnerable older adults will need assessment by a primary care provider and require close monitoring to ensure benefit without compromising safety.

Interventions

Suggestions for exercise programs are based on the patient's medical history, focusing on both cardiovascular problems and musculoskeletal problems such as degenerative joint disease or musculoskeletal pain. Exercise programs should include endurance, strength, balance, and flexibility components (Resnick et al, 2006):

▶ *Endurance* exercises include continuous movement involving large muscle groups that is sustained for a minimum of 10 minutes. These types of exercises increase breathing and heart rate and improve the health of the heart, the lungs and the circulatory system. Examples of endurance exercises are swimming, bicycling, walking briskly, tennis, dancing, and gardening (mowing and raking). Initially, endurance exercises should be for a short duration and gradually increased.

▶ *Strength training* (resistance) exercises build muscles and increase muscle strength by moving or lifting against some type of resistance such as hand or ankle weights or resistance bands. The exercises should be performed at least twice a week.

▶ *Balance* exercises improve standing and gait and help prevent falls. Tai chi exercises have been shown to be of benefit for older people (Box 10-11).

▶ *Flexibility* exercises keep the body limber and increase range of motion. These exercises should be performed at least 3 days a week. Yoga is another form of exercise that can be practiced regardless of one's condition.

Nonambulatory older people can also engage in physical activity and may benefit the most from an exercise program in terms of function and quality of life. "Muscle weakness and atrophy are probably the most functionally relevant and reversible aspects to exercise in nonambulatory older adults" (Resnick et al, 2006, p. 2). Upper extremity cycling, marching in place, stretching, range of motion, water-based activities, and chair yoga are examples of exercises for nonambulatory older adults. For older adults in nursing homes, participation in self-care activities improves functioning and also contributes to greater staff, family, and resident satisfaction (Resnick et al, 2008). The Res-Care Intervention, a self-efficacy based approach to restore and/or maintain the residents' physical function can be used as a model for restorative care in nursing homes (Resnick et al, 2008).

The older person may be able to integrate activity into daily life rather than doing a specific exercise. Examples are walking to the store instead of driving, golfing, swimming, hiking, raking leaves, and gardening. Those limited to institutional facilities should also be encouraged to increase the amount of walking. First it may be only from the bed to the bathroom; then, with time, down the hall; and eventually around the total facility or even outside. Restorative walking programs and other exercise programs should be an integral activity in all long-term care institutions.

Where there is a need for especially low-intensity exercise, the person can work for 2 to 3 minutes, rest for 2 to 3 minutes, and continue this pattern for 15 to 20 minutes. Some examples of moderate-intensity activity include washing and waxing the car for 45 to 60 minutes, washing windows or floors for 45 to 60 minutes, gardening for 35 to 40 minutes, wheeling one's self in a wheelchair for 30 to 40 minutes, walking 2 miles in 30 minutes, or swimming laps or water aerobics for 20 minutes (www.americangeriatrics.org/education/falls.shtml).

The Centers for Disease Control and Prevention provides an excellent resource, *Growing Stronger: Strength Training for Older Adults* (www.cdc.gov/nccdphp/dnpa/physical/growing_stronger/index.htm).

| Box 10-11 | Evidence-Based Practice: Influence of Intense Tai Chi Training on Physical Performance and Hemodynamic Outcomes in Transitionally Frail Older Adults |

Purpose

This study explores the extent and time course over which tai chi (TC) affects measures of physical performance and cardiovascular function in older adults who are becoming frail.

Sample and Setting

The study included 311 participants ranging in age from 70 to 97 (M 80.9) who were living in 20 independent congregate living facilities in the greater Atlanta area.

Method

A 48-week randomized trial was provided to 291 women and 20 men who were transitionally frail (older than 70 years old and had fallen at least once in the past year). Participants were randomized to either TC exercise or wellness education (control) interventions. Physical performance (gait speed, reach, chair-rises, 360-degree turn, picking up an object from the floor, and single limb support) and hemodynamic outcomes (heart rate and blood pressure) were obtained at baseline and after 4, 8, and 12 months.

Results

The TC training had a positive impact on body mass index, systolic blood pressure, and heart rate as well as on chair rises. Fall occurrences were also reduced. Positive outcomes became apparent after 4 or 8 months of training and persisted through completion of the intervention.

Implications

TC exercise programs have positive benefits for frail older adults, including improved cardiovascular performance, decreased falls, and increased functional ability, and these benefits are demonstrated after at least 4 months of training.

Data from Wolf S et al: The influence of intense tai chi training on physical performance and hemodynamic outcomes in transitionally frail older adults, *J Gerontol A Biol Sci Med Sci* 61A(2):184-189, 2006.

The National Institute on Aging offers educational materials on exercise and aging including on-line video demonstrations of exercise (http://nihseniorhealth.gov/exercise/exercisestotry/01.html). Examples of strength training exercises are presented in Figure 10-1.

Exercise Prescription

As noted earlier, the majority of older adults do not exercise regularly. Motivational interventions are important when encouraging older adults to begin an exercise program and should be continued to insure ongoing adherence. Resnick et al (2006) suggest that emphasizing the immediate outcomes or benefits that can be expected from regular exercise (improvement of current health and quality of life) is important. These authors further suggest an "exercise prescription" that explains the type of exercises the person should do on a regular basis. A list of safety tips for exercise should also be provided (www.easyforyou.info/).

The following seven-step approach to implementing an exercise program may help older adults stay motivated to continue (Resnick, 2003):

1. Education
2. Exercise prescribing
3. Goal identification
4. Exposure to the exercise behavior
5. Role models
6. Verbal encouragement
7. Verbal reinforcement and rewards

Suggestions for exercise programs for older adults are presented in Box 10-12.

IMPLICATIONS FOR GERONTOLOGICAL NURSING AND HEALTHY AGING

This chapter has looked separately at the need for rest and sleep and the need for activity. In summary, it is apparent that each area influences the function of the other. The quality and the overall perception of life can

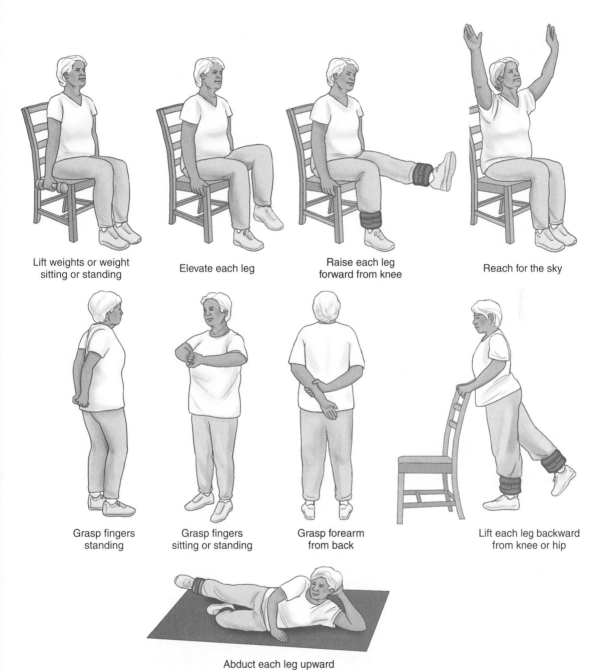

Lift weights or weight
sitting or standing

Elevate each leg

Raise each leg
forward from knee

Reach for the sky

Grasp fingers
standing

Grasp fingers
sitting or standing

Grasp forearm
from back

Lift each leg backward
from knee or hip

Abduct each leg upward

Fig. 10-1 Examples of strength-training exercises. (*Modified from Centers for Disease Control and Prevention. Growing stronger: strength training for older adults: Exercises: stage 1. Accessed 6/30/06 from www.cdc.gov/nccdphp/dnpa/physical/growing_stronger/exercises/index.htm.*)

Box 10-12	Suggestions for Exercise Programs for Older Adults

- Provide appropriate screening before beginning an exercise program.
- Provide information on the benefits of exercise, emphasizing short-term benefits such as sleeping better.
- Clarify the misconceptions associated with exercise (fatigue, injury).
- Assess for declines in function, and discuss how exercise can minimize these declines.
- Assess barriers to exercise and how to overcome them.
- Provide an "exercise prescription" that specifies what exercises the person should perform and how often. Include daily and long-term goals.
- Goals should be specific and achievable, and should match the older person's perceived needs and health and cognitive abilities, as well as their interests.
- Provide choices as to types of exercises, and design the program so that the person can do it at home or elsewhere when formal training ends.
- Provide self-monitoring methods to assist in visualizing progress.
- Group-based programs and exercising with a buddy may be more successful.
- Try to make the program fun and entertaining (walking with favorite music, socializing with friends).
- Discuss potential side effects of exercise and any symptoms that should be reported.
- Share stories about your own personal exercise program and the benefits.
- Follow up frequently on progress, and provide reinforcement.
- Begin with low-intensity physical activity for sedentary older adults.
- Initiate low-intensity activities in short sessions (less than 10 minutes), and include warm-up and cool-down components with active stretching.
- Progression from low to moderate intensity is important to obtain maximum benefits, but activity level changes should be instituted gradually.
- Lifestyle activities (e.g., raking, gardening) can build endurance when performed for at least 10 minutes.

Data from Cress M, Buchner D, Prohaska T et al: Best practices for physical activity programs and behavior counseling in older adult populations, *J Aging Phys Act* 13(1):61-74, 2005; Jitramontree N: *Evidence-based protocol. Exercise promotion: walking in elders,* Iowa City, Iowa, 2001, University of Iowa Gerontological Nursing Interventions Research Center, Research Dissemination Core; Schneider JK, Eveker A, Bronder D et al: Exercise training program for older adults: incentives and disincentives for participation, *J Gerontol Nurs* 29(9):21-31, 2006; Struck B, Ross K: Health promotion in older adults: prescribing exercise for the frail and home bound, *Geriatrics* 61(5):22-27, 2006; Resnick B, Ory M, Rogers M, Page P, Lyle RM et al: Screening for and prescribing exercise for older adults, *Geriatr Aging* 9(3):174-182, 2006.

be augmented when the nurse monitors these specific functions and provides support or assistance according to identified problems. Gerontological nurses must be knowledgeable about age-related changes in sleep and activity and the effect of lifestyle on these changes. Many older people may have misconceptions about sleep and exercise, and the nurse can assess beliefs and understanding and provide education to enhance optimal wellness.

Assessment of sleep, the chosen level of activity, and the design of interventions must be grounded in evidence-based knowledge and applied to meet the needs of each unique individual. Common practices such as the use of hypnotics for sleep without a thorough assessment or being confined to a wheelchair because there is no one to help maintain walking skills lead to disabling and preventable problems for older people. Adequate sleep and activity are essential

to physical, emotional, and cognitive functioning. Poor sleep and decline in functional capacity affect the ability to perform activities of daily living, compromise independence, and lead to disability and illness. Improvement of function is possible for even the most frail elder, and gerontological nurses must incorporate the health promotion activities discussed in this chapter into any plan of care for an older adult.

APPLICATION OF MASLOW'S HIERARCHY

Sleep and activity needs must be met not only to maintain biological integrity, but also to meet higher-level needs such as safety and security, belonging and attachment, self-esteem and self-efficacy, and self-actualization and transcendence. The older adult would not survive if these needs were not met independently or with the assistance of others. Ineffective sleep, rest, and activity patterns contribute to depression, loneliness, and loss of independence and self-esteem, as well as physical and cognitive illnesses. Maintaining adequate sleep and activity allows the older person to continue to find fulfillment in activities, and in life itself, despite limitations that may be associated with aging and illness.

KEY CONCEPTS

▶ Many chronic conditions often interfere with the quality and quantity of sleep. Rest and sleep are restorative, recuperative, and necessary for the preservation of life. Sleep is a barometer of health and can be considered one of the vital signs.

▶ Complaints of sleep difficulties should be thoroughly investigated and not attributed to age. Nonpharmacological interventions should always be considered in any plan of care to improve sleep.

▶ Activity is an indication of an individual's health and wellness; inability to exercise, do physical work, or perform activities of daily living is one of the first indicators of decline.

▶ Lack of physical activity increases the risk for many medical conditions experienced by elders. Exercise can be done by elders who are ambulatory, chairbound, or bedridden and should include endurance exercises, strength training, balance exercises, and flexibility exercises.

▶ The benefits of exercise are that it maintains functional ability, enhances self-confidence and self-sufficiency, decreases depression, improves one's general lifestyle, maintains mental functional capacity, and decreases the risk of medical problems.

▶ Exercise counseling and an exercise prescription should be included in assessment of all older adults.

ACTIVITIES AND DISCUSSION QUESTIONS

1. What age-related changes affect rest, sleep, and activity in older adults?
2. How would you assess an elder for adequacy or inadequacy of rest, sleep, and activity?
3. Develop an exercise prescription for an older adult residing in the community.
3. Discuss the nursing interventions to promote rest, sleep, and activity.
4. Develop a nursing care plan using wellness and North American Nursing Diagnosis Association (NANDA) diagnoses.

RESOURCES

Websites

National Center on Sleep Disorders Research
www.nhlbi.nih.gov/sleep

NIH Senior Health (exercises for older adults)
http://nih.seniorhealth.gov/exercise

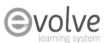

For additional resources, please visit evolve.elsevier.com/Ebersole/gerontological.

REFERENCES

Alessi C, Martin J, Webber A et al: Randomized controlled trial of a nonpharmacological intervention to improve abnormal sleep/wake patterns in nursing home residents, *Jour Am Geriatr Soc* 53(5):803-810, 2005.

American Geriatrics Society: *Falls prevention in older people*, 2001. Accessed 10/11/08 from www.americangeriatrics.org/education/cp_index.shtml.

Boeve BF, Silber MH, Ferman TJ: REM sleep behavior disorder in Parkinson's disease and dementia with Lewy bodies, *J Geriatr Psychiatry Neurol* 17(3):146-157, 2004.

Brooks P, Peever J: Glycinergic and GABA$_A$–mediated inhibition of somatic motor neurons does not mediate rapid eye movement sleep motor atonia, *J Neurosci* 28(14):3535-3545, 2008.

Buckle J: Clinical aromatherapy: therapeutic uses for essential oils, *Adv Nurse Pract* 10(5):67-68, 2002.

Cefalu C: Evaluation and management of insomnia in the institutionalized elderly, *Ann Long-Term Care* 12(6):25-32, 2004.

Centers for Disease Control and Prevention: *Older adults receiving exercise counseling*, 2007. Accessed 10/11/08 from: www.cdc.gov/Features/dsExerciseCounseling/

Chaperon C, Farr L, LoChiano E: Sleep disturbance of residents in a continuing care retirement community, *J Gerontol Nurs* 33(10):21-28, 2007.

Colcombe S, Erickson K, Scalf P et al: Aerobic exercise training increases brain volume in aging humans, *J Gerontol A Biol Sci Med Sci* 61A(11):1166-1171, 2006.

Fahlman M, Topp R, McNevin N et al: Structured exercise in older adults with limited functional ability: assessing the benefits of an aerobic plus resistance training program, *J Gerontol Nurs* 33(6):32-39, 2007.

Ferrucci L, Simonsick E: A little exercise, *J Gerontol A Biol Sci Med Sci* 61A(11):1154-1156, 2006.

Fiatarone M, O'Neill E, Ryan M et al: Exercise training and nutritional supplementation for the physical frailty in very elderly people, *N Engl J Med* 330(25):1769-1755, 1994.

Hughes S, Prohaska T, Rimmer J, Heller T: Promoting physical activity among older people, *Generations* 29(2):54-59, 2005a.

Hughes S, Williams B, Molina A et al: Characteristics of physical activity programs for older adults: results of a multisite survey, *Gerontologist* 45(5):667-675, 2005b.

Kochar J, Fredman L, Stone K, Cauley J: Sleep problems in elderly women caregivers depend on the level of depressive symptoms: results of the caregiver-study of osteoporotic fractures, *J Am Geriatr Soc* 55(12):2002-2009, 2007.

McCurry S, Gibbons L, Logsdon R et al: Nighttime insomnia treatment and education for Alzheimer's disease: a randomized, controlled trial, *J Am Geriatr Soc* 53(5): 793-802, 2005.

Missildine K: Sleep and the sleep environment of older adults in acute care settings, *JGN* 34(6):15-21, 2008.

National Sleep Foundation: *Sleep in America*, 2006. Accessed 10/6/08 from www.sleepfoundation.org

La Reau R, Benson L, Watcharotone K: Examining the feasibility of specific nursing interventions to promote sleep in hospitalized elderly patients, *Geriatr Nurs* 29(3):197-206, 2008.

Resnick B: Exercise for older adults: what to prescribe and how to motivate, *Caring for the Ages* 4(1):8-12, 2003.

Resnick B, Ory M, Rogers M et al: Screening and prescribing exercise for older adults, *Geriatr Aging* 9(3):174-182, 2006. Accessed 7/8/08 from www.medscape.com/viewarticle/535189_print.

Resnick B, Petzer-Aboff, I, Galik G: Barriers and benefits to implementing a restorative care intervention in nursing homes, *J Am Med Dir Assoc* 9(7):102-108, 2008.

Resnick B, Simpson M, Bercovitz A et al: Pilot testing of the restorative care intervention: impact on residents, *J Gerontol Nurse* 32(3): 39-47, 2006.

Reuben D, Herr K, Pacala J: *Geriatrics at your fingertips 2006-2007*, ed 8, New York, 2006, American Geriatrics Society.

Struck BD, Ross KM: Health promotion in older adults: prescribing exercise for the frail and homebound: *Geriatrics* 61(5):22-7, 2006.

Subramanian S, Surani S: Sleep disorders in the elderly, *Geriatrics* 62(12):10-32, 2007. Accessed 12/17/07 from http://geri.com/geriatrics/content/printContentPopup.jsp?id=477152.

U.S. Department of Health and Human Services: *Healthy people 2010*, ed 2, Washington, DC, 2000, U.S. Government Printing Office.

Voelker R: Behavioral strategies restore sleep for patients with dementia, *CNS Senior Care* 6(4), 2007.

Winkelman J, Allen R, Tenzer P, Hening W: Restless legs syndrome: nonpharmacologic and pharmacologic treatments, *Geriatrics* 62(10):13-16, 2007.

Zee P, Bloom H: Understanding and resolving insomnia in the elderly, *Geriatrics (Suppl May):* 1-12, 2006.

Promoting Healthy Skin and Feet

GLOSSARY

Debride To remove dead or infected tissue, usually of a wound.

Emollient An agent that softens and smoothes the skin.

Eschar Black, dry, dead tissue.

Hyperemia Redness in a part of the body caused by increased blood flow, such as in area of an infection.

Maceration Tissue that is over-hydrated and subject to breakdown.

Slough Dead tissue that has become wet, appearing as yellow to white and fibrous.

Tissue tolerance The amount of pressure a tissue (skin) can endure before it breaks down, as in a pressure sore.

Xerosis Very dry skin.

THE LIVED EXPERIENCE

I can't thank you enough for helping me with my feet. I have been to the podiatrist, but no one has made them, and me, feel so good. I feel like I can walk forever now—you are an angel.

Tom, age 86

Gerontological nurses have an instrumental role in promoting the health of the skin and the feet of the persons who seek their care. Both are sometimes overlooked when dealing with other, more immediately life-threatening problems. However, preservation of the integrity of the skin and the functioning of the feet is essential to well-being. In order to promote healthy aging, the nurse needs information about common problems encountered by the elderly and skill in developing effective interventions for both acute and chronic conditions.

INTEGUMENT

The skin is the largest organ of the body, and has at least seven physiological functions (Box 11-1). Exposure to heat, cold, water, trauma, friction, and pressure notwithstanding, the skin's function is to maintain a homeostatic environment. Healthy skin is durable, pliable, and strong enough to protect the body by absorbing, reflecting, cushioning, and restricting various substances and forces that might enter and alter its function; yet it is sensitive enough to relay subtle messages to the

Box 11-1	Physiological Function of the Skin

- Protects underlying structures
- Regulates body temperature
- Serves as a vehicle for sensation
- Stores fat
- Is a component of the metabolism of salt and water
- Is a site for two-way gas exchange
- Is a site for the production of vitamin D when exposed to sunlight

brain. When the integument malfunctions or is overwhelmed, discomfort, disfigurement, or death may ensue. However, the nurse can both promptly recognize and help to prevent many of the sources of danger to a person's skin in the promotion of the best possible health. Tips for maintaining healthy skin can be found in Box 11-2.

Many skin problems are seen as we age, both in health and when compromised by illness or mobility limitations. The skin problems seen in older adults are

Box 11-2	Tips for Healthy Skin

- Watch for any break in the skin, and initiate treatment as soon as possible.
- For those with diabetes or PVD, consult a health care provider promptly if skin break occurs.
- Use a humidifier if necessary to keep room humid.
- When bathing, use tepid water only; and limit time in the water, which dehydrates skin.
- Use only mild skin cleaners without perfume or lanolin. Apply to damp skin after bathing or washing.
- Pat dry; do not rub.
- Do not add bath oil to water to minimize risk of slipping.
- Apply moisturizers as often as necessary to maintain continuous coverage.
- Choose clothing made of soft cotton or other nonabrasive materials.
- Drink several glasses of water every day to maintain systemic hydration.
- Protect skin from exposure to cold temperatures.

PVD, Peripheral vascular disease.

influenced by the environment and age-related changes (see Chapter 6). The most common skin problems of aging are xerosis (dry skin), pruritus, seborrheic keratosis, herpes zoster, and cancer. Those who are immobilized or medically fragile, such as residents of nursing facilities, are at risk for fungal infections and pressure ulcers, both major threats to wellness.

Common Skin Problems

Xerosis

Xerosis is extremely dry, cracked, and itchy skin. Xerosis and pruritus (see next section) are the most common skin problems for persons living in nursing homes (Norman, 2003). It occurs primarily in the extremities, especially the legs, but can affect the face and the trunk as well. The thinner epidermis of older skin makes it less efficient, allowing more moisture to escape. Inadequate fluid intake worsens xerosis as the body will pull moisture from the skin in an attempt to combat systemic dehydration (see Chapter 6).

Exposure to environmental elements such as artificial heat, decreased humidity, use of harsh soaps, and frequent hot baths or hot tubs contributes to skin dryness (called a "winter itch"). Nutritional deficiencies and smoking lead to dehydration of the outer layer of the epidermis. Hospitals and nursing homes accelerate the development of xerosis through routine bathing, use of drying soap, prolonged bed rest, and the action of bed linen on the patient's skin. For persons with incontinence, the skin must be protected from both the burning of urine or feces and from excess dryness that arises from the frequent washing and drying that is necessary.

Dry skin may be just dry skin, but it may also be a symptom of more serious systemic disease (e.g., diabetes mellitus, hypothyroidism, renal disease) or dehydration.

Pruritus

One of the consequences of xerosis is *pruritus*, that is, itchy skin. It is a symptom, not a diagnosis or disease, and is a threat to skin integrity because of the attempts to relieve it by scratching. It is aggravated by perfumed detergents, fabric softeners, heat, sudden temperature changes, pressure, vibration, electrical stimuli, sweating, restrictive clothing, fatigue, exercise, and anxiety.

Pruritus also may accompany systemic disorders such as chronic renal failure, biliary or hepatic disease, and iron deficiency anemia. Intense nocturnal itching is a primary sign of scabies, which occurs with some frequency in nursing home facilities or sites of communal living. The gerontological nurse should always listen carefully to the patient's ideas of why the pruritus is occurring and what relieves it and what aggravates it.

Keratoses

There are two types of keratoses, seborrheic and actinic (discussed in the cancer section to follow). *Seborrheic keratosis* is a benign growth that appears mainly on the trunk, the face, the neck, and the scalp as single or multiple lesions found especially in men. One or more lesions are present on nearly all adults older than 65 years. An individual may have dozens of these benign lesions. Seborrheic keratosis is a waxy, raised, verrucous lesion, flesh-colored or pigmented in varying sizes (Figure 11-1). The lesions have a "stuck on" appearance, as if they can be scraped off. Seborrheic keratoses may be removed by a dermatologist for cosmetic reasons. A variant seen in darkly pigmented persons occurs mostly on the face and appears as numerous small, dark, possibly tag-like lesions (see www.dermatlas.com).

Herpes Zoster

Herpes zoster (HZ), or shingles, is a viral infection frequently seen in older adults. The peak incidence occurs between ages 50 and 70 years. The lifetime risk of all people is 10% to 20% (Habif, 2005). Immunosuppressed elders and those with histories of chicken pox (varicella) are at greatest risk. However HZ can occur in healthy people as well. It always occurs along a nerve pathway, or *dermatome*. The more dermatomes involved, the more serious the infection, especially if it involves the head. When the eye is affected it is always a medical emergency. Most HZ occurs in the thoracic region (66% of cases); 10% to 20% are trigeminal, 10% to 20% are cervical, 5% to 10% are lumbar, and fewer than 5% are sacral (Habif, 2005). In most cases, the severity of the infection increases with age.

The onset may be preceded by chills, fever, gastrointestinal disturbance, malaise, and pain or paresthesias. Before diagnosis, the person may complain of headache, photophobia, and malaise. Occasionally, local lymphadenopathy is present but no fever (Habif, 2005). The area where the eruption *will* occur is burning, painful, or tender and is a predictive sign.

During the healing process, clusters of papulovesicles develop along a nerve pathway. The lesions themselves eventually rupture, crust over, and resolve. Scarring may result, especially if scratching or poor hygiene leads to a secondary bacterial infection. HZ is infectious until it becomes crusty. HZ may be very painful and pruritic, and as many as 20% of elderly patients may have postherpetic neuralgia (PHN) lasting weeks or months after resolution of the acute infection. The pain of PHN has been very difficult to control and can significantly affect one's quality of life (see Chapter 16).

Photo Damage of the Skin

Although exposure to sunlight is necessary for the production of vitamin D, the sun is also the most common causes of skin damage and skin cancer. With the accumulated years of sun exposure, the risk is significantly increased for older adults. The damage (photo or solar damage) comes from prolonged exposure to ultraviolet (UV) light from the environment or in tanning booths. Although the amount of sun-induced damage varies with skin type and genetics, much of the associated damage is preventable. Ideally, preventive measures begin in childhood, but clinical evidence has shown that some improvement can be achieved at anytime by limiting sun exposure and using sunscreens regularly.

Skin Cancers

It is believed that there are more than 1 million new unreported cases of basal cell and squamous cell cancer a year. Most of these are curable; the type with the greatest

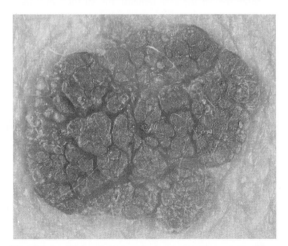

Fig. 11-1   Seborrheic keratosis in an older adult. *(From Habif TP:* Clinical dermatology: a color guide to diagnosis and therapy, *ed 4, St Louis, 2004, Mosby.)*

potential to cause death is melanoma, of which 62,480 new cases were expected in 2008 (American Cancer Society [ACS], 2008). Melanoma is most often seen in light-skinned persons.

Persons with a history of sunburns, use of tanning beds, skin cancer, or exposure to carcinogenic materials, or with sun sensitivity or a depressed immune system are at particular risk. Increasing age along with a history of sun exposure increases one's risk even further.

Actinic Keratosis

Actinic keratosis is a precancerous lesion which may become a squamous cell carcinoma (Mayo Clinic, 2007). It is directly related to years of overexposure to UV light. Risk factors are older age and fair complexion. It is found on the face, the lips, and the hands and forearms, areas of chronic sun exposure in everyday life. Actinic keratosis is characterized by rough, scaly, sandpaper-like patches, pink to reddish-brown on an erythematous base (Mayo Clinic, 2007). Lesions may be single or multiple; they may be painless or mildly tender. The person with actinic keratoses should be monitored by a dermatologist every 6 to 12 months for any change in appearance of the lesions. Early recognition, treatment, and removal of this lesion is easy and important. Removal is aimed at preventing the possible conversion to a malignant lesion.

Basal Cell Carcinoma

Basal cell carcinoma is the most common malignant skin cancer. It affects up to 800,000 Americans a year (Skin Cancer Foundation, 2006). It is slow-growing, and metastasis is rare. A basal cell lesion can be triggered by extensive sun exposure, especially burns, chronic irritation, and chronic ulceration of the skin. It is more prevalent in light-skinned persons. It usually begins as a pearly papule with prominent telangiectasis (blood vessels) or as a scar-like area with no history of trauma. Basal cell carcinoma is also known to ulcerate. It may be indistinguishable from squamous cell carcinoma and is diagnosed by biopsy. Early detection and treatment are necessary to minimize disfigurement.

Squamous Cell Carcinoma

Squamous cell carcinoma is the second most common skin cancer. However, it is aggressive and has a high incidence of metastasis if not identified and treated promptly. Squamous cell cancer is more prevalent in fair-skinned, elderly men who live in sunny climates and is usually found on the head, the neck, or the hands. Individuals in their mid-sixties who have been or are chronically exposed to the sun (e.g., persons who work out of doors, are athletes, etc.) are prime candidates for this type of cancer. Less common causes include chronic stasis ulcers, scars from injury, and exposure to chemical carcinogens, such as topical hydrocarbons, arsenic, and radiation. The lesion begins as a firm, irregular, fleshy, pink-colored nodule that becomes reddened and scaly, much like actinic keratosis, but it may increase rapidly in size. It may also be hard and wart-like with a gray top and horny texture, or it may be ulcerated and indurated with raised, defined borders. Because it can appear so differently, it is often overlooked or thought to be insignificant. The best advice to give older patients, especially those who live in sunny climates, is that they should be regularly screened by a dermatologist.

Melanoma

A neoplasm of melanocytes, melanoma is the least common skin cancer but has a high mortality rate because of its ability to metastasize quickly. Blistering sunburns before the age of 18 are thought to damage Langerhans' cells, which affect the immune response of the skin and increase the risk for a later melanoma. The legs and backs of women and the backs of men are the most common sites. Two thirds of melanomas develop from preexisting moles; only one third arise alone. Melanoma has a classical multicolor, raised appearance with an asymmetrical, irregular border. It may appear to be of any size, but the surface diameter is not necessarily reflective of the size beneath the surface, similar in concept to an iceberg. It is treatable if caught very early, before it has a chance to invade surrounding tissue. If the nurse finds any questionable lesions, the individual should be referred to a dermatologist immediately. The "ABCD" approach to assessing such potential lesions is used (Box 11-3).

Box 11-3	ABCD Rules of Melanoma

Asymmetry: One half does not match the other half.
Border irregularity: The edges are ragged, notched, or blurred.
Color: The pigment is not uniform in color, having shades of tan, brown, or black, or a mottled appearance with red, white, or blue areas.
Diameter: The diameter is greater than the size of a pencil eraser or increasing in size.

IMPLICATIONS FOR GERONTOLOGICAL NURSING AND HEALTHY AGING

The gerontological nurse is in the perfect position to promote healthy skin in older adults. In doing so, quality of life and comfort can be significantly improved.

Xerosis

Since one of the major causes of xerosis is age-related changes, the nurse attends to environmental prevention and treatment and provides expert skin care. Maintaining an environment of about 60% humidity is a start. The challenge is to find ways to rehydrate the epidermis, especially the outer layer or the corneum stratum.

The skin can only be hydrated with water. Topical skin products can help retain natural moisture in the skin. Most lubricants such as creams, lotions, and emollients work by trapping moisture and are most effective when applied to towel-patted, damp skin immediately after a bath. Bath oils and other hydrophobic preparations may also be used to hold in moisture. Light mineral oil is equally as effective as and more economical than commercial brands. However, oils poured directly into a tub or shower increase the risk for falls. It is safer and more effective to apply the oil directly to the moist skin. Water-laden emulsions without perfumes or alcohol are best.

To prevent excessive loss of moisture and natural oil during bathing, only tepid water temperatures and superfatted soaps or skin cleansers without hexachlorophene or alcohol should be used. Products such as Cetaphil, Basis, Dove, Tone, and Caress soaps or Jergens, Neutrogena, or Oil of Olay bath washes are effective in helping to prevent the loss of the protective lipid film from the skin surface. Deodorant soaps and detergents contain alcohol as drying agents and should be avoided except in places such as the axilla and the groin.

In cases of extreme dryness, petroleum jelly can be applied to affected areas before bed and the skin will be smoother and moister in the morning. Oils and ointments with zinc oxide are designed to coat the skin and replace the skin's natural oil barrier. This approach is often used to prevent excoriations from feces or urine. However these can only be used on clean skin.

Pruritus

When xerosis leads to pruritus, the goal is to reduce and hopefully alleviate the itching. If rehydration of the stratum corneum is not sufficient to control itching, cool compresses, or oatmeal or Epsom salt baths may be helpful. Failure to control the itching increases the risk for eczema, excoriations, cracks in the skin, inflammation, and infection arising from the usually linear excoriations from scratching. The nurse should be alert to signs of infection, rough, scaly, or flaky skin, and accompanying pruritus anywhere on the body.

Cancer

The nurse also has an active role in the prevention and early recognition of skin cancers. This role may include working with community awareness and education programs, screening clinics, and direct care. In promoting skin health, the nurse is vigilant in observing skin for the changes that require further evaluation.

Age-related skin changes, such as thinning and diminished melanocytes, significantly increase the risk for solar damage and subsequent skin cancer. By far the most important preventive nursing intervention is to educate the adults regarding the risks of photo and smoke damage. Preventive strategies include the use of sunscreens and protective clothing and limiting sun exposure (see Box 11-4).

Box 11-4   Sun Protection Recommendations

- Avoid the midday sun (10 AM to 3 PM) when the ultraviolet radiation is most intense.
- Use sunscreen daily (if going outside) regardless of the weather in sunny or potentially sunny regions.
- For partial protection, wear clothing that covers the exposed areas of the skin and a broad-brimmed hat to protect the face and the top of head, especially if working outside in sunny regions.
- Select and use a sunscreen with a sun protection factor (SPF) of 15 or higher. Apply before sun exposure, and reapply periodically after perspiring heavily or swimming.
- Avoid getting sunburned, and limit sun expose at all times.
- Be aware of reflection from sand, snow, and water, which will intensify the radiation.
- Avoid sun if taking photosensitizing drugs such as the tetracyclines.
- Avoid sunscreens with para-aminobenzoic acid (PABA) if allergic to procaine, sulfonamides, or hair dyes, because of cross-sensitization.
- Avoid tanning beds and sun lamps.

Secondary prevention is in the form of early diagnosis. Following a thorough clinical screening, the elder and the intimate partner can be taught to perform regular "checks" of each other's skin, watching for signs of change and the need to contact a primary care provider or dermatologist promptly. For the person with keratosis and multiple freckles (nevi) photographing the body parts may be a useful reference. The adage "when it doubt, get it checked" is an important one.

Herpes Zoster

The majority of the care and treatment of the person with herpes zoster is medical, with prompt initiation of antiviral medications and optimal pain management. Nursing care includes providing emotional support during the outbreak and education regarding reducing secondary infections and cross-contamination. Weeping and ruptured vesicles should be kept covered with an absorbent yet nonadherent or damp product. If the product, such as a $4'' \times 4''$ gauze, adheres, warm normal saline can be applied to the gauze until the body releases it. Hands should be washed after contact as well as bedding, towels, and clothing.

Vascular Insufficiency and the Skin

Hypertension and diabetes are extremely common problems for persons as they age (see Chapters 17 and 20), and especially for persons of color. One possible complication of both of these is peripheral vascular disease (PVD) and for many, serious skin infections and lesions that follow, from mild stasis dermatitis to ulceration and gangrene. The two types of vascular insufficiency are arterial (also called peripheral artery disease [PAD] or lower-extremity artery disease [LEAD]) and venous (VI). In promoting healthy aging, the nurse is aware of the signs of insufficiency and can quickly take steps to minimize the most harmful sequelae. In caring for the person with vascular insufficiency it is of utmost importance to protect the limb and the skin from further injury.

Skin Problems Associated with Cardiovascular Problems

Arterial Insufficiency: Peripheral Artery Disease (PAD)

PAD is the most common type of PVD and affects 8 to 12 million Americans, or 12% to 20% of the population over 65. The incidence of PAD increases with age. The person with PAD is 4 to 5 times more at risk for a myocardial infarction or a stroke than those without PAD (American Heart Association, 2007). It is often caused by enlarging atherosclerotic plaques, which lead to ischemia of the limb and can lead to severe infections and limb loss. Many persons with PAD, either diagnosed or not, complain of pain or muscle fatigue with exercise. In more severe cases the lower-extremity can be extremely painful when walking or when the legs are elevated (called "intermittent claudication"). The pain is only relieved when the legs are returned to a dependent position (to increase arterial flow downward) or when the person stops walking and rests, thus eliminating the extra circulatory demands made by exercise (Table 11-1). Risk factors include obesity, coronary artery disease, smoking, hyperlipidemia, hypertension, and diabetes or a family history of the same (American Heart Association, 2007).

The slightest trauma to a lower extremity (LE), such as bumping the side of a wheelchair, can result in an arterial ulcer, which is very difficult and sometimes impossible to heal without surgical intervention. Pain is a very significant problem, the ulcer increasing the pain already arising from the insufficiency.

Venous Insufficiency

VI is usually a consequence of a deep venous thrombosis (DVT) occurring at some time in the past. The most important risk factors are uncontrolled diabetes and venous hypertension with impaired functioning of the valves within the veins. Venous ulcers, also called stasis ulcers, are a major complication.

Edema of the LE may be the first sign of VI and can become particularly troublesome and affect functioning. Later there is a brownish discoloration of the skin in the lower half of the extremity from leakage of iron from the red blood cells. In individuals with dark-pigmented skin, the discoloration is darker than the surrounding tissue.

Skin tissue becomes vulnerable to insignificant trauma, such as an insect bite or the pressure of snug, elastic-topped ankle socks. These or other events can precipitate venous ulcer formation, or ulceration can develop spontaneously.

Such ulcerations can be painful and are always difficult to heal. Although they are most often found over the outer malleolus, they can become quite extensive. The characteristics of venous ulcers are summarized in Table 11-1. In one study, patients with venous leg ulceration reported their greatest problems to be pain, difficulty with outdoor mobility, and difficulty finding appropriate and comfortable footwear (Heinen et al, 2006).

Table 11-1 Comparison of Arterial and Venous Insufficiency of the Lower Extremities

CHARACTERISTICS	ARTERIAL	VENOUS
Ulcer location	Between or tips of toes Over phalangeal heads and on heels Lateral malleolus or pretibial area (for diabetic patients), over metatarsal heads, on side or sole of foot	Lower calf and ankle especially the medial malleolus
Ulcer characteristics	Well-defined edges Black or necrotic tissue Deep, pale base Nonbleeding	Uneven edges Ruddy granulation tissue Superficial Bleeding
Pain	Exceedingly painful with elevation Relieved with dependency Chronic pain Constant severe pain with complete occlusion	Deep muscle pain if deep vein thrombosis develops Relieved by elevation
Pulses	Absent or weak	Normal
Associated changes in leg and foot	Thin, shiny, dry skin Thickened toenails Absence of hair growth Temperature variations (cooler if there is no cellulitis) Elevational pallor Dependent rubor Atrophy or no change in limb size	Firm edema Reddish brown discoloration of skin, especially of shin Evidence of healed ulcers Dilated and tortuous superficial veins

IMPLICATIONS FOR GERONTOLOGICAL NURSING AND HEALTHY AGING

The most important aspect of caring for the person with vascular insufficiency is to ensure that the proper diagnosis is made and treatment is consistent with it. To promote the health of the lower extremities the nurse stays alert for the signs of potential problems and takes prompt action to minimize tissue damage. If ulcers develop, treatment must be consistent with evidence-based practice. The nurse also helps elders reduce risk factors whenever possible, such as encouraging smoking cessation and careful control of hypertension. The nurse helps reduce the incidence of ulcerations with aggressive steps to protect an affected limb from accidental injury.

A complaint of lower-extremity pain at rest necessitates prompt referral to a health care provider such as a vascular surgeon. Since the symptoms and problems associated with PAD are the result of ischemia of the extremity, interventions that promote circulation are helpful, such as finding ways for the person to dangle his or her feet. In the long-term care setting, all caregivers must recognize that the patient or resident who is not "complying" with instructions to elevate the LE may be refusing because elevation—even that of lying down in bed—may cause sudden and severe pain. A person may be more comfortable sleeping in a recliner where the feet may remain at least somewhat dependent. If an ulcer develops, the best that can be done may be to prevent it from worsening. The wound is kept warm and covered (see Table 11-1). Compression is always contraindicated.

In contrast, compression is the mainstay of the nursing interventions associated with VI. The care goals are maximizing function, relieving edema, and treating the venous stasis ulcers as needed. Treatment usually consists of a combination of therapies, such as leg elevation whenever the person is sitting and elastic support stockings worn during waking hours. Although the stockings are usually considered uncomfortable, wearing them should nonetheless be encouraged. They are now available in an assortment of colors, including skin tones that are more acceptable than the traditional white.

For maximal effect, support stockings should be put on before the person gets out of bed. They should extend to the top of the leg and "rolling" prevented, since constriction is increased at the roll. When putting on elastic stockings, it is sometimes helpful for both men and women to first put on nonrestrictive knee-high nylon stockings (not pantyhose). The rougher support hose can then more easily be pulled on over the hose. This method calls for minimal energy expenditure and promotes independence.

Treatment of the venous ulcer includes managing the exudate and again, preventing worsening. It may never heal. Fortunately, not everyone has accompanying pain.

Skin Problems of Particular Concern for Persons in Nursing Facilities

Owing to the debilitated state of many of the persons who reside in long-term care settings, they are at particular risk for the development of fungal skin infections and pressure ulcers. We do not usually think of healthy aging and pressure ulcers at the same time. However, consistent with the wellness approach described in Chapter 1, there is another way to view the gerontological nurse's promotion of healthy aging, namely, preventing and treating impairments in skin integrity: "Wellness is a state of being and feeling that one strives to achieve through effective health practices."

Candidiasis (*Candida albicans*)

The fungus *Candida albicans* (referred to as "yeast") is present on the skin of healthy persons of any age. However, under certain circumstances and in the right environment a fungal infection can develop. Persons who are obese, malnourished, receiving antibiotic or steroid therapy, or have diabetes are at increased risk. *Candida* grows especially well in areas that are moist, warm, and dark, such as in skinfolds, in the axilla and the groin, and under pendulous breasts. It can also be found in the corners of the mouth associated with the chronic moisture of angular cheilitis. In the vagina we also call it a "yeast infection." If this is found in an older woman, it may mean that her diabetes either has not yet been diagnosed or is in poor control.

Inside the mouth a *Candida* infection is referred to as "thrush" and is associated with poor hygiene and immunocompromise, such as those with long-term steroid use (e.g., because of chronic obstructive pulmonary disease), who are receiving chemotherapy, or who test positive for or are infected with human immunodeficiency virus (HIV) or acquired immunodeficiency

syndrome (AIDS). In the mouth, candidiasis appears as irregular, white, flat to slightly raised patches on an erythematous base that cannot be scraped off. The infection can extend down into the throat and cause swallowing to be painful. In severely immunocompromised persons the infection can extend down the entire gastrointestinal tract.

On the skin, *Candida* is usually maculopapular, glazed, and dark pink in persons with less pigmentation and grayish in persons with more pigmentation. If it is advanced the central area may be completely red and/or dark, and weeping with characteristic bright red and/or dark satellite lesions (distinct lesions a short distance from the center). At this point the skin may be edematous, itching, and burning.

The best approach to managing fungal infections is to prevent them, and the key to prevention is limiting the conditions that encourage fungal growth. Prevention is prioritized for persons who are obese, bedridden, incontinent, or diaphoretic. In contrast to the treatment of dry skin, attention is given to the adequacy of the drying of target areas of the body after bathing, prompt management of incontinent episodes, and the use of loose-fitting cotton clothing and cotton underwear (and changing it when damp) and avoidance of incontinence products that are tight or have plastic that touches the skin.

One of the best ways to dry hard-to-reach, vulnerable areas is with a hair dryer set on low. A folded, dry washcloth or cotton sanitary pad can be placed under the breasts or between skinfolds to promote exposure to air and light. Cornstarch should never be used because it promotes the growth of *Candida* organisms. Optimizing nutrition and glycemic control are also important.

The goal of treatment is to eradicate the infection. This includes not only the use of prescribed antifungal medication, but also the active involvement of the nurse to reduce or eliminate the conditions that created the problem. The affected area of the skin must be cleansed carefully and dried thoroughly before antifungal preparations are applied. A mild soap or cleansing agent, such as Cetaphil, should be used. Antifungal preparations come in powders, creams, and lotions. Since the latter two trap moisture, the powder is recommended. They are usually needed for 7 to 14 days or until the infection is completely cleared. Antifungal medications include miconazole (Micatin), clotrimazole (Lotrimin), nystatin (Mycostatin), and econazole (Spectazole). Treatment of oral *Candida* infection includes mouth swishing and swallowing with an antifungal suspension and/or sucking on antifungal troches. Angular cheilitis is treated with a topical antifungal ointment to the corners of the mouth. If the *Candida* cannot be eliminated in the usual course of therapy, it may be necessary to use ketoconazole or fluconazole systemically for a prescribed period.

Pressure Ulcers

According to the National Pressure Ulcer Advisory Panel (2007), a pressure ulcer is "localized injury to the skin and/or underlying tissue usually over a bony prominence, as a result of pressure, or pressure in combination with shear and/or friction." As tissue is compressed, blood is diverted and blood vessels are forcibly constricted by the persistent pressure on the skin and underlying structures; thus cellular respiration is impaired and cells die from ischemia and anoxia. Intervention at any point in this development can stop the advancement of the pressure ulcer. Reducing the number of pressure ulcers for persons in nursing facilities is an objective of *Healthy People 2010* (Box 11-5).

Just how much pressure can be endured by tissue (tissue tolerance) is highly variable from body location to location and person to person. Tissue tolerance is inversely affected by moisture, amount of pressure, friction, shearing, and age and is directly related to malnutrition, anemia, and low arterial pressure.

The prevalence of pressure ulcers is quite high in later life. Approximately 25% of all persons over 70 have at least one at any point in time (Sommers et al, 2007). Persons with pressure ulcers are found in all settings, including intensive care units (Shahin et al, 2008). Those who are at the greatest risk for the development of an ulcer are the frail, the nonambulatory, and persons with neurological impairments.

Pressure ulcers can develop anywhere on the body but are seen most frequently on the posterior aspects, especially the sacrum, the heels, and the greater trochanters (Lyder, 2006). Secondary areas of breakdown include the lateral condyles of the knees and the ankles. The pinna of the ears is another area subject to breakdown, as are the elbows and the scapulae. If one is lying prone, the knees, the shins, and the pelvis sustain undue pressure.

Heels are particularly apt to develop pressure ulcers, since they are small surfaces that receive a high degree of pressure. In many cases, heel ulcers are inevitable in the presence of peripheral vascular insufficiency combined with immobility. In the acute care setting, patients who are supine for prolonged periods, such as during surgical procedures, may exit the operating room with newly acquired pressure ulcers.

Pressure ulcers are costly to treat, and extended separation from friends and loved ones may be necessary during treatment. For many, an ulcer will prolong recovery and extend rehabilitation. Complications include the need for grafting or amputation, sepsis, or even death, and may lead to legal action by the individual or his or her representative against the caregiver. In the acute care setting the cost of treatment of hospital-acquired ulcers is no longer covered, and the facility must absorb all of the cost.

It is difficult to predict which individuals will develop pressure ulcers, and it is even more difficult to restore skin integrity once it has been broken. The two most important predictive factors are severity of illness and involuntary weight loss owing to poor nutritional status, especially dehydration, hypoproteinemia, and vitamin deficiencies. Other important indicators of increased risk are impaired sensory feedback systems, which prevent discomfort from being noticed, and impaired mobility or immobilization by restraint or sedation. However, most pressure ulcers are considered preventable.

The development of pressure ulcers is a dynamic process that makes constant vigilance and reassessment necessary. The Braden Scale (Bergstrom et al, 1994) and the Norton Scale (Norton, 1996) are risk assessment tools used frequently in the clinical setting in an attempt to identify persons at high risk for pressure sores.

Box 11-5	*Healthy People 2010: Pressure Ulcers*

- **Objective 1-16:** Reduce the proportion of nursing home residents with a current diagnosis of pressure ulcers.
- **Baseline (1997):** 16 per 1000 residents
- **Target:** 8 diagnoses per 1000 residents

From U.S. Department of Health and Human Services: *Healthy People 2010: national health promotion and disease prevention objectives,* Washington, DC, 2000, The Department. Available at http://www.healthypeople.gov/document/html/tracking/od01.htm#longterm. Accessed 10/25/08.

IMPLICATIONS FOR GERONTOLOGICAL NURSING AND HEALTHY AGING

In all settings nurses, working with patients and significant others, are the persons who are the most responsible for the prevention and treatment of pressure ulcers and other interruptions in skin integrity. Nurses must be able to implement preventive measures as well as identify early signs and initiate appropriate interventions to prevent further skin breakdown and to promote healing. Failure to do this jeopardizes the health and life of the person. The nurse alerts the health care provider of the need for prescribed treatments, recommends treatments, and administers and evaluates the changing status of the wound(s) and adequacy of treatments.

Assessment

Assessment begins with a detailed head-to-toe skin examination and analysis of laboratory findings. Laboratory values that have been correlated with risk for the development and the poor healing of pressure ulcers include those that reflect anemia and poor nutritional status.

Visual and tactile inspection of the entire skin surface with special attention to bony prominences is essential. Inspection is best accomplished in nonglare daylight or, if that is not possible, with focused lighting; special attention should be directed to affected areas when an individual uses orthotic devices such as corsets, braces, prostheses, postural supports, splints, slings, or casts.

The nurse looks for any interruption of skin integrity or other changes, including redness or hyperemia; if pressure is present, it should be relieved and the area reassessed in 1 hour. In darker-pigmented persons, redness may not be observed. Instead it is necessary to look for induration, darkening, or a shadowed appearance of the skin and to feel for warmth or a boggy texture to the affected tissue compared with the surrounding tissue. Pressure areas should be palpated for changes in temperature and tissue resilience. Blisters or pimples with or without hyperemia and scabs over weight-bearing areas in the absence of trauma should be considered suspect.

Ulcers are assessed with each dressing change for worsening, with a detailed assessment repeated on a weekly, biweekly, and as needed basis in the home or the long-term care or rehabilitation setting (Box 11-6). The purpose is to specifically and carefully evaluate the effectiveness of treatment. If there are no signs of healing from week to week or worsening is seen, then either the treatment is insufficient or the wound has become infected; in both cases, treatment must be changed (Box 11-7).

Pressure Ulcer Classification

Pressure ulcers are classified according to the scale developed and updated by the National Pressure Ulcer Advisory Panel (2007) ranging from a suspected injury, to stages 1 through 4 and "unstageable" wounds

---

Box 11-6	Key Aspects of Assessment of a Pressure Ulcer

1. Location and exact size (width, depth, length)
2. Condition of the surrounding tissue
3. Condition of the wound edges: for example, smooth and white or irregular and pink
4. Wound bed: warmth, moisture, color, odor, amount, and color of exudate

---

Box 11-7	Examples of Complications of Pressure Ulcers

- Local infection of wound or surrounding tissue
- Extension of the infection to the bone: osteomyelitis
- Systemic infection: septicemia
- Extended period when acute and chronic medical and nursing care is necessary
- Tetanus
- Loss of function from a disfiguring wound

(Figure 11-2). The ulcer is always classified by the highest stage "achieved," and reverse staging is never used. This means that the wound is documented at the stage representing the maximum damage and depth that has occurred. As the wound heals, it fills with granulation tissue composed of endothelial cells, fibroblasts, collagen, and an extracellular matrix. Muscle, subcutaneous fat, and dermis are not replaced. A stage IV pressure sore that is healing does not revert to stage III and then stage II. It remains defined as a healing (it is hoped) stage IV pressure ulcer. Wounds that are covered in black (eschar) or yellow fibrous (slough) necrosis cannot be staged because it is not possible to determine the condition of the underlying wound bed. These wounds are documented as "unstageable." Once the dead tissue has been removed (debrided) the wound can be staged.

Finally, careful and detailed documentation of the condition of the skin is required. The PUSH tool (Pressure Ulcer Scale for Healing) provides a detailed form that covers all aspects of assessment, but contains only three items and takes only a short time to complete (Gardner et al, 2005). Most institutions have special forms or screens on their computer software

Stage I

Erythema not resolving within thirty (30) minutes of pressure relief. Epidermis remains intact. REVERSIBLE WITH INTERVENTION.

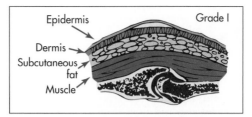

Stage II

Partial-thickness loss of skin layers involving epidermis and possibly penetrating into but not through dermis. May present as blistering with erythema and/or induration; wound base moist and pink; painful; free of necrotic tissue.

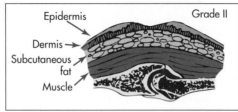

Stage III

Full-thickness tissue loss extending through dermis to involve subcutaneous tissue. Presents as shallow crater unless covered by eschar. May include necrotic tissue, undermining, sinus tract formation, exudate, and/or infection. Wound base is usually not painful.

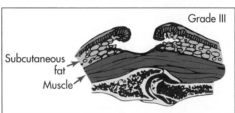

Stage IV

Deep tissue destruction extending through subcutaneous tissue to fascia, possibly involving muscle layers, joint, and/or bone. Presents as a deep crater. May include necrotic tissue, undermining, sinus tract formation, exudate, and/or infection. Wound base is usually not painful.

Unstageable

A wound that is covered by eschar or slough, preventing the visualization of the wound bed.

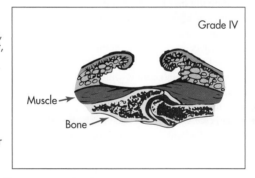

Fig. 11-2   Pressure sore development.

for recording the skin assessment. For those persons with ulcers, photographic documentation is highly recommended both at the onset of the problem and at intervals during its treatment (Ahn and Salicido, 2008). The reader is referred to the web site www.npuap.org for more information.

Interventions

The goal of nurses is to help maintain skin integrity against the various environmental, mechanical, and chemical assaults that are potential causes of breakdown. The goals are consistent with the most basic of Maslow's Hierarchy, one of meeting physiological needs. In promoting healthy aging of all persons, nurses focus on prevention, taking action to eliminate friction and irritation to the skin such as from shearing; reduce moisture so that tissues do not macerate; and displace body weight from prominent areas to facilitate circulation to the skin (Lyder, 2006). The nurse should be familiar with the types of supportive surfaces and types of dressings so the most effective products are used. The nurse should assess the frequency of position change, adding pillows so that skin surfaces do not touch, and establish a turning schedule if needed and patient is agreeable to this.

Box 11-8	Promoting Wound Healing

- Keep wound warm at all times
- Keep clean and moist at all times
- Protect from further injury
- Promptly absorb exudate and fill dead space with a biofriendly material
- Do not subject tissue to caustic products (e.g., Betadine)

Nutritional intake should be monitored, as well as the serum albumin, hematocrit, and hemoglobin levels. Diets high in protein, carbohydrates, and vitamins are necessary to maintain and promote tissue growth. The helpfulness of supplemental amino acids such as arginine, glutamine, and cysteine has not been supported by research (Lyder, 2006). If appetite is lacking, appetite stimulants may be prescribed. The nurse promotes nutritional health by ensuring that dining time is a pleasant experience for the person. This may be contrary to the usual practice in some nursing homes, but doing so has improved the nutrition of high risk elders (Chapter 8).

Realistically, it is not always possible to prevent interruptions in skin integrity caused by overwhelming conditions, especially in the long-term care setting. Fortunately, the state of the science of wound care is well developed, and evidence-based guidelines are available. Sources of information include the websites of the National Pressure Ulcer Advisory Panel (www.npuap.org) and the National Association of Wound, Ostomy and Continence Nurses (www.nwocns.org).

Although a full discussion of the treatment options and indications for their use in the nursing care and treatment of pressure ulcers is beyond the scope of this text, key points in the promotion of healing can be found in Box 11-8.

Consultation with a wound care specialist is advisable for wounds that are extensive or nonhealing. Specialized nurses such as enterostomal therapists or nurse practitioners who may work with wound centers or surgeons provide consultation in nursing homes, offices, or clinics.

HEALTHY FEET

Feet influence one's physical, psychological, and social well-being. Feet carry one's body weight, hold the body erect, coordinate and maintain balance in walking, and must be rigid yet loose and adaptable enough to conform to changing walking surfaces. Little attention is given to one's feet until they interfere with walking and moving and ultimately the ability to remain independent.

Nurses and people in general have a fairly strong negative reaction to having contact with others' feet. It is aesthetically unpleasant to many. Yet promoting healthy feet and good care of the feet can alleviate disability, pain, and decrease the risk for falling. It is for these reasons that this text emphasizes the importance of feet to the well-being of the elderly.

Common Foot Problems

The human foot is a complex structure with many bones, joints, tendons, muscles, and ligaments. Some foot irregularities and problems are genetically inherited; however, many problems occur because of the shoes we wear, wear and tear, and misuse of feet. Shoe styles affect the foot, the hip, and the leg.

Older feet, subjected to a lifetime of stress, may not be able to continue to adapt, and inflammatory changes in bone and soft tissue can occur. Foot health and function may reflect systemic disease or give early clues to physical illness (Figure 11-3). Sudden or gradual changes in the condition of the nails or the skin of the feet or the appearance of recurring infections may be precursors of more serious health problems.

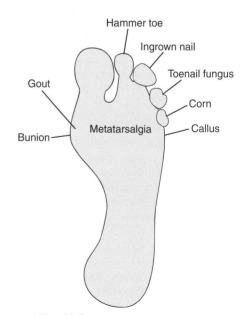

Fig. 11-3   Common foot problems.

Rheumatological disorders such as the different forms of arthritis usually affect other joints but can also affect the feet (see Chapter 18). Gout occurs most often in the joint of the great toe but is a systemic disease (see Chapter 18). Both diabetes and PVD commonly cause problems in the lower extremities that can quickly become life-threatening.

Major abnormalities occur gradually. Without proper care and treatment, these conditions become disabling and threatening to the person's mobility and independence. Care of the foot takes a team approach, including the person, the nurse, the podiatrist, and the person's primary health care provider. Nurses have the opportunity to promote healthy aging by applying their knowledge of the common problems of the feet and their skills in foot care.

Corns, Calluses, and Bunions

Corns and *calluses* are both growths of compacted skin that occur as a result of prolonged pressure, usually from ill-fitting, tight shoes. Corns are cone-shaped and develop on the top of the toe joints from the rubbing of the shoe on the joint. Soft corns form between opposing surfaces of the toes from prolonged squeezing. Both can interfere with the ability to walk and wear shoes comfortably. Once formed, continued pressure on the corn will cause pain. Unless the friction and pressure are relieved, they will continue to enlarge and cause increasing pain.

Many elders self-treat corns and calluses by following what they or their parents have done for years. Over-the-counter preparations may remove the corn temporarily but may also burn the surrounding healthy tissue. Chemical burns and ulcerations from these products can result in the loss of toes or a leg for the person with diabetes, with neurological impairment, or with poor circulation in the LE. Some people use razor blades and scissors to removed the affected tissue; this is very dangerous and is never recommended. Oval corn pads, moleskin, or lamb's wool, with a hole cut in the center for the corn, can be used for more proper treatment. This can be placed around the corn, protecting it from pressure without restricting circulation to healthy tissue. Moleskin is a skin-protective product available in the foot care section of pharmacies and hiking supply stores. Moleskin adheres for several days or longer but should be removed when it becomes wet or excessively soiled. Removing moleskin from the feet should be done slowly to prevent tearing of skin. For persons prone to calluses, daily lubrication of the feet is very important. For persons with PVD and diabetes foot care should only be performed by a trained nurse, doctor, or podiatrist.

Irritation from soft corns between the toes can be eased by loosely wrapping small amounts of lamb's wool around the involved toe, or cotton balls can be placed between the toes. Newer pads of a gel type are also useful to protect against friction and pressure.

Mild corns may resolve themselves when pressure is removed and the offending shoes are replaced by others with a better fit. Larger or resistant corns may need surgical removal by a podiatrist. Corns are not usually removed from high-risk persons, such as those with diabetes or PVD, because of the risk of poor wound healing at the surgical site.

Bunions are bony deformities that also develop from long-standing squeezing together of the first (great) and second toes. Bony prominences develop over the medial aspect of the joint of the great toe and, at times, at the lateral aspect of the fifth metatarsal head (the joint of the little toe and called a *tailor bunion* or a *bunionette*). There may be a hereditary factor in their development. Walking can be markedly compromised with any of these. Bunions may be treated with corticosteroid injections or antiinflammatory pain medications. A custom-made shoe should be considered. Shoes that provide forefront space (e.g., running shoes) work well. Surgery is a possibility.

The nurse promotes comfort by working with the person to find shoes that will properly support and protect the foot and not worsen the deformity or problem. At the time of this writing Medicare covered the cost of orthotic shoes once a year for persons with diabetes.

Hammer Toes

A *hammer toe* is permanently flexed with a claw-like appearance; the condition is a result of muscle imbalance and pressure from the big toe slanting toward the second toe. The toe then contracts, leaving a bulge on top of the joint. It is aggravated, again, by poor-fitting shoes and is often seen in conjunction with bunions (Meadows, 2006). This condition limits the ability to walk and restricts balance and comfort. As with bunions, treatment includes professional orthotics or specially designed protective devices; properly fitting, nonconstricting shoes; and/or surgical intervention.

Fungal Infections

Fungal infections are very common on the aging foot, and the incidence increases with age (Habif, 2005). It may affect the skin of the foot as well as the nails. Nail fungus, or *onychomycosis,* is characterized by

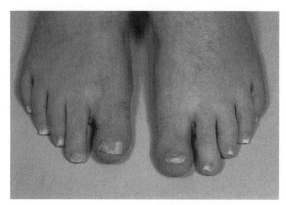

Fig. 11-4 Onchomycosis: yellowing, crumbling, and thickening of the toenails. *(From Bolognia J, Jorizzo JL, Rapini R:* Dermatology, *St Louis, 2003, Mosby.)*

Box 11-9	Essential Aspects of Foot Assessment

Observation of Mobility
- Gait
- Use of assistive devices
- Footwear type and pattern of wear

Past Medical History
- Neuropathies
- Musculoskeletal limitations
- PVD
- Vision problems
- History of falls
- Pain affecting movement

Bilateral Assessment
- Color
- Circulation and warmth
- Pulses
- Structural deformities
- Skin lesions
- LE edema
- Evidence of scratching
- Rash or excessive dryness
- Condition and color of toenails

PVD, Peripheral vascular disease; *LE,* lower-extremity.

degeneration of the nail plate with color changes to yellow or brown and opaque, brittleness, and thickening of the nail (Figure 11-4). A fine powdery collection of fungus forms under the center of the nail, separating the layers and pushing it up, causing the sides of the nail to dig into the skin like an ingrown toenail. Culturing is the only definitive way to diagnose onychomycosis. Hands should be washed each time feet with a fungal infection are handled. When nails are involved, cure is difficult to impossible because of the limited circulation to the nails. Several oral medications are available, but all are expensive and of limited effectiveness, are taken for long periods of time (3 to 12 months), and are potentially toxic to the liver and heart.

The fungal infection of the foot (*Tinea pedis*) is due to many of the same causes as *Candida* elsewhere on the body. *Tinea pedis* is treated similarly to any other fungal infections. Feet, especially between the toes, should be kept dry and clean and regularly exposed to sun and air. Topical application of antifungal powders, in addition to the hygiene measures already noted, is the usual treatment. If exacerbated by diabetes, glycemic control is an additional goal.

IMPLICATIONS FOR GERONTOLOGICAL NURSING AND HEALTHY AGING

The gerontological nurse is an advocate for promoting the best foot health possible. Foot care is a prime factor in the maintenance of mobility and independence. Nursing care of person with foot problems should be directed toward optimal comfort and function, removing possible mechanical irritants, and decreasing the likelihood of infection. The nurse has the important function of assessing the feet for clues of functional ability and their owner's well-being—not just bathing and applying lotion to the feet (Box 11-9). Nurses can identify potential and actual problems and make referral to or seek assistance as needed from the primary care provider or podiatrist for any changes in the feet.

Gerontological nursing care includes observation of gait, postural deformities, physical limitations, position of the foot with the heel strike, and the type of shoe worn and its condition, including sole wear. Inspect feet for irritation, abrasions, and other lesions; check for hazards to the maintenance of adequate circulation to the lower extremities and the existing circulatory status; and observe the individual's general mobility. Periodic assessment of the feet is especially important for persons with diabetes, heart disease, PVD, and thyroid or renal conditions as well as any neurological impairment, such as reduced or absent sensation resulting from a stroke.

Care of the Toenails

Care of the feet and nails of persons in the long-term care setting falls to the nurse. Poor close vision, difficulty bending, obesity, or increased thickness makes self-care difficult. Normal nails that become too long will begin to interfere with stockings, hose, or shoes. Ideally, toenails should be trimmed after the bath or shower when they are softened, but if this is not possible, soaking the feet for 20 to 30 minutes before care is sufficient. They should be clipped straight across and even with the top of the toe, with the edges filed slightly to remove the sharpness but not to the point of rounding (Figure 11-5). Diabetic foot care should only be done by the podiatrist or the registered nurse (RN) with some experience, with special care to prevent accidental damage or trauma to the skin. Diabetic nail care can never be delegated to the licensed practical nurse (LPN) or certified nurse assistant (CNA). Persons with diabetes or peripheral neuropathy should never have pedicures from commercial establishments.

Nails that are neglected will become long and curved. This type of nail is known as *ram's horn* because of its appearance. Hard, thickened nails indicate inadequate nutrition to the nail matrix because of trauma or poor circulation. Once the nail becomes thickened, it will remain so. Nails that are thick and hard split easily, causing trauma to the matrix, pain, and possibly infection. Any attempt by the nurse or other caregiver to cut these nails may result in further damage to the matrix or precipitate an infection. These conditions should be brought to the attention of a podiatrist.

An ingrown toenail is a fragment of nail that pierces the skin at the edge of the nail. Often this problem is a consequence of the hypertrophy of the nail with onychomycosis, of improper cutting of the nail, or of pressure exerted on the toes by tight hosiery or shoes.

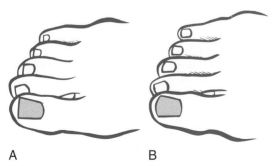

Fig. 11-5 Cutting toenails. **A,** Correct angle and shape. **B,** Incorrect angle and shape.

Ingrown toenails should be referred to the podiatrist because of the risk of infection. Temporary relief can be provided by inserting a small piece of cotton under the affected nail corner.

Nursing interventions include assisting the older person to understand the necessity of appropriate footwear and to obtain it. Shoes should be new enough to provide support and should not have excessive sole wear, especially in any one area. For persons with diabetes or other neurological impairments, the shoes should cover and protect the foot entirely without pressure areas. For persons with arthritis, firm soles are more comfortable than soft soles and may decrease pain associated with walking (Meadows, 2006).

Shoes should be functional, that is, cover, protect, and stabilize the foot and provide maximum toe space. They must also be the right size. One foot is usually larger than the other, and feet lengthen slightly with age and are largest in the afternoons. Shoes should be fitted to the largest foot, and afternoon purchases are advised. There should be about a half inch of space (a "thumb's width") from the longest toe to the tip of the shoe while the person is standing. Shoes should provide enough forefoot space laterally and dorsally with a wide toe box and comfortable fit, such as that found in ultralight walking shoes and running shoes. Fabric shoes are not recommended for persons with diabetes or PVD. Low-heeled shoes place less stress on the legs and back than completely flat shoes and are ideal for comfort.

Slip-on shoes are helpful for those who are unable to bend or lace shoes, but care must be taken that the person will not accidentally "slip out" of the shoe, which can lead to a fall. Velcro closures are useful for those who have limited finger dexterity.

Custom-made shoes, although expensive, may be necessary for persons with bunions or any other deformity. These come in a broad range of prices. Medicare will cover the cost of one pair of orthotic shoes per year for persons with diabetes when purchased from an approved vendor.

▶ KEY CONCEPTS

▶ The skin is the largest and most visible organ of the body; it has multiple roles in maintaining one's health.

▶ Maintaining adequate moisture and skin lubrication will reduce the incidence of xerosis and other skin problems.

▶ The best way to minimize the risk of skin cancer is to avoid prolonged sun and smoke exposure.

▶ Prompt treatment of the persons with a herpes zoster infection is needed to decrease the risk of postherpetic neuralgia.

▶ The problems of the skin and the feet may reflect systemic disease.

▶ Mobility is fundamental to independence; therefore care of the feet and toenails is an important area for the gerontological nurse.

▶ A pressure ulcer is documented by stage, which reflects the greatest degree of tissue damage; and as it heals, reverse staging is not appropriate.

▶ A pressure ulcer that is covered in dead tissue (eschar or slough) cannot be staged until it has been debrided.

▶ Darkly pigmented persons will not display the "typical" erythema of a stage I pressure ulcer or early PVD, therefore closer vigilance is necessary.

▶ Persons with PVD, diabetes, or peripheral neuropathy are at special risk for serious skin problems.

ACTIVITIES AND DISCUSSION QUESTIONS

1. Describe the common skin and foot problems an older adult is more likely to experience.
2. What is the nurse's responsibility in health promotion related to maintaining skin integrity?
3. List several interventions that apply to skin care and to foot care.
4. Develop a nursing care plan using wellness and North American Nursing Diagnosis Association (NANDA) diagnoses.

RESOURCES

Educational Materials

Guidelines, educational information, and professional opportunities with the Wound, Ostomy and Continence Nurses Society (www.wocns.org)

Materials and tools available from the National Pressure Ulcer Advisory Panel (www.npuap.org)

Patient and professional information available at the National Institute of Arthritis, Musculoskeletal and Skin Diseases (www.nih.gov/niams)

Photos and information about a range of skin problems (www.dermatlas.com)

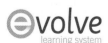

For additional resources, please visit evolve.elsevier.com/Ebersole/gerontological.

REFERENCES

Ahn C, Salicido RS: Advances in would photography and assessment methods, *Adv Skin Wound Care* 21(2):94-95, 2008

American Cancer Society (ACS): *Cancer facts & figures 2008*, Atlanta, 2008, The Society.

American Heart Association: *Peripheral Artery Disease (PAD)*, September 6, 2007. Accessed 4/19/08 from www.americanheart.org.

Bergstrom N, Allman R, Alvarez OM et al: *Treatment of pressure ulcers. Clinical practice guideline no. 15, AHCPR pub no. 95-0652,* Rockville, Md, 1994, U.S. Department of Health and Human Services, Public Health Service, Agency for Health Care Policy and Research.

Gardner SE, Frantz RA, Bergquist S, Shin CD: A prospective study of the pressure ulcer scale for healing (PUSH). *J Gerontol Series A* 60:93-97, 2005.

Habif TP: *Skin disease: diagnosis and treatment*, ed 2, St. Louis, 2005, Mosby.

Heinen MM, Persoon A, van de Kerkhof P et al: Ulcer-related problems and health care needs in patients with venous leg ulcerations: a descriptive, cross-sectional study, *Int J Nursing Studies* 44(8):1296-1303, 2006.

Lyder C: Effective management of pressure ulcers, *Adv Nurse Pract* 14(7):32-40, 2006.

Mayo Clinic: *Actinic keratosis*, January 4, 2007. Accessed 4/19/08 from www.mayoclinic.com.

Meadows M: *Taking care of your feet,* 2006, U.S. Food and Drug Administration. Accessed 4/18/08 from www.fda.gov.

National Pressure Ulcer Advisory Panel: *Pressure ulcers stages revised*, February 2007. Accessed 4/19/08 from www.npuap.org.

Norman RA: Xerosis and pruritus in the elderly: recognition and management, *Dermatol Ther* 16(3):254-259, 2003.

Norton D: Calculating the risk: reflections on the Norton Scale, *Adv Wound Care* 9(6):38-43, 1996.

Shahin ES, Dassen T, Halfens RJ: Incidence, prevention and treatment of pressure ulcers in intensive care patients: a longitudinal study, *Int J Nurs Stud* 2008 in press, corrected proof available online April 8, 2008, DOI:10.1016/i.iijnurstu.2008.02.011.

Skin Cancer Foundation (SCF): About melanoma; about squamous cell; about basal cell carcinoma, 2006. Accessed 4/19/08 from www.skincancer.org.

Sommers MS, Johnson SA, Beery TA: *Diseases and disorders: a nursing therapeutics manual*, ed 3, Philadelphia, 2007, F.A. Davis.

12

Maintaining Mobility and Environmental Safety

LEARNING OBJECTIVES

Upon completion of this chapter, the reader will be able to:

- Discuss the effects of impaired mobility on general function and quality of life.
- Specify risk factors for impaired mobility.
- Identify older adults at risk for falls and list several measures to reduce fall risk.
- Understand the effects of restraints and discuss appropriate alternatives for safety promotion.
- Identify factors in the environment that contribute to the safety and security of the older person.
- Relate strategies for protecting the older person from injury and accidents in the home and in the community.
- Develop a nursing care plan appropriate for an elder at risk of falling.

GLOSSARY

Orthostatic (postural) hypotension A drop in blood pressure occurring when a person assumes an upright position after being in a lying-down position.
Proprioception Sensations from within the body regarding spatial position and muscular activity.

Sarcopenia Loss of skeletal muscle mass, strength, and function.
Syncope Brief lapse in consciousness caused by transient cerebral hypoxia.

THE LIVED EXPERIENCE

After that fall last year when I slipped on the urine in the bathroom, I feel so insecure. I find myself taking small, shuffling steps to avoid falling again, but it makes me feel awkward and clumsy. When I was younger, I never worried about falling, but now I'm so afraid I will break a bone or something.

Betty, age 75

MOBILITY, SAFETY, AND SATISFACTION

Mobility is the capacity one has for movement within one's environment, both the immediate one and the larger-scale. In infancy, moving about is the major mode of learning and interacting with the environment.

In old age, one moves more slowly and purposefully, sometimes with more forethought and caution. Throughout life, movement remains a significant means of personal contact, sensation, exploration, pleasure, and control.

This chapter focuses on maintaining maximal mobility both in health and in the presence of various disorders, the assessment of gait and mobility status, the effects of restraints, measures to promote safety without the use of restraints, causes and consequences of falls in older adults, fall risk reduction, and aids and interventions that are useful when mobility is impaired. Specific information will be provided to promote a safe environment for older adults in all settings. Issues related to transportation and driving as essential aspects of environmental mobility are also included. Activity and exercise are discussed in Chapter 10 and bone and joint problems affecting mobility are discussed in Chapter 18.

Mobility and Agility

Mobility and comparative degrees of agility are based on muscle strength, flexibility, postural stability, vibratory sensation, cognition, and perceptions of stability. Aging produces changes in muscles and joints, particularly of the back and the legs. Strength and flexibility of muscles decrease, and to a somewhat lesser extent endurance also decreases, especially if there is a decrease in activity as one ages. Movements and range of motion become more limited. Normal wear and tear reduce the smooth cartilage of joints. Movement is less fluid as one ages, and joints change as regeneration of tissue slows and muscle wasting occurs. Proper management of chronic illnesses and maintenance of healthy lifestyles forestalls the onset of mobility limitation in old age.

Sarcopenia, a loss of skeletal muscle mass, strength, and function thought to be related to aging, contributes to mobility impairments and disability and is a marker of frailty (Janssen, 2006). Limitations in mobility are approximately 3 times greater in older women and 2 times greater in older men with sarcopenia (Yeom et al, 2008). Findings from studies in the United Kingdom suggest that "prenatal and postnatal development of muscle fibers and muscle growth during puberty may have critical, or at least sensitive, effects on musculoskeletal aging and risk of frailty" (Kuh, 2007).

Some gait changes thought to be associated with aging include a narrower standing base, wider side-to-side swaying when walking, slowed responses, a greater reliance on proprioception, diminished arm swing, and increased care in gait. Steps are slower, and there is a decrease in step height (lifting of the foot when taking a step). These changes are less pronounced in those who remain active and at a desirable weight. A sedentary lifestyle, excess weight, and smoking are associated with mobility problems (Yeom et al,

2008). Health promotion programs to address these factors will contribute to improving mobility and functional status among older adults. Exercise and strength training, even for frail elders, improve mobility and function (Chapter 10). Various degrees of immobility are often temporary or permanent consequences of illness. Falls and fractures often bring about periods of immobility. Consequences of immobility are shown in (Box 12-1).

On a broader scale, elders frequently have limited environmental mobility because of a lack of transportation or loss of a driver's license. In summary, many normal and abnormal changes affect the fluidity and comfort of movement and the capacity for involvement with one's surroundings. Impairment of mobility is highly associated with poor outcomes in older people (Morley et al, 2003). Maintenance of mobility and safety for older adults is one of the most important components of gerontological nursing.

Healthy People 2010 (U.S. Department of Health and Human Services, 2000) contains goals and objectives that relate to mobility and safety concerns for older adults (Box 12-2).

Disorders Affecting Mobility

Common conditions that accompany the normal changes of aging, as well as disorders that occur more frequently in older adults, merit special attention. Osteoporosis, gait disorders, Parkinson's disease, strokes, and arthritic conditions markedly affect movement and functional capacities (see Chapters 18 and 21). Mobility may also be limited by paresthesias; amputations;

Box 12-1	Consequences of Immobility

- Dehydration
- Bronchial pneumonia
- Contractures
- Constipation
- Pressure ulcers
- Incontinence
- Hypothermia
- Iatrogenic complications
- Disability
- Institutionalization
- Loss of independence
- Isolation and depression

Box 12-2 | **Goals and Objectives of *Healthy People 2010*: Mobility and Safety**

- Reduce deaths from falls.
- Reduce hip fractures among older adults.
- Eliminate racial disparities in the rate of total knee replacement.
- Prevent illness and disability related to arthritis and other rheumatic conditions and osteoporosis.
- Decrease the proportion of all adults with chronic joint symptoms who have difficulty in performing two or more personal care activities, thereby preserving independence.
- Increase the proportion of adults ages 18 and older with arthritis who seek help if they experience personal and emotional problems.
- Increase the proportion of adults who have seen a health care provider for chronic joint symptoms.
- Increase the proportion of persons with arthritis who have had effective, evidence-based arthritis education as an integral part of the management of their condition.
- Increase the mean number of days without severe pain among adults who have chronic joint symptoms.
- Reduce the proportion of adults with osteoporosis.
- Reduce the proportion of adults who are hospitalized for vertebral fractures associated with osteoporosis.

From U.S. Department of Health and Human Services: *Healthy People 2010: national health promotion and disease prevention objectives,* Washington, DC, 2000, The Department.

---

neuromotor disturbances; fractures; foot, knee, and hip problems; and illnesses that deplete one's energy. Many elders in their later years have some of these afflictions, with women significantly outnumbering men in this respect.

FALLS AND FALL RISK REDUCTION

Defining a Fall

A fall has been defined in the literature as unintentionally coming to rest on a lower area such as the ground or floor (Buchner et al, 1993). A recent study (Zecevic et al, 2006) comparing the definition of a fall and reasons for falls among seniors, health care providers, and the research literature suggested that the word *fall* is interpreted in many different ways. Often the terms *slips, trips,* and *falls* are used interchangeably. Exactly what constitutes a fall for reporting procedures in institutions is problematic and can lead to inconsistencies in data (Zecevic et al, 2006). Therefore it is important to define a fall in words that seniors understand and to use an operational definition of falls in all research and fall-reporting data. Further recommendations from the study included asking older people about falls that did not result in injury and assessing the circumstances of a fall, near fall, mishap, or misstep as important information for prevention of future falls.

Falls: A Significant Geriatric Syndrome

Among older adults, falls are the leading cause of injury deaths and the most common cause of nonfatal injuries and hospital admissions for trauma (Centers for Disease Control [CDC], 2006a). Falls are a significant public health problem, and the rates of fall-related deaths among older adults has risen significantly over the past decade (Stevens et al, 2006) (Box 12-3). The federal government and many groups involved in health in aging have made fall risk reduction a major initiative.

All falls in the nursing home setting are considered sentinel events and must be reported to the Centers for Medicare & Medicaid Services (CMS). In response to rising fall-related sentinel events in health care organizations, the Joint Commission (JC) has established National Patient Safety Goals (NPSG) for fall reduction in all JC-approved institutions across the health care continuum (Capezuti et al, 2008). The National Center for Injury Prevention and Control and the National Resource Center for Safe Aging provide valuable information on falls and fall risk–reduction programs useful for older people and professionals (see Resources at the end of the chapter and on the Evolve site).

Falls are a symptom of a problem, although they become the focus of a problem when they occur.

Box 12-3	Statistics on Falls and Fall-Related Concerns

- One third of people older than 65 years fall at least 1 time each year, and about half of those fall repeatedly.
- Falls account for 40% of nursing home admissions annually (Tideiksaar, 2005).
- Of those who fall, 20% to 30% suffer moderate to serious injuries such as hip fractures or head traumas (Centers for Disease Control and Prevention, 2006a).
- Traumatic brain injuries accounted for 46% of fatal falls among older adults (Stevens et al, 2006).
- More than half of deaths related to falls occurred within the home (Staats, 2008).
- Up to 20% of hospitalized patients and 45% of those in long-term care facilities will fall. In these settings, injury rates are considerably higher with 10% to 25% of institutional falls resulting in fracture, laceration, or the need for hospital care (American Geriatrics Society, 2001).
- Men are more likely to die from a fall. After adjusting for age, the fall fatality rate in 2004 was 49% higher for men than for women (Centers for Disease Control and Prevention, 2006a).
- Rates of fall-related fractures among older adults are more than twice as high for women as for men. White women have significantly higher rates of fall-related hip fractures than black women (Stevens et al, 2006).
- More than 95% of hip fractures among older adults are caused by falls.
- Between 18% and 33% of older patients with hip fractures die within 1 year of their fracture.
- Up to 25% of adults who lived independently before their hip fracture have to stay in a nursing home for at least a year after their injury (Magaziner et al, 2000).
- Direct care costs related to falls are estimated at more than $20 billion and are projected to rise to over $34 billion by 2030 (Chang et al, 2004; Quigley, 2005).

Falls are rarely benign in older people. The etiology of falls is multifactorial; falls may indicate neurological, sensory, cognitive, medication, or musculoskeletal problems or impending physical illness. The cause of a fall is usually an interaction between an environmental factor, such as a wet floor, and an intrinsic factor, such as limited vision, cognitive impairment, or gait problems. In institutional settings, iatrogenic factors such as limited staffing, lack of toileting programs, and restraints and side rails also interact to increase fall risk. Frail older people with mobility and functional impairments are at the greatest risk of falls (Tideiksaar, 2005).

Factors Contributing to Falls

After age 65, individuals fall most frequently because of external reasons; however, with increasing age, internal and locomotor reasons become increasingly prevalent. Some fall risk factors increase proportionally as one ages:

- ▶ disturbances in visual acuity
- ▶ cognitive impairment
- ▶ postural hypotension
- ▶ cardiac arrhythmias
- ▶ uncontrolled diabetes
- ▶ depressive symptoms
- ▶ lower-extremity weakness
- ▶ gait disturbances
- ▶ use of four or more prescription medications

Abnormal gait affects 20% to 50% of people over age 65 and increases susceptibility to falls. Arthritis of the hip and the knee and foot deformities are common causes of gait disturbances and instability (Rubenstein and Trueblood, 2004). Those who fall more often tend to be women, more functionally impaired, and taking more medications. Episodes of acute illness or exacerbations of chronic illness are times of high fall risk (Tinetti, 2003). In inpatient settings, root causes of patient falls were attributed to inadequacies in the following: patient assessment (accounting for 70% of patient falls); communication (accounting for more than 60% of patient falls); and environmental safety and security (accounting for 50% of patient falls) (Gray-Micelli, 2008). A relationship may exist between urinary tract infections and falls, particularly in nursing home patients with dementia. One study noted that insomnia is a fall risk factor in institutionalized elders who may get out of bed during the night while drowsy and fall (Avidan et al, 2005). Table 12-1 presents fall risk factors.

Even if a fall does not result in injury, falls contribute to a loss of confidence that leads to reduced physical activity, increased dependency, and social withdrawal (Rubenstein et al, 2003). Fear of falling

Table 12-1 Fall Risk Factors for Elders

CONDITIONS	SITUATIONS
Sedative and alcohol use, psychoactive medications, diuretics, anticholinergics, antidepressants	Urinary incontinence, urgency, nocturia
Four or more medications	Environmental hazards
Unrelieved pain	Recent relocation, unfamiliarity with new environment
Previous falls and fractures	Inadequate response to transfer and toileting needs
Female, 80 years or older	Assistive devices used for walking
Acute and recent illness	Inadequate or missing safety rails, particularly in bathroom
Cognitive impairment (delirium, dementia)	Poorly designed or unstable furniture
Diabetes	High chairs and beds
Dehydration	Uneven floor surfaces
Weakness of lower extremities	Glossy, highly waxed floors
Abnormalities of gait and balance	Wet, greasy, icy surfaces
Unsteadiness, dizziness, syncope	Inadequate visual support (glare, low wattage bulbs, lack nightlights)
Foot problems	General clutter
Depression, anxiety	Inappropriate footwear
Decreased vision or hearing	Pets that inadvertently trip an individual
Fear of falling	Electrical cords
Postural hypotension	Loose or uneven stair treads
Postprandial drop in blood pressure	Throw rugs
Skeletal and neuromuscular changes that predispose to weakness and postural imbalance	Reaching for a high shelf
Functional limitations in self-care activities	Inability to reach personal items, lack of access to call bell or inability to use
Wheelchair-bound	Side rails, restraints
Decreased weight	Lack of staff training in fall risk–reduction techniques
Inability to rise from a chair without using the arms	
Slow walking speed	

Data from: NIA/NIH Senior Health: Falls and older adults, 2006, Accessed April 1, 2008 from http://nihseniorhealth.gov/falls/causesandriskfactors/01.html; Feinsod F et al: Reducing fall risk in long-term care residents through the interdisciplinary approach, *Ann Long-Term Care* 13(7):25-33, 2005; Rubinstein T, Alexander N, Hausdoff J: Evaluating fall risks in older adults: steps and missteps, *Clin Geriatr* 11(1):52-61, 2003; Tinetti ME, Speechley J, Ginter SF: Risk factors for falls among elderly persons living in the community, *N Engl J Med* 319(26): 1701-1707, 1988.

("fallophobia") may restrict an individual's life space (area in which an individual carries on activities). Fear of falling is an important predictor of general functional decline and a risk factor for future falls. Frequent falls contribute significantly to the downward spiral in frail older people (Morley, 2002). Nursing staff may also contribute to fear of falling in their patients by telling them not to get up by themselves or using restrictive devices to keep them from independently moving about (Resnick, 2002). More appropriate nursing responses would be to assess fall risk and design individual prevention interventions and safety plans that enhance mobility and independence and decrease fall risk.

IMPLICATIONS FOR GERONTOLOGICAL NURSING AND HEALTHY AGING

Assessment

A comprehensive assessment, including attention to the conditions and situations noted above, and nursing observations of function, are essential in assessing fall risk. The nurse is most likely to have had extended opportunities to observe the elder's functioning, whether in the community or in an institution. Families' observations also provide important data. Older people may be reluctant to share information about falls for fear of losing independence, so the gerontological nurse must use judgment and empathy in eliciting information about falls, assuring the person that there are many modifiable factors to increase safety and help maintain independence.

Assessment is an ongoing process that includes "multiple and continual types of assessment, reassessment, and evaluation following a fall or intervention to prevent a fall. Assessment includes 1) assessment of the older adult patient at risk; 2) nursing assessment of the patient following a fall; 3) assessment of the environment and other situational circumstances upon admission and during hospitalization; and 4) assessment of the older adult's knowledge of falls and their prevention, including willingness to change behavior if necessary, to prevent falls" (Gray-Micelli, 2008, p. 164).

Fall Risk Assessment

A variety of fall risk assessment instruments are available, and those that have been evaluated for reliability and validity should be used in institutional settings rather than creating new instruments (Gray-Micelli, 2008). Fall risk assessments provide general information about a person's risk factors but must be used in combination with additional individual assessment so that appropriate fall risk–reduction interventions can be developed and modifiable risk factors identified and managed. Additional research is needed to develop valid, reliable instruments to differentiate levels of fall risk in various settings.

The Hendrich II Fall Risk Model (Figure 12-1) is an example of an instrument that has been validated with skilled nursing and rehabilitation populations (Miller, 2008). The Morse Fall Scale (Morse et al, 1989) is also widely used in hospitals and other inpatient settings (www.va.gov/NCPS/CogAids/FallPrevention/index.html#). In the nursing home setting, the Minimum Data Set (MDS) calls for information about a history of falls and hip fractures in the last 180 days, and the fall-related resident assessment protocol (RAP) provides an excellent overview of fall risk and fall assessment. Box 12-4 presents fall RAP triggers identified on the MDS 2.0. See Chapter 5 for discussion of MDS.

The American Geriatrics Society (AGS, 2001) recommends that all persons over 65 years be asked at least once a year about falls. A history of falls is an important predictor of future falls, and any older person who reports a fall should be observed using the Get-Up-and-Go Test (Mathias et al, 1986) (Figure 12-1). This test is a practical assessment tool for older people that can be adopted in any setting (Resnick et al, 2001). The client is asked to rise from a straight-backed chair, stand briefly, walk forward about 10 feet, turn, walk back to the chair,

turn around, and sit down. Performance is graded on a 5-point scale from 1 (normal) to 5 (severely abnormal). The quality of the movement is assessed for impaired balance. A score of 3 or higher suggests high risk for falling.

An older person who is seen after a fall, who demonstrates abnormalities of gait or balance and impaired performance on the Get-Up-And-Go Test, or who has had recurrent falls should have a comprehensive fall evaluation (CFE) (Box 12-5). The MDS also includes a balance assessment and functional assessment for older adults residing in long-term care facilities.

Environmental Assessment

Assessment of home safety and environmental factors should also be included in a comprehensive fall assessment of community-dwelling elders. Environmental barriers often discourage ambulation in various settings. In the outside environment, steps and curbs may be too high. Buses, subway trains, elevators, revolving doors, and escalators may move too rapidly for the slower-moving older person to enter and exit comfortably. Thus the individual may find the interactional world gradually shrinking as a result of factors that are beyond his or her control. In the UK, road signs indicate areas of caution where older people may be crossing, similar to signs found in the US for children. It sends a message that older people's safety on the roads is important. Fortunately, in the past 2 decades, the government has made a concerted effort to encourage the elimination of environmental barriers for the disabled, and this has had a beneficial effect on older adults as they negotiate the environment.

Home safety assessment should include fall and injury risk, as well as fire and crime risk assessment. An evidence-based home safety assessment tool developed by Tanner (2003) includes fall and injury risk, as well as fire and crime risk assessment (Box 12-6). Older adults with Alzheimer's may present with additional risk factors for fall and other injuries. Hurley and colleagues (2004) describe a home safety/injury model for persons with Alzheimer's disease and their caregivers that addresses the physical environment and caregiver competence. Table 12-2 provides suggestions for assessment of safety in the home environment. Environmental safety is further discussed later in this chapter.

Assessment After a Fall

Incomplete analysis of the reasons for a fall can result in repeated incidents. It is essential that nurses evaluate each older adult's risk for falls. Postfall assessments (PFAs) are

Hendrich II Fall Risk Model™			
Confusion Disorientation Impulsivity		4	
Symptomatic Depression		2	
Altered Elimination		1	
Dizziness Vertigo		1	
Male Gender		1	
Any Administered Antiepileptics		2	
Any Administered Benzodiazepines		1	
Get Up & Go Test			
Able to rise in a single movement – No loss of balance with steps		0	
Pushes up, successful in one attempt		1	
Multiple attempts, but successful		3	
Unable to rise without assistance during test (OR if a medical order states the same and/or complete bed rest is ordered) * If unable to assess, document this on the patient chart with the date and time		4	
A Score of 5 or Greater = High Risk		**Total Score**	

Fig. 12-1 The Hendrich II Fall Risk Model, a fall risk assessment tool recommended by the Hartford Institute for Geriatric Nursing. ©2007 AHI of Indiana Inc. All Rights Reserved. US Patent (US20050182305) has been allowed. Reproduction and use prohibited except by written permission from AHI of Indian Inc.

essential to prevention of future falls and implementation of risk-reduction programs, particularly in institutional settings (Gray-Micelli et al, 2005). If the older adult cannot tell you about the circumstances of the fall, information should be obtained from staff or witnesses. The purpose of the PFA is to identify the underlying cause of the fall and assist in implementing appropriate individualized risk-reduction interventions. "Components of the PFA are typically routinely performed by professional nurses in all patient settings, although this evaluation may be limited according to the completeness of the questions and examination included on the tool used" (Gray-Micelli, 2008, p. 176). Standard "incident report" forms do not provide adequate postfall assessment information. Box 12-7 presents provides information for a PFA that can be used in health care institutions.

Box 12-4	Fall-Related Resident Assessment Protocol Triggers Identified on the MDS 2.0

Alzheimer's disease or other dementia
Arthritis
Cane, walker, crutch
Cardiac dysrhythmia
Cardiovascular, psychotropic, or diuretic
  medications
Decline in cognition
Decline in functional status
Delirium
Device or restraint
Dizziness, vertigo, syncope
Fracture of hip, history of falls
Incontinence
Hemiplegia or hemiparesis
Hypotension
Impaired hearing or vision
Joint pain
Loss of arm or leg movement
Manic depression
Missing limb
Osteoporosis
Pacemaker
Parkinson's disease
Seizures
Unstable chronic or acute condition
Unsteady gait
Wandering

MDS, Minimum Data Set.
Adapted from Buckwalter K, Katz I, Martin H: Guide to the prevention and management of falls in the elderly, II, *CNS Long-Term Care* 3(2 Spring):31, 2004.

Restraints and Side Rails

Restraints have been used historically for the "protection" of the client and for the security of the client and staff. Restraints may be physical or chemical. A physical restraint is defined as "any manual method or physical or mechanical device, material, or equipment attached or adjacent to the individual's body that the individual cannot remove easily which restricts freedom of movement or normal access to one's body" (www.cms.gov).

Chemical restraints have come under careful scrutiny, both legal and ethical, in recent years. Chemical restraints are considered the use of medication, particularly psychotropics, under any of the following conditions (Tideiksaar, 1998):

▶ Given without specific indications
▶ Given in excessive doses and affecting functioning
▶ Used as sole treatment without using behavioral interventions
▶ Administered for the convenience of the staff

Physical restraints were originally used to control the behavior of individuals with mental illness considered to be dangerous to themselves or others (Evans and Strumpf, 1989). Some common reasons for restraining patients today include prevention of falls, altered mental status, prevention of harming self or others, wandering, agitation, and prevention of interference with treatment. The problem of restraint use was first brought to the forefront of nursing attention by a request from Doris Schwartz, one of the gerontological nursing pioneers, for information from practicing nurses regarding their observations and concerns about restraint usage. In the intervening time, and largely through the efforts of Schwartz, her colleagues, and substantial nursing research, the use of restraints has been drastically reduced.

To date, there is no evidence in the literature documenting the efficacy of physical restraints in maintaining safety, preventing disruption of treatment, or controlling behavior. In fact, research over the past 20 years, primarily in long-term care settings, has shown that the practice of physical restraint is ineffective and hazardous (Capezuti et al, 2008). Physical restraints, intended to prevent injury, do not protect patients from falling, wandering, or removing tubes and other medical devices. Physical restraints may actually exacerbate many of the problems for which they are used and can cause serious injury as well as emotional and physical problems.

Physical restraints are associated with higher mortality rates, injurious falls, nosocomial infections, incontinence, contractures, pressure ulcers, agitation, and depression. Although prevention of falls is most frequently cited as the primary reason for using restraints, restraints do not prevent serious injury and may even increase the risk of injury and death. Injuries occur as a result of the patient attempting to remove the restraint or attempting to get out of bed. "The most common mechanism of restraint-related death is by asphyxiation—that is, the person is suspended by a restraint from a bed or chair and the ability to inhale is inhibited by gravitational chest compression" (Capezuti et al, 2008, p. 168).

Box 12-5 | **Recommended Components of Clinical Assessment and Management for Older Persons Living in the Community Who are at Risk for Falling**

Assessment And Risk Factor

Circumstances of previous falls*

Medication use
- High-risk medications (e.g., benzodiazepines, other sleeping medications, neuroleptics, antidepressants, anticonvulsants, or class IA antidysrhythmics)*,†,‡
- Four or more medications‡

Vision
- Acuity <20/60
- Decreased depth perception
- Decreased contrast sensitivity
- Cataracts

Postural blood pressure (after ≥5 minutes in a supine position, immediately after standing, and 2 minutes after standing)‡
≥20 mm Hg (or ≥20%) drop in systolic pressure, with or without symptoms, either immediately upon standing or after 2 minutes of standing

Balance and gait†,‡
- Patient's report or observation of unsteadiness
- Impairment on brief assessment (e.g., the Get-Up-and-Go Test or performance-oriented assessment of mobility)

Targeted neurological examination
- Impaired proprioception*
- Impaired cognition*
- Decreased muscle strength†,‡

Targeted musculoskeletal examination: examination of legs (joints and range of motion) and examination of feet*

Targeted cardiovascular examination†
- Syncope
- Arrhythmia (if there is known cardiac disease, an abnormal electrocardiogram, and syncope)

Home-hazard evaluation after hospital discharge†,‡

Management

Changes in environment and activity to reduce the likelihood of recurrent falls
Review and reduction of medications

Ample lighting without glare; avoidance of multifocal glasses while walking; referral to an ophthalmologist

Diagnosis and treatment of underlying cause, if possible; review and reduction of medications; modification of salt restriction; adequate hydration; compensatory strategies (e.g., elevation of head of bed, rising slowly, or dorsiflexion exercises); pressure stockings; pharmacological therapy if the previously listed strategies fail

Diagnosis and treatment of underlying cause, if possible; reduction of medications that impair balance; environmental interventions; referral to physical therapist for assistive devices and for gait and progressive balance training

Diagnosis and treatment of underlying cause, if possible; increase in proprioceptive input (with an assistive device or appropriate footwear that encases the foot and has a low heel and thin sole); reduction of medications that impede cognition; awareness on the part of caregivers of cognitive deficits; reduction of environmental risk factors; referral to physical therapist for gait, balance, and strength training

Diagnosis and treatment of the underlying cause, if possible; referral to physical therapist for strength, range of motion, and gait and balance training and for assistive devices; use of appropriate footwear; referral to podiatrist

Referral to cardiologist; carotid-sinus massage (in the case of syncope)

Removal of loose rugs and the use of nightlights, nonskid bathmats, and stair rails; other interventions as necessary

*Recommendation of this assessment is based on observational data that the finding is associated with an increased risk of falling.

†Recommendation of this assessment is based on one or more randomized controlled trials of a single intervention.

‡Recommendation of this assessment is based on one or more randomized controlled trials of a multifactorial intervention strategy that included this component.

From Tinetti M: Preventing falls in elderly persons, *N Engl J Med* 348(1), 42-49, 2003.

Box 12-6	Evidence-Based Practice: Assessing Home Safety in Homebound Older Adults

Purpose
The study explored safety risks for vulnerable homebound elders.

Sample and Setting
The study focused on 208 homebound adults (60 years of age and over), living in rural areas in northern Alabama, who were assessed for safety risks within their own homes.

Method
Registered nurse students conducted the home safety assessments in two 1-hour home visits over a 4-week period using a 57-item home safety assessment instrument modified from several existing tools. There were subscales of the instrument: risk for falls (external and internal factors); history of falls; risk for injury; use of personal precautions; risk and preparation for fire and disasters; and risk for crime. Individual item responses were analyzed based on frequency of responses. Total subscale analyses were examined with an ordinal scale range of no, low, moderate, and high risk.

Results
The subscale with the highest level of risk was risk for falls (external) with 44% of the participants scoring at moderate to high risk levels for falls. Of the participants, 49% had experienced a fall, and 50% or more reported previous falls and the use of medications that cause dizziness. Further findings: 41% of the participants did not have grab bars around the shower and/or bath and the toilet in the bathroom, an important safety feature to prevent falls; 28% were poorly prepared to respond to fire or disaster; 11% had been a victim of crime at home, and 34% considered themselves a moderate to high risk for crime.

Implications
Conducting home safety assessments to prevent injury is an important nursing responsibility. Home safety assessments should be multifaceted and include internal and external risk for falls, history of near falls and past falls, use of personal precautions, risk and preparation for fire and disasters, and risk for crime. Following identification of risks, specific plans to minimize risk must be implemented and evaluated.

Data from Tanner E: Assessing home safety in homebound older adults, *Geriatr Nurs* 24(3):250-254, 256, 2003.

Table 12-2   Assessment and Interventions of the Home Environment for Older Persons

PROBLEM	INTERVENTION
BATHROOM	
Getting on and off toilet	Raised seat; side bars; grab bars
Getting in and out of tub	Bath bench; transfer bench; hand-held shower nozzle; rubber mat; hydraulic lift bath seat
Slippery or wet floors	Nonskid rugs or mats
Hot water burns	Check water temperature before bath; set hot water thermostat to 120° F or less Use bath thermometer
Doorway too narrow	Remove door and use curtain; leave wheelchair at door and use walker
BEDROOM	
Rolling beds	Remove wheels; block against wall
Bed too low	Leg extensions; blocks; second mattress; adjustable-height hospital bed
Lighting	Bedside light; night-light; flashlight attached to walker or cane
Sliding rugs	Remove; tack down; rubber back; two-sided tape
Slippery floor	Nonskid wax; no wax; rubber-soled footwear; indoor-outdoor carpet
Thick rug edge or doorsill	Metal strip at edge; remove doorsill; tape down edge
Nighttime calls	Bedside phone; cordless phone; intercom; buzzer; lifeline

Table 12-2   Assessment and Interventions of the Home Environment for Older Persons—cont'd

PROBLEM	INTERVENTION
KITCHEN	
Open flames and burners	Substitute microwave; electrical toaster oven
Access to items	Place commonly used items in easy-to-reach areas; adjustable-height counters, cupboards, and drawers
Hard-to-open refrigerator	Foot lever
Difficulty seeing	Adequate lighting; utensils with brightly colored handles
LIVING ROOM	
Soft, low chair	Board under cushion; pillow or folded blanket to raise seat; blocks or platform under legs; good armrests to push up on; back and seat cushions
Swivel and rocking chairs	Block motion
Obstructing furniture	Relocate or remove to clear paths
Extension cords	Run along walls; eliminate unnecessary cords; place under sturdy furniture; use power strips with breakers
TELEPHONE	
Difficult to reach	Cordless phone; inform friends to let phone ring 10 times; clear path; use answering machine and call back
Difficult to hear ring	Headset; speaker phone
Difficult to dial numbers	Preset numbers; large button and numbers; voice-activated dialing
STEPS	
Cannot manage	Stair glide; lift; elevator; ramp (permanent, portable, or removable)
No handrails	Install at least on one side
Loose rugs	Remove or nail down to wooden steps
Difficult to see	Adequate lighting; mark edge of steps with bright-colored tape
Unable to use walker on stairs	Keep second walker or wheelchair at top or bottom of stairs
HOME MANAGEMENT	
Laundry	Easy to access; sit on stool to access clothes in dryer; good lighting; fold laundry sitting at table; carry laundry in bag on stairs; use cart; use laundry service
Mail	Easy-to-access mailbox; mail basket on door
Housekeeping	Assess safety and manageability; no-bend dust pan; lightweight all-surface sweeper; provide with resources for assistance if needed
Controlling thermostat	Mount in accessible location; large-print numbers; remote-controlled thermostat
SAFETY	
Difficulty locking doors	Remote-controlled door lock; door wedge; hook and chain locks
Difficulty opening door and knowing who is there	Automatic door openers; level doorknob handles; intercom at door
Opening and closing windows	Lever and crank handles
Cannot hear alarms	Blinking lights; vibrating surfaces
Lighting	Illumination 1 to 2 feet from object being viewed; change bulbs when dim; adequate lighting in stairways and hallways; night-lights

Continued

Table 12-2   Assessment and Interventions of the Home Environment for Older Persons—cont'd

PROBLEM	INTERVENTION
LEISURE	
Cannot hear television	Personal listening device with amplifier; closed captioning
Complicated remote	Simple remote with large buttons; universal remote control; voice control–activated remote control; clapper
Cannot read small print	Magnifying glass; large-print books
Book too heavy	Read at table; sit with book resting on lap pillow
Glare when reading	Place light source to right or left; avoid glossy paper for reading material; black ink instead of blue ink or pencil
Computer keys too small	Replace keyboard with one with larger keys

Modified from Rehabilitation Engineering Research Center on Aging (RERC-Aging), Center for Assistive Technology, University at Buffalo.

Box 12-7   Postfall Assessment Suggestions

History
Description of the fall from the individual or witness
Individual's opinion of the cause of the fall
Circumstances of the fall (trip or slip)
Individual's activity at the time of the fall
Presence of comorbid conditions, such as a previous stroke, Parkinson's disease, osteoporosis, seizure disorder, sensory deficit, joint abnormalities, depression, or cardiac disease
Medication review
Associated symptoms, such as chest pain, palpitations, lightheadedness, vertigo, fainting, weakness, confusion, incontinence, or dyspnea
Time of day and location of the fall
Presence of acute illness

Physical Examination
Vital signs: postural blood pressure changes, fever, or hypothermia
Head and neck: visual impairment, hearing impairment, nystagmus, bruit
Heart: arrhythmia or valvular dysfunction
Neurological signs: altered mental status, focal deficits, peripheral neuropathy, muscle weakness, rigidity or tremor, impaired balance
Musculoskeletal signs: arthritic changes, range of motion (ROM), podiatric deformities or problems, swelling, redness or bruises, abrasions, pain on movement, shortening and external rotation of lower extremities

Functional Assessment
Observe and inquire about the following:
Functional gait and balance: observe resident rising from chair, walking, turning, and sitting down
Balance test, mobility, use of assistive devices or personal assistance, extent of ambulation, restraint use, and prosthetic equipment
Activities of daily living: bathing, dressing, transferring, and toileting

Environmental Assessment
Staffing patterns, unsafe practice in transferring, delay in response to call light
Faulty equipment
Use of bed and chair alarms
Call light within reach
Wheelchair and bed locked
Adequate supervision
Clutter; walking paths not clear
Dim lighting
Glare
Uneven flooring
Wet, slippery floors
Poorly fitting seating devices
Inappropriate footwear
Inappropriate eye wear

The use of restraints is a source of great physical and psychological distress to older adults and may intensify agitation and contribute to depression. The following quotes from a qualitative study on restraints by Strumpf and colleagues (1992, p. 126) illustrate:

"I felt like a dog and cried all night. It hurt me to have to be tied up. I felt like I was nobody, that I was dirt. It makes me cry to talk about it. The hospital is worse than a jail."

"I don't remember misbehaving, but I may have been deranged from all the pills they gave me. Normally, I am spirited, but I am also good and obedient. Nevertheless, the nurse tied me down, like Jesus on the cross, by bandaging both wrists and ankles. . . . It felt awful, I hurt and I worried. Callers, including men friends, saw me like that and I lost something. I lost a little personal prestige. I was embarrassed, like a child placed in a corner for being bad. I had been important . . . and to be tied down in bed took a big toll . . . I haven't forgotten the pain and the indignity of being tied."

Restrictions on restraint usage dictated by the Omnibus Reconciliation Act (OBRA) provide specific guidelines for restraint use in long-term care facilities. All long-term care facilities must comply with statements from the Federal Register (1991) that relate to physical and chemical restraints and abuse (Box 12-8). The combination of research-based clinical evidence, increased knowledge about restraint alternatives, advocacy groups' efforts, and changed standards and regulations concerning restraints has contributed to a significant reduction in restraint use (Eliopoulos, 2005).

Box 12-8   Statements on Use of Restraints and Abuse

The resident has the right to be free from any physical or chemical restraints imposed for purposes of discipline or convenience, and not required to treat the resident's medical symptoms. The resident has the right to be free from verbal, sexual, physical, and mental abuse, corporal punishment, and involuntary seclusion.

The facility must develop and implement written policies and procedures that prohibit mistreatment, neglect, and abuse of residents.

The facility must ensure that the resident's environment remains as free of accidental hazards as possible, and that each resident receives adequate supervision and assistance devices to prevent accidents.

From V56187 Fed. Reg. Step 26, p. 48825, 1991.

Restraint-free care is now the standard of practice and an indicator of quality care in all health care settings although transition to that standard is still in progress, particularly in acute care settings. An evidence-based practice guideline for restraint use in acute care with a decision algorithm has been developed by Park and Hsiao-Chen Tang (2007) (Figure 12-2). Flaherty (2004) remarked that a "restraint-free environment should be held as the standard of care and anything less is substandard. The fact that it is done in some European hospitals (deVries et al, 2004) and in some U.S. hospitals, even among delirious patients (Flaherty et al, 2003), and some nursing facilities (Gatz, 2000; Makowski et al, 2000) should be evidence enough that it can be done everywhere" (p. 919).

With the movement toward freedom from restraints and the promotion of the least restrictive environment, the establishment of safety plans is essential. Removing restraints without careful attention to safety promotion and effective alternative strategies can jeopardize safety. Many of the suggestions on safety and fall risk reduction in this chapter can be used to promote a safe and restraint-free environment. Implementing best practice nursing in restraint-free care calls for recognition, assessment, and intervention for physical and psychosocial concerns contributing to patient safety, knowledge of restraint alternatives, interdisciplinary teamwork, and institutional commitment. The use of advanced practice nurse consultation in implementing alternatives to restraints has been most effective (Bourbonniere and Evans, 2002; Capezuti, 2004). Fall risk reduction and alternative strategies to restraints are presented in Boxes 12-9 and 12-10.

Side Rails. The use of side rails is also coming under scrutiny through nursing research. Historically, side rails have been used to prevent falling from the bed, but this practice is being replaced by careful evaluation of their use. Side rails are no longer viewed as simply attachments to a patient's bed but may be considered restraints with all the accompanying concerns just discussed. When side rails impede the person's desired movement or activity, they meet the definition of a restraint. Evaluation of the proper use of side rails before applying them is necessary. Elizabeth Capezuti, a gerontological nurse researcher, has extensively studied the use of side rails and bed-related fall outcomes, as well as individualized safety interventions. An instrument for evaluating the use of side rails can be found at www.nursing.upenn.edu/centers/hcgne/gero_tips/PDF_files/Evaluation_of_Siderail_Usage.pdf.

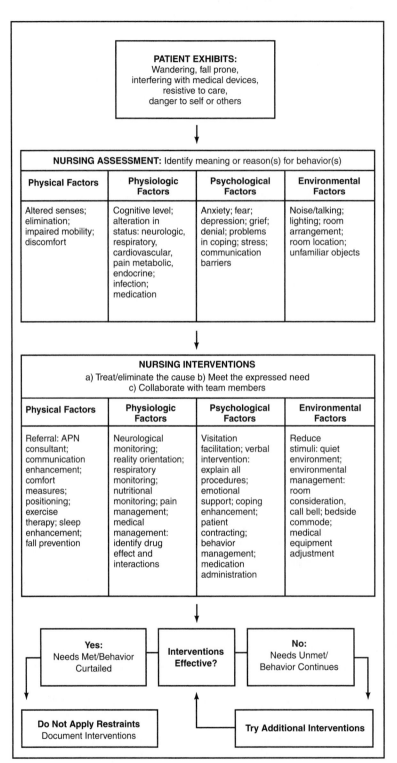

Fig. 12-2 Decision algorithm: behavior management and restraint-free care. *(From: Park M, Hsiao-Chen Tang J: Evidence-based guidelines: changing the practice of physical restraint use in acute care, J Gerontol Nurs 33[2]:9-16, 2007.)*

Box 12-9	Fall Risk Reduction and Alternative Strategies to Restraints

- Work with the interdisciplinary team; nurses cannot manage these complicated challenges alone.
- Lower the bed to the lowest level, or use a bed that is especially designed to be low to the floor.
- Use concave mattress.
- Use bed boundary markers to mark edges of bed such as mattress bumpers, rolled blanket, or "swimming noodles" under sheets.
- Place soft floor mat or a mattress by the bed to cushion any falls.
- Use water mattress to reduce movement to edge of bed.
- Have person at risk sleep on mattress on the floor.
- Remove wheels from bed.
- Clear the floor of debris, excessive furniture; make sure it is not wet or slippery.
- Place nonskid strips on floor next to bed; ensure that floors are nonskid
- Place call bell within reach, and make sure the patient can use it—attach call bell to garment.
- Provide visual reminders to encourage the patient to use call bell.
- Use night lights in room and bathroom.
- Use identification bracelet or door sign to indicate patients at risk for falling.
- Inform all staff of fall risk, and put fall risk and fall risk–reduction interventions on care plan.
- Involve family and all staff in fall risk–reduction education and activities.
- Identify on Kardex and call bell console those patients at high risk.
- Assess ambulation ability; refer to physical therapy for walking and/or strengthening.
- Have ambulation devices within reach, and make sure patient knows how to use them properly.
- Use bed, chair, or wrist alarms (the best alarm tells you only that there is an emergency; still need frequent checks, supervised areas). Apply patient-worn sensor (lightweight alarm worn above the knee that is position-sensitive).
- Keep person in supervised area or room within view of the nursing station.
- Check for orthostasis (systolic drop greater than 20 mm Hg systolic and/or greater than 10 mm Hg after 2 minutes of standing).
- If the person is able, he or she should walk at every opportunity possible. If the patient walked in or could walk before hospitalization, make every effort to keep the patient walking during hospitalization.
- Establish toileting plan, and take the person to the bathroom frequently.
- Have the person use bedside commode.
- Make sure the person knows the location of the bathroom—leave door open so he or she can see the toilet, or put a picture of a toilet on the door; clear path to bathroom.
- Know sleeping patterns—if the person is usually up during the night, get him or her up in a chair and keep at nursing station.
- Use bolsters, lap buddies.
- Do frequent bed checks, especially in evening and at night.
- Be especially alert at change-of-shift times.
- Understand that very few people spend all day in bed; activity is necessary.
- Use upper half side rails only.
- Provide diversional activities (catalogues, puzzles, busy box).
- Wedge cushions in wheel chairs or materials that promote sitting in an upright position without restraints (occupational therapy can be helpful in this area).
- Have the person sit in a reclining geriatric chair, chair with a deep seat, bean bag chair, rocker—keep close to nurses' station in the chair
- Arrange for family and/or sitter to be with the person, especially at high-risk times.
- If the person wears glasses, hearing aid, or dentures, see that they are worn.
- Have purse (empty or without harmful items or important papers or money) in bed with the person, if a woman
- Have the person sleep with shoes on or rubber-soled slippers or socks with nonskid treads.
- Ensure that pain is well managed.
- If the person is (or has been) married, line spouse's side of the bed with pillows or bolsters.
- Provide trapeze to enhance mobility in bed.
- Provide grab bars in bathroom and shower, shower chair with suction bottom.
- Provide elevated toilet seat.
- Have the person wear clothing that is easy to pull down for toileting.
- Create a grid with masking tape on floor in front of doorway, use black half-rug, and camouflage exit doors with wallpaper, window treatments, etc., if the person is wandering or trying to exit.
- Place stop sign on exit door.
- Use a behavior log to track when the person is trying to get up, and/or when he or she seems agitated.
- Provide hip protectors, helmets, and arm pads.

Box 12-10	Restraint Alternatives: Dealing with Tubes, Lines, and Other Medical Devices

- Preoperative teaching and showing the tubes and explaining may be effective in decreasing anxiety about devices.
- Use guided exploration and a mirror to help patient understand what is in place and why.
- Provide comfort care to the site—oral and nasal care, anchoring of tubing, topical anesthetic on site.
- First question: "Is the device really necessary?" Remove as soon as possible. Foley catheters should be used only if patient needs intensive output monitoring or has an obstruction.
- Weigh risks and benefits of restraint versus therapy. Are alternatives available—replace intravenous (IV) tubing with heparin lock, deliver medications intramuscularly (IM), consider intermittent IV administration or hypodermoclysis.
- Use camouflage: clothing or elastic sleeves, temporary air splint (occupational therapy [OT] can be helpful), skin sleeves to prevent IV tube dislodgement.
- Use mitts instead of wrist restraints; roll belts instead of vest restraints.
- Use diversional activity aprons (zipping-unzipping, threading exercises, dials and knobs), busy box, or therapeutic activity kit (www.hartfordign.org/trythis).
- Hide lines by placing in unobtrusive place; place tubing behind patient out of his or her view; have patient wear long sleeves or double surgical gowns with cuffs to prevent access.
- Hang IV bags behind the patient's field of vision.
- Nasogastric (NG) tubes—replace with percutaneous endoscopic gastrostomy (PEG) tube if necessary but obtain comprehensive speech therapy (ST) swallowing evaluation. If NG tube is used, use as small a lumen as possible to minimize irritation; consider taping with occlusive dressings.
- Cover PEG tube or abdominal incisions and other tubes with abdominal binder, sweat pants.
- For men with Foley catheters—shave area just above pubis, and tape catheter to pubis. NEVER secure catheter to leg (causes discomfort and can cause a fistula). Run tubing around back and down leg to a leg bag. Patient should wear underpants and pajama pants.
- Take restraints off while working with patient.
- Use modified soft collar for tracheotomy protection.

Interventions

Programs to reduce fall risk aim to eliminate or reduce remediable risk factors (Nnodim and Alexander, 2005). The most successful approaches to fall risk reduction include education of clinicians about fall risk reduction, multifactorial assessment, and interventions directed at the identified risk factors (Tinetti et al, 2003; Tinetti et al, 2008). These approaches have been shown to reduce the occurrence of falling by 25% to 39% (Tinetti, 2003). Fall risk–reduction programs are a shared responsibility of all health care providers caring for older adults. They also call for the individual (and informal and formal caregivers) to be educated in all aspects of environmental hazards and to become aware that falling may be an indication of other underlying problems.

Choosing the most appropriate interventions to reduce the risk of falls depends on appropriate assessment at various intervals depending on the person's changing condition. A "one size fits all" (Capezuti, 2004, p. 461) approach is not effective, and further research is needed to determine the type, the frequency, and the timing of interventions best suited for specific populations (e.g., community-living older adults, hospitalized older adults, institutionalized elders, and ethnically diverse elders) (Quigley, 2005). Box 12-11 presents an innovative fall risk–reduction program in an acute care facility. A Nursing Standard of Practice Protocol: Fall Prevention can be found at http://consultgerirn.org/topics/falls/want_to_know_more).

The AGS provides excellent resources for professionals and patients on falls in older adults, including the "Guideline for the Prevention of Falls in Older Persons" and "A Patient's Guide to Preventing Falls" (www.americangeriatrics.org). The American Medical Directors Association also provides a practice guideline regarding falls and fall risk in long-term care (www.amda.com). The AGS Panel on Falls Prevention (2001) recommends the following interventions:

▶ Gait training and correct use of assistive devices
▶ Medication review (particularly psychotropics)

Box 12-11	The Ruby Slipper Fall Intervention Program

Nurse Ginny Goldner of St. Joseph's Hospital in Tucson, Arizona, started the "Ruby Slipper" program to identify patients at risk for falling and to help prevent falls in elderly patients. Patients at risk for falls wear red socks with nonskid treads so that anyone, from a housekeeper to a head nurse, who sees them walking around or trying to get out of bed will know to stay with them until they are safely back in bed. Education on fall risk reduction, identification of patients at high risk, and Ruby Slipper rounds on high-risk patients to see if they need anything, such as to go to the bathroom, are included in the program as well. The program has reduced patient falls by nearly 75%. Ginny was awarded the March of Dimes Arizona Innovation and Creativity Nurse of the Year Award for the program.

Data from Arizona Hospital and Healthcare Association, www.azhha.org. For information, contact Ginny Goldner RN, MS at (520) 873-3722 or email vgoldner@carondelet.org.

▶ Exercise programs that include balance training
▶ Assessment and treatment of postural hypotension and cardiovascular disorders
▶ Environmental hazard modification
▶ Staff education

The panel also recommends a facilitated home safety assessment for all older persons at risk for falls.

Exercise. The relationship between exercise and fall risk reduction is strong, particularly combined with balance training, for elders in the community. Although the best type, duration, and intensity of exercise have not been determined, exercise programs must be at least 10 weeks in duration, must be individualized, and must include balance training for benefit. Group exercises may also be effective. Further research is needed to evaluate the effect of exercise in long-term care settings, as well as the effect of programs such as *tai chi chuan* (see Chapter 10).

Environmental Modifications. Environmental modifications alone have not been shown to reduce falls, but when included as part of a multifactorial program, they may be of benefit in risk reduction. However, a home safety assessment conducted by an occupational therapist after hospital discharge resulted in significant fall risk reduction in a group of older patients (AGS, 2001).

Medication Review. Reduction of medications is an important component of effective fall-reducing programs in both community-based and long-term care studies. Medications, including over-the-counter (OTC) and herbals, should be reviewed and limited to those that are absolutely essential. Risk of falls increases with the use of four or more medications, particularly neuroleptics and benzodiazepines (both long- and short-acting).

Behavior and Education Programs. As a single strategy, behavior and education programs do not reduce falls but are recommended as part of multifactorial intervention programs. Information should be provided to the older person, to health care professionals, and to caregivers on fall risk factors and fall risk–reduction strategies. There are many excellent sources of information available for both consumers and professionals on interventions to reduce fall risk (see Resources at the end of the chapter and at evolve.elsevier.com/Ebersole/gerontological).

Assistive Devices. Research on multifactorial interventions including the use of assistive devices has demonstrated benefits in fall risk reduction. It is important to provide instruction and supervision on the correct use of assistive devices. If you think your client could benefit from an assistive device, consult specialists and rehabilitation therapists. Assist the client in obtaining a written prescription for the assistive device because Medicare may cover up to 80% of the cost of the device; other insurance coverage varies.

Many devices are available that are designed for specific benefits. When the correct device is obtained, the older person will need assistance in learning how to use it correctly. This should be provided by specialists in physical therapy. Nurses working with older adults with assistive devices can supervise correct use. New technologies such as canes that "talk" and provide feedback to the user are developing, and continued research is needed to evaluate their effectiveness (Gray-Micelli, 2008). In general, the following principles should be observed with use of assistive devices:

▶ Place your cane firmly on the ground before you take a step, and do not place it too far ahead of you. Put all of your weight on your unaffected leg, and then move the cane and your affected leg a comfortable distance forward. With your weight supported on both your cane and your affected leg, step through with your unaffected leg.
▶ Always wear low-heeled, nonskid shoes.
▶ When using a cane on stairs, step up with the stronger leg and down with the weaker leg. Use the cane as support when lifting the weaker leg. Bring the

cane up to the step just reached before climbing another step. When descending, place the cane on the next step down, move the disabled leg down, and then move the good leg down.

▶ When using a walker, stand upright and lift or roll the walker with both hands a step's length ahead of you. Lean slightly forward and hold the arms of the walker for support. Step toward it with the weaker leg and then bring the stronger leg forward. Do not climb stairs with a walker.

▶ Every assistive device must be adjusted to individual height; the top of the cane should align with the crease of the wrist.

▶ Choose a size and shape of cane handle that fits comfortably in the palm; like a tight shoe, it will be a constant irritant if it is not properly fitted.

▶ Cane tips are most secure when they are flat across the bottom and have a series of concentric rings. Replace tips frequently, because they wear out and a worn tip is insecure.

▶ Wheelchairs are a necessary adjunct at some level of immobility. These can be used in a healthful way and without demeaning the individual. The various types of motorized chairs can be handled with ease and provide a great deal of independence for wheelchair users. It is important that a professional evaluate the wheelchair for proper fit and provide training on proper use and safety. Often, physical and occupational therapists can assist in wheelchair mobility programs. At one Veterans Affairs Medical Center, the physical therapy department routinely offered driving and safety classes for users of motorized wheelchairs and scooters.

Other Interventions. Other potential interventions include assessment and treatment of osteoporosis to reduce fracture rates (see Chapter 18). Older people with osteoporosis are more likely to experience serious injury from a fall. The use of hip protectors for prevention of hip fractures in high-risk individuals may be considered, but further research is needed to determine their effectiveness (Kiel et al, 2007). Compliance has been a concern related to the ease of application and getting them off quickly enough for toileting (Gray-Micelli, 2008).

Formal vision assessment is also an important intervention to identify remediable visual problems. Although a significant relationship exists between visual problems and falls and fractures, little research has been conducted on interventions for visual problems as part of fall risk–reduction programs. Poor visual acuity, reduced contrast sensitivity, decreased visual field, cataracts, and use of nonmiotic glaucoma medications have all been associated with falls.

ENVIRONMENTAL SAFETY

A safe environment is one in which one is capable, with reasonable caution, of carrying out activities of daily living (ADLs) and instrumental activities of daily living (IADLs), as well as the activities that enrich one's life, without fear of attack, accident, or imposed interference. It is the job of nurses and other health team members to ensure, to the greatest extent possible, a safe environment for individuals within their care in the institution or in the home. Table 12-2 provides assessment and interventions of the home environment.

Vulnerability to environmental risks increases as people become less physically or cognitively able to recognize or cope with real or potential hazards. Older adults and their caregivers need to be knowledgeable about risks and interventions to avoid unsafe behaviors and situations.

Vulnerability to Environmental Temperatures

Given the nation's growing problems with supply and costs of energy, many older adults are exposed to temperature extremes in their own dwellings. Environmental temperature extremes pose a serious risk to older persons with declining physical health. Preventive measures entail paying attention to impending changes of season, as well as strategies to protect the individual against extremes of temperature. Early intervention in extreme temperature exposure is crucial because excessively high or low body temperatures further impair thermoregulatory function and can be lethal.

Neurosensory changes in thermoregulation delay or diminish the older person's awareness of temperature changes and may impair behavioral and thermoregulatory responses to dangerously high or low environmental temperatures (Chapter 6). Many of the medications taken by older people affect thermoregulation by affecting the ability to vasoconstrict or vasodilate, both of which are thermoregulatory mechanisms. Other drugs inhibit neuromuscular activity, suppress metabolic heat generation, or dull awareness (e.g., tranquilizers, pain medications). Alcohol is notorious for inhibiting thermoregulatory function by affecting vasomotor responses in either hot or cold weather.

Economic, behavioral, and environmental factors may combine to create a dangerous thermal environment in which older persons are subjected to temperature extremes from which they cannot escape or that they cannot change. Caretakers and family members should be aware that persons are vulnerable to temperature extremes if they are unable to shiver, sweat, control blood supply to the skin, take in sufficient liquids, move about, add or remove clothing, adjust bedcovers, or adjust the room temperature. A temperature that may be comfortable for a young and active person may be too cold or too warm for a frail elder.

Economic conditions often play a role in determining whether an older person living in the community can afford air conditioning or adequate heating. More older people die from excessive heat than from hurricanes, lightning, tornadoes, floods, and earthquakes combined (CDC, 2006b). In 2003, a record heat wave in Europe claimed an estimated 30,000 lives; 14,000 died in France alone (Sykes, 2005; Schwartz et al, 2006). Trends toward global warming will increase the risks of extreme heat–related events in the future. Local governments and communities must coordinate response strategies to protect the older person. Strategies may include providing fans and opportunities to spend part of the day in air-conditioned buildings, and identification of high-risk older people.

Hyperthermia

When body temperature rises above normal ranges because of environmental or metabolic heat loads, a clinical condition called heat illness, or hyperthermia, occurs. Hyperthermia is a temperature-related illness and is classified as a medical emergency. Annually, there are numerous deaths among elders from temperature extremes, and these could be almost entirely prevented with education and caution. Although most of these problems occur in the home among individuals who do not have air conditioning during temperature extremes, older adults with multiple physical problems residing in institutions may be especially vulnerable to temperature changes. Elders with cardiovascular disease, diabetes, or peripheral vascular disease and those taking certain medications (anticholinergics, antihistamines, diuretics, beta blockers, antidepressants, antiparkinsonian drugs) are at risk. Interventions to prevent hyperthermia when ambient temperature exceeds 90° F (32° C) are presented in Box 12-12.

Hypothermia

Hypothermia is a medical emergency necessitating comprehensive assessment of neurological activity, oxygenation, renal function, and fluid and electrolyte balance. The term *hypothermia* literally means "low heat," but it is used clinically to describe core temperatures below 35° C (95° F). Two situations tend to produce hypothermia: (1) a healthy individual is exposed

---

Box 12-12   Interventions to Prevent Hyperthermia

- Drink 2 to 3 L of cool fluid daily.
- Minimize exertion, especially during the heat of the day.
- Stay in air-conditioned places, or use fans when possible.
- Wear hats and loose clothing of natural fibers when outside; remove most clothing when indoors.
- Take tepid baths or showers.
- Apply cold wet compresses, or immerse the hands and feet in cool water.
- Evaluate medications for risk of hyperthermia.
- Avoid alcohol.

From Ebersole P, Hess, P, Touhy T et al: *Toward healthy aging: human needs & nursing response,* ed 7, St. Louis, 2008, Mosby.

---

to severely cold environmental conditions for a prolonged period; or (2) a person with impaired thermoregulatory ability is left without protection in a room with temperatures that may be comfortable for a younger person. The more severe the impairment or prolonged the exposure, the less thermoregulatory responses can defend against heat loss.

Older people are particularly predisposed to hypothermia because the opportunity for heat loss frequently coexists with the decline in heat generation and conservation responses. Such coexistence occurs frequently among persons who are homeless or cognitively impaired, those injured in falls or with other trauma, and persons with cardiovascular, adrenal, or thyroid dysfunction. Other risk factors include excessive alcohol use, exhaustion, poor nutrition, inadequate housing, and the use of sedatives, anxiolytics, phenothiazines, and tricyclic antidepressants.

Unfortunately, a dulling of awareness accompanies hypothermia, and persons experiencing it rarely recognize the problem or seek assistance. For the very old and frail, environmental temperatures below 65° F (18° C) may cause a serious drop in core body temperature to 95° F (35° C) or less. Factors that increase the risk of hypothermia are numerous, as shown in Box 12-13.

Under normal temperature conditions, heat is produced in sufficient quantities by cellular metabolism of food, the friction produced by contracting muscles, and the flow of blood. Paralyzed or immobile persons lack the ability to generate significant muscle heat by muscle

Box 12-13   Factors that Increase the Risk of Hypothermia in Older Adults

Thermoregulatory Impairment
Failure to vasoconstrict promptly or strongly on exposure to cold
Failure to sense cold
Failure to respond behaviorally to protect oneself against cold
Diminished or absent shivering to generate heat
Failure of metabolic rate to rise in response to cold

Conditions that Decrease Heat Production
Hypothyroidism, hypopituitarism, hypoglycemia, anemia, malnutrition, starvation
Immobility or decreased activity (e.g., stroke, paralysis, parkinsonism, dementia, arthritis, fractured hip, coma)
Diabetic ketoacidosis

Conditions that Increase Heat Loss
Open wounds, generalized inflammatory skin conditions, burns

Conditions that Impair Central or Peripheral Control of Thermoregulation
Stroke, brain tumor, Wernicke's encephalopathy, subarachnoid hemorrhage
Uremia, neuropathy (e.g., diabetes, alcoholism)
Acute illnesses (e.g., pneumonia, sepsis, myocardial infarction, congestive heart failure, pulmonary embolism, pancreatitis)

Drugs that Interfere with Thermoregulation
Tranquilizers (e.g., phenothiazines)
Sedative-hypnotics (e.g., barbiturates, benzodiazepines)
Antidepressants (e.g., tricyclics)
Vasoactive drugs (e.g., vasodilators)
Alcohol (causes superficial vasodilation; may interfere with carbohydrate metabolism and judgment)
Others: methyldopa, lithium, morphine

From Worfolk JB: Keep frail elders warm, *Geriatr Nurs* 18(1):7-11, 1997.

activity and become cold even in normal room temperatures. It is important to closely monitor body temperature in older people and pay particular attention to lower than normal readings. Older people with some degree of thermoregulatory impairment are, when exposed to cold temperatures, at high risk for hypothermia if they undergo surgery, are injured in a fall or accident, or are lost or left unattended in a cool place. Persons who are emaciated and have poor nutrition lack insulation, as well as fuel for metabolic heat-generating processes, so they may be chronically mildly hypothermic. Box 12-14 lists factors and situations that may induce low basal body temperature in elders.

IMPLICATIONS FOR GERONTOLOGICAL NURSING AND HEALTHY AGING

Recognition of clinical signs and severity of hypothermia is an important nursing responsibility. Nurses are responsible for keeping frail elders warm for comfort and prevention of problems. It is important to closely monitor body temperature in older people and pay particular attention to both lower and higher readings compared with a person's baseline. The potential risk of hypothermia makes prevention important and early recognition vital.

Detecting hypothermia among home-dwelling older people is sometimes difficult, because unlike in the clinical setting, no one is measuring body temperature. For persons exposed to low temperatures in the home or the outdoors, confusion and disorientation may be the first overt signs. As judgment becomes clouded, a person may remove clothing or fail to seek shelter, and hypothermia can progress to profound levels. For this reason, regular contact with home-dwelling elders during cold and very hot weather is crucial. For those with preexisting alterations in thermoregulatory ability, this surveillance should include even mildly cool weather. Specific interventions to prevent hypothermia are shown in Box 12-15.

Box 12-14	Factors Associated with Low Body Temperature in Older Adults

Aging

Increases risk of thermoregulatory dysfunction
Increases risk of acute and chronic conditions that predispose to hypothermia

Low Environmental Temperature

Risk of hypothermia increases below 65° F.

Thinness and Malnutrition

Very thin people have less thermal insulation, higher surface area/volume ratios
Prolonged malnutrition can decrease the metabolic rate by 20% to 30%

Poverty

Increases risk of thinness and malnutrition, inadequate clothing, low environmental temperature secondary to poor housing conditions and inadequate heat

Living Alone

Associated with poverty, delayed detection of hypothermia, delayed rescue if person falls

Nocturia and Night Rising

Associated with falls; if rescue delayed and person lies immobilized for a long time, hypothermia may develop as heat is conducted away from the body to the cold floor

Orthostatic Hypotension

An indicator of autonomic nervous system impairment; dizziness and postural instability are associated with falls

From Worfolk JB: Keep frail elders warm, *Geriatr Nurs* 18(1): 7-11, 1997.

Vulnerability to Natural Disasters

Natural disasters such as hurricanes, tornadoes, floods, and earthquakes claim the lives of many people worldwide each year. In addition, human-made or human-generated disasters include chemical, biological, radiological, and nuclear terrorism and food and water contamination. The events of September 11, 2001 have prompted much thought and planning related to human-generated disasters.

Older people are at great risk during and after disasters, and the older population has the highest casualty rate during disaster events when compared to all other age groups (Burnett et al, 2008). The tragedies that occurred during Hurricane Katrina in 2005 highlighted the serious consequences of disasters on older people, both those in the community and those living in institutions. Before Katrina, older people comprised 15% of the population in New Orleans, but after the event accounted for 70% of the dead (Campbell, 2008). Fifty-six percent of the evacuees at the Astrodome following Katrina were 65 years of age or older. "Although most healthy older people will be able to cope with the effects of a disaster, there is a large number of vulnerable older adults who are at risk for short- and long-term adverse outcomes. These include, but are not limited to, elders who depend on others for daily functioning; those with limited mobility; those who are socially isolated, cognitively impaired, or institutionalized; and those with a prior exposure to an extreme or prolonged traumatic stressor (e.g., refugees from terrorist regimes or Holocaust survivors)" (Brown, 2008, p. 21).

IMPLICATIONS FOR GERONTOLOGICAL NURSING AND HEALTHY AGING

Gerontological nurses must be knowledgeable about disaster preparedness and assist in the development of plans to address the unique needs of older adults, as well as educate fellow professionals, older adult clients, and community agencies about disaster preparedness. Burnett et al (2008) reported on a rapid triage tool, the Seniors Without Families Team (SWiFT), to identify the needs of older adults both before and after a disaster. The authors of the tool reported that "if a simple assessment had been administered to the city's elderly before Katrina struck, planning officials would have known that 65% of this population would not be able to transport themselves during an evacuation and could have made evacuation plans that would have reduced the number of lives lost" (Burnett et al, 2008, p. 15). Comprehensive planning is necessary to respond to the needs of the aging population in emergency situations around the world (Barratt, 2008). Lach and colleagues (2005) provide excellent information for nurses considering disaster planning for older people. Additional resources can be found at the end of this chapter and at evolve.elsevier.com/Ebersole/gerontological.

TRANSPORTATION

Even though one is physically able to move about, there may be many hindrances to full use of public space. Available transportation is a critical link in the ability of

Box 12-15	Nursing Interventions to Prevent Cold Discomfort and the Development of Accidental Hypothermia in Frail Elders

Desired Outcomes
- Hands and limbs warm
- Body relaxed, not curled
- Body temperature >97° F
- No shivering
- No complaints of cold

Interventions
- *Maintain a comfortably warm ambient temperature* no lower than 65° F. Many frail elders will require much higher temperatures.
- *Provide generous quantities of clothing and bedcovers.* Layer clothing and bedcovers for best insulation. Be careful not to judge your patient's needs by how you feel working in a warm environment.
- *Limit time patients sit by cold windows* to short periods in which they are warmly dressed.
- *Provide a head covering* whenever possible—in bed, out of bed, and particularly out-of-doors.
- Cover patients well during bathing. The standard—a light bath blanket over a naked body—is not enough protection for frail elders.
- *Cover naked patients with heavy blankets for transfer to and from showers;* dry quickly and thoroughly before leaving shower room; cover head with a dry towel or hood while wet.
- *Dry wet hair quickly* with warm air from an electric dryer. Never allow the hair of frail elders to air-dry.
- *Use absorbent pads* for incontinent patients rather than allowing urine to wet large areas of clothing, sheets, and bedcovers. Avoid skin problems by changing pads frequently, washing the skin well, and applying a protective cream.
- *Provide as much exercise as possible* to generate heat from muscle activity.
- *Provide hot, high-protein meals and bedtime snacks* to add heat and sustain heat production throughout the day and as far into the night as possible.

From Worfolk JB: Keep frail elders warm, *Geriatr Nurs* 18(1):7-11, 1997.

the elderly to remain independent and functional. The lack of accessible transportation may contribute to other problems, such as social withdrawal, poor nutrition, or neglect of health care. Even when a municipal transportation service is available, elders may not use it. Urban buses and subways not only are physically hazardous, but also are often dangerous. A "crisis in mobility" exists for many older people because of the lack of an automobile, an inability to drive, limited access to public transportation, health factors, geographical location, or economic considerations. Culturally and ethnically diverse older people may experience more difficulty getting around than older whites, and rural residents may experience more difficulty than urban residents.

Older persons may desire increased contact with friends and relatives; however, even more crucial is the need to reach medical services, shopping areas, and service agencies. If mobility is hampered, both security and the sense of belonging to the mainstream of society may be blocked. The emphasis on a "barrier-free" (structurally revised) transportation system and reduced fares has been helpful to many older people, but some cannot avail themselves of public transportation because of physical disability or residence in a high-crime area.

County, state, or federally subsidized transportation is being provided in certain areas to assist older people in reaching social services, nutrition sites, health services, emergency care, medical care, recreational centers, mental health services, day care programs, physical and vocational rehabilitation, continuing education, and library services. Although transportation can often be found for special needs, it is virtually impossible to locate transportation for pleasure or recreation. Senior centers offer a wide range of activities for older people, as well as transportation services. Nurses can refer older people to local service and aging-related organizations, such as area agencies on aging, for information on resources and financial assistance for services.

Driving

Driving is one of the instrumental activities of daily living (IADL) for most elders because it is essential in obtaining necessary resources. Assessments of functional capacities often neglect this important activity. Evaluation should include whether an individual can drive, feels safe while driving, and has a driver's license. Renouncing the mobility and independence afforded by driving one's own car has many psychological ramifications, as well as inconveniences. Giving up driving is a major loss for an older person both in terms of independence and pleasure, as well as feelings of competence and self-worth. Many older people depend on driving in order to maintain their basic needs, and the inability to drive can cause depression and isolation. For many, alternate transportation is not readily available, and consequently, they may continue driving beyond the time when it is safe.

The leading cause of accidental death among persons older than 65 years is a motor vehicle accident; for those older than 75 years, motor vehicle accidents are the second leading cause of death after falls. Drivers aged 65 and older who sustain injuries in motor vehicle crashes are more likely to die from their injuries than are younger drivers (Staats, 2008). Age-related changes in driving skills, including vision changes, cognitive impairment, and various medical illnesses and functional impairments, are all factors related to driving safety for older adults. Older adults with dementia are 2.4 to 4.7 times more likely to be involved in a driving accident than age-matched noncognitively impaired individuals (Siberski, 2008).

Driver's license renewal procedures vary from state to state and, to help ensure the safety of older drivers, may include accelerated renewal cycles, renewal in person rather than electronically or by mail, and vision and road tests (www.iihs.org/laws/state_laws/older_drivers.html). The issues of driving in the older adult population are the subject of a great deal of public discussion. Many older drivers and their families struggle with issues related to continued safety in driving, and families struggle with when and how to tell older people they are no longer safe to drive.

IMPLICATIONS FOR GERONTOLOGICAL NURSING AND HEALTHY AGING

Health care providers should encourage open discussion of issues related to driving with the older person and his or her family and should identify impairments that affect safe driving, correct them when possible, and offer alternatives for transportation. Vehicle adaptations, sensory aids, elder driving training, and driving assessment programs are helpful in promoting safe driving (Gilfillan and Schwartzberg, 2005; Perkinson et al, 2005). Jett and colleagues (2005) provide useful strategies from a qualitative study involving guided interviews with participants for counseling people with dementia regarding driving (Box 12-16).

A mnemonic, SAFE DRIVE (McGregor, 2002), addresses key components by which to screen older drivers. The components include the following:

S Safety record
A Attention skills
F Family report
E Ethanol use
D Drugs
R Reaction time
I Intellectual impairment
V Vision and visuospatial function
E Executive functions

The American Medical Association, in partnership with the National Highway Traffic Safety Administration, provides the *Guide to Assessing and Counseling*

Box 12-16	Action Strategies Used to Bring About Driving Cessation
Imposed Type	**Involved Type**
Report person to Division of Motor Vehicles for possible license suspension	All family members and individual meet, discuss the situation, and come to a mutual agreement of the problem
Use of deception or threats such as false keys, disabling the car, saying car was stolen	Dialog is ongoing from the earliest signs of cognitive impairment about the eventuality of the need to stop driving
Attempts to order or control, such as provider writing a prescription, commands from children to stop driving	Arrangements are made for alternative transportation plans that are available when needed and acceptable to the individual

From Jett K et al: Imposed versus involved: different strategies to effect driving cessation in cognitively impaired older adults, *Geriatr Nurs* 26(2):111-116, 2005.

Older Drivers that includes step-by-step plans for assessing older driver safety. Other resources can be found at the end of the chapter and at evolve.elsevier.com/Ebersole/gerontological.

In summary, the capacity to move about on two legs, horses, and wheeled vehicles has been portrayed from the earliest recorded time. The gerontological nurse can be significant in facilitating this most fundamental human need and can assist older people in moving as far as their reach extends and as far as our imagination will allow.

APPLICATION OF MASLOW'S HIERARCHY

Movement is integral to the attainment of all levels of need as conceived by Maslow. Needs met by maintaining mobility include basic biological function, activity, security, social contacts, pride, and dignity. Thus maintaining mobility is an exceedingly important issue. Restrictions of mobility affect older people's ability to meet basic needs, their independence, and their ability to enjoy a sense of belonging and to maintain desired activities.

▶ KEY CONCEPTS

▶ Mobility provides opportunities for exercise, exploration, and pleasure and is the crux of maintaining independence.
▶ Ease of mobility is thought to be the most visible measure of one's overall health and survival capacity.
▶ Changes with aging in bones, muscles, and ligaments affect one's balance and gait and increase instability.
▶ Gait disorders are often an obvious index of systemic problems and should be investigated thoroughly.
▶ A thorough nursing assessment must include assessment of fall risk, balance, and gait, as well as intrinsic, extrinsic, and iatrogenic factors.
▶ Implementation of fall risk–reduction interventions is one of the most important proactive considerations to preserve health and function for the elderly.
▶ Physical restraints are not appropriate for "safety" and increase injuries related to falls. Restraint-free care, fall risk–reduction interventions, and a safe environment are essential to best practice care for elders.
▶ Transportation for the elderly is critical to their physical, psychological, and social health.

▶ ACTIVITIES AND DISCUSSION QUESTIONS

1. Put your shoes on the wrong feet, and then ask another student to analyze your gait.
2. Borrow a pair of bifocals from someone, and then attempt to go up and down stairs.

3. Evaluate the safety of your living quarters, using Table 12-2 as a guide.
4. Discuss your activities that increase your vulnerability to falls.
5. Discuss falls you have had and their consequences. Consider how it might have been different if you were 80 years old.
6. Obtain a wheelchair, and sit in it for 20 minutes with a restraining belt around your waist. Discuss your feelings with a partner. Reverse the process with your partner.
7. Discuss the various reasons why you might need to ensure safety for a hospitalized elder, and identify several alternatives that might be appropriate.

▶ RESOURCES

Websites
National Center for Injury Prevention and Control
Tool kit to prevent senior falls
www.cdc.gov/ncipc/pub-res/toolkit/toolkit.htm

National Institute on Aging
Age Page Health Information: Preventing Falls and Fractures, Crime and Older People, Hyperthermia, Hypothermia, Older Drivers
website: www.niapublications.org

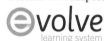

For additional resources, please visit evolve.elsevier.com/Ebersole/gerontological.

▶ REFERENCES

American Geriatrics Society (AGS), British Geriatrics Society, and American Academy of Orthopaedic Surgeons Panel on Falls Prevention: Guideline for the prevention of falls in older persons, *J Am Geriatr Soc* 49(5):664-672, 2001.

Avidan A, Fries B, James M et al: Insomnia and hypnotic use recorded in the minimum data set as predictors of falls and hip fractures in Michigan nursing homes, *J Am Geriatr Soc* 53(6):955-962, 2005.

Barratt J: International perspectives on aging and disasters, *Generations* 21(4):5760, 2008.

Bourbonniere M, Evans LK: Advanced practice nursing in the care of frail older adults, *J Am Geriatr Soc* 50(12):2062-2076, 2002.

Brown L: Issues in mental health care for older adults after disasters, *Generations* 31(4):21-26, 2008.

Buchner DM, Hornbrook MC, Kutner NG et al: Development of the common data base for the FICSIT trials, *J Am Geriatr Soc* 41(3):297-308, 1993.

Burnett J, Dyer C, Pickins S: Rapid needs assessments for older adults in disasters, *Generations* 31(4):10-15, 2008.

Campbell J: Applying the "disaster lens" to older adults, *Generations* 31(4):5-7, 2008.

Capezuti E: Building the science of falls-prevention research, *J Am Geriatr Soc* 52(3):461-462, 2004.

Capezuti E, Zwicker D, Mezey M, Fulmer T: *Evidence-based geriatric nursing protocols for best practice,* ed 3, NewYork, 2008, Springer.

Centers for Disease Control and Prevention, National Center for Injury Prevention and Control: *Web-based Injury Statistics Query and Reporting System (WISQARS)* [online], (2006a). Available at www.cdc.gov/ncipc/wisqars. Accessed 7/1/08.

Centers for Disease Control and Prevention: Heat-related deaths—United States, 1999-2003, *MMWR Morbidity and Mortality Weekly Report* 55(29):796-798, 2006b.

Chang J, Morton SC, Rubenstein LZ et al: Interventions for the prevention of falls in older adults: systematic review and meta-analysis of randomized clinical trials, *BMJ* 328(20):68-684, 2004.

deVries OJ, Ligthart GJ, Nikolaus T, on behalf of the participants of the European Academy of Medicine of Ageing—Course III: Differences in period prevalence of the use of physical restraints in elderly inpatients of European hospitals and nursing homes [Letter], *J Gerontol Med Sci* 59(9)9:922-923, 2004.

Eliopoulos C: *Gerontological nursing,* Philadelphia, 2005, Lippincott Williams & Wilkins.

Evans LK, Strumpf NE: Tying down the elderly: a review of the literature on physical restraint, *J Am Geriatr Soc* 37(1):65-74, 1989.

Federal Register: VG6187 Fed Reg, (Sept. 26, 1991), p. 48825.

Flaherty J: Zero tolerance for physical restraints: difficult but not impossible, *J Gerontol A Biol Sci Med Sci* 59A(9): M919-920, 2004.

Flaherty JH, Tariq SH, Raghavan S et al: A model for managing delirious older inpatients, *J Am Geriatr Soc* 51(7):1031-1035, 2003.

Gatz D: Moving to a restraint-free environment, *Balance* 4(6):12-15, 2000.

Gilfillan C, Schwartzberg J: Addressing the at-risk older driver, *Clin Geriatr* 13(8):27-34, 2005.

Gray-Micelli D: Preventing falls in acute care. In Capezuti E, Zwicker D, Mezey M, Fulmer T, editors: *Evidence-based geriatric nursing protocols for best practice,* New York, 2008, Springer.

Gray-Micelli D, Johnson J, Strumpf N: A stepwise approach to a comprehensive post fall assessment, *Ann Long-Term Care* 13(12):16-24, 2005.

Hurley A, Gauthier A, Horvath K et al: Promoting safer home environments for persons with Alzheimer's disease: the home safety/injury model, *J Gerontol Nurs* 30(6):43-51, 2004.

Janssen I: Influence of sarcopenia on the development of physical disability: the cardiovascular health study, *J Am Geriatr Soc* 54(1):56-62, 2006.

Jett K, Tappen R, Roselli M: Imposed versus involved: different strategies to effect driving cessation in cognitively impaired older adults, *Geriatr Nurs* 26(2):111-116, 2005.

Kiel D, Magaziner J, Zimmerman S: Efficacy of a hip protector to prevent hip fracture in nursing home residents: the HIP PRO randomized controlled trial, *JAMA* 298(4): 413-422, 2007.

Kuh D and the New Dynamics of Ageing (NDA) Preparatory Network: A life course approach to healthy aging, frailty, and capability, *Jour Gerontol* 62A(7):717-721, 2007.

Lach H, Langan J, James D: Disaster planning: are gerontological nurses prepared? *J Gerontol Nurs* 31(11):21-28, 2005.

Magaziner J, Hawkes W, Hebel S et al: Recovery from hip fracture in eight areas of function, *J Gerontol A Biol Sci Med Sci*, 55(9):M487-M488, 2000.

Makowski TR, Maggard W, Morley JE: The Life Care Center of St. Louis experience with subacute care, *Clin Geriatr Med* 16(4):701-724, 2000.

Mathias S, Nayak US, Isaacs B: Balance in elderly patients: the "get up and go" test, *Arch Phys Med Rehabil* 67(6): 387-389, 1986.

McGregor D: Driving over 65: proceed with caution, *J Gerontol Nurs* 28(8):221-226, 2002.

Miller C: *Nursing for wellness in older adults,* Philadelphia, 2008, Lippincott Williams & Wilkins.

Morley J: A fall is a major event in the life of an older person, *J Gerontol A Biol Sci Med Sci* 57(8):M492-M495, 2002.

Morley JE, Flaherty JH, Thomas DR: Geriatricians, continuous quality improvement, and improved care for older persons, *J Gerontol A Biol Sci Med Sci* 58(9): M809-M812, 2003.

Morse J, Morse R, Tylko S: Development of a scale to identify the fall-prone patient, *Can J Aging* 8(4):336-377, 1989.

Nnodim J, Alexander N: Assessing falls in older adults, *Geriatrics* 60(10):24-29, 2005.

Park M, Hsiao-Chen Tang J: Evidence-based guidelines: changing the practice of physical restraint use in acute care, *J Gerontol Nurs* 33(2):9-16, 2007.

Perkinson M, Berg-Weger M, Carr D et al: Driving and dementia of the Alzheimer type: beliefs and cessation strategies, *Gerontologist* 45(5):676-685, 2005.

Quigley P: Research agenda on the risk and prevention of falls: 2002-2007, *J Rehabil Res Dev* 42(1):vii-x, 2005.

Resnick B: In Henkel G: Beyond the MDS: team approach to falls assessment, prevention and management, *Caring for the Ages* 3(4):15-20, 2002.

Resnick B, Corcoran M, Spellbring A: Gait and balance disorders. In Adelman AM, Daly MP, editors: *Twenty common problems in geriatrics,* New York, 2001, McGraw-Hill.

Rubenstein T, Alexander N, Hausdoff J: Evaluating fall risk in older adults: steps and missteps, *Clin Geriatr* 11(1):52-61, 2003.

Rubenstein L, Trueblood P: Gait and balance assessment in older persons, *Ann Long-Term Care* 12(2):39-46, 2004.

Schwartz B, Parker C, Glass T, Hu H: Global environmental change: what can health care providers and the environmental health community do about it now? *Environ Health Perspect* 43(3):325-334, 2006.

Siberski J: Knowing when to brake: older adults and driving, *Aging Well* 1(1):36-39, 2008.

Staats D: Health promotion in older adults: what clinicians can do to prevent accidental injuries, *Geriatrics* 63(4): 12-17, 2008.

Stevens J, Ryan G, Kresnow M: Fatalities and injuries from falls among older adults—United States, 1993-2003 and 2001-2005, *MMWR Morbidity and Mortality Weekly Report* 50(45):1221-1224 2006.

Strumpf N, Wagner L, Evans L, Patterson J: *Reducing restraints: individualized approaches to behavior*, Huntington Valley, Pa, 1992, The Whitman Group.

Sykes K: A healthy environment for older adults: the aging initiative of the Environmental Protection Agency, *Generations* 29(2):65-69, 2005.

Tanner EK: Assessing home safety in homebound older adults, *Geriatr Nurs* 24(4):250-256, 2003.

Tideiksaar R: *Falls in older adults,* Baltimore, 1998, Health Professions Press.

Tideiksaar R: *Falls in older persons: prevention and management,* ed 3, Baltimore, 2005, Health Professions Press.

Tinetti ME: Preventing falls in elderly persons, *N Engl J Med* 348(1):42-49, 2003.

Tinetti ME, Baker DI, King M et al: Effect of dissemination of evidence in reducing injuries from falls, *N Engl J Med* 359(3):252-261, 2008.

U.S. Department of Health and Human Services: *Healthy People* 2010. *national health promotion and disease prevention objectives,* Washington, DC, 2000, The Department.

Yeom H, Fleury J, Keller C: Risk factors for mobility limitation in community-dwelling older adults: a social ecological perspective, *Geriatr Nurs* 29(2):133-140, 2008.

Zecevic A, Salmoni A, Speechley N, Vandervoot A: Defining a fall and reasons for falling: comparisons among the views of seniors, health care providers, and the research literature, *Gerontologist* 46(3):367-376, 2006.

Assessment Tools in Gerontological Nursing

Upon completion of this chapter, the reader will be able to:

- Discuss the advantages and disadvantages of the use of standardized assessment tools in gerontological nursing.
- Contrast the three types of formats used in the collection of assessment data.
- Describe the range of tools that may be used in the comprehensive gerontological assessment.
- Begin to develop the skills needed to select an evidence-based and appropriate tool for a specific situation and use it correctly.
- Identify key differences in assessing older adults and younger adults.

ADLs, Activities of daily living Those tasks necessary to maintain one's health and basic personal needs.

IADLs, Instrumental activities of daily living Those tasks necessary to maintain one's home and independent living.

Report-by-proxy One person (the proxy) answering questions or providing information for another person, based on the first person's knowledge of the second person.

ASSESSMENT TOOLS IN GERONTOLOGICAL NURSING

Gerontological nurses conduct skilled and detailed assessments of and with the persons who entrust themselves to their care. The process of assessing older adults is strikingly different from that with younger adults in that it is more complex, more detailed, and takes much longer to complete. More often, partial or problem-oriented assessments are done. If comprehensive assessment is needed, this is usually performed by a nurse-led interdisciplinary health care team.

The health assessment is composed of a number of parts, which will be reviewed in this chapter. Assessment includes the collection of physical data as well as integration of biological, psychosocial, and functional information. Assessment is at all levels of Maslow's Hierarchy. Questions regarding genetic background in this age group have most relevance as they relate to Alzheimer's disease, stroke, diabetes, and several types of cancer.

Assessment of the older adult requires special abilities: to listen patiently, to allow for pauses, to ask questions that are not often asked, to obtain data from all available sources, and to recognize normal changes of aging (see Chapter 6). Assessment of older adults takes more time because of their increased medical and social complexity and must be paced according to the stamina of both the person and the nurse. The quality and speed of the assessment derive from an art born of experience. Novice nurses should neither be expected nor expect themselves to do this proficiently but should expect to see both their skills and the amount of information obtained increase over time. According to Benner (1984), assessment is a task for the expert. However, an expert is not always available. By following some basic guidelines and learning how to use select assessment tools, reasonably reliable data may be obtained by nurses at all skill levels.

Over the years, nurses and others have developed tools to facilitate and standardize the collection of assessment data. A number of the tools used in the gerontological setting are presented here. The use of tools will increase the likelihood of obtaining more reliable data. This of course is followed by the analysis of the data and determination of the nursing diagnoses reflecting the person's needs. In the nursing process, the development of nursing interventions follows the analysis. By accomplishing them both, the nurse contributes to the nation's goal of increasing the quality of life lived for all Americans and the health of older adults (U.S. Department of Health and Human Services [USDHHS], 2005) (see www.healthypeople.gov/About/goals.htm).

Assessment tools exist that can broadly categorize physical health, motor capacity, manual ability, self-care ability, more complex instrumental abilities, and cognitive and social function. Assessments are completed in every nursing setting. In most settings, standardized formats are used routinely, especially in the switch from written medical records to electronic databases (especially see discussion of Minimum Data Set [MDS] and Outcomes and Assessment Information Set [OASIS] in Chapter 5). Which assessments are done depends both on the setting and the purpose. Sometimes these tools come directly from the gerontological literature, and other times they are modified to meet the particular needs of the setting.

There are three approaches used for collecting assessment data: self-report, report-by-proxy, and observation. In the self-report format, questions are either asked directly or the person is expected to respond to written questions about his or her health status. Abilities tend to be overestimated with this approach. This information is obtained indirectly when a report-by-proxy approach is used; that is, the nurse asks another person, such as a staff nurse, aide, spouse, or child to report their observations and beliefs. This format is used extensively with persons who are cognitively impaired and tends to underestimate the person's abilities and health. In the observational approach the nurse collects and records the data as she or he has measured and observed the person's health status using objective parameters.

The usual physical examination and performance-based functional assessments are examples of observational measures. Observation and the use of tools are probably the most accurate but are limited in that they only represent a snapshot in time.

Certain guidelines should be followed regardless of the type or format of tool used:

▶ Whenever possible, collect the data at a time when the patient is at his or her best.
▶ If a standard tool is being used, be sure it is used correctly; training may be required.
▶ To avoid biasing the response, do not direct the way the question is answered.
▶ Explore for more information only if it is needed to complete the assessment.
▶ Approach questions that are more personal, such as sexual functioning, in a matter-of-fact but nonetheless sensitive manner.
▶ Record the responses accurately, using the patient's own words where possible; do not analyze at the same time the data are being collected. For example, if the patient says "I have a runny nose," this is not recorded as "Patient has a cold."

Ideally, assessment tools should be used to gather baseline data before the older adult has a health crisis. Periodically, the person can be reassessed using the same tools. For example, a person who has an altered mental status as a result of an illness or medication should be reassessed later to determine if his or her status has gotten better or worse.

The Health History

The initiation of the health history marks the beginning of the nurse-client relationship and the assessment process. It begins with a review of what the person reports as a problem, known as the chief complaint. This is considered objective data that is written in the patient's own words. In an older adult this complaint is much more likely to be vague and less straightforward. For example, it is not unusual for the person to complain "I just don't feel well."

The health history is best collected either verbally in a face-to-face interview or using the interview to review a written history completed by the patient or patient's proxy beforehand. The latter method is usually much faster than the former, although it should never be used if the person has limited vision, questionable reading level, reduced language fluency, or limited English proficiency. Written histories provide reliable information only when the person's reading level is adequate for the documents used. If the elder has limited language proficiency, a trained medical interpreter is needed and the interview will generally take about twice as long.

Any health history form or interview should include a patient profile, a past medical history, a review of symptoms and systems, a medication history (prescribed and over-the-counter products such as herbals and dietary supplements), a family history for clues to genetic influences, and a social history. The social history includes current living arrangements, economic resources to meet current health-related or food expenses, amount of family and friend support, and community resources available if needed. Finally, if functional status is measured by observation, by self-report, or by proxy.

To meet the needs of our increasingly diverse population of elders, the use of questions related to the explanatory model (see Chapter 4; Kleinman, 1980) is recommended to complement the health history (Box 4-4). The responses will better enable the nurse to understand the elder and plan appropriate and effective interventions.

When a more comprehensive assessment is indicated, additional information is collected, often with well-established tools. Additional areas include cognitive abilities, education, psychological well-being; caregiver stress or burden; and patterns of health and health care. Areas or problems frequently not addressed by the care provider or mentioned by the elder but that should be addressed are sexual dysfunction, depression, incontinence, musculoskeletal stiffness, alcoholism, hearing loss, and memory loss or confusion. For discussion and assessment of alcohol use and abuse see Chapter 24. Although not usually conducted by a nurse, a driving assessment may be recommended any time there is a question of ability. Careful and thorough documentation of the history will help to maximize the quality of care provided (see Chapter 5).

Physical Assessment

The next step in the health assessment includes the evaluation of vital signs and laboratory results followed by the physical assessment. In younger persons, nurses usually learn to conduct a complete "head-to-toe." The techniques used in the physical exam are applicable to any age group; however, because of the complexity of the older adult, a head-to-toe exam is more difficult and can be excessively time-consuming and burdensome. When performing a physical assessment the geronto-

logical nurse must be able to quickly prioritize what is the most necessary to know (based on the chief complaint) and work from there. When the chief complaint is not known, such as with persons with moderate to advanced dementia or with expressive aphasia, a more thorough assessment is necessary.

Fortunately we have a number of excellent assessment tools at our disposal. These have been primarily developed for those who are very frail and for those who are exhibiting signs or symptoms of some of the most common conditions affecting older adults. Several tools are discussed or referred to in this chapter. We ask the reader to note that these serve only as examples of what is available. For a list of additional evidence-based tools, visit www.hartfordign.org and the *Try This Series*. Another potential source for tools can be found at www.ncgnp.org. Finally, with the current volume of materials available on the Internet, additional information about the use of and research related to any of the tools discussed in this chapter can easily be found.

Comprehensive Assessment for the Frail and Medically Complex Elder

FANCAPES is a model for a comprehensive yet prioritized assessment that is especially useful for the frail elder. It emphasizes the determination of very basic needs and the individual's functional ability to meet these needs independently; these are the needs that form the most basic level of Maslow's Hierarchy. The acronym *FANCAPES* represents *F*luids, *A*eration, *N*utrition, *C*ommunication, *A*ctivity, *P*ain, *E*limination, and *S*ocialization. It can be used in all settings, may be used in part or whole depending on the need, and is easily adaptable to functional pattern grouping if nursing diagnoses are used. The nurse obtains comprehensive information in each section, guided by the questions provided below.

F–Fluids

What is the current state of hydration? Does the person have the functional capacity to consume adequate fluids to maintain optimal health? This includes the ability to sense thirst, mechanically obtain the needed fluids, swallow them, and excrete them.

A–Aeration

Is the person's oxygen exchange adequate for full respiratory functioning? This means the ability maintain an oxygen saturation of at least 96% in most situations. Is supplemental oxygen required, and if so, is it possible for the person to obtain it? What is the respiratory rate and depth at rest and during activity, talking, walking, and exercise and while performing activities of daily living? What sounds are auscultated, palpated, and percussed, and what do they suggest? For the older persons it is particularly important to carefully assess lateral and apical lung fields.

N–Nutrition

What mechanical and psychological factors are affecting the person's ability to obtain and benefit from adequate nutrition? What is the type and amount of food consumed? Does the person have the ability to bite, chew, and swallow? What impact is the oral health status or periodontal disease having? For edentulous persons, do their dentures fit properly and are they worn? Does the person understand the need for special diets? Has this diet been designed so that it is consistent with the person's eating and cultural patterns? Can the person afford the special foods needed, if any? If the person is at risk for aspiration, including those who are tube fed, have preventive strategies been taught? For more detailed assessments of nutrition measures, see Chapter 8.

C–Communication

Is the person able to communicate his or her needs adequately? Do the persons who provide care understand the patient's form of communication? What is the person's ability to hear in various environments? Are there any environmental situations in which understanding of the spoken word is inadequate? If the person depends on lip-reading, is his or her vision adequate? Is the person able to clearly articulate words that are understandable to others? Does the person have either expressive or receptive aphasia, and if so has a speech therapist been made available to the person and significant others? What is the person's reading and comprehension levels? (Assume it is no greater than fifth grade if unknown.) (See Chapter 7.)

A–Activity

Is the person able to participate in the activities necessary to meet basic needs such as toileting, grooming, and meal preparation? How much assistance is needed, if any, and is someone available to provide this if needed? Is the person able to participate in activities that meet higher levels of needs such as belonging (e.g., church attendance) or finding meaning in life? What are the person's ability to feed, toilet, dress, and groom; to prepare meals; to dial the telephone; and to

voluntarily move about with or without assistive devices? Does the person have the coordination, balance, ambulatory skills, finger dexterity, grip strength, and other capacities necessary to participate fully in day-to-day life?

P–Pain

Is the person experiencing physical, psychological, or spiritual pain? Is the person able to express pain and the desire for relief? Are there cultural barriers between the nurse and the patient that make the assessment of or expression of pain difficult? How does the person customarily attain pain relief (see Chapter 16)?

E–Elimination

Is the person having difficulty with bladder or bowel elimination? Is there a lack of control? Does the environment interfere with mechanical elimination and related personal hygiene; for example, are toileting facilities adequate and accessible? Are any assistive devices used, and if so, are they available and functioning? If there are problems, how are they affecting the person's social functioning?

S–Socialization and Social Skills

Is the person able to negotiate relationships in society, to give and receive love and friendship, and to feel self-worth?

Functional Assessment

Whereas the emphasis of FANCAPES is on physical needs, a full functional assessment is broader. A thorough functional assessment will help the gerontological nurse promote healthy aging by doing the following:

▶ Identifying the specific areas in which help is needed or not needed
▶ Identifying changes in abilities from one period to another
▶ Assisting in the determination of the need for specific service(s)
▶ Providing information that may be useful in determining the safety of a particular living situation

The major tools used in functional assessment are those that assess the individual's ability to perform the tasks needed for self-care (i.e., those needed to maintain one's health) and separately, those tasks needed for independent living. Self-care activities are known as ADLs, or activities of daily living. ADLs are most often identified as eating, toileting, ambulation, bathing, dressing, and grooming. Three of these tasks (grooming, dressing, bathing) entail higher cognitive function than the others.

The instrumental activities of daily living, or IADLs, such as cleaning, yard work, shopping, and money management are tasks needed for independent living. The successful performance of IADLs calls for a higher level of cognitive and physical functioning than the ADLs. For persons with dementia, the progressive loss of abilities begins with IADLs and progresses to the ADLs. The nurse must keep in mind that the willingness and skill to perform specific ADLs and IADLs are influenced by the social and cultural factors unique to the person.

Numerous tools are available that describe, screen, assess, monitor, and predict functional ability. Generally, the assessment does not break down a task into its component parts, such as picking up a spoon or cup or swallowing water, when assessment of eating is done; instead, eating is seen as a total task. Most of the tools result in a score of some kind—a rating of the person's ability to do the task alone, with assistance, or not at all. The ratings are done by self-report, proxy, or observer as noted above. The tools are useful in that they serve the purposes noted above. However, most of the time the use of ratings is not sensitive enough to show small changes in function. The *Katz Index* (Katz et al, 1963) developed in 1963 serves as a basic framework for most of the measures of ADLs since that time. There are several versions of the Katz Index; one is based on a 3-point scale and allows one to score client performance abilities as independent, assistive, dependent, or unable to perform. Another version of the tool assigns 1 point to each ADL that can be completed independently and a zero (0) if unable to perform these activities. Scores will range from a maximum of 6 (totally independent) to 0 (totally dependent) (Wallace and Shelkey, 2007) A score of 4 indicates moderate impairment, whereas 2 or less indicates severe impairment (Table 13-1). This scoring puts equal weight on all activities, and the determination of a cutoff score is completely subjective. Despite these limitations, the tool is useful because it creates a common language about patient function for all caregivers involved in planning overall care and discharge.

The *Barthel Index* (Mahoney and Barthel, 1965) is commonly used in rehabilitation settings to measure the amount of physical assistance required when a person can no longer carry out ADLs. It has proven to be especially useful as a method of documenting improvement of a patient's ability. The Barthel Index ranks the functional status as either independent or dependent and then allows for further classification of independent into intact or limited, and dependent into needing a helper or unable to do the activity at all. Training in the correct use and scoring of this tool is required.

The *Functional Independence Measure (FIM)* is widely used and the most comprehensive functional assessment tool for rehabilitation settings. It includes measure of ADLs, mobility, cognition, and social functioning. It was developed through the work of a number of experts and has been thoroughly tested. Ordinarily the tool is completed through the joint efforts of the interdisciplinary team and used for both planning and evaluation of progress. Considerable training is required to accurately use the FIM (Granger and Hamilton, 1993); however, its use is encouraged.

The IADLs are considered to be more complex activities necessitating higher functioning than the ADLs. The original scoring tool for IADLs was developed by Lawton and Brody (1969). Again, both the original tool and the subsequent variations use the self-report, proxy, and observed formats with the three levels of functioning (independent, assisted, and unable to perform). The pros and cons of using these are the same as the measures of ADLs. Box 13-1 gives an example of a self-rated instrument for IADLs.

The ADLs and IADLS can also be measured using performance tools. These tools overcome the problems associated with self-report and proxy report and yield more objective measurement of performance. They take longer to conduct, and again the cutoffs are subjective and arbitrary. The three performance tests related to mobility are simple and quick: the ability to stand with feet together in a side-by-side manner and in a tandem and semitandem position, a timed walk of 8 feet, and a timed rise from a chair and return to a seated position, repeated 5 times (Box 13-2).

When assessing both functional status and cognitive abilities, slightly different tools are indicated. The *Blessed Dementia Score* (Blessed et al, 1968) is a 22-item tool scored from 0 to 27. The higher the score, the greater the degree of dementia. This tool incorporates aspects of ADLs, IADLs, memory, recalling events, and finding one's way outdoors. The *Clinical Dementia Rating Scale* (Morris, 1993) and the *Global Deterioration Scale* (Reisberg et al, 1982) also assess both functional and cognitive abilities are used to stage dementia. Determining the functional and cognitive stage of the dementia can allow the nurse to provide considerable anticipatory teaching to both the family and other caregivers.

Table 13-1   Katz Index of Independence in Activities of Daily Living

ACTIVITIES (0 OR 1 POINT)	INDEPENDENCE (1 POINT)	DEPENDENCE (0 POINTS)
	NO supervision, direction, or personal assistance	WITH supervision, direction, personal assistance, or total care
BATHING Points: _____	(1 point) Bathes self completely or needs help in bathing only a single part of the body such as the back, the genital area, or disabled extremity.	(0 points) Needs help with bathing more than one part of the body, or getting in or out of the tub or shower. Requires total bathing.
DRESSING Points: _____	(1 point) Gets clothes from closets and drawers and puts on clothes and outer garments complete with fasteners. May have help tying shoes.	(0 points) Needs help with dressing self or needs to be completely dressed.
TOILETING Points: _____	(1 point) Goes to toilet, gets on and off, arranges clothes, cleans genital area without help.	(0 points) Needs help transferring to the toilet or cleaning self, or uses bedpan or commode.
TRANSFERRING Points: _____	(1 point) Moves in and out of bed or chair unassisted. Mechanical transferring aids are acceptable.	(0 points) Needs help in moving from bed to chair or requires a complete transfer.
CONTINENCE Points: _____	(1 point) Exercises complete self-control over urination and defecation.	(0 points) Is partially or totally incontinent of bowel or bladder.
FEEDING Points: _____	(1 point) Gets food from plate into mouth without help. Preparation of food may be done by another person.	(0 points) Needs partial or total help with feeding or requires parenteral feeding.
TOTAL POINTS = _____	6 = High (patient independent)	0 = Low (patient very dependent)

From Katz S et al: Progress in the development of the index of ADL, *Gerontologist* 10(1):20-30, 1970.

Mental Status Assessment

As persons enter their 80's and 90's their risk for impaired cognitive abilities increases. With increases in age there is an increased rate of dementing illnesses, such as Alzheimer's. Cognitive ability is also easily threatened by any disturbance in health. Indeed, altered or impaired mental status may be the first sign of anything from a heart attack to a urinary tract infection. The gerontological nurse must be aware of the basic tools that are used in the assessment of mental status, especially cognitive abilities and mood. See also a discussion of assessment of delirium in Waszynski and Petrovic (2008) and Chapter 21.

Cognitive Measures

Mini-Mental State Examination. The tool that is most used is the *Mini-Mental State Examination (MMSE)* by Folstein and colleagues (1975). The MMSE is a 30-item instrument that is used to screen for cognitive deficiencies and is one of the factors in the determination of a diagnosis of dementia or delirium. It tests orientation, short-term memory and attention, calculation ability, language, and construction. To ensure that the results of this test are valid and reliable, it must be administered exactly as it is written. It cannot be given to persons who cannot see or write or who are not proficient in English. A score of 30 suggests no impairment, and a score of 24 or less suggests potential dementia; however,

Box 13-1	Instrumental Activities of Daily Living

1. Telephone:
    I: Able to look up numbers, dial, and receive and make calls without help
    A: Able to answer phone or dial operator in an emergency but needs special phone or help in getting number or dialing
    D: Unable to use telephone
2. Traveling:
    I: Able to drive own car or travel alone on bus or taxi
    A: Able to travel but not alone
    D: Unable to travel
3. Shopping:
    I: Able to take care of all shopping with transportation provided
    A: Able to shop but not alone
    D: Unable to shop
4. Preparing meals:
    I: Able to plan and cook full meals
    A: Able to prepare light foods but unable to cook full meals alone
    D: Unable to prepare any meals
5. Housework:
    I: Able to do heavy housework (e.g., scrub floors)
    A: Able to do light housework but needs help with heavy tasks
    D: Unable to do any housework
6. Medication:
    I: Able to take medications in the right dose at the right time
    A: Able to take medications but needs reminding or someone to prepare them
    D: Unable to take medications
7. Money:
    I: Able to manage buying needs, write checks, pay bills
    A: Able to manage daily buying needs but needs help managing checkbook, paying bills
    D: Unable to manage money

I, Independent; *A,* assistance needed; *D,* dependent.

From *Multidimensional Functional Assessment Questionnaire,* ed 2, 1978, by Duke University Center for the Study of Aging and Human Development with permission of Duke University.

adjustments are needed for educational level. In the long-term care setting, the MMSE is administered by either the nurse or the social worker as part of the collection of period data for the MDS (Minimum Data Set) (see Chapter 5).

Clock Drawing Test. The *Clock Drawing Test,* which has been used since 1992 (Mendez et al, 1992; Tuokko et al, 1992), is a screening tool that helps identify those with cognitive impairment and that is used as a measure of severity. It requires some manual dexterity to complete. It would not be appropriate to use with individuals with any limitations in the use of their dominant hand. A person is presented with either a blank piece of paper or a paper with a circle drawn on it. He or she is then asked to draw the face of a clock so that it says 2:40 or some other time. Scoring is based on both the position of the numbers and the position of the hands (Box 13-3). This tool does not establish criteria for dementia, but if performance on the clock drawing is impaired, it suggests the need for further investigation and analysis. Another evidence-based version of this measure is Royall's CLOX (Kennedy, 2007).

The Mini-Cog. The Mini-Cog was developed as a tool that could establish cognitive status more quickly, without the equipment needed for the MMSE and the limitations of educational adjustments. It is the evidenced-based tool now recommended (Doerflinger and Carolan, 2007). It combines one aspect of the MMSE (short-term memory recall) with the test of executive function of the Clock Drawing Test. It has been found to be highly sensitive to diagnosing dementia (Borson et al, 2000) and as a predictor of delirium in older hospitalized persons (Brodaty et al, 2006; Alagiakrishnan et al, 2007).

Mood Measures

The above-mentioned tools are measures of cognitive ability. Other tools are needed to assess mood, especially to determine the presence or absence of depression, a common and too often unrecognized problem in older adults. Persons with untreated depression are more functionally impaired and will have prolonged hospitalizations and nursing home stays, lowered quality of life, and perhaps shortened length of life (see Chapter 24). Persons with depression may appear as if they have dementia, and many persons with dementia are also depressed. The interconnection between the two calls for skill and sensitivity in the nurse to ensure that elders receive the most appropriate and effective care possible. For a discussion of depression assessment in Chinese elders, see Wu and Kelley (2007). See Chapter 21 for further discussion of cognitive assessment.

Geriatric Depression Scale. The *Geriatric Depression Scale (GDS),* developed by Yesavage and colleagues (1983) is used for mood measurement. It is a

Box 13-2 Functional Performance Tests

Standing Balance
Instructions: semitandem stand.* The nurse:

a. First demonstrates the task.
(The heel of one foot is placed to the side of the first toe of the other foot.)

b. Supports one arm of the older adult while he or she positions the feet as demonstrated above. The elder can choose which foot to place forward.

c. Asks if the person is ready, then releases the support and begins timing.

d. Stop timing when the older adult moves the feet or grasps the nurse for support or when 10 seconds have elapsed.
*Start with the semitandem stand. If it cannot be done for 10 seconds, then the **side-by-side** test should be done.
If the semitandem can be accomplished for the requisite 10 seconds, carry out the full tandem stand following the same instructions as above, except the **full tandem** calls for placing the heel of one foot directly in front of the toes of the other foot.

Scoring	Full tandem	Semitandem	Side-by-side
0	_____	<10 seconds or unable	<10 seconds or unable
1	_____	<10 seconds or unable	10 seconds
2	<3 seconds or unable	10 seconds	_____
3	3 to 9 seconds	10 seconds	_____
4	10 seconds	10 seconds	_____

Standing Balance score: _____

Walking Speed
Instructions: The nurse:

a. Sets up an 8-foot walking course with an additional 2 feet at both ends free of any obstacles.

b. Places an 8-foot rigid carpenter's ruler to the side of the course.

c. Instructs the older adult to "walk to the other end of the course at your normal speed, just like walking down the street to go to the store." Assistive devices should be used if needed.

d. Times two walks. **The fastest of the two is used as the score.**

Scoring

0	Unable
1	>5.6 seconds
2	4.1 to 5.6 seconds
3	3.2 to 4 seconds
4	<3.2 seconds

Walking Speed score: _____

Chair Stands
Instructions: The nurse:

a. Places a straight-backed chair next to a wall.

b. Asks the older adult to fold the arms across the chest and stand up from the chair 1 time. If successful, the nurse goes on to Step c.

c. Asks the older adult to stand and sit 5 times as quickly as possible.

d. Times from the initial sitting position to the final standing position at the end of the fifth stand.

Scores are for the five rise-and-sits only. If the older adult performs fewer than five repetitions, the score is 0.

Scoring

0	Unable
1	>16.6 seconds
2	13.7 to 16.5 seconds
3	11.2 to 13.6 seconds
4	<11.2 seconds

Chair Stands score: _____ **Total of all performance tests (0-12)** _____

Modified from Guralnik JM, Simonsic EM, Ferrucci L et al: A short physical performance battery assessment of lower extremity function: association with self-reported disability and prediction of mortality and nursing home admission, *J Gerontol A Biol Sci Med Sci* 49(2):M85-M94, 1994; and Bennett JA: Activities of daily living: old-fashioned or still useful? *J Gerontol Nurs* 25(5):22-29, 1999.

Box 13-3   Clock Drawing Test

Instructions
On a blank piece of paper:
   Ask the elder to draw a circle.
   Ask the elder to place the numbers 1-12 inside the circle as for a clock.
   Ask the elder to place the hands at 3:45.

Scoring
Draws closed circle	Score 1 point
Places numbers in correct position	Score 1 point
Includes all 12 correct numbers	Score 1 point
Places hands in correct position	Score 1 point

Interpretations
Errors such as grossly distorted contour or extraneous markings are rarely produced by cognitively intact persons.

Clinical judgment must be applied, but a low score indicates the need for further evaluation.

Data from Mendez MF, Ala T, Underwood KL: Development of scoring criteria for the clock drawing task in Alzheimer's disease, *J Am Geriatr Soc* 40(11):1095-1099, 1992; Tuokko H, Hadjistaropoulost T, Miller J et al: The clock test: a sensitive measure to differentiate normal elderly from those with Alzheimer disease, *J Am Geriatr Soc* 40(6):579-584, 1992.

30-item tool designed for gerontological patients and is based almost entirely on psychological factors. The GDS has been extremely successful in determining depression because it deemphasizes physical complaints, sex drive, and appetite, those things most affected by medications. It is viewed as a more accurate measure of depression in the elderly than other tools. It cannot be used in persons with dementia or cognitive impairment. An updated, shorter 15-item version is now available at www.hartfordign.org (Kurlowicz and Greenberg, 2007). (See Appendix 24-A.)

Assessment of Social Supports

A comprehensive assessment of an older adult would be incomplete without an evaluation of social networks and support. Assessment of social supports considers an individual's surrounding network of intimates, friends, and family and their ability to provide companionship and assistance in times of need. Tools to adequately measure social networks have been in development for a number of years. However, the many nuances and configurations of social support networks make standardized measurements difficult. One tool that has shown some usefulness is the Family APGAR. Although it was designed for younger families, it has potential for use with elders and their families.

Family APGAR

The *Family APGAR* (Smilkstein et al, 1982; Table 13-2) addresses five specific family functions: *A*daptation, *P*artnership, *G*rowth, *A*ffection, and *R*esolution. A score of fewer than 3 out of a possible 10 points indicates a highly dysfunctional family (at least as perceived by the person). A 4- to 6-point score suggests moderate family dysfunction. These results alone should not be considered definitive for family dysfunction. The APGAR tool is useful in the following situations:

▶ Interviewing a new patient
▶ Interviewing a person who will be caring for a chronically ill family member
▶ Following adverse events (death, diagnosis of cancer, etc.)
▶ When the patient history suggests family dysfunction

If an elder has more intimate social relationships with friends than with the spouse or family or is without family or spouse, the Friend APGAR should be used. The questions are the same as in the Family APGAR but with the word *Friend* substituted for *Family*.

An additional value of this instrument is the ability to assess the caregiver's perception of emotional support and social supports with a new diagnosis of Alzheimer's disease in a relative. There are also a number of tools specifically designed to measure the burden of the caregiver role; for example, see Figure 13-1, available at www.hartfordign.org (see also Chapter 24).

Environmental and Safety Assessment

Environmental safety is an issue at all ages. For persons with limitations in cognition, mobility, vision, or hearing or at risk for a fall-related injury, safety is especially important. Nurses in every setting are responsible for promoting the safety of the persons under their care. For a discussion of an excellent tool to assess hearing in the older adult see Chapter 3 and *Try This* #12 A Brief Healing Loss Screener (www.hartfordign.org) (Demers, 2007).

The most commonly used tools related to safety are administered by home health nurses and occupational

Table 13-2   The Family APGAR

The following questions have been designed to help us better understand you and your friends.

Friends are nonrelatives from your school or community with whom you have a sharing relationship.

The following questions have been designed to help us better understand you and your family. You should feel free to ask questions about any item in the questionnaire.

"Family" is the individual(s) with whom you usually live. If you live alone, consider family as those with whom you now have the strongest emotional ties. Comment space should be used if you wish to give additional information or if you wish to discuss the way the question applies to your family. Please try to answer all questions.

For each question, check only one box

	Almost always	Some of the time	Hardly ever		Almost always	Some of the time	Hardly ever
I am satisfied that I can turn to my friends for help when something is troubling me.	☐	☐	☐	I am satisfied that I can turn to my family for help when something is troubling me.	☐	☐	☐
Comments:				Comments:			
I am satisfied with the way my friends talk over things with me and share problems with me.	☐	☐	☐	I am satisfied with the way my family talks over things with me and shares problems with me.	☐	☐	☐
Comments:				Comments:			
I am satisfied that my friends accept and support my wishes to take on new activities or directions.	☐	☐	☐	I am satisfied that my family accepts and supports my wishes to take on new activities or directions.	☐	☐	☐
Comments:				Comments:			
I am satisfied with the way my friends express affection, and respond to my emotions, such as anger, sorrow, or love.	☐	☐	☐	I am satisfied with the way my family expresses affection, and responds to my emotions, such as anger, sorrow, or love.	☐	☐	☐
Comments:				Comments:			
I am satisfied with the way my friends and I share time together.	☐	☐	☐	I am satisfied with the way my family and I share time together.	☐	☐	☐
Comments:				Comments:			

Who lives in your home?* List by relationship (e.g., spouse, significant other,†child, or friend).

Please check below the column that best describes how you now get along with each member of the family listed.

Relationship	Age	Sex	Well	Fairly	Poorly
_____	___	___	☐	☐	☐
_____	___	___	☐	☐	☐
_____	___	___	☐	☐	☐

Table 13-2 The Family APGAR—cont'd

If you don't live with your own family, please list below the individuals to whom you turn for help most frequently. List by relationship (e.g., family member, friend, associate at work, or neighbor).			Please check below the column that best describes how you now get along with each person listed.		
Relationship	Age	Sex	Well	Fairly	Poorly
_____	_____	_____	☐	☐	☐
_____	_____	_____	☐	☐	☐
_____	_____	_____	☐	☐	☐

*If you have established your own family, consider home to be the place where you live with your spouse, children, or significant other; otherwise, consider home as your place of origin (e.g., the place where your parents or those who raised you live).

†"Significant other" is the partner you live with in a physically and emotionally nurturing relationship, but to whom you are not married.

From Smilkstein G, Ashworth C, Montano D: Validity and reliability of the family APGAR as a test of family function, *J Fam Pract* 15(2): 303-311, 1982.

therapists. In general they consist of lists of potential dangers and the status of the danger (present or absent) and provide suggestions or an opportunity for planning to reduce the potential dangers. Often nurses think of safety related to the risk for falling, but fire hazards, poisoning, and problems with temperature (hypothermia or hyperthermia) exist as well. Unfortunately many older persons who have lived in their homes for many years are also in potential danger because of increased crime and victimization. See also Chapter 12 for a more detailed discussion of mobility and environmental safety.

Integrated Assessments

In some cases an integrated approach is used rather than a collection of separate tools and assessments. The most well known is the *Older American's Resources and Service (OARS)* (Pfeiffer, 1979). The *Comprehensive Assessment and Referral Evaluation* tool was designed for assessment of functional status and mental health (Gurland et al, 1983). These and other tools were taken into consideration in the development of the MDS currently used in skilled nursing facilities and the *OASIS System* in the home care setting (see Chapter 5). All these tools are quite comprehensive and therefore quite lengthy. Once completed, they serve as a resource for a detailed plan of care.

Older American's Resources and Service

The classic *OARS instrument* was designed to evaluate ability, disability, and the capacity level at which the person is able to function. It is set up in such a manner in

that each of five subscales may be used separately. The five subscales include social resources, economic resources, physical health, mental health, and ability to perform ADLs. The person's functional capacity in each area is rated on a scale of 1 (excellent) to 6 (completely impaired). At the conclusion of the assessment a cumulative impairment score (CIS) is established, which can range from the most capable (6) to total disability (30). This aids in establishing the degree of need and the resources required for both daily living and quality of healthy life. Information considered in each domain includes the following. Similarities between some aspects of the subscales of the OARS and Maslow's Hierarchy can be found.

Social Resources. The social resources dimension addresses the social skills and the ability to negotiate and make friends. Is the person able to seek help from friends, family, and strangers? Is there a caregiver available if needed? Who is it, and how long is the person available? Does the individual belong to any social network or group, such as a special interest or church group? How are belonging needs met?

Economic Resources. Data about monthly income and sources (Social Security, Supplemental Security Income, pensions, income generated from capital) are needed to determine the adequacy of income compared with the cost of living and food, shelter, clothing, medications, and small luxury items. This information can provide insight into the client's relative standard of living and point out areas of need that might be alleviated by use of additional resources unknown to the elder.

I am going to read a list of things that other people have found to be difficult. Would you tell me if any of these apply to you? (Give examples.)

	Yes = 1	No = 0
Sleep is disturbed (e.g., because is in and out of bed; wanders around at night)		
It is inconvenient (e.g., because helping takes so much time; it's a long drive over to help)		
It is a physical strain (e.g., because of lifting in and out of a chair; effort or concentration is required)		
It is confining (e.g., helping restricts free time; cannot go visiting)		
There have been family adjustments (e.g., because helping has disrupted routine; there has been no privacy)		
There have been changes in personal plans (e.g., had to turn down a job; could not go on vacation)		
There have been other demands on my time (e.g., from other family members)		
There have been emotional adjustments (e.g., because of severe arguments)		
Some behavior is upsetting (e.g., because of incontinence; has trouble remembering things; accuses people of taking things)		
It is upsetting to find has changed so much from his/her former self (e.g., he/she is a different person than he/she used to be)		
There have been work adjustments (e.g., because of having to take time off)		
It is a financial strain		
Feeling completely overwhelmed (e.g., because of worry about _____; concerns abourt how to manage)		
TOTAL SCORE (Count yes responses. Any positive answer may indicate a need for intervention in that area. A score of 7 or higher indicates a high level of stress.)		

Fig. 13-1   Caregiver strain index. *(From Robinson BC: Validation of a caregiver strain index, J Gerontol 38[3]:344-348, 1983. Copyright The Gerontological Society of America.)*

Mental Health. Consideration is given to intellectual function, the presence or absence of psychiatric symptoms, and the amount of enjoyment and interaction the person gets from life.

Physical Health. Diagnoses of major and common diseases of older persons, the type of prescribed and over-the-counter medications the person is taking, and the person's perception of his or her health status are the basis of evaluation. Excellent physical health includes participation in regular vigorous activity, such as walking, dancing, or biking at least twice each week, and preferably daily. Seriously impaired physical health is determined by the presence of one or more illnesses or disabilities that are severely painful or life-threatening, or necessitate extensive care.

Activities of Daily Living. The ADLs included in the OARS are walking, getting in and out of bed, bathing, combing hair, shaving, dressing, eating, and getting to the bathroom on time by oneself. The IADLs measured include tasks such as dialing the telephone, driving a car, hanging up clothes, obtaining groceries, taking medications, and having correct knowledge of their dosages.

Fulmer SPICES

The *Fulmer SPICES*, an overall assessment tool of older adults (Wallace and Fulmer, 2007), has proved reliable and valid in use in later life whether in health or illness; in acute, skilled nursing, long-term care facilities; or at home. The acronym *SPICES* refers to six common syndromes of the elderly that require nursing interventions: *S*leep disorders, *P*roblems with eating or feeding, *I*ncontinence, *C*onfusion, *E*vidence of falls, and *S*kin breakdown. Nurses are encouraged to make a 3 × 5 card with this acronym on it and carry it with them to use as a reference when caring for older adults (see www. hartfordign.org). It is a system for alerting the nurse of the most common problems that occur in the health and well-being of the older adult, particularly those who have one or more medical conditions.

IMPLICATIONS FOR GERONTOLOGICAL NURSING AND HEALTHY AGING

Whether the nurse is working with a standardized tool or creating one, the goal is always to collect data that are the most accurate and to do so in the most efficient, yet caring manner possible. The use of tools serves as a way to organize the collected data necessary for assessment and makes it possible to compare the data from time to time. As noted above, each tool has strengths and weaknesses. A number of factors complicate assessment of the older adult. These include the difficulty of differentiating the effects of aging from those originating from disease, the coexistence of multiple diseases, the underreporting of symptoms by older adults, atypical presentation or nonspecific presentation of illness, and the increase in iatrogenic illnesses.

Overdiagnosis or underdiagnosis occurs when the normal age changes are not considered; these include both physical changes and psychosocial changes. Underdiagnosis is far more common in gerontological nursing. Many symptoms or complaints are ascribed to normal aging rather than a health problem that may be developing. Assessing the older adult with multiple chronic conditions is also a challenge. Symptoms of one condition can exacerbate or mask symptoms of another. The gerontological nurse is challenged to provide the highest

level of excellence in the care of the elderly. If a particular tool will facilitate the achievement of this goal, it should be used. If the tool serves little purpose and is burdensome to either the nurse or the patient, it should be avoided or replaced. When approaching assessment from a wellness perspective Maslow's Hierarchy provides a useful framework.

KEY CONCEPTS

▶ Assessment of the physical, cognitive, psychosocial, and environmental status is essential to meeting the specific needs of the older adult and implementing appropriate interventions.

▶ Whether the data for an assessment tool are collected by self-report, by report-by-proxy, or through nurse observation will affect the quality and quantity of the data.

▶ Knowledge of how to use a particular gerontological assessment tool is needed to accurately administer it.

▶ Comorbidity of many older adults complicates obtaining and interpreting assessment data.

ACTIVITIES AND DISCUSSION QUESTIONS

1. What is the importance of the measurement of ADLs and IADLs in older adults?

2. For each ADL, develop a plan of interventions that you would institute to compensate for ADL deficits and that would still foster an elder's independence as much as is realistic.

3. What makes an assessment tool effective?

4. What tool or tools would be most appropriate for assessing an elder in the community, in the hospital, in long-term care, or in day care? Give your rationale for the choices.

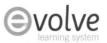
learning system

For additional resources, please visit evolve.elsevier.com/Ebersole/gerontological

REFERENCES

Alagiakrishnan K, Marrie T, Rolfson D et al.: Simple cognitive testing (Mini-Cog) predicts in-hospital delirium in the elderly, *J Am Geriatr Soc*, 55(2), 314-316, 2007.

Benner P: *From novice to expert*, Menlo Park, CA, 1984, Addison-Wesley.

Blessed G, Tomlinson BE, Roth M: The association between qualitative measures of dementia and of senile change in the cerebral grey matter of elderly subjects, *Br J Psychiatry* 114(512):797-811, 1968.

Borson S, Scanlan J, Brush M et al: The Mini-Cog: a cognitive "vital signs" measure for dementia screening in multilingual elderly, *Int J Geriatr Psych* 15(11):1021-1027, 2000.

Brodaty H, Low L, Gibson L, Burns K: What is the best dementia screening instrument for general practitioners to use? *Am J Geriatr Psychiatry* 14:391-400, 2006.

Demers K: Hearing loss in older adults—A brief hearing loss screener. The Hartford Institute for Geriatric Nursing, *Try This Series #12.2007*. Available at: http://www.hartfordign.org/Resources/Try_This_Series. Accessed 10/20/08.

Doerflinger D, Carolan M: Mental status assessment of older adults: the Mini-Cog. The Hartford Institute for Geriatric Nursing, *Try This Series #3.2007*. Available at: http://www.hartfordign.org/Resources/Try_This_Series. Accessed 10/20/08.

Folstein MF, Folstein SE, McHugh PR: Mini-mental state: a practical method for grading the cognitive state of patients for the clinician, *J Psychiatr Res* 12(3):189-198, 1975.

Fulmer T: The geriatric nurse specialist role: a new model, *Nurs Manage* 22(3):91-93, 1991.

Granger CV, Hamilton BB: The Uniform Data System for Medical Rehabilitation: report of first admissions for 1991, *Am J Phys Med Rehabil* 72(1):33-38, 1993.

Gurland B, Kuriansky J, Simon R: The Comprehensive Assessment and Referral Evaluation (CARE)—rationale, development, and reliability. *Int J Aging Devel* 8(1):9-42, 1983.

Katz S, Ford AB, Moskowitz RN et al: Studies of illness in the aged: the index of ADL: a standardized measure of biological and psychosocial function, *JAMA* 185:914-919, 1963.

Kennedy GJ: Brief evaluation of executive dysfunction: An essential refinement in the assessment of cognitive impairment. The Hartford Institute for Geriatric Nursing, *Try This Series # D3.2007*. Available at: http://www.hartfordign.org/Resources/Try_This_Series. Accessed 10/20/08.

Kleinman A: *Patient and healers in the context of culture: an exploration of the borderland between anthropology, medicine, and psychiatry,* Berkeley, 1980, University of California Press.

Kurlowicz L, Greenberg S: The Geriatric Depression Scale (GDS). The Hartford Institute for Geriatric Nursing, *Try This Series #4.2007*. Available at: http://www.hartfordign.org/Resources/Try_This_Series. Accessed 10/20/08.

Lawton MP, Brody EM: Assessment of older people: self-maintaining and instrumental activities of daily living, *Gerontologist* 9(3):179-186, 1969.

Mahoney FI, Barthel DW: Functional evaluation: the Barthel Index, *Md State Med J* 14:61-65, 1965.

Mendez MF, Ala T, Underwood KL: Development of scoring criteria for the Clock Drawing Task in Alzheimer's disease, *J Am Geriatr Soc* 40(11):1095-1099, 1992.

Morris JC: The clinical dementia rating (CDR): current version and scoring rules, *Neurology* 43(11):2412-2414, 1993.

Pfeiffer E: *Physical and mental assessment—OARS.* Workshop Intensive, Western Gerontological Society, San Francisco, April 28, 1979.

Reisberg B, Ferris S, deLeon MJ et al: The global deterioration scale for assessment of primary progressive dementia, *Am J Psychiatry* 139(9):1136-1139, 1982.

Smilkstein G, Ashworth C, Montano D: Validity and reliability of the family APGAR as a test of family function, *J Fam Pract* 15(2):303-311, 1982.

Tuokko H, Hadjistaropoulost T, Miller J et al: The clock test: a sensitive measure to differentiate normal elderly from those with Alzheimer disease, *J Am Geriatr Soc* 40(6):579-584, 1992.

U.S. Department of Health and Human Services (USDHHS): *Healthy People* 2010. The *cornerstone of prevention.* Washington, DC, 2005, U.S. Government Printing Office. Available at www.healthypeople.gov/Publications/Cornerstone.pdf. Accessed 7/12/08.

Wallace M, Fulmer T: Fulmer SPICES: an overall assessment tool for older adults. The Hartford Institute for Geriatric Nursing, *Try This Series #1.2007*. Available at: http://www.hartfordign.org/Resources/Try_This_Series. Accessed 10/20/08.

Wallace M, Shelkey M: Katz Index of Independence in activities of daily living. The Hartford Institute for Geriatric Nursing, *Try This Series #2.2007*. Available at: http://www.hartfordign.org/Resources/Try_This_Series. Accessed 10/20/08.

Waszynski CM, Petrovic K: Nurses' evaluation of the confusion assessment method: a pilot study, *J Gerontol Nurs* 34(4):49-56, 2008.

Wu CM, Kelley LS: Choosing an appropriate depression assessment tool for Chinese older adults, *J Gerontol Nurs* 33(8):12-22, 2007.

Yesavage JA, Brink TL, RoseT et al: Development and validation of a geriatric depression screening scale: a preliminary report, *J Psychiatr Res* 17(1):37-49, 1982-1983.

Safe Medication Use for Older Adults

LEARNING OBJECTIVES

Upon completion of this chapter, the reader will be able to:

- Explain age-related pharmacokinetic changes.
- Discuss potential use of chronotherapy for the older adult.
- Describe drug use patterns and their implications for the older adult.
- Explain the roles of elder, caregiver, and social network in ensuring medication adherence.
- List interventions that can help promote medication adherence by the elder.
- Identify diagnoses or symptoms for which psychotropic drugs are prescribed.
- Discuss issues concerning psychotropic medication management in the elderly population.
- Develop a nursing care plan for patients prescribed psychoactive medications.

GLOSSARY

Adverse reaction A harmful, unintended reaction to a drug.

Bioavailability The amount of drug that becomes available to effect changes in target tissues.

Biotransformation A series of chemical alterations of a drug occurring in the body.

Half-life The time it takes after administration to inactivate half of a drug.

Iatrogenic An adverse result of something that is done or given to a person in the context of providing care.

Potentiation The strengthening of the effect of one or more substances (e.g., food or another drug) when they are used in combination.

Regimen A scheduled plan for the taking of medications, such as twice a day, with food, etc.

Side effect A consequence of a drug or procedure other than that for which it is used (e.g., dry mouth).

Target tissue Tissue or organ intended to receive the greatest concentration of a drug or to be most affected by the drug.

Therapeutic window The range of the plasma concentration of a drug within which it is safe and effective.

THE LIVED EXPERIENCE

It is so hard to keep track of my medications. I try arranging them in little cups to take with each meal, but then there are the ones that I take at odd times. Those are the easiest to forget. I get really confused and think sometimes I have taken them twice. I really wish I didn't have to take so many pills, but I'm not sure what would happen if I stopped any of them. I don't even know why I'm taking most of them.

Geraldo, hypertensive, diabetic, and having cardiac problems

In the United States, persons 65 years of age and older are the largest users of prescription and over-the-counter (OTC) medications. Making up only 12% of the population, they consume 30% of the prescribed medications or a range somewhere between 0 and 13 prescription drugs per person, and about 40% of OTC medications or other supplements such as herbs (Steinman et al, 2006; Gallagher et al, 2007). Residents of long-term care facilities take the most medications of all. Elders accumulate prescriptions as they accumulate chronic diseases and number of health care providers (Green et al, 2007).

Unfortunately, the number of adverse drug reactions increases with the number of medications used. Adverse drug reactions (ADRs) have been found to be a notable cause for hospitalization as well as a cause of iatrogenic mortality and morbidity for those already hospitalized (Perri et al, 2005). This has been found to occur not only in the United States but in countries as far ranging as Brazil (Passarelli et al, 2005) and Germany (Junius-Walker et al, 2007).

How elders use their prescribed medicines and other bioactive products depends on many factors related to the person's own unique characteristics, situations, beliefs, understanding about illness, functional and cognitive status, perception of the necessity of the drugs, severity of symptoms, reactions to the medications, finances, access, and alternatives, and the compatibility of such products with their lifestyle. From the perspective of Maslow's Hierarchy of Needs, drugs impinge on many levels. When used appropriately, prescription medications can enhance one's quality of life at every level. When they are used inappropriately, they threaten all levels of the Hierarchy, especially the most basic level of physiological stability. At times, even when drugs are used appropriately, they may adversely affect the elder's health and well-being.

Gerontological nurses have a responsibility to help minimize the risks of medication use in the persons who receive their care. A review of the changes in pharmacokinetics, the pharmacodynamics, and issues in drug use are presented in this chapter. The final section deals with the use of psychotropic agents. These are frequently prescribed to frail elders with the potential for both great benefit and significant risk.

PHARMACOKINETICS

The term pharmacokinetics refers to the movement of a drug in the body from the point of administration as it is absorbed, distributed, metabolized, and finally, excreted. It is important for gerontological nurse to understand how pharmacokinetics may differ in older adults (Figure 14-1). There is no conclusive evidence of an appreciable change in overall pharmacokinetics with aging. However there are several changes with aging (see Chapter 6) that may have an effect. This chapter is not intended to replace a pharmacology text, but to supplement it for the key points of intersection between medication use and the aging process.

Absorption

In order for a drug to be effective it must be absorbed, into the blood stream. The amount of time between the administration of the drug and its absorption depends on a number of factors, including the route of introduction (i.e., intravenous, oral, parenteral, transdermal, or rectal), bioavailability, and the amount of drug that passes into the body. The drug is delivered immediately to the blood stream with administration by intravenous route, and quickly with parenteral and transdermal routes and through mucous membranes such as the rectum and the oral mucosa. Orally administered drugs are absorbed the most slowly through the gastrointestinal track.

There are a number of normal age-related physiological changes that have implications for differences in both the prescribing and the administration of medications for older adult. The commonly seen diminished gastric pH will retard the action of acid-dependent drugs. Delayed stomach emptying may diminish or negate the effectiveness of short-lived drugs that could become inactivated before reaching the small intestine. The absorption of some enteric-coated medications, which are specifically meant to bypass stomach absorption, may be delayed so long that their action begins in the stomach and may produce gastric irritation or nausea. Absorption is also influenced by changes in gastrointestinal motility. If there is increased motility in the small intestine, drug effect is diminished because of shortened contact time and therefore decreased absorption and effectiveness. Conversely, slowed intestinal motility can increase the contact time and therefore the amount absorbed and the drug's effect. This increases the risk for adverse reactions or unpredictable effects.

Many medications commonly taken by older adults can also affect the absorption of other drugs. Antispasmodic drugs slow gastric and intestinal motility. In some instances the ingested drug's action may be useful, but when there are other medications involved, it is necessary to consider the problem of drug absorption alterations due to drug-drug interaction. Antacids or

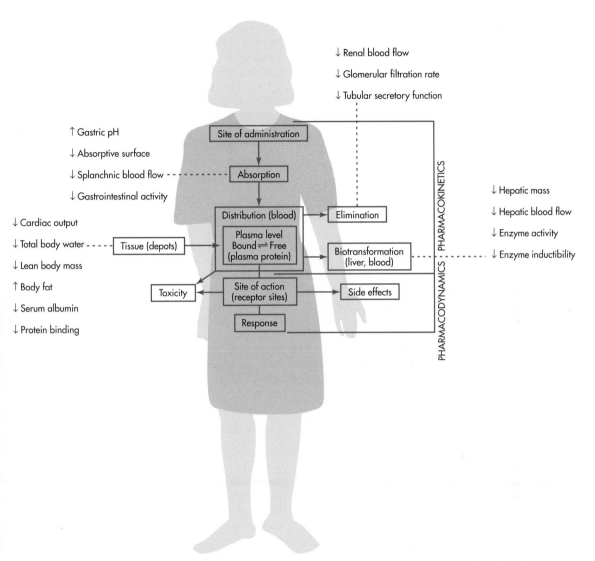

Fig. 14-1 Physiological changes of aging and the pharmacokinetics and pharmacodynamics of drug use. *(Data from Kane RL, Ouslander JG, Abrass IB:* Essentials of clinical geriatrics, *New York, 1984, McGraw-Hill; Lamy PP: Hazards of drug use in the elderly: commonsense measures to reduce them,* Postgrad Med *76(1):50-53, 1984; Vestal RE, Dawson GW: Pharmacology and aging. In Finch CE, Schneider EL, editors:* Handbook of biology and aging, *New York, 1985, Van Nostrand Reinhold; Roberts J, Tumer N: Pharmacodynamic basis for altered drug action in the elderly,* Clin Geriatr Med *4(1):127-149, 1988; Montamat SC, Cusack BJ, Vestal RE: Management of drug therapy in the elderly,* N Engl J Med *321(5):303-309, 1989.)*

iron preparations affect the availability of some drugs for absorption by binding the drug with elements and forming chemical compounds. Drug-food interactions may either decrease or increase the amount absorbed. For example when a bisphosphonate such as Fosamax is taken with food of any kind, the absorption is reduced to only a few milligrams, and therefore the drug has no effect on the target organ, the bones.

Distribution

Once a drug is absorbed it must be transported to the receptor site on the target organ to have any effect. Distribution depends on the availability of plasma protein in the form of lipoproteins, globulins, and especially albumin. As drugs are absorbed, they bind with the protein and are distributed throughout the body. Normally, a predictable percentage of the absorbed drug is inactivated as it is bound to the protein. The remaining free drug is available in the blood stream and has therapeutic effect when an effective concentration is reached in the plasma. Many older adults have an insignificant reduction in the serum albumin level. In others, especially those with prolonged illness or malnutrition (such as residents in skilled nursing facilities), the serum albumin may become dramatically diminished. When this occurs, toxic levels of available free drug may accumulate unpredictably, especially of highly protein-bound medications with narrow therapeutic windows, such as phenytoin and salicylates (Gulick and Jett, 2008).

Potential alterations of drug distribution in late life are related to changes in body composition, particularly decreased lean body mass, increased body fat, and decreased total body water (see Figure 14-1). Decreased body water leads to higher serum levels of water-soluble drugs, such as digoxin, ethanol, and aminoglycosides. Adipose tissue nearly doubles in older men and increases by one half in older women; therefore drugs that are highly lipid-soluble are stored in the fatty tissue, extending and possibly elevating the drug effect (Masoro and Austed, 2003). This includes drugs such as lorazepam, diazepam, chlorpromazine, phenobarbital, and haloperidol (Haldol).

Metabolism

Biotransformation is the process by which the body modifies the chemical structure of the drug. Through this process the compound is converted to a metabolite that is later more easily excreted. A drug will continue to exert a therapeutic effect as long as it remains in either its original state or as an active metabolite. Active metabolites retain the ability to have a therapeutic effect, as well as the same or a greater chance of causing adverse effects. For example, the metabolites of acetaminophen (Tylenol) can cause liver damage with higher dosages (>4 gm/24 hr or more than four extra-strength products). The duration of drug action is determined by the metabolic rate and is measured in terms of half-life, or how long the drug remains active in the body.

The liver is the primary site of drug metabolism. With aging, the liver's activity, mass, volume, and blood flow are reduced (see Chapter 6). These changes result in a potential decrease in the liver's ability to metabolize drugs such as benzodiazepines (e.g., the tranquilizer lorazepam [Ativan]). These changes result in a significant increase in the half-life of these drugs. For example, the half-life of diazepam (Valium) in a younger adult is about 37 hours, but in an older adult extends to as long as 82 hours. If the dose and timing are not adjusted, the drug can accumulate, and the administration of a single dose can have significantly more effects than in a younger person. In most situations the use of Valium is contraindicated (Fick et al, 2003).

Excretion

Drugs and their metabolites are excreted in sweat, saliva, and other secretions but primarily through the kidneys. However, since kidney function declines significantly in aging, so does the ability to excrete or eliminate drugs in a timely manner. The considerably decreased glomerular filtration rate leads to prolongation of the half-life of drugs, or the amount of time required to eliminate the drug, again presenting opportunities for accumulation and increasing the potential for toxicity or other adverse events (see Chapter 6). Although renal function cannot be estimated by the serum creatinine level, it can be approximated by the calculation of the creatinine clearance (see below). Reductions in dosages for renally excreted drugs (e.g., allopurinol, vancomycin) are needed when the creatinine clearance is reduced.

Estimated Creatinine Clearance (The Cockcroft-Gault Equation):

$$\frac{(140 - age) \times wt\ (kg)\ (if\ female, \times 0.85)}{(serum\ creatinine \times 72)}$$

For alternative calculations also see: http://nkdep.nih.gov/professionals/gfr_calculators

Gomella LG and Haist SA: Clinician's Pocket Reference. New York: McGraw Hill, 2007.

Pharmacodynamics

Pharmacodynamics refers to the interaction between a drug and the body (see Figure 1-1). The older the person gets, the more likely there will be an altered or unreliable response of the body to the drug. Although it is not always possible to explain the change in response, several mechanisms are known. The aging process causes a decreased response to beta-adrenergic receptor stimulators and blockers; decreased baroreceptor sensitivity; and increased sensitivity to a number of medications, especially anticholinergics, benzodiazepines, narcotic analgesics, warfarin (Coumadin), and the cardiac drugs diltiazem and verapamil (Briggs, 2005). If food-drug interactions occur, the problems are worsened. For example, drinking grapefruit juice at the same time as one takes a "statin" such as Lipitor or any number of antibiotics may cause an unreliable response. There is also a growing body of knowledge about the interaction of herbal preparations and currently prescribed medications. For example, ginkgo biloba is commonly thought to enhance cognitive function. However it will increase the potential for bleeding when an anticoagulant is used at the same time (Youngkin, 2008) (see Table 14-1). In addition to the expected dry mouth, drugs with anticholinergic properties

Table 14-1   Selected Herb-Medication Interactions

HERB	MEDICATION	COMPLICATION	NURSING ACTION
Garlic	Warfarin sodium, or any anticoagulant or antiplatelet drug NSAIDs such as ketoprofen Anticlotting drugs such as streptokinase and urokinase	Risk of bleeding increases	Advise client not to take without provider approval
	Antimetabolite such as cyclosporine	Risk of less effective response	Advise against use
	Insulin or oral hypoglycemic agent such as pioglitazone or tolbutamide	Serum glucose control may improve, lowering the amount of antidiabetic medication needed	Monitor blood glucose levels
Ginkgo	Aspirin Heparin sodium Warfarin sodium	Risk of bleeding increases	Teach client not to take without approval of provider
	Antidiabetic drugs Insulin Glimepiride, metformin, and other oral drugs for DMT2	May alter blood glucose levels	Monitor blood glucose closely
	Antidepressants MAOIs, SSRIs	May cause abnormal response or decrease effectiveness	Advise not to take with these drugs
	Antihypertensives Nifedipine	May cause increased effect	Monitor blood pressure
Ginseng	Insulin and oral antidiabetic drugs	Blood glucose levels may be altered	Monitor blood glucose levels; monitor for hyperglycemia, hypoglycemia
	Anticoagulants and antiplatelet drugs	May increase bleeding	Advise use with caution
	MAOIs	Headaches, tremors, mania	Advise against use
	Immunosuppressants	May interfere with action	Advise against use
	Stimulants	May cause additive effect	Advise against use

(Continued)

Table 14-1   Selected Herb-Medication Interactions—cont'd

HERB	MEDICATION	COMPLICATION	NURSING ACTION
Green tea	Warfarin sodium	May alter anticoagulant effects	Advise against use
	Stimulants	May cause additive effect	Advise to use with care
Hawthorn	Digoxin	May cause a loss of potassium, leading to drug toxicity	Monitor blood levels
	Beta blockers and other drugs lowering blood pressure and improving blood flow	May be additive in effects	Monitor blood pressure meticulously; advise that this concern extends to erectile dysfunction drugs also
St. John's wort	"Triptans" such as sumatriptan, zolmitriptan	May increase risks of serotonergic adverse effects, serotonin syndrome, cerebral vasoconstriction	Advise against use
	HMG-CoA reductase inhibitors	May decrease plasma concentrations of these drugs	Monitor levels of lipids
	MAOIs	May cause similar effects as with use with any SSRI	Advise against use
	Digoxin	Decreases the effects of the drug	Advise against use
	Alprazolam	May decrease effect of drug	Advise against use
	Amitriptyline	May decrease effect of drug	Advise against use
	Efavirenz and other anti-HIVs	May decrease drug level	Advise against use
	Ketoprofen	Photosensitivity	Advise sun block use
	Tramadol and some SSRIs	May increase risk of serotonin syndrome	Advise against use
	Olanzapine	May cause serotonin syndrome	Advise against use
	Paroxetine	Sedative-hypnotic intoxication	Advise against use
	Theophylline Albuterol	Increases metabolism; decreases drug blood level	Monitor drug effects
	Warfarin	May decrease anticoagulant effect	Advise against use
	Amlodipine	Lowers efficacy of calcium channel	Advise against use
	Estrogen or progesterone	May decrease effect of hormones	Advise that this effect may occur

DMT2, Diabetes mellitus type 2; HIV, human immunodeficiency virus; HMG-CoA, 3-hydroxy-3-methylglutaryl coenzyme A; MAOIs, monoamine oxidase inhibitors; NSAIDs, nonsteroidal antiinflammatory drugs; SSRIs, selective serotonin reuptake inhibitors.
Adapted by Yougkin E: The use of herbal supplements in late life. In Ebersole P, Hess P, Touhy T, et al. Toward healthy aging, 2008, St. Louis, Mosby. From Basch E, Ulbricht C: Natural standard herb & supplement handbook: the clinical bottom line, St Louis, 2005, Mosby; Jellin JM (ed.): Natural medicines comprehensive database, 2006, (website): www.naturaldatabase.com/. Accessed 11/15/06; NDH pocket guide to drug interactions, Philadelphia, 2002, Lippincott, Williams & Wilkins; Wilson BA, Shannon MT and Shields KM: Nurses drug guide, Upper Saddle River, NJ, 2004, Pearson Prentice Hall; Yoon SL, Schaffer SD: Herbal, prescribed, and over-the-counter drug use in older women: prevalence of drug interactions, Geriatr Nurs 27(2):118-129, 2006.

can cause confusion and urinary retention (Miller, 2008). The use of benzodiazepines is associated with an increased risk for accidental injury, and they are on the "do-not-use" list for older adults (Fick et al, 2003).

CHRONOPHARMACOLOGY

Another factor that affects both pharmacokinetics and pharmacodynamics appears to be the normal biorhythms of the body and the differences in these rhythms in men and women. The relationship of biological rhythms to variations in the body's response to drugs is known as chronopharmacology. Although it has not yet been explored in the elderly, chronopharmacology is a developing science that may lead to more effective drug therapy (Bruguerolle, 2007). The best time to administer medications, is now being considered in light of the biorhythms of various physiological processes.

As noted on page 232, absorption depends on gastric acid pH, the level of motility of the gastrointestinal tract, and blood flow. All have been shown to have biorhythmical variations. Distribution of protein-bound drugs depends on albumin and glycoproteins produced by the liver. During the day, albumin levels are high, but they are low in the early-morning. Drug metabolism is also biorhythmical. Oxidation, hydrolysis, decarboxylation, and demethylation by liver enzymes demonstrate rhythmic variations. Renal elimination depends on kidney perfusion, glomerular filtration, and urine acidity and has shown rhythmic variation. The brain, the heart, and blood cells have also been found to have varied rhythmicity, resulting in a cyclical response for beta blockers, calcium channel blockers, angiotensin-converting enzyme (ACE) inhibitors, nitrates, and other, similar drugs. Drugs such as Fosamax and Actonel must be taken on arising in the morning for maximum effectiveness (Bruguerolle, 2007). Table 14-2 shows some of the rhythmical influences on diseases and physiological processes.

The potential for decreasing individual doses of medications and/or the frequency of administration for elders is the primary benefit of chronopharmacologically based therapy. Both decreases may ultimately improve the therapeutic effect and decrease toxic effects and may improve patient adherence to a medication regimen. In addition, chronotherapeutics may provide financial benefit to the patient by reducing the overall medication expense if lower or fewer doses are needed.

Table 14-2 Rhythmical Influences on Disease and Physiological Processes

DISEASE OR PROCESS	RHYTHMICAL INFLUENCE
Allergic rhinitis	Symptoms worse in the morning
Arterial blood pressure	Circadian surge—morning hours
Asthma	Greatest respiratory distress overnight (during sleeping)
	Symptoms peak in early morning (4 to 5 AM)
Blood plasma	Plasma volume falls at night, thus hematocrit increases
Cancer	Tumor cells proliferate when normal cell miosis is low
Cardiac disease	Angina, myocardial infarction, thrombolytic stroke occur in the first 4 hours after waking (peak 9 AM) (through 10 PM)
	(Prinzmetal's angina—during sleep)
Catecholamines	Increase in early morning
Fibrinolytic activity	Increase in early morning
Platelet activation	May result from abnormality in circadian rhythm, which affects cortisol levels, body temperature, sleep-wake cycle
Gastric system	Gastric acid secretion peaks every morning (2 to 4 AM); circannual variability—incidence of gastric ulcers greater in winter
Osteoarthritis	Pain more severe in morning
Potassium excretion	Lowest in morning; highest in late afternoon
Rheumatoid arthritis	Pain more severe in late afternoon
Systemic insulin	Highest in afternoon

MEDICATION ISSUES AND OLDER ADULTS

Polypharmacy

Although there is controversy about how many drugs are "too many," polypharmacy is the term used to indicate multiple drug use, and usually this implies the use of some drugs that are duplicated or unnecessary (Figure 14-2). Junius-Walker and colleagues (2007) define polypharmacy as taking more than five medications at the same time. In their study of German elders, the average number of prescribed medications was 3.7 and the average number of over-the-counter (OTC) bioactive products was 1.4. They also found that almost 27% of those surveyed took over five medications; and, as the number increased, so did the likelihood of inclusion of inappropriate medications (ineffective, duplicative, or not indicated). Polypharmacy may occur "accidentally" if an existing drug regimen is not considered when new medications are prescribed or any number of the thousands of OTC preparations and supplements are added to the prescribed medications. The two major concerns with polypharmacy are the increased risk for drug interactions and the increased risk for adverse events.

Drug Interactions

The more medications a person takes, the greater the possibility that one or more of them will interact with each other, with an herbal product, with a nutritional supplement, with food, or with alcohol. When two or more medications or foods are given together or close

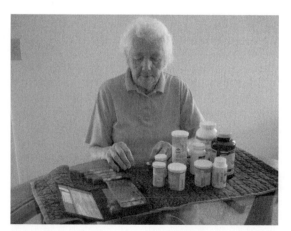

Fig. 14-2   Polypharmacy. *(Courtesy Shannon Perry, Phoenix, AZ.)*

together, the drugs may potentiate one another, or make one or both either more or less effective.

An interaction may result in altered pharmacokinetic activity or alterations in the absorption, distribution, metabolism, or excretion of one or any of the medications. Absorption can be delayed by drugs exerting an anticholinergic effect. Tricyclic antidepressants act in this manner to decrease gastrointestinal motility and interfere with the absorption of other drugs. More than one drug may compete to simultaneously occupy the necessary binding receptors, preventing one or the other from reliably reaching the target organs and creating a varied bioavailability of one or both.

Interference with enzyme activity may alter metabolism and cause drug deficiencies or toxic and adverse responses from altered renal tubular function. Outside the body, interactions can occur any time that two medications or foods are mixed together before administration. For example, when delivering medications through a feeding tube, giving each one separately takes more time than is usually feasible. In haste the nurse may crush and deliver all of them simultaneously. The appropriate administration requires that the nurse know not only which medications are "crushable" but also which can be administered together. For example, Fosamax and the other bisphosphonates must be taken with a full glass of water 1 hour before any other medication, beverage, or food is ingested.

In pharmacodynamic interactions, one drug alters the patient's response to another drug without changing the pharmacokinetic properties. This can be especially dangerous for older adults when two or more drugs with the same effect are additive, that is, together they are more potent than each one taken separately. Unless attention is paid to what the overall drug list includes, when each drug is administered, and what other products are taken, a harmful situation of polypharmacy will occur. The nurse decreases the likelihood of this happening by monitoring the medications he or she administers and by encouraging the persons under their care to do the same. Although there is much that is unknown about the use of herbs and other bioactive substances, as studies are completed, the nurse will need to learn more and more about potential adverse reactions and interactions in order to safely manage medications.

Adverse Drug Reactions

An adverse drug reaction (ADR) or adverse drug event (ADE) is an unwanted pharmacological effect, ranging from a minor annoyance to death and including allergic reactions. ADRs can sometimes be predicted from the pharmacological action of the drug (e.g., bone marrow depression from cancer chemotherapy; bleeding from Coumadin). Predictable ADRs can also occur when a patient is started on a drug at a dosage that is inappropriately high or one that necessitates laboratory monitoring and adjustment that is not done (e.g., lithium, Coumadin).

ADRs occur in all settings in which one takes or is administered medications. Page and Ruscin (2006) found that 31.9% of the elders studied experienced at least one ADR while hospitalized. In a study conducted in Brazil, this number increased to 46.2% (Passarelli et al, 2005) It is important to note that 60% of these adverse events were related to errors in monitoring, a responsibility that falls heavily on nurses. Among the most common drugs that led to adverse reactions are cardiac, diuretics, nonopioid pain relievers, hypoglycemic agents and anticoagulants (Budnitz et al, 2007). All of these are frequently prescribed to older adults. Because of the large number of medications taken by most older adults in long-term care settings and their frequently altered nutritional and fluid status, the risk for adverse reactions is of special concern to nurses working in this setting.

The use of medications thought to be inappropriate for use in older adults (Table 14-3) has also been found to increase the risk for ADRs and related hospitalizations. Even one inappropriate medication, such as ibuprofen or propoxyphene (Darvon products such as Darvocet), has the potential to increase this risk (Perri et al, 2005). It has been estimated that overall 49% of persons taking inappropriate medications are admitted to the hospital in connection with these medications, or 16% of all admissions are related to the taking of inappropriate-medications (Gallagher et al, 2007).

ADRs are not always predictable. An elderly patient who is well controlled on a stable dose of a drug may undergo a change in his or her physiology or environment and the body's response to the drug may be altered (e.g., levothyroxine [Synthroid]). Changes in diet can also have a profound impact on drug effect. For example, decreased fluid intake can cause lithium toxicity and increased intake of leafy green vegetables will counteract the anticoagulant effects of Coumadin and aspirin (Miller, 2008). Some drugs interfere with the body's ability to regulate temperature (e.g., antipsychotics, stimulants) such that hot weather can lead more easily to heat stroke (Semla et al, 2008). Other drugs are photosensitizing,

Table 14 -3 Examples of Drugs Considered Inappropriate for the Elderly

DRUG	CONCERN
Alprazolam (Xanex)	Rapid addiction, prolonged sedation effects, potential for confusion and falling. Long-acting benzodiazepine
Amitriptyline (Elavil)	Strong anticholinergic and sedating properties, little effect on depression. With low does, sometimes effective for neurogenic pain
Chlorpropamide (Diabinese)	Long lasting, danger of hypoglycemia increased in elderly
Cimetine (Tagamet)	Significant risk for ADR with many substances and medications
Cyclobenzaprine (Flexeril)	Anticholinergic side effects, sedation, weakness
Diazepam (Valium)	Long-acting benzodiazepines produce prolonged sedation, increasing fall risk and confusion risk (see alprazolam)
Diphenhydramine (Benedryl)	Excessive sedation, dry mouth, urinary retention, confusion
Dipyridamole (Persantine)	Orthostatic hypotension
Disopyramide (Norpace)	May induce heart failure, strongly anticholinergic
Doxepin (Sinequan)	Strong anticholinergic and sedating properties
Meperidine (Demerol)	Metabolite accumulation in elderly, can cause tremors and seizures
Oxybutynin (Ditropan)	Strongly anticholinergic, confusion
Propoxyphene and combinations containing propoxyphene (such as Darvocett)	No analgesic advantage over acetaminophen Side effects are similar to narcotics
Temazepam (Restoril)	Confusion, prolonged half-life

Adapted from multiple sources, all based on: Fick DM, Cooper JW, Wade WE, et al: Updating the Beers criteria for potentially inappropriate medication use in older adults: results of a US consensus panel of experts, *Arch Intern Med* 163(22):2716-2724, 2003. Updated list can be found at http://www.dcri.duke.edu/ccge/curtis/beers.html. Accessed 10/19/08.

and an increase in sun exposure can lead more quickly to sunburn than expected (e.g., sulfa drugs, antidepressants, and many antipsycotics) (Semla et al, 2008). Older adults who have decreased fluid intake because of illness or because they cannot get to fluids, or who have inadequate intake during hot weather, may quickly become volume depleted and develop increased sensitivity to the orthostatic hypotensive effects of alpha blockers (e.g., phenothiazines, terazosin) or even toxicity (Gulick and Jett, 2008).

One of the most troublesome ADRs for the older adult is drug-induced delirium and confusion. Polypharmacy with several psychoactive drugs exerting anticholinergic actions is perhaps the greatest precipitator of delirium as an adverse reaction. Too often delirium goes unrecognized as an ADR and instead is viewed as a worsening of preexisting dementia or even new-onset dementia (see Chapter 21). Any time there is a change in one's cognitive abilities, the possibility of drug effect must be thoroughly evaluated. See Box 14-1 for a partial list of drugs with the potential to adversely affect cognitive functioning.

Another common adverse effect seen in older adults is lethargy, especially with the use of a number of the cardiovascular agents and antidepressants. Like confusion, lethargy can also be misinterpreted as a symptom of the worsening of cardiac, respiratory, or neurological conditions rather than as an ADR.

Among other troublesome effects are those related to sexual functioning. Although they are not detailed here, many medications interfere with or contribute to sexual dysfunction for adults of any age. The categories that are most responsible are cardiovascular drugs (some antihypertensives and ACE inhibitors) and psychotropic drugs (antidepressants, phenothiazines).

Misuse of Drugs

The more drugs taken, the more likely misuse will occur. Forms of drug misuse include overuse, underuse, erratic use, and contraindicated use. Misuse can occur for any number of reasons, from inadequate skills of the nurse or the prescriber, to misunderstanding of instructions, or to inadequate funds to purchase prescribed medications. Although this is often referred to as noncompliance or nonadherence, "misuse" is a term that is more descriptive of what is happening. Despite the addition of Medicare D (see Chapter 22), a medication coverage program, financial concerns can still be significant when the "donut-hole" is reached, or that interval during which there is no coverage (Jett and Resnick, 2005). For older adults not eligible for coverage, such as recent immigrants, the cost of necessary medication may be prohibitive.

As early as 1994, Wilcox and others identified 20 drugs that were considered inappropriate for elders, including controversial cardiovascular agents (propranolol, methyldopa, reserpine). Since that time Fick and colleagues (2003) have worked further to develop the original Beers' (1997) list identifying drugs that carry higher-than-usual risk when used in older adults. The use of this list has been adopted by nursing home regulators, and the list has been used as a measure of quality. When one of the listed "inappropriate" medications is prescribed in the long term care setting the overwhelming benefit of its use must be documented by the prescriber. The Beers list has been recommended as a "best practice" by the Hartford Institute of Geriatric Nursing (Molony, 2003).

Misuse by patients may be accidental, such as happens through misunderstanding or inability to read labels or understand instructions, or it may be deliberate, such as in an attempt to make a prescription last longer for financial reasons or because of beliefs that the dose is either too low or too high. For a striking example of misunderstandings and cultural differences between prescribers and patients, the reader is referred to the book by Anne Fadiman (1998), *The Spirit Catches You and You Fall Down*.

When a patient is labeled as noncompliant, the nurse and other health care personnel may become exasperated

---

Box 14-1	Common Medications with the Potential to Cause Cognitive Impairment

Alcohol
Analgesics
Anticholinergics
Antidepressants
Antihistamines
Antiparkinsonian agents
Antipsychotics
Benzodiazepines
Beta blockers
Digitalis, Lanoxin
Diuretics
Muscle relaxants
Sedatives, hypnotics

and angry at the individual for his or her failure to follow the established plan of care. In an attempt to help and do what they think is best for the patient, the nurse and other care providers tend to forget or ignore that one cannot and will not comply with a prescription or treatment plan under certain circumstances, such as when it is incompatible with the person's day-to-day life. For example, the individual cannot follow the instruction "take medication 3 times per day with meals" if he or she eats only two meals each day.

Memory failures associated with nonadherence to medication regimens are of two general types: forgetting the way to take medications correctly and "prospective" recall failure, which is failure to remember to take medication at the correct times (Miller, 2008). The more frequently a medication must be taken, the less anyone will comply. With more and more medications coming in once-daily dosing rather than 3 or 4 times each day, we can expect more people to take their medications as instructed.

Problems with health literacy also limit the ability to correctly take medications (see Chapter 7). Many older adults, especially those from minority groups, have low levels of literacy; written instructions should be at the third-grade level or below (see www.clearcommunica-tion.com). Limitations in vision will interfere with the reading of instructions, especially of bottle labels. One can ask the pharmacist to use large type or symbols. The practice of nurses and doctors giving rapid-fire directions is not effective when addressing most persons, especially those with hearing impairments or the normal age-related need for slightly slower verbalizations; and the use of ambiguous terms such as "slowly increase" or "only in moderation" leads to further difficulties.

Unfortunately, it is also common for the nurse to explain the treatment and give directions concerning medications when the patient is physically uncomfortable or is about to be discharged from a care facility; to explain in English even when the person has limited English proficiency; or to explain in a noisy or busy place. Background noise can significantly reduce understandability of speech for those with normal age-related hearing loss (see Chapter 8).

The individual must first comprehend and be committed to the treatment. The care provider must be able to communicate the information in a way that compensates for language differences and physical-sensory and cognitive changes so that the person understands. The person also must accept the need for the medication as it is prescribed to be willing to follow the treatment plan. The elder must be able to use what has been learned to obtain the prescribed medication, apply instructions, and adjust to the regimen.

IMPLICATIONS FOR GERONTOLOGICAL NURSING AND HEALTHY AGING

Assessment

The initial step in ensuring that elders use drugs safely and effectively is to conduct a comprehensive drug assessment. Although in some settings a clinical pharmacist collects the medication history, more often it is completed through the combined efforts of the licensed or registered nurse and the prescribing health care provider (a physician or a nurse practitioner).

In the ideal situation, it is best to use a "brown bag approach," or to ask the person to bring in all medications and other products they are currently taking in a bag. As each container is removed from the bag, the person is asked how he or she actually takes the medicine rather than depending on how the prescription is written, to begin to determine possible misunderstandings or misuse. An alternative method is a 24-hour medication recall, such as "Tell me everything you have taken in the last 24 hours." Two final approaches are associated with the review of systems or problems. These questions will be something like, "What do you take for your heart? circulation? breathing?" Or, if you know the person's major health problems, you may say, for example, "What do you take for headaches?" or "What do you use for indigestion?" Without the bag of medications or a list of some kind, patients often answer some of the above questions with descriptions (e.g., "a little blue pill" or "a bad-tasting one"), but it is a start.

As the nurse learns the herbs, supplements, and OTC and prescribed medications that are taken, the assessment can continue. There is a great deal of information that is needed, but it is vital to promoting the health of the person and healthy aging. See Box 14-2 for examples of the information needed in a comprehensive medication history for all substances taken. Through this assessment the nurse can learn of discrepancies between the prescribed dosage and the actual dosage, potential drug-drug and food-drug interactions, and potential or actual ADRs.

Monitoring and Evaluation

A significant part of the gerontological nurse's responsibilities is to monitor and evaluate the effectiveness of prescribed treatments and observe for signs of problems

Box 14-2	Components of a Comprehensive Medication Assessment

Medications taken and prescribed, as described by patient, with names, doses, and frequency

Diagnosis associated with each medication

Belief regarding effectiveness and necessity of medications

Over-the-counter preparations, with doses, frequency, and reason taken

Herbals, with doses, frequency, and reason taken

Nutritional supplements, with doses, frequency, and reason taken

Medication-related problems, such as side effects, difficulty with adherence

Ability to pay and obtain prescription medications

Source of prescriptions

Persons involved in decision making regarding medications

Use of other drugs, such as tobacco or nicotine in gum, patch, or smoking

Use of social drugs, such as alcohol and caffeine, and nonprescription drugs

Drugs borrowed from others

Recently discontinued drugs

History of allergies, interactions, and adverse drug reactions

Strategies used to remember when to take drugs as prescribed

Identification of malnutrition and hydration status

Recent drug blood levels as appropriate

Recent measurement of liver and kidney functioning

(ADRs, etc.)—either from a change in condition or what are known as iatrogenic complications (problems that are the result of something we have done or given to the person). Monitoring and evaluating involve making astute observations and documenting those observations, noting changes in physical and functional status (e.g., vital signs, performance of activities of daily living, sleeping, eating, hydrating, eliminating) and mental status (e.g., attention and level of alertness, memory, orientation, behavior, mood, emotional display and affect, content and characteristics of interactions). Monitoring also means ensuring that blood levels are measured as they are needed; such as scheduled thyroid-stimulating hormone (TSH) levels for all persons taking thyroid replacement, international normalized ratios (INRs) for all persons taking warfarin, or periodic

hemoglobin A_{1c} levels for all persons with diabetes. Care of a patient also means that the nurses promptly communicate their findings of potential problems to the patient's nurse practitioner or physician. The reader is referred to a geriatric pharmacology reference text for more detailed and thorough information. This information may also be available from specialized clinical pharmacists.

Patient Education

Usually the nurse is responsible for educating patients about medication use. Ideally, the nurse empowers the person to participate fully in goal setting and treatment planning (Box 14-3). Education relating to safe medication use can be accomplished on an individual basis or in small groups. Elders should be encouraged to exercise the right to question and know what they are taking, how it will affect them, and the alternatives available to them as a part of their basic rights. Pamphlets and booklets written in lay terms and in appropriate language and reading level should be available. If there are none that are appropriate, the nurse can be creative and develop a booklet or information sheet that will meet the patient's needs. Information is best presented in a bulleted format rather than in paragraph form. Type should be large and boldface.

Because of the complex needs of the older patient, education can be particularly challenging. The following tips may be helpful when the goal of the nurse is to promote healthy aging:

1. *Key persons*: Find out who, if anyone, manages the person's medications, helps the person, or assists with decision making; when applicable and with the elder's permission, make sure that the helper is present when any teaching is done.

2. *Environment:* Minimize distraction, and avoid competing with television or others demanding the patient's attention; make sure the person is comfortable and is not hungry, thirsty, tired, too warm or too cold, in pain, or in need of the toilet.

3. *Timing:* Provide the teaching during the best time of the day for the person, when he or she is most alert, engaged, and energetic. Keep the education sessions short and succinct.

4. *Communication:* Ensure that you will be understood. Make sure the elders have their glasses or hearing aids on if they are used. Use simple and direct language, and avoid medical or nursing jargon (e.g., "intake"). Remain respectful at all times, and do not allow negative stereotypes to cloud communication.

Box 14-3	Empowering the Patient for Safe Medication Practices: What Elders Should Know about Taking Their Medications

- What is the name of each drug?
- What is the purpose of each drug?
- What is the dose per administration?
- What is the number of doses every day?
- What is the best time to take the medication?
- How should the medication be taken?
- Can the medication be taken with other drugs?
- Which medications can and cannot be taken together?
- Are any special techniques, devices, or procedures necessary to administer the medication?
- For how long should the medication be taken?
- What are the common side effects?
- If side effects occur: What should the elder do? What changes in administration are necessary? When should the drug be stopped? When should the physician or pharmacist (or both) be called?
- What can be done at home to monitor for a therapeutic drug response?
- What should be done if a dose is missed?
- How many refills are allowed?
- How should the medication be stored?
- What are the nonprescription preparations that should not be used with the present drug therapy?
- Take all medications prescribed unless the physician states otherwise.
- Stop taking the medication and report if any new or unusual problems occur, such as shortness of breath, nausea, diarrhea, vomiting, sleepiness, dizziness, weakness, skin rash, or fever.
- Never take medication prescribed for another person.
- Do not take any medication more than 1 year old or past the expiration date on the container.
- Store medications in a safe place, preferably the kitchen, rather than the bathroom, where moisture from bathing, especially showers, may affect the medicine.
- Do not keep medicines, especially sedatives and hypnotics, on the bedside stand, because when you are sleepy, you may forget that you have already taken the medication earlier.
- Do not place different medicines in the same container.
- Take a sufficient supply of all medicines in their individual containers when traveling away from home.
- Use a chart to keep track of medications.

Encourage questions. If the person is blind, Braille instructions may be available.

5. *Reinforce teaching:* Provide memory aids to reinforce teaching. Have actual medications or containers handy to visually illustrate directions. For persons who can read, use written charts and lists with large letters and simple language. For persons who cannot read, charts with pictures of the medications and symbols for times of the day or color coding can be used, such as a moon for evening use or a drawing of silverware for "with meals." If food is required with the medication or must be avoided, this should be indicated on the charts. Weekly calendars with pockets for medications indicating day, time, and date can be used; or a daily tear-off calendar to remind the elder to take daily medication can be used. Clear envelopes or sandwich bags contain-

ing the medication can be affixed to the dated square on a daily basis; each envelope or bag should state the name of the drug and dose and times it is to be taken that day. Commercial drug boxes are available for single or multiple doses by the day, week, or month, and some have alarms. Some pharmacies are equipped to fill prescriptions using such containers. After discharge from a hospital or nursing home, a follow-up phone call can help with assessing accurate medication usage or other problems with medications. A nurse's home visit to patients at high risk for problems, such as those with cognitive deficits or those with many medications for new conditions, reinforces medication information and provides assessment information.

6. *Evaluate teaching:* Have the patient repeat back instructions, including names of medications, purposes,

side effects, times of administration, and method for remembering to take the medicines and to mark off their ingestion.

7. *Avoiding drug interactions*: Patients should be taught to obtain all their medications from the same pharmacy if possible. This will allow the pharmacist to monitor for drug duplications and interactions. When elders have no prescription drug coverage, they may need to shop around for the best prices, and this does increase the risk for problems. Additional information about recognizing and responding to early signs of ADR may save lives.

Medication Administration

Most elders self-administer their own medications; others receive them from family, friends, or health care professionals. In nursing homes the administration of medications occupies nearly all of the "medication" nurses' time. In assisted living facilities, medication administration is an optional service and available only if permitted by local laws. Regardless of the setting or the persons involved, several skills are needed for safe administration.

Because of the high rate of arthritis and other debilitating conditions, it may be difficult or impossible for the person to remove a cap or break a tablet. If no children will have access to the medications, the patient can request alternative bottle caps that are easier to open. Either the person or the nurse can also ask the pharmacist to pre-break the pills or dispense a smaller dose. Pill cutters are commercially available but still call for fine motor dexterity to place the pill for cutting in the correct place.

Most medications are taken orally. Many tablets and capsules are difficult to swallow because of their size or because they stick to the tongue, especially if the mouth is dry. Administration of a drug in liquid form is sometimes preferable and allows for flexible dosing; concentrations can be varied so that quantities of solution can be prepared and taken by the teaspoon, tablespoon, or ounce, simple and commonly used household measurements. Since household spoons vary greatly in actual volume, the nurse should ensure that the elder is using an accurate measure. Crushing tablets or emptying the powder from capsules into fluid or food should not be done unless specified by the pharmaceutical company or approved by a pharmacist, because it may interfere with the effectiveness of the drug (causing either underdose or toxicity) or create problems in administration, as well as injure the mouth or gastrointestinal tract.

Some people have difficulty swallowing capsules. The person can be advised to place capsules on the front of the tongue and swallow a fluid; this should wash it to the back of the throat and down. Other persons do better with pills or capsules when taken with a semisolid food, such as applesauce, chocolate syrup, or peanut butter—as long as the substances do not interact.

Enteric-coated, extended-release, or sustained-released products are all used to allow absorption at different places in the gastrointestinal tract. These should never be crushed, broken, opened, or otherwise altered before administration. However, since the formulation of medications is rapidly changing, the reader is advised to contact a clinical pharmacist, consult a very current drug handbook or package inset (found in Physician's Desk References, or PDRs) for the changing list of "do-not-crush" products.

The transdermal patch, also called the transdermal delivery system (TDDS), is one of the newer approaches to medication administration, and more and more medications are being transformed to be administered by this route. The TDDS provides for a more constant rate of drug absorption and eliminates concern for gastrointestinal absorption variation, gastrointestinal tolerance, and drug interaction. TDDSs are not recommended for persons who are noticeably underweight because absorption is unpredictable owing to the reduced body fat. Box 14-4 provides guidelines for the use of TDDSs.

PSYCHOTROPIC MEDICATIONS

Psychotropic medications are those that alter brain chemistry, emotions, and behavior. They include antipsychotics (neuroleptics), antidepressants, mood stabilizers, antianxiety agents (*anxiolytics*), and sedative-hypnotics. This section of the chapter provides an overview of psychotropic medications used to treat symptoms that occur in disorders of behavior, cognition, arousal, and mood in the gerontological population. A section is devoted to treating the movement disorders that may occur as a side effect from the use of antipsychotics.

In 1987 the Health Care Finance Administration mandated that residents of long-term care settings may only be prescribed psychotropic drugs for specific diseases or symptoms and that the use be monitored, reduced, or eliminated when possible. Prescribing physicians and nurse practitioners may exceed the recommended doses only if documentation reasonably explains the rationale for the benefit of the higher dose in restoring function or preventing dangerous behavior

Box 14-4	Guidelines for Transdermal Delivery Systems

Administration
1. Confirm appropriate patient and order
2. Know the proper place for administration if specified
3. Remove previous patch
4. Prepare clean and smooth skin surface with similar lean-to-fat tissue ratio
5. Rotate locations of patches
6. Wear gloves and wash hands before and after contact with patch.
7. Open package taking care not to touch the active side of the patch
8. Never cut or alter patch as packaged
9. Press smooth patch firmly for 10 seconds for secure contact

Side Effects
1. Observe for rash at application site
2. Notify prescriber as soon as possible

Disposal
1. Using gloves, fold sticky edges together
2. Dispose in a closed garbage can to keep away from pets and children

(Omnibus Budget Reconciliation Act [OBRA], 1987). A patient should be prescribed a psychotropic medication only after thorough medical, psychological, and social assessments are done. These should be done quickly to enable the patient to receive the appropriate treatment as soon as possible. Pharmacological interventions should always be supplemented by nonpharmacological measures such as counseling. Nursing assessment before medication intervention contributes knowledge and baseline information that can optimize the patient's medical and psychological improvement. Issues to consider include the patient's medical status (and other medications that might interact with psychotropics), mental status, ability to carry out activities of daily living, and ability to participate in social activities and maintain satisfying relationships with others, as well as the potential for patient or caregiver compliance with any pharmacological or nonpharmacological recommendations.

The gerontological nurse, especially one working in a long-term care setting, is likely to care for older adults with psychiatric problems, especially depression, anxiety, and psychosis. The rate of depression for elderly persons living in the community is estimated at about 20%, increasing to about 50% for those living in long-term care settings (Pollock and Reynolds, 2000). Anxiety is also common and when treated with benzodiazepines increases the older person's risk for adverse effects and drug interactions. Unfortunately the use of psychotherapy is very limited, first because of the rarity of persons with a specialty training in gerontological psychiatry or counseling, and second because of the very low reimbursement rates established by Medicare.

Finally a small group of elders, especially those with neurological conditions or dementia, may develop psychosis at some time in their illnesses. Psychosis is also seen in delirium from an infection or from an ADR and in the few elders with schizophrenia or Lewy body dementia. Persons with psychoses are often treated with antipsychotics that call for special attention and skills from the gerontological nurse in cooperation with a psychiatrist or a psychiatric nurse practitioner specializing in geriatrics. (See Chapter 21.)

Antidepressants

Antidepressants, as the name implies, are drugs used to treat depression. In the past, the major drugs used were monoamine oxidase inhibitors (MAOIs) and tricyclic antidepressants (TCAs), especially amitriptyline (Elavil) and doxepin (Sinequan). These drugs required high doses to be effective and had a significant side effects and adverse effects such as dry mouth, constipation, sedation and urinary retention. Since the development of the newer drugs, such as selective serotonin reuptake inhibitors (SSRIs) and NSSRIs (nonselective serotonin reuptake inhibitors), MAOIs and TCAs are rarely seen for psychotropic use, nor should they be used for the treatment of depression in older adults.

The SSRIs (e.g., Zoloft, Prozac, Lexapro) and NSSRIs have been found to be highly effective, with minimal or manageable side effects, and are the drugs of choice for use in older adults. Most of these cause initial problems with nausea or a dry mouth. One side effect of the SSRIs that does not resolve with time, if experienced, is sexual dysfunction. The NSSRIs and other antidepressants, such as Effexor, Wellbutrin, and trazodone, are less likely to cause this problem and may be preferred by elders who are sexually active. Wellbutrin has also been found to reduce nicotine cravings, and the combined effect may be very helpful to some; it cannot be used for persons with a history of seizures. Most older adults are sensitive to these medications and may find significant relief from depression at low doses. Although it sometimes takes time to find the optimal dose, the nurse can help the elder monitor target symptoms and advocate for continued dose adjustments or changes until relief is obtained rather than the depression being simply reduced. (See Chapter 24.)

Antianxiety Agents

Drugs used to treat anxiety are referred to as anxiolytics or *antianxiety agents.* These agents include benzodiazepines, buspirone (BuSpar), and beta blockers. Antihistamines, especially diphenhydramine (Benadryl), are often used but not recommended owing to their anticholinergic effects. The decision to treat anxiety pharmacologically is based on the degree to which the anxiety interferes with the person's ability to function and subjective feelings of discomfort.

Although they are usually contraindicated, the most frequently used agents are benzodiazepines. Despite the fact that benzodiazepines have been available for almost 30 years, only minimal research has been done in the elderly (Madhusoodanan and Bogunovic, 2004). What we do know is that older adults metabolize these drugs slowly, so they persist in the blood stream for long periods and can easily reach toxic levels. Side effects include drowsiness, dizziness, ataxia, mild cognitive deficits, and memory impairment. Signs of toxicity include excessive sedation, unsteady gait, confusion, disorientation, cognitive impairment, memory impairment, agitation, and wandering. Because these symptoms resemble dementia, people can easily be misdiagnosed once they start taking benzodiazepines.

Benzodiazepines are highly addicting yet very popular because of their quick sedating effects for the highly anxious person. However, because of the problems noted above they should be avoided except in extreme cases. If necessary, lorazepam (Ativan) appears to be the least problematic, when prescribed in very low doses and for short periods. It has the shortest half-life of the benzodiazepines and no active metabolites.

Buspirone is a safer alternative. Although a side effect is dizziness, this is often dose-related and resolves with time. Buspirone is not addicting and has an additive effect to some of the SSRIs, so lower doses can be used. No effect is felt by the patient or observed by the nurse for 5 to 7 days, and the drug may be mistakenly discontinued because of its apparent lack of effect. Buspirone is best used for chronic anxiety and is not indicated for acute needs. (See Chapter 24.)

Antipsychotics (Neuroleptics)

The term "psychosis" covers a range of thinking and behavioral disorders that are based on responses of the ill person to a private reality—a reality that may be distressing and problematic for the patient and those around him or her. Characteristically, psychosis occurs in schizophrenia but can also occur in mania, depression, delirium, dementia, and paranoid states. Psychosis manifests itself as delusional thinking and hallucinations, both of which can cause extreme anxiety and bizarre behavior. Antipsychotics, formerly known as *major tranquilizers* and now known as *neuroleptics,* are drugs used to treat psychotic symptoms.

Unfortunately neuroleptics are often misused by caregivers and health care providers in an attempt to control troublesome behaviors, and too often they are used without a careful assessment of the underlying cause of the behavior. Inappropriate use of antipsychotic medications may mask a reversible cause for the psychosis, such as infection, dehydration, fever, electrolyte imbalance, an ADR, or a sudden change in the environment (Bullock and Saharan, 2002).

When used appropriately and cautiously in true psychosis, antipsychotics can provide a person with relief from what may be frightening and distressing symptoms. When used, drugs with the lowest side effects profile and at the lowest dose possible should be prescribed. In most states the prescribing and use of antipsychotics in long-term care settings is carefully monitored.

There are different classes and potencies of antipsychotics. Strong antipsychotics (high potency), such as haloperidol (Haldol), are less sedating but cause more extrapyramidal reactions. The elderly are susceptible to developing extrapyramidal reactions, particularly neuroleptic-induced parkinsonian symptoms. Weak antipsychotics (low potency), such as chlorpromazine (Thorazine), are sedating and cause orthostatic hypotension, thereby increasing the risk for falls. Anticholinergic effects also include dry mouth, constipation, urinary retention, hypotension, and confusion. Careful nursing observation is essential for monitoring side effects and drug interactions whenever any of these medications are given (see Chapter 24).

Persons who take neuroleptics cannot tolerate excess environmental heat due to their effects on the thermoregulatory section of the brain. Even mild elevations of core temperature can result in liver damage called *neuroleptic malignant syndrome.* The problem is more likely to occur during hot weather. The person taking neuroleptics must avoid or be protected from hyperthermia by ensuring a cool environment. Appropriate preventive interventions include adequate hydration, activity in a cool area away from direct sunlight, and use of a fan or sponge bath if overheating should occur. The patient may or may not communicate his or her discomfort from the heat, so assessment of body temperature is essential. Any circumstance resulting in dehydration greatly increases the risk of heatstroke with the morbidity and mortality increasing with age. Diuretics, coffee, alcohol, lithium, and uncontrolled diabetes decrease vascular volume, thereby decreasing the body's ability to sweat. Anticholinergics inhibit sweating and lead to further heat retention.

Movement Disorders

While neuroleptic malignant syndrome is not commonly seen, the most significant potential side effects of antipsychotics are movement disorders, also referred to as *extrapyramidal syndrome (EPS)* reactions. These include acute dystonia, akathisia, parkinsonian symptoms, and tardive dyskinesia.

Acute Dystonia. An acute dystonic reaction is an abnormal involuntary movement consisting of a slow and continuous muscular contraction or spasm. Involuntary muscular contractions of the mouth, jaw, face, and neck are common. The jaw may lock (trismus), the tongue may roll back and block the throat, the neck may arch backward (opisthotonos), or the eyes may close. In an oculogyric crisis, the eyes are fixed in one position. Often this creates a feeling of needing to look up constantly without the ability to make the eyes come down. Dystonias can be painful and frightening. An acute dystonic reaction may occur hours or days following antipsychotic medication administration, or after dosage increases, and may last minutes to hours.

Akathisia. Akathisia refers to the compulsion to be in motion and may occur at any time during therapy. Patients describe feeling restless, being unable to be still, having an unrelenting desire to move, and feeling "like crawling out of my skin." Often this symptom is mistaken for worsening psychosis instead of the ADR that it is. Pacing, aimless walking, fidgeting, shifting weight from one leg to the other, and marked restlessness are characteristic behaviors for a person experiencing akathisia.

Parkinsonian Symptoms. The use of neuroleptics may cause a collection of symptoms that mimic Parkinson's disease. A bilateral tremor (as opposed to a unilateral tremor in true Parkinson's), bradykinesia, and rigidity may be seen, which may progress to the inability to move. The patient may have an inflexible facial expression and appear bored and apathetic and be mistakenly diagnosed as depressed. More common with the higher-potency antipsychotics, parkinsonian symptoms may occur within weeks to months of the initiation of antipsychotic therapy.

Caregivers or others unfamiliar with these EPS reactions often become alarmed. Although frightening, acute dystonia is not usually dangerous and is quickly relieved by anticholinergic medication, such as benztropine (Cogentin), trihexyphenidyl (Artane), or diphenhydramine (Benadryl), providing relief within minutes if given intravenously, within 10 to 15 minutes if given intramuscularly, and within 30 minutes if given orally. These medications should be readily available to treat an EPS reaction for all persons taking antipsychotics. Although they are not recommended for use in the elderly, anticholinergics and amantadine (Symmetrel), a dopamine agonist, are sometimes prescribed to prevent dystonic reactions, but because of slow onset of action, they are not used for acute treatment.

Tardive Dyskinesia. When neuroleptics have been used continuously for at least 3 to 6 months, patients are at risk for the development of the irreversible movement disorder of *tardive dyskinesia (TD)*. Both low- and high-potency agents are implicated (Miller, 2008). Symptoms of TD usually appear first as wormlike movements of the tongue; other facial movements include grimacing, blinking, and frowning. Slow, maintained, involuntary twisting movements of limbs, trunk, neck, face, and eyes (involuntary eye closure) have been reported. There is no treatment that reverses the effect of TD; therefore it is essential that the nurse is attentive for early detection so that the health care provider can make prompt changes to the psychotropic regimen.

Response to treatment is the most important consideration when psychotropics are taken. Subjective patient comments about feelings and symptoms and objective observations about the patient's behavior are important data for evaluating the effectiveness of a drug. Several tools are available to help the nurse monitor the patient taking antipsychotics. The Abnormal Involuntary Movement Scale (AIMS), which was designed by the National Institute of Mental Health (NIMH, 1976), should be used before therapy and after initiation of therapy. Other tools used for research on and monitoring of movement disorders include the Barnes Rating Scale for Drug-Induced Akathisia (Barnes, 1989) and the Simpson-Angus Rating Scale for EPS (Simpson and Angus, 1970).

Mood Stabilizers

Mood stabilizers are the group of agents used for the treatment of bipolar disorders, which is seen as uncontrollable fluctuations in mood from one extreme to another which affect the person's day-to-day life. Symptoms of a severe manic phase many include confusion, paranoia, labile affect, pressured speech and flight of ideas, morbid or depressive content of thought, increased psychomotor activity resembling agitated depression, and altered orientation and attention span. However, instead many have periods of hypomania characterized by significantly increased energy and movement and somewhat diminished judgment. For the older adult in the long-term setting the symptoms of bipolar disorders are easily confused with others. For example wandering is common for persons with moderate dementia as is emotional liability.

The nurse who is caring for a patient with a bipolar disorder or who is taking a mood stabilizer should seek guidance from the person's psychiatrist regarding specific strategies to enhance the person's quality of life and which laboratory testing is required for monitoring. If the patient is taking lithium, this is especially important. Lithium interacts with other medications and certain foods and has a narrow therapeutic window. For example, a low-salt diet will elevate the lithium level, and a high-salt diet will decrease it. Likewise, thiazide diuretics and nonsteroidal antiinflammatory drugs (NSAIDs) will elevate the serum lithium level. Side effects include the following: confusion, disorientation, and memory loss; flattening of T waves on the electrocardiogram; polyuria and polydipsia; nausea, vomiting, and diarrhea; fine resting tremor; benign goiter; and ataxia.

IMPLICATIONS FOR GERONTOLOGICAL NURSING AND HEALTHY AGING

All the medications presented in this chapter have indications, side effects, interactions, and individual patient reactions. The nurse's advocacy role includes education for the patient and the family or the caregiver. Further, the nurse must determine whether side effects are minimal and tolerable or serious. Asking the patient produces subjective data; and observing the patient's interactions, behavior, mood, emotional responses, and daily habits provides objective data. From this compilation of data, patient problems can be delineated, nursing diagnoses developed, outcome criteria planned, and interventions initiated.

Medications occupy a central place in the lives of many older persons; cost, acceptability, interactions, unacceptable side effects, and the need to schedule medications appropriately all combine to create many difficulties. Although nurses, with the exception of advanced-practice nurses, do not prescribe medications, we believe that their having a basic understanding of issues specific to the safe administration and consumption of medications in the elderly will reduce the use of inappropriate medications and allow the nurse to observe more closely for adverse side effects and interactions. In the role of educator, the nurse might also increase adherence through personally and culturally appropriate instructions.

The gerontological nurse is a key person in ensuring that the medication use is appropriate, effective, and as safe as possible. The knowledgeable nurse is alert for potential drug interactions and for signs or symptoms of ADRs. The nurse promotes the actions necessary to prevent drugs from becoming toxic and to treat toxicity promptly should it occur. Nurses in the long-term care setting are responsible for monitoring the overall health of the residents, including being alert for the need for laboratory tests and other measures to ensure correct dosage of several medications (e.g., Coumadin, vancomycin, thyroxin). The nurse must give prompt attention to changes in physiological function that are either the result of the medication regimen or are affected by the regimen, such as potassium level to minimize the likelihood of adverse and toxic reactions. The nurse is often the person to initiate assessment of medication use, evaluate outcomes, and provide the teaching needed for safe drug use and self-administration. In most settings the nurse is also in a position to influence the timing of prescribed doses so residents might more easily benefit from the findings from the developing knowledge of chronopharmacology (Barry et al, 2007). In all settings, a vital nursing function is to educate patients and to ensure that they understand the purpose of, the side effects of, and the time to call the provider regarding their medications.

▶ KEY CONCEPTS

▶ As we age, the way our body responds to medications changes.

▶ Any medication has side effects. The therapeutic goal is to reduce the targeted symptoms without undesirable side effects.

▶ Drug-drug and drug-food incompatibilities are an increasing problem of which nurses must be aware.

▶ Polypharmacy is one of the most serious problems of elders today, and this is usually the first area to investigate when adverse physiological events occur.

▶ Drug misuse may be triggered by prescriber practices, individual self-medication, individual physiology, altered biodegradability, nutritional and fluid states, and inadequate assessment before prescribing.

▶ Nurses must consider the occurrence of a possible adverse medication effect immediately if a change in the person's condition is observed; including mental status changes in an individual who is normally alert and aware or increasing confused. Many drugs cause temporary cognitive impairment in older persons.

▶ Chronotherapy that uses biorhythms of the body for the most effective medication therapy has the potential to decrease dose, frequency, and cost of medication regimens and to improve adherence to drug therapy.

▶ The side effects of psychotropic medications vary significantly; thus these medications must be selected and prescribed for the older adult with care. This increases the nurse's responsibility in the administration and monitoring of these medications.

▶ The response of the elder to treatment with psychotropic medications should show reduced distress, clearer thinking, and more appropriate behavior.

▶ It is always expected that pharmacological approaches augment rather than replace nonpharmacological approaches.

▶ Older adults are particularly vulnerable to developing movement disorders (extrapyramidal symptoms, parkinsonism symptoms, akathisia, dystonias) with the use of antipsychotics.

▶ The Omnibus Budget Reconciliation Act (OBRA) restricts the use of psychotropic drugs in the long-term care setting unless they are truly needed for specific disorders and to maintain or improve function.

▶ Any time a behavior change is noted in a person, reversible causes must be sought and treated before medications are used.

▶ Dosages of medications must be carefully titrated for the individual, and the individual's responses must be accurately and consistently recorded.

ACTIVITIES AND DISCUSSION QUESTIONS

1. What are the age-related changes that occur in pharmacokinetics of the older adult?
2. What is meant by *chronotherapeutics,* and how applicable is it to elders? Explain your answer.
3. What are the drug use patterns of the elderly, and what can be done to correct or improve them?

4. Explain the role of the elder, the care provider, and the social network in medication adherence.
5. List a variety of measures that the nurse can suggest to assist older adults with their medication use and adherence to a medication regimen.
6. What are the most troublesome side effects of antipsychotic medications?
7. Mrs. J. is calling out repeatedly for a nurse; other patients are complaining, and you simply cannot be available for long periods to quiet her. Considering the setting and the OBRA guidelines, what would you do to manage the situation?

RESOURCES

Websites
www.nimh.nih.gov
The latest information on the use of psychotropic drugs

www.alzheimers.org
Information about drugs used for Alzheimer's disease

www.hartfordign.org
An excellent review of "Beers' Criteria for Potentially Inappropriate Medication Use in the Elderly" in their "Try This" section

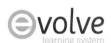

For additional resources, please visit evolve.elsevier.com/Ebersole/gerontological.

REFERENCES

Barry PJ, O'Keefe N, O'Connor K, O'Mahony D: Inappropriate prescribing in the elderly: a comparison of the Beers criteria and the improved prescribing in the elderly tool (IPET) in acutely ill elderly hospitalized patients, *J Clin Pharm Ther* 31(6):617-626, 2007.

Beers MH: Explicit criteria for determining potentially inappropriate medication use by the elderly: an update, *Arch Intern Med* 157(14):1531-1536, 1997.

Briggs GC: Geriatric issues. In Younkgin E, Sawin KJ, Kissinger J, Israel D, editors: *Pharmacotherapeutics: a primary care guide,* Upper Saddle River, NJ, 2005, Prentice-Hall.

Bruguerolle B: Clinical chronopharmacology in the elderly, *Chronobiol Int* 25(1):1-15, 2007.

Budnitz DS, Shehab N, Kegler SR, Richards CL: Medication use leading to emergency department visits for adverse drug events in older adults, *Ann Intern Med* 147(11): 755-765, 2007.

Bullock R, Saharan A: Atypical antipsychotics: experience and use in the elderly, *Int J Clinic Prac* 56(7):515-525, 2002.

Fadiman A: *The spirit catches you and you fall down,* New York, 1998, Farrar, Straus and Giroux.

Fick DM, Cooper JW, Wade WE et al: Updating the Beers criteria for potentially inappropriate medication use in older adults: results of a US consensus panel of experts, *Arch Intern Med* 163(22):2716-2724, 2003.

Gallagher PF, Barry PJ, Ryan C et al: Inappropriate prescribing in an acutely ill population of elderly patients as determined by Beers' criteria, *Age Aging* 37(1):96-101, 2007.

Green JL, Hawley JN, Rask KJ: Is the number of prescribing physicians an independent risk factor for adverse drug events in an elderly outpatient populations? *Am J Geriatr Pharmacother* 5(1):31-39, 2007.

Gulick G, Jett K: Geropharmacology. In Ebersole P et al, editors: *Toward healthy aging: human needs and nursing response*, ed 7, St. Louis, 2008, Mosby.

Jett K, Resnick B: *Medicare Part D Drug Benefit: tips for nurses.* Available at http://www.consultgerirn.org/advocacy/medicare_part_d_drug_benefit_tips_for_nurses/. Accessed 10/19/08

Junius-Walker U, Theile G, Hummers-Pradier E: Prevalence and predictors of polypharmacy among older primary care patients in Germany, *Fam Pract* 24(1):14-19, 2007.

Madhusoodanan S, Bogunovic OJ: Safety of benzodiazepine use in the geriatric population, *Expert Opin Drug Saf* 3(5):485-493, 2004.

Masoro EJ, Austed SN, editors: *Handbook of biology and aging,* ed 5, San Diego, 2003, Academic Press.

Miller CA: *Nursing for wellness in older adults,* ed 5, Philadelphia, 2008, Wolters Kluwer Health.

Molony SL: Beers' criteria for potentially inappropriate medication use in the elderly, *J Geront Nurs* 29(11):6-7, 2003.

National Institute of Mental Health (NIMH), Psychopharmacology Research Branch: Abnormal involuntary movement scale. In Guy W, editor: *ECDEU assessment manual for psychopharmacology,* revised, Rockville, MD, 1976, The Institute.

Omnibus Budget Reconciliation Act (OBRA) of 1987, Washington, DC, 1987, US Government Printing Office. House of Representatives, 100th Congress, 1st Session, Report 100-391.

Page PL 2nd, Ruscin JM: The risk of adverse drug events and hospital-related morbidity and mortality among older adults with potentially inappropriate medication use, *Am J Geriatr Pharmacother* 3(3):205-210, 2006.

Passarelli MC, Jacob-Filho W, Figueras A: Adverse drug reactions in an elderly hospitalized population: inappropriate prescription is a leading cause, *Drugs Aging* 22(9):767-777, 2005.

Perri M 3rd, Menon AM, Deshpande AD et al: Adverse outcomes associated with inappropriate drug use in nursing homes, *Ann Pharmacother* 39(3):405-411, 2005.

Pollock G, Reynolds CF III: Depression in late life. *Harvard Mental Health Letter, Harvard Health Online* 2000. Accessed December 11, 2008 from www.health.harvard.edu/medline/Mental/M0900b.html.

Semla TP, Beizer JL, Higbee MD: *Geriatric dosage handbook,* ed 8, Cleveland, 2008, Lexi-Comp, Inc.

Spiers MV, Kutzik DM: A multidimensional framework for understanding medication adherence in the elderly: a prescription for rethinking, Unpublished paper, 1995.

Steinman MA, Landefeld CS, Rosenthal GE et al: Polypharmacy and prescribing quality in older people, *J Am Geriatr Soc* 54(10):1516-1523, 2006.

Wilcox SM, Himmelstein DU, Woolhandler S: Inappropriate drug prescribing for the community dwelling elderly, *JAMA* 272(4):292-296, 1994.

Youngkin E: The use of herbs and supplements in late life. In Ebersole P, Hess P, Touhy T et al, editors: *Toward healthy aging: human needs and nursing response*, ed 7, St. Louis, 2008, Mosby.

Living with Chronic Illness

LEARNING OBJECTIVES

Upon completion of this chapter, the reader will be able to:

- Define chronic illness and explain the differences between chronic illness and acute illness.
- Explain the concept of wellness in chronic illness.
- Discuss explanatory models of chronic illness.
- Discuss the factors that influence the experience of chronic illness.
- Relate strategies that have been used successfully to maintain maximal function and increase an individual's ability for self-care.
- Discuss nursing interventions to maximize wellness in the presence of chronic illness.

GLOSSARY

Trajectory The path followed by a body or an event moved along by the action of certain forces.
Exacerbation A worsening. In medicine, exacerbation may refer to an increase in the severity of a disease or its signs and symptoms.

Exorbitant Exceeding that which is usual or proper.

THE LIVED EXPERIENCE

"Because you understand my disease, you don't understand me. To understand that I am ill does not mean that you understand how I experience my illness. I am unique. I think and feel and behave in a combination that is unique to me. You do not understand me because you have a label for my disease or a plan for my treatment. It is not my disease or treatment that you need to understand. It is me. This could happen to you. . . . You are just a diagnosis away from being a patient."

(Jevne, 1993, p. 121)

CHRONIC ILLNESS

Scope of the Problem

The rising prevalence and associated costs of chronic illness is a global health concern. Chronic illness accounts for over half the global health burden (World Health Organization, 2005). By 2020, estimates are that chronic illness will account for nearly 80% of worldwide disease. In the United States, an estimated 133 million Americans experience at least one chronic illness, and by 2030, this number is expected to reach 170 million (American Hospital Association, 2007; Astin and Closs, 2007).

Three out of four U.S. health care dollars are spent to care for individuals with chronic illnesses, and costs are expected to increase from $125 million annually in 2000 to $171 million in 2030 (Partnerships for Solutions, 2001; American Hospital Association 2007). Chronic illnesses also exact significant personal costs and burden due to diminished quality of life for both the individual and his or her family and significant others.

This chapter discusses chronic illness and the implications for gerontological nursing and healthy aging. Information on specific chronic illnesses and associated symptoms can be found in Chapters 16, 17, 18, 19, 20, and 21.

Definition of Chronic Illness

Chronic illnesses are "conditions that last a year or more and require ongoing medical attention and/or limit activities of daily living (Hwang et al, 2001, p. 268). From a nursing perspective, "chronic illness is the irreversible presence, accumulation, or latency or disease states or impairments that involve the total human environment for supportive care and self-care, maintenance of function and prevention of further disability" (Curtin and Lubkin, 1995, pp. 6-7).

Chronic Illness and Aging

Many factors influence the rapid rise in the number of individuals with chronic illnesses including the aging of the population, advances in medical sciences in extending the life span and in treating illness, and a rise in some chronic conditions such as asthma and diabetes in younger people (Partnerships for Solutions, 2001). Life expectancy for Americans was 47 years in 1900. Life expectancy at birth hit a new record high in 2006 of 78.1 years. Record high life expectancy was recorded in that year for both white and black males (76 years and 70 years, respectively) as well as for white and black females (81 years and 76.9 years) (Centers for Disease Control and Prevention [CDC] National Center for Health Statistics Office, 2008a).

At this time, a longer life often means living longer with a chronic illness, especially for the longer-lived women. Illnesses such as human immunodeficiency virus (HIV)/acquired immunodeficiency syndrome (AIDS), cancer, and Alzheimer's are becoming chronic illnesses to live with for extended periods. Much remains to be learned about the distribution, the risk factors, and effective measures to prevent or delay the onset of chronic conditions.

Chronic illnesses are common among older adults. About 88% of older adults have at least one chronic illness, and 50% have at least two (Zauszniewski et al, 2007). By the time a person has lived 50 years, he or she is likely to have at least one chronic condition. It may be slight arthritis at the site of an old football injury, hypertension, diabetes mellitus, obesity, or any one of a number of illnesses. The most common chronic condition for all ages is sinusitis, whereas for persons older than 65 years, the most common chronic conditions are arthritis and hypertension (Figure 15-1). Chronic illnesses in older people can be categorized as follows:

1. Nonfatal chronic illness—conditions such as osteoarthritis or hearing or vision problems. These contribute to disability and increased health care costs, but most individuals can live with them for many years

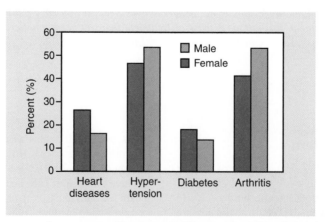

Fig. 15-1   Percentage of persons ages 65 years and older reporting selected chronic conditions, by sex, United States, 2002-2003. *(Data from National Health Interview Survey. Redrawn from the Data Warehouse on Trends in Health and Aging. Accessed 7/1/06 from www.cdc.gov/nchs/agingact.htm.)*

2. Serious, eventually fatal chronic conditions— cancers, organ system failures, dementia, strokes
3. Frailty—a condition in which the body has little reserves left and any disturbance can cause multiple health conditions and costs (Larsen, 2006). Frailty is discussed later in the chapter.

For the older adult, the presence or absence of a chronic illness is not as important as its effect on one's functioning. The effect may be as little as an inconvenience or as great as an impairment of one's ability to perform activities of daily living (ADLs), or instrumental activities of daily living (IADLs) (Figure 15-2). Limitations in ability to perform ADLs and IADLs occur more frequently among individuals over the age of 75, but recent trends show that the disability rate among older adults has declined and the incidence of chronic disability has dropped dramatically. However, the health disparities that exist for many minority populations and the obesity epidemic have the potential to reduce these gains (CDC, 2007) (see Chapter 4).

Prevention

Research has shown that chronic illness and poor health are not inevitable consequences of aging. Many chronic illnesses are preventable through lifestyle choices or early detection and management of risk factors. Many also can be managed with medical treatment and/or improved diet and exercise. Health promotion activities and attention to healthy lifestyle habits can postpone and reduce morbidity for older people. The term *compressed morbidity,* discussed by Fries (1989), refers to the postponement of illness and disability caused by chronic illness and is a key public health goal (Morley and Flaherty, 2002). Key strategies for improving the health of older people are presented in Box 15-1.

Eliminating three risk factors—poor diet, inactivity, and smoking—would prevent 80% of heart disease and stroke, 80% of type 2 diabetes, and 40% of cancer (American Hospital Association, 2007). Public health efforts have traditionally focused on physical health, but health and well-being includes physical and mental health. The promotion of cognitive health is an emerging public health priority and an essential feature of health-related quality of life (CDC, 2007) (see Chapter 21).

Public health efforts can help individuals avoid preventable illness and disability as they age. The nation's goals, as published in *Healthy People 2010,* are to increase the span of healthy life for all persons and to decrease disparities in health outcomes among population subgroups (U.S. Department of Health and Human

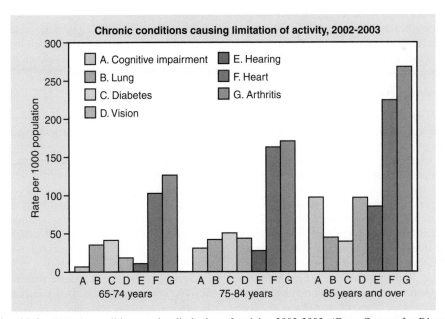

Fig. 15-2   Chronic condition causing limitation of activity, 2002-2003. *(From Centers for Disease Control and Prevention, National Center for Health Statistics,* Health, *United States, 2005, Figure 20. Redrawn from www.cdc.gov.)*

Box 15-1	Key Strategies for Improving the Health of Older People

1. Healthy lifestyle behaviors
2. Injury prevention
3. Delivery of culturally appropriate clinical preventive services
4. Immunization and preventive screenings
5. Self-management techniques for those with chronic illnesses

Modified from U.S. Department of Health and Human Services (USDHHS), Centers for Disease Control and Prevention (CDC), *Healthy aging: preventing disease and improving quality of life among older Americans,* Washington, DC, 2006, U.S. Government Printing Office; Lang J, Moore M, Harris A, Anderson L: Healthy aging: priorities and programs of the Centers for Disease Control and Prevention, *Generations* 29(2):24-29, 2005.

Services [USDHHS], 2000). It is expected that these goals will or can be achieved through improved strategies to effectively treat health problems and through the increased use of preventive health strategies for all persons, regardless of age, ethnicity, and income.

As a result of these efforts, we have the potential to live longer and perhaps in better health than our parents. A focus on healthy aging requires the nurse to implement health promotion and disease prevention activities in the care of people of all ages.

Acute Versus Chronic Illness

Chronic disorders and acute illness cannot really be separated, because so many conditions are intricately intertwined; acute disorders have chronic sequelae, and many of the commonly identified chronic disorders tend to intermittently flare up into acute problems and then to go into remission.

Acute illnesses are those that occur suddenly and often without warning (e.g., stroke, myocardial infarction, hip fracture, or infection) and with signs and symptoms related to the disease process itself. These are usually treated aggressively when they occur and end in a relatively short time. Without treatment, or even with treatment, acute problems in late life can quickly become the cause of death. At other times, the sequelae of the acute episode is a new or exacerbated chronic condition.

A chronic illness continues indefinitely, is managed rather than cured, and necessitates that the individual

"learn to live with it" (Lundman and Jansson, 2007, p. 109). By definition, it is always present although not always visible. If not triggered by an acute event, the onset may be insidious and identified only during a health screening. Symptoms of the effects of the illness, including disabilities, may not appear for years. For example, the person with hypertension develops enough heart damage to cause an acute episode of heart failure.

The person with a chronic illness may have episodic exacerbations or remain in remission with no symptoms for a long time (Larsen, 2006). People with chronic illnesses often continue to work and perform their usual activities early in their diseases. Later, and with increasing age, the effects of the limitations increase. Many elders have several chronic disorders simultaneously (comorbidities) and have great difficulty managing the complexity of the overlapping and often contradictory demands. The term comorbidity refers to the presence of coexisting conditions in an individual (Larsen, 2006).

Symptoms of chronic illness interfere with many normal activities and routines, make medical regimens necessary, disrupt patterns of living, and frequently make it necessary for the individual to make significant lifestyle changes. Physical suffering, loss, worry, grief, depression, functional impairment, and increased dependence on family or friends for support are among the negative consequences of chronic illnesses (Warshaw, 2006; Lundman and Jansson, 2007). One of the greatest fears of older people is being dependent on others as a result of chronic illness (Zauszniewski et al, 2007).

Frailty Syndrome

Frailty is an independent geriatric syndrome that may be seen in older people with multiple comorbidities. Frailty is "a stage of age-related physiologic vulnerability, resulting from impaired homeostatic reserve and a reduced capacity of the organism to withstand stress" (Fried et al, 2001, p. M146). Frailty includes both physical and mental decline and leads to an increased risk for morbidity and mortality (Hartford Institute for Geriatric Nursing, 2008). Frailty has also been linked to acute illness, falls, and institutionalization (Espinoza and Walston, 2005).

Seven percent of older people are classified as frail; however, the prevalence of frailty increases up to 40% in persons aged 80 years and over. With the dramatic increase in the oldest-old population, frailty is becoming increasingly common (Fried et al, 2004). Being female or African American and having less education and lower income are also associated with frailty (Young, 2003).

Factors responsible for the pathogenesis of frailty include sarcopenia and related metabolic pathogenic factors, atherosclerosis, cognitive impairment, and malnutrition (Morley et al, 2002). Weight loss, fatigue, muscle weakness, slow or unsteady gait, and declines in activity are signs and symptoms of frailty (Hartford Institute for Geriatric Nursing, 2008).

Frailty often goes unnoticed and the symptoms attributed to the aging process. The identification of frailty in its early stage is important because interventions may prevent functional decline and other negative consequences. Interventions are aimed at maintaining homeostatic balance. Resistance and balance exercises, aggressive nutritional support, treatment of depression, delirium, diabetes, osteoporosis, and hypertension, appropriate social support, aggressive treatment of pain, and treatment of early cognitive impairment may improve outcomes for the frail older person.

Care Delivery System

The current health care system, with its focus on immediate medical needs such as accidents, severe injury, and sudden bouts of illness, does not meet the needs of individuals with chronic illness, nor does it support health promotion and disease prevention (Partnerships for Solutions, 2001). "We have a 'sick' care system rather than a 'healthy' care system" (American Hospital Association, 2007).

"The health care system is based on a component style of care in which each component of the system is reimbursed independently, i.e., hospital visit, home care, skilled nursing facility care. Each component of the system views the client from its narrow window of care. No one entity, practice, institution, or agency is managing the entire disease, and certainly not managing the illness experience of the client and family. No one is responsible for the overall care of the individual, just their own independent component, and with that approach higher costs may occur" (Larsen, 2006, p. 4).

Health insurance coverage for preventive health care services and rehabilitation, long-term, and home care needed by individuals with chronic illnesses is often limited. A growing concern is the number of adults in the United States who are uninsured. Adults without health insurance are more than twice as likely to visit the emergency department or be hospitalized for a chronic condition as those with insurance

(American Hospital Association, 2007). Whereas Medicare covers the cost of some preventive services, coverage for long-term care focuses primarily on recovery from the acute phase of an illness. Chapters 22 and 26 discuss health care costs and funding for older people as well as transitions in care across the continuum.

Health care providers also lack training, education, and skills to care for the growing numbers of people with chronic illnesses. Most education programs for health care workers focus on episodic care in acute care settings (Astin and Closs, 2007). The World Health Organization (2005) report *Preparing a healthcare workforce for the 21st century: The challenge of chronic conditions* presents a training model and competencies in the care of individuals with chronic illness for all health care workers (Box 15-2).

Wellness in Chronic Illness

High-level wellness is an integrated method of functioning that maximizes the individual's unique potential (Dunn, 1972). Physical manifestations of chronic illness are often multiple and serious but need not kill the spirit or define the person. The wellness approach suggests that every person has an optimal level of functioning to achieve a good and satisfactory existence (well-being). Even in chronic illness and dying, an optimum level of wellness and well-being is attainable for each individual.

The wellness continuum picks up where the traditional medical model leaves off. Instead of a downward negative trajectory for the health of the older adult, focused on deterioration, the wellness model rises and moves in a positive direction. The individual may reach plateaus in his or her ascension to a higher-level wellness. The person may also regress because of an illness event, but the event can be a stimulus for growth and a return to moving up the wellness continuum (Chapter 1). Wellness is not given to a person; rather, it is a state of being and feeling that one strives to achieve through motivation and health practices. An individual must work hard to achieve wellness, just as he or she must work hard to perform competently at a job.

The greatest factor in establishing wellness is adaptation. To achieve maximization of life satisfaction, adaptation of lifestyle is necessary. What is wellness in the face of chronic illness? Results of a qualitative study (Hodges et al, 2001) using art to explore the perceptions of nurses, students, and the elderly about living with a chronic

Box 15-2	Competencies to Improve Care for Chronic Conditions

1. Patient-Centered Care
- Interviewing and communicating effectively
- Assisting changes in health-related behaviors
- Supporting self-management
- Using a proactive approach

2. Partnering
- Partnering with patients
- Partnering with other providers
- Partnering with communities

3. Quality Improvement
- Measuring care delivery and outcomes
- Learning and adapting to change
- Translating evidence into practice

4. Information and Communication Technology
- Designing and using patient registries
- Electronic patient records
- Using computer technologies
- Communicating with partners

5. Public Health Perspective
- Providing population-based care
- Systems thinking
- Working across the care continuum
- Working in primary health care–led systems

Data from: World Health Organization: *Preparing a health care workforce for the 21st century: the challenge of chronic conditions,* World Health Organization, 2005. Accessed 6/19/08 from www.who. int/chp/knowledge/publications/workforce_report.pdf.

illness offer insight. Whereas nurses and students viewed chronic illness negatively, the elderly talked about the importance of hope, a steadfast refusal to give up, and a commitment to going forward in spite of limitations. As one 70-year-old woman stated, "If you stop, you're done" (p. 394). Building on the courage of older adults coping with chronic illnesses, disabilities, and other losses is a good starting point for gerontological nurses.

THEORETICAL FRAMEWORKS FOR CHRONIC ILLNESS

Several theoretical frameworks have been used to understand the effect of chronic illness and organizing the nurse's response to calls from persons with chronic illness: Maslow's Hierarchy of Needs, the Chronic Illness Trajectory (Strauss and Glaser, 1975; Corbin and Strauss, 1988; Woog, 1992), and the Shifting Perspectives Model (Paterson, 2001).

Maslow's Hierarchy of Needs

Maslow's Hierarchy of Needs ranks needs from the most basic, namely those related to the maintenance of biological integrity, to the most complex, or those associated with self-actualization. According to this theory, the higher-level needs cannot be met without first meeting the lower-level needs. In other words, moving toward healthy aging is an evolving and developing process. A wellness approach centers on assisting older people to meet as many of Maslow's defined needs as possible (Figure 15-3). As basic-level needs are met, the satisfaction of higher-level needs is possible, with ever-deepening richness to life regardless of one's age or illnesses. The nurse prioritizes care from the most essential basic needs to those things we think of as associated with quality of life. Ensuring that the needs are met at any of the levels is significantly more complex for a person with a chronic condition.

As people's basic needs are met, they will feel safe and secure. They will likely sleep better and feel more comfortable interacting with others. While interacting with others, people begin to meet their need of belonging. The nurse works to create environments in which meaningful relationships and activities can remain a part of the elder's life in the presence of a chronic health problem. A person whose basic needs are met, who feels safe and secure, and who has a sense of belonging will also have self-esteem and self-efficacy. In other words, people will accept and honor who they are and feel that they have some personal power and self-confidence; they will know that they are important as people and that they inherently have value.

Finally, Maslow's highest level of wellness is that of self-actualization. Self-actualization is seen as people reaching out beyond themselves and finding meaning in their lives, a sense of fulfillment. This sense of self and meaning if often challenged with the diagnosis of a chronic illness, and as a disability develops or progresses, the sense of self may be doubted. The sensitive gerontological nurse is in the perfect position to help older adults to adapt to the changes in their lives and perhaps find new joys and new meaning. Figure 15-4 depicts a diabetes wellness perspective using Maslow's Hierarchy of Needs.

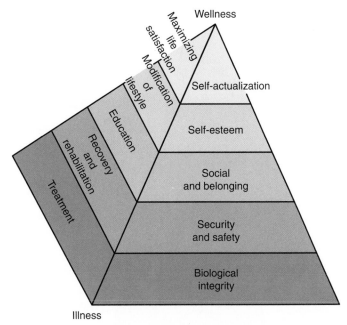

Fig. 15-3 Correlation between illness-wellness continuum and Maslow's hierarchy of needs. *(Developed by Patricia Hess.)*

Chronic Illness Trajectory

The trajectory model of chronic illness, originally conceptualized by Anselm Strauss and Barney Glaser (1975), has long aided health care providers to better understand the realities of chronic illness. Later, Corbin and Strauss (1988) presented a view of chronic illness as a trajectory that traces a course of illness forward through eight phases. In its entirety, a chronic illness may include a preventive phase (pretrajectory), a definitive phase (trajectory onset), a crisis phase, an acute phase, a stable phase, an unstable phase, and a downward and a dying phase (Table 15-1). The shape and stability of the trajectory is influenced by the combined efforts, attitudes, and beliefs held by the elder, family members and significant others, and the involved health care providers. Key points of the model are based on the theoretical assumptions listed in Box 15-3.

The patient's perceptions of needs met and basic biological functional limitations are paramount to predicting movement along the illness trajectory (Corbin and Strauss, 1992). Maslow's concept of five major levels of needs that affect function and self-perception fits well with the Corbin-Strauss model. In this respect,

our wellness approach largely hinges on assisting the elder in meeting as many of Maslow's defined needs as possible at any given time. These efforts enhance the individual's potential for remaining on a plateau or gaining ground in any of the trajectory phases.

The Shifting Perspectives Model of Chronic Illness

The chronic illness trajectory model described above views living with a chronic illness as a progression of phases in which the person follows a predictable trajectory. The Shifting Perspectives Model (Paterson, 2001), derived from a synthesis of qualitative research findings, views living with chronic illness as an ongoing, continually shifting process in which the person moves between the perspectives of wellness in the foreground or illness in the foreground.

This model is more reflective of an "insider" perspective on chronic illness as opposed to the more traditional "outsider" view. Further, this model provides a change in perspective from the traditional approach of patient-as-client to one of client-as-partner in care, and focuses on health within illness rather than loss and burden (Larsen at el, 2006, p. 40). People's

Potential Problems

Unattainable without resolution
   of lower level needs

Intimacy compromised
   by condition, medications,
   or emotions;
   may see self as different,
   not normal like others

Lifestyle or pattern changes;
   participation limited, diet
   restricted, socialization
   influenced

Infection prone; possible
   hypoglycemic reactions,
   ketoacidosis, diminished
   sensations (neuropathy)

Physiological disruption of
   metabolism (specifically
   glucose); increased risk of
   cardiovascular, renal, and
   neurological sensory problems

Needs

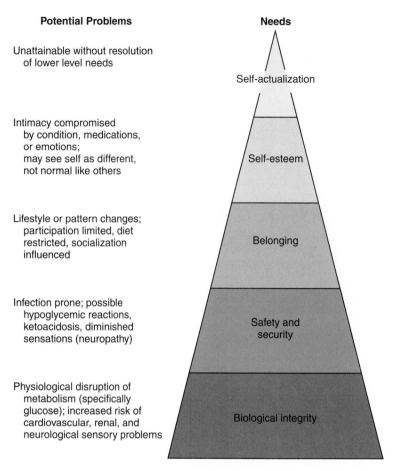

Self-actualization

Self-esteem

Belonging

Safety and
security

Biological integrity

Strategies to Meet Needs

Growth continued within
   the individual's perspective

Emphasis on the abilities, not the
   limitations; open discussion on
   sexuality and sex; explanation
   of approaches to sexual
   gratifications in light of drug,
   physical, and emotional
   influences

Education about normalcy in
   social situations such as dining
   out, social drinking, diet
   planning, and food choices;
   discussion and illustration
   about positive lifestyle pattern
   adjustments

Rehabilitation and recovery:
   teach necessary skills, activities,
   knowledge needed to feel safe
   and secure—skin care, use of
   syringe, actions to take with
   signs and symptoms, ways to
   independently or with
   appropriate help accomplish
   necessary tasks

Treatment provided with
   methods to control and
   monitor physiological state and
   meet needs—insulin or oral
   antihyperglycemic agents,
   urine testing, adequate
   balanced nutrition, exercise, etc.

Fig. 15-4   Diabetes wellness perspective.

perspective of the chronic illness is neither right nor wrong but is a reflection of their needs and situation. How people perceive the chronic illness at any given time influences how they interpret and respond to the disease, themselves, caregivers, and situations affected by the illness (Paterson, 2001; Lindqvist et al, 2006).

Chronic illness contains elements of both illness and wellness, and people with chronic illness live in the "dual kingdoms of the well and the sick" (Donnelly, 1993, p. 6). The illness in the foreground perspective is characterized by a focus on sickness and the suffering, loss, and burden the illness causes. The illness in the foreground perspective occurs when people are newly diagnosed, when new disease-related symptoms appear, or during an acute phase of the illness. This perspective has a protective function, may assist in conserving energy, and helps a person learn more about the illness and try to adjust and come to terms with it (Paterson, 2001).

Shifts toward the illness in the foreground perspective occur when there are perceived threats to control (signs of disease progression, lack of skills to manage the symptoms, disease-related stigma, interactions with others that emphasize dependence and hopelessness). Return to the wellness perspective calls for courage and resilience as well as the development of strategies and resources to adjust to the changes. Nurses can assist by understanding the person's perspective and providing education and support. The shift from illness to wellness is an active process triggered by the need to return to the wellness perspective.

In the wellness in the foreground perspective, the focus is centered more on the self than the disease and its consequences. The illness becomes part of who a person is but it does not define the person. The illness is seen as an opportunity for growth and meaningful changes in relationships with the environment and

Table 15-1   The Chronic Illness Trajectory: Definitions of Phases and Goals

PHASE	DEFINITION
1. Pretrajectory	Before the illness course begins, the preventive phase, no signs or symptoms present
2. Trajectory onset	Signs and symptoms are present, includes diagnostic period
3. Crisis	Life-threatening situation
4. Acute	Active illness or complications that require hospitalization for management
5. Stable	Illness course—symptoms controlled by regimen
6. Unstable	Illness course—symptoms not controlled by regimen but not requiring hospitalization
7. Downward	Progressive deterioration in physical and/or mental status characterized by increasing disability and/or symptoms
8. Dying	Immediate weeks, days, hours preceding death

Examples of goals that nurses might establish include the following:

1. To assist the client in overcoming a plateau during a comeback phase by increasing adherence to a regimen so that he or she might reach the highest level of functional ability possible within limits of the disability
2. To assist a client in making the attitudinal and lifestyle changes needed to promote health and prevent disease
3. To assist a client who is in a downward trajectory make the adjustments and readjustments in biography and everyday life activities that are necessary to adapt to increasing physical deterioration
4. To assist the client who is in an unstable phase to gain greater control over symptoms that are interfering with his or her ability to carry out everyday activities
5. To assist a client in maintaining illness stability by finding a way to blend illness management activities with biographical and everyday life activities

Goals can be broken down into specific client-oriented objectives. Built into the objectives are the criteria that will be used to evaluate the effectiveness of each intervention. What is important here is to look at what takes place in the process (the steps) of working toward a goal, as well as the end to be reached, and to be realistic about what can be achieved in what time period, taking into consideration the desires, wants, and abilities of the client and the family.

From Woog P: *Chronic illness trajectory framework: the Corbin and Strauss nursing model,* New York, 1992, Springer.

others. This perspective is fostered by learning as much as possible about the illness, creating supportive environments, paying attention to one's own patterns of response to the illness, and sharing one's knowledge of the disease with others.

With this perspective, one is able to focus on the emotional, spiritual, and social aspects of life while still attending to disease management and the effects of the illness on one's life. Results of a study of men with advanced prostate cancer suggested that having the wellness perspective in the foreground was a desirable state, and the men were reluctant to describe themselves as ill (Lindqvist et al, 2006). Health care professionals who see the person with chronic illness as sick, focusing only on the disease and its symptoms, may not provide opportunities or support for wellness.

Paterson (2001) suggests that the shifting perspectives model calls for understanding the person's perspective and the reasons the person varies in his or her attention to symptoms; the nurse must support persons with either perspective. This model may be compared to working toward self-actualization in Maslow's hierarchy while also meeting the lower level basic needs. The person shifts between a wellness and an illness perspective depending on the moment and the needs and demands of living with a chronic illness. At any point in time, one may take precedence over the other, but the goal is to move toward the highest level of well-being even in the presence of illness.

IMPLICATIONS FOR GERONTOLOGICAL NURSING AND HEALTHY AGING

Chronic illnesses are illnesses to live with, and nursing's response is one of long-term caring. The focus of treatment for chronic illness is seldom on cure, but rather on care for the person. This kind of nursing requires a different focus from acute care nursing, where the emphasis is on attention to immediate and life-threatening needs and attempts to cure. "Chronic health problems are not fixable with shiny new technology, and do not promise the suspense, exhilarating hope, and

Box 15-3	Key Points in the Chronic Illness Trajectory Framework

- The majority of health problems in late life are chronic.
- Chronic illnesses may be lifelong and entail lifetime adaptations.
- Chronic illness and its management often profoundly affect the lives and identities of both the individual and the family members or significant others.
- The acute phase of illness management is designed to stabilize physiological processes and promote a recovery (comeback) from the acute phase.
- Other phases of management are designed primarily to maximize and extend the period of stability in the home, with the help of family and augmented by visits to and from health care providers and other members of the rehabilitation and restoration team.
- Maintaining stable phases is central in the work of managing chronic illness.
- A primary care nurse is often in the role of coordinator of the multiple resources that may be needed to promote quality of life along the trajectory.

dramatic ending that acute medical crises often do. They simply continue day after day, often invisible or misunderstood" (Hodges et al, 2001, p. 390).

Assessment

Assessment of the elder with a chronic illness involves the selection of appropriate tools, ongoing evaluation of responses and outcomes, careful observation, periodic monitoring, alert watchfulness, and most importantly, discussion and collaboration with elders about their perceptions and the meaning their illness has for them. In the case of chronic illness and the great variability in presentation and impact on individual lifestyle, adequate assessment is critical. In chronic illness, assessment focuses on function and how the chronic illness affects function.

Functional assessments strive to identify the quantity and quality of disability in chronic illness. These assessments, although sometimes not specific to the medical treatment regimen, are often a good measure of the patient's response and adaptation to chronic health problems. Disability assessment helps identify

the gap between the existing patient self-care abilities and needed self-care resources. The difference between these two (existing abilities and needed resources) identifies areas where nursing care should focus. In this approach to assessment we are embracing the idea of an illness as chronic; patients can achieve various degrees of adaptation, and as nurses we can help maximize their function and therefore their quality of life. Chapter 13 discusses comprehensive assessment and assessment instruments.

Since many people with chronic illness manage their conditions in a community setting and may need assistance from caregivers, assessment must also focus on the ability of family or significant others to assist and cope with caregiving. Chapter 23 presents a discussion of the caregiving role.

Interventions

Interventions in the care of chronically ill individuals must take into consideration the client's emotional responses, perspectives on the illness, individual needs, self-care ability, support from family and friends, and available resources, as well as the trajectory experience. Chronic illness affects all aspects of a person's life, and interventions must be holistic in focus. Eliopoulos (2001, p. 480) states, "The success to which a chronic condition is managed can make the difference between a satisfying lifestyle, in which control of the illness is but one routine component, and a life controlled by the demands of the illness." Nursing roles in the care of persons with chronic illnesses are presented in Box 15-4.

Caring

Caring has historically formed the foundation of nursing. The concept of caring has been studied by many nursing scholars. Sister Simone Roach's (1992) "5 C's" of caring offer a framework for understanding the meaning of caring. According to Roach, the 5 C's are a way of understanding what the nurse is doing when he or she is caring, and they provide a comprehensive view of caring. The 5 C's are as follows:

▶ Competence: having the ability and skills to provide required nursing care
▶ Compassion: a sensitivity to the pain and brokenness of others
▶ Conscience: moral awareness, practicing within the moral framework, doing what "ought" to be done, and advocating for conditions of justice

Box 15-4	Nursing Roles in Caring for Persons with Chronic Illness

- Listen to the story, and come to know the person and what gives him or her meaning in life.
- Provide education about the illness and its management.
- Provide ongoing assessment with a focus on prevention of complications.
- Relieve symptoms that interfere with function and quality of life.
- Help clients set realistic goals and expectations.
- Focus on potential rather than limitations.
- Teach the skills required for effective self-care.
- Ensure delivery of needed care and support for both the person and the family or significant others.
- Encourage verbalization of feelings.
- Provide support for losses and facilitate the grieving process.
- Provide access to resources.
- Refer appropriately and when needed.
- Assist in helping the chronically ill person balance the effects of treatment on quality of life.
- Maintain hope through development of caring, reciprocal relationships, and hopeful environments.
- Assist to die with dignity and comfort.

▶ Commitment: staying with the person on the journey; nursing as a lifelong commitment and way of life; doing the work of nursing because you want to, not because you have to

▶ Confidence: inspiring trust through the nurse's caring

All of the 5 C's must be actualized in caring. In other words, being competent in skills without compassion or being compassionate without adequate skills and knowledge does not demonstrate caring. Older adults with chronic illnesses are not seeking cure; rather, they need care of the highest quality. Practicing within this framework, nurses bring expertise in caring to meet the needs of older adults with chronic illnesses. Nursing's response of caring brings this expertise to assist people in adapting, continuing to grow, and attaining a level of wellness and wholeness despite chronic illnesses and functional limitations. "The nurse-client relationship is integral to the care of people living with a chronic illness" (Giddings et al, 2007, p. 564). Gerontological nurses know that understanding and

caring for older adults with chronic illnesses and long-term disabilities requires close caring relationships and accompanying the person on their journey, day after day, with hope, courage, and joy.

Special Considerations in Chronic Illness

Regardless of the nature of chronic problems, there are special considerations that almost universally need attention and must be addressed actively by nurses. It is not sufficient to wait until the client brings up the topic. The following discussion addresses several of these, not as a comprehensive coverage of the topics, but as a touchstone for further examination and discussion. Pain, which is common in some conditions, is discussed in Chapter 16, and sexuality is discussed in Chapter 23. Complementary therapies, are often useful in the management of chronic illness. Information about complementary and alternative resources can be found in Chapter 16 and at www.nccam.nih.gov.

Fatigue

Fatigue is a common complaint of persons living with chronic illness. The fatigue experienced in chronic illness is different from the normal feeling of being tired in connection with activity. This type of fatigue affects every aspect of the person's life and may interfere with performing ADLs as well as performing in family and societal roles (Berquist et al, 2006). It is often variable and unpredictable and either ignored or incorrectly assumed to be an inevitable part of the aging process. Instead, fatigue may be a symptom of the illness, a side effect of a medication, or a symptom of depression, or all of these.

The goal of nursing intervention is to find ways to decrease fatigue and assist in managing its effects on daily life (Berquist et al, 2006). The most important intervention is to validate the reality and debilitating effects of the disorder if and when it occurs. Assessment instruments are available to assess fatigue and may be useful. Nurses may also ask clients to rate their level of fatigue on a scale of 1 to 10 (Berquist et al, 2006). It is also important to assess for and treat depression that may be superimposed on the fatigue of chronic illness.

Discussing patterns of fatigue and identifying the precipitants is important. Gerontological nurses may encourage the person with a chronic illness to keep a health diary. The health diary may assist in developing self-awareness regarding perception and management of a chronic illness. It is also helpful to emphasize the wisdom of the body and balance rest and activity within limitations to help conserve energy for activities that are most important or necessary. Energy to enjoy life's activities becomes more precious with advancing age. Chronic problems tax the level of energy one has "in the bank."

The diary may also assist the nurse in understanding the experience of the illness from the patient's perspective so that interventions can be tailored to this person's unique journey. Interventions for the person with fatigue include strategies for energy conservation, appropriate balance of exercise and rest, and adequate nutrition (Box 15-5). Nurses should listen carefully to what is most important to the older adult, as well as what responses are most useful. People with chronic illnesses are really the "experts" on managing their illnesses and lifestyle.

Grieving

Grieving the loss of independence, control, status, activities, social roles, appearance, comfort, and the loss of one's identity as a healthy person may occupy much of one's time initially when adapting to a chronic illness,

---

Box 15-5	Interventions for Fatigue

- Set priorities, and make a list of daily activities identifying which are essential, desirable, transferable, and optional.
- Delegate activities and learn to accept help as needed.
- Anticipate needed resources and determine the most efficient way to carry out important activities
- Act during times of peak energy.
- Pace activities by planning for rest and activity, breaking big tasks into smaller, more manageable ones, spreading activities out over the day and week, and resting for short periods before activity.
- Use relaxation strategies such as visual imagery, music, and massage.
- Exercise appropriately to increase muscle strength and endurance. Consult with physical therapist for specific therapeutic exercises, depending on type of illness.
- Consume a healthy, nutritious diet and maintain normal body weight.

Data from: Berquist S, Neuberger G, Jamison M: Altered mobility and fatigue. In Lubkin I, Larsen P, editors: *Chronic illness: impact and interventions*, ed 6, Sudbury, MA, 2006, Jones & Bartlett

---

particularly if the onset has been abrupt and the loss interferes directly with a major source of one's pleasure. As the mother with a handicapped newborn mourns the loss of the visualized "perfect" infant, the elder may begin to memorialize the "perfect" self that no longer exists. In fact, the perfection of the earlier image of the self may grow far beyond the reality that existed.

A recent study describing the losses experienced by persons with severe, chronic physical illness and the occurrence of chronic sorrow (Ahlstrom, 2007), revealed that losses are a significant part of life, constantly present (Box 15-6). Losses were often associated with periods of sorrow. Chronic sorrow, experienced by 53% of the participants, was cyclical in nature, alternating with periods of happiness and satisfaction.

Nursing interventions for loss and grief are to encourage the person to talk about their losses, provide support through active listening, and recognize the stages of grief that may be occurring. Clearly, response to losses and grief reactions will be highly individual, depending on the significance of the loss to the individual and the number of additional losses with which the individual is attempting to cope. It is important to come to know the person and what is most meaningful in their life to understand the impact of losses. The number and recent occurrence of other losses in the life of the individual may have depleted psychic reserves (see Chapter 25).

There often seems to be a subversive sense of failure or weakness in individuals who have developed a chronic disorder, as if they could will it away by strength of mind, determination, and courage. The suffering a chronic illness entails is compounded by a sense of responsibility for remaining healthy, especially in the current wellness climate. There is often the persistent thought that hard work and adherence to a strict treatment regimen will bring about cure, and when that does not occur, a sense of shame develops. This is a serious problem that is deeply rooted in the work ethic that has been so cultivated in the older generation, and it may affect an elder's willingness to seek and accept help.

Given these tendencies, it is imperative that the nurse not overtly or covertly reinforce the client's sense of personal failure. Living with a chronic illness is a process that is continually changing as one adapts to the grief over the lost self and learns to embrace the needs of the emerging self.

Fostering Self-Care

In the day-to-day life of the person with chronic illness, self-care skills are of the greatest importance. Nurse theorist Dorothea Orem has provided a useful

| Box 15-6 | Evidence-Based Practice: Experience of Loss and Chronic Sorrow in Persons with Severe Chronic Illness |

Purpose

The aim of the study was to describe losses narrated by persons afflicted with severe chronic physical illness and to identify the occurrence of chronic sorrow.

Sample and Setting

The study investigated 30 participants in Sweden with severe, disabling physical disease or injury between the ages of 18 and 64 years who had personal assistance in their daily lives for at least 3 months.

Method

A qualitative study with an abductive approach of analysis, including both inductive and deductive interpretations. Participants were interviewed twice, and there was an independent assessment of the deductive results concerning chronic sorrow.

Results

All of the participants had experienced repeated physical, emotional, and social losses. Most common were loss of "bodily function," "loss of relationship," "loss of autonomous life," "loss of life imagined," and "loss of identity," which included the loss of human worth, dignity, and a changed self-image. Sixteen of the 30 participants were assessed to be in a state of chronic sorrow with respect to one criterion of chronic sorrow: "loss experience, ongoing or single event."

Implications

Persons with severe chronic illness often experience recurring losses that are consistent with the phenomenon of chronic sorrow. Nursing interventions include active listening, being patient, and allowing time for expression of feelings. Knowledge of the existence of chronic sorrow will assist nurses to support these persons in a sensitive and appropriate way.

Reference: Ahlstrom G: Experience of loss and chronic sorrow in persons with severe chronic illness, *J Nurs Healthcare Chron Illness* in association with *J Clin Nurs* 16(3a):76-83, 2007.

language and taxonomy for both understanding and responding to the call from persons with self-care needs (1980, 1995).

According to Orem, each person has self-care needs called *universal self-care requisites*. Each person also develops self-care capacity, or the ability to meet theses requisites. However, under some circumstances, the needs exceed the person's capacity to meet them and a self-care deficit ensues in which the person is unable to carry out basic functions without assistance. These deficits are primarily the result of pathophysiological disorders that impinge on neuromuscular, musculoskeletal, or sensory integrity, but they can also have a psychological or spiritual origin.

Nursing interventions include assessment of self-care abilities and deficits. The appropriate approach is highly individualized and may involve changing the environment, modifying the treatment, or teaching the individual strategies to compensate for the pathophysiological changes. It may also involve teaching others how to provide the needed care or teaching the person how to direct the provision of care by others.

Prevention of Iatrogenic Disturbances

While the nurse is working to reduce the complications of the chronic illness itself, a secondary risk increases—that of iatrogenesis (a complication or by-product of the health care intervention or environment itself). The emphasis has largely been on control of the potentially deleterious effects of hospitalization (see Chapters 2 and 26), yet iatrogenesis can develop in any setting (Box 15-7). Sometimes, the treatment of the illness can be more devastating than the illness itself.

The person may become incontinent with the addition of a potent diuretic, not because of a new physiological problem but from the increase in urinary frequency without an increase in access to toileting facilities. A new medication can cause depression, poor appetite, fatigue, or erectile dysfunction while

Box 15-7	Common Iatrogenic Problems Associated with an Institutional Stay

- Loss of mobility because of insufficient ambulation
- Incontinence because of inattention when needed; sometimes becomes a permanent problem
- Confusion or delirium caused by medications, treatments, anesthesia, and translocation
- Pressure ulcers caused by immobility and reduced sensation
- Dehydration caused by limited access to fluids
- Fluid overload caused by improper use of intravenous fluids
- Nosocomial infections caused by infectious agents in surroundings
- Urinary tract infections caused by catheter usage
- Upper respiratory tract infections caused by immobility and shallow breathing and aspiration of oral secretions
- Fluid and electrolyte imbalances caused by medications and treatments
- Falls because of unfamiliar environment, weakness, and positional instability
- Impaired sleep because of treatments and environment
- Malnutrition caused by anorexia and insufficient assistance in eating

improving control of the underlying illness. Elders with some functional impairments may find themselves completely dependent during an acute illness.

Whenever a negative change is likely or occurs after an intervention, the nurse can be proactive in working with the person and the care team in identifying the potential or actual effect and assessing treatment from a benefit-burden perspective. The goal is to treat the illness-related problems without compromising function and quality of life. Chapters 2 and 26 discuss some models to prevent iatrogenesis in hospitalized elders.

Assistive Technology

Advances in all types of technology hold promise for improving quality of life, decreasing the need for personal care services, and enhancing independence and the ability to live safely at home. *Assistive technology* refers to any device or system that allows a person to perform a task independently or that makes the task easier and safer to perform. Health care technologies, telemedicine, mobility and ADL aids, and environmental control systems (smart houses) (see www. futurehealth.rochester.edu) are some examples of assistive technology (see Chapter 12 for discussion of mobility and ADL aids). *Gerotechnology* is the term used to describe assistive technologies for older people and is expected to significantly influence how we live in the future.

A new technology is the growing field of telemedicine including remote electronic monitoring of patients. Already found in more rural settings, telemedicine offers exciting possibilities in the home or other setting, reducing health care costs and promoting self-management of illness. A home health nurse may see a patient discharged home after an acute exacerbation of heart failure. The nurse completes a thorough assessment, records it on a handheld computer, and automatically transmits it to other nurses and to the health care provider. A specialized chair is placed in the home, and the elder is instructed to sit on it each morning. Automated blood pressure, pulse, and weight are taken at the preset time, and the information is sent directly to the home health office and the provider's office over the patient's phone line. The home health nurse is quickly alerted to potential problems, including a "missed chair appointment," and the provider can make rapid changes to the medical plan as needed.

Telemedicine offers exciting possibilities for nursing at both the generalist and advanced-practice levels. An even more interesting example of telemedicine via robotics is being tested at a long-term care facility in California. Companion, a 5-ft, 5-inch tall 200-pound robot with a camera, microphone, and video screen, is being used to enable a physician to examine residents and interact with family members and staff at the bedside (Brunk, 2008).

In hospitals and long-term care facilities, devices being used include wireless pendants to track people's movements, load cells built into beds to create an alert when the person gets out of bed as well as to monitor sleep and weight patterns, and bed lifts that assist the person to go from lying down to standing up with the push or a button. Electronic health records are another technology that will improve care and are particularly important for people with chronic illnesses that make multiple providers and care across settings necessary.

The Center for Aging Services Technologies (CAST) is an international coalition of more than

400 technology companies, aging-services organizations, businesses, research universities, and government representatives working together under the auspices of the American Association of Homes and Services for the Aging (AAHSA) to develop new technology solutions to improve the quality of care while reducing health care costs. According to the CAST website (www.agingtech.org/about.aspx), "Technology already has transformed our lives—from email to MP3s and from online shopping to cell phones. It is time now for technology to transform the experience of aging." CAST provides a video, "Imagine the Future of Aging," illustrating the kinds of technologies that will be available to support an older person living at home (www.agingtech.org/imagine_video.aspx).

As baby boomers and future generations age, comfort with technology will be increased and people will seek opportunities for better, safer, and more independent living in ways not yet imagined. At this time, assistive technologies can be cost prohibitive for many older people, but with further development they may become more accessible and affordable for more people.

Models of Chronic Illness Care

Many efforts are under way to improve care for persons with chronic illness by providing cost-effective and care-efficient services that improve outcomes and quality of life. The traditional medical care model and models of public health have not been effective in dealing with the complexity of chronic illness. Although not all people with a chronic illness experience high care needs, the cost of care for those who do is rising exorbitantly, and funding is becoming increasingly limited. The costs of chronic illness (more than 75% of total medical expenditures), access to care, quality outcomes, and patient satisfaction remain issues of concern (Chin et al, 2006). Almost half of Americans living with chronic illness reported that the cost of care is a financial burden; 89% have difficulty in obtaining adequate health insurance; and 72% report having difficulty getting necessary care from health care providers (Chin et al, 2006).

People with chronic illnesses often have to navigate a system that requires them to coordinate several disparate financing and delivery systems themselves, making it more difficult to obtain the full range of appropriate services. People who need access to different programs are likely to find that each program has different eligibility criteria and sets of providers, and that there is little communication or coordination between providers. As a result, the health care delivery system for those with chronic illnesses is complex and confusing, and care is often fragmented, less effective, and more costly (Partnerships for Solutions, 2003). A summary of the challenges in care of the older person with a chronic illness is presented in Box 15-8.

Managed care, case management, disease management, evidence-based protocols for disease management, care coordination, collaborative models of self-management, and programs such as the Program of All-Inclusive Care for the Elderly (PACE) are examples of models being used. The Centers for Medicare & Medicaid Services (CMS) is also conducting and evaluating projects involving disease management and case management designed to improve quality and outcomes of care for older adults with chronic illnesses (www.cms.hhs.gov/demoprojectsevalrpts/). Another resource with a focus on developing exemplary models of chronic illness care is the Building Health Systems for People with Chronic Illnesses (BHS), a national initiative funded by the Robert Wood Johnson Foundation (www.partnershipsforsolutions.org).

The goal of these efforts is to build an integrated system to ensure that services meet the needs of individuals with chronic illnesses in a cost-effective manner. Elements essential to new models of care include coordination of care, identification of risk, improved access, prevention and health promotion, use of evidence-based protocols to manage illness, holistic

---

Box 15-8   Challenges in the Care of the Older Person with a Chronic Illness

- Long-term and uncertain nature of the illness
- Costs associated with care
- Little coordination of care across the continuum
- Inadequate funding for preventive and long-term care
- Lack of health care professionals with expertise in geriatrics and chronic care
- Acute and episodic focus in medical care and in reimbursement
- Growing numbers of uninsured and continued disparities in health care outcomes for racially and culturally diverse individuals
- Need for active partnership between the individual and family and significant others and the health care provider

approaches, interdisciplinary focus, management of transitions across the continuum, and a collaborative approach encouraging self-management of the illness in a partnership between the person living with the chronic illness and health care professionals (Chin et al, 2006; Warshaw, 2006) (see Box 15-2).

Results of a randomized controlled trial of a collaborative care model for older adults with Alzheimer's disease (Callahan et al, 2006) demonstrated a significant improvement in the quality of care and in behavioral and psychological symptoms of dementia among primary care patients and their caregivers without significantly increasing the use of antipsychotics or sedative-hypnotics. The model used care management by an interdisciplinary team led by an advanced-practice nurse. Nurses, both at the generalist and advanced-practice level, are particularly well suited to take lead roles in care of individuals with chronic illness.

Small-Group Approaches to Chronic Illness

Early affiliation with a group confronting similar issues may help some individuals with chronic illnesses with their adaptation to the altered role requirements and provide shared strategies for coping. Small group meetings are among the most effective and economical ways of assisting individuals in meeting informational and psychosocial needs. They can also be designed to provide family support and counseling. Self-help groups can be seen as support systems, consumer participant systems, expressive-social influence groups, or homogeneously identified therapeutic groups. Support groups provide the opportunity to obtain information and share similar experiences and perspectives. Facilitating adjustment to new roles and activities and facilitating redefinition of self and meanings constitutes a large part of working with groups.

There are many support services and opportunities for group work available from organizations devoted to particular chronic illnesses (e.g., Alzheimer's Association, American Heart Association, Parkinson's Disease Foundation) as well as many opportunities on the Internet. Suggestions can be found in the resources section of many chapters in this book and at evolve.elsevier.com/Ebersole/gerontological.

Rehabilitation and Restorative Care

Many individuals experiencing chronic illness will require short- or long-term rehabilitation and restorative care. The focus of rehabilitation and restorative care is to capitalize on the individual's needs and strengths in a manner that will help him or her achieve the highest practicable level of function. "Rehabilitation seeks to improve the individual's quality of life in any way, no matter how small, in relation to physical, emotional, or spiritual well-being; and ultimately return that individual to a residence of his choice and at minimal personal risk. This implies integration into society plus support in and by the community" (Williams, 1993, p. 361).

Rehabilitation services take place in acute care, outpatient care, rehabilitation and skilled care facilities, and in the home. Restorative care follows the same principles of rehabilitative care, with the focus of the former on maintenance and the latter on improvement. In the skilled nursing facility setting, the existence of restorative nursing programs for ADLs, toileting, range of motion (ROM), ambulation, and feeding contributes to restoration or maintenance of function.

Considerations In Planning Rehabilitation Care

The rehabilitative plan often begins in the acute care setting and continues into long-term care settings, the community, and persons' homes. The following issues are considered in the planning:

1. The person is in a crisis when admitted to the hospital, and personal strengths are not always evident or easily assessed.
2. Multidisciplinary discharge planning must begin upon admission, and a nurse or case manager should be assigned to each client who will need rehabilitation.
3. Rehabilitation focuses on abilities, not disabilities. It maximizes strengths and supports limitations.
4. A quick discharge to home or nursing facility will occur whenever possible; for the frail elder, this may occur sooner than he or she is ready for the level of activity required in a specialized rehabilitation setting.

Comprehensive interdisciplinary assessment is critical to the rehabilitation plan, which involves working alongside the elder and family (Box 15-9). The total assessment includes a comprehensive biopsychosocial history, functional assessment, and a plan of care with long- and short-term goals. Weekly interdisciplinary team-patient-family conferences are held to evaluate the person's progress, revise goals as needed, and develop discharge plans. Chapter 26 provides additional information on rehabilitative and restorative care and transitional care.

Box 15-9	Members of the Rehabilitation Care Team

- Rehabilitation nurse specialist
- Physical therapist
- Occupational therapist
- Speech therapist
- Social worker
- Discharge planner
- Psychologist
- Prosthetist and orthotist
- Audiologist
- Physician, nurse practitioner
- Vocational rehabilitation specialist
- Person in rehabilitation
- Person's significant others

IMPLICATIONS FOR GERONTOLOGICAL NURSING AND HEALTHY AGING

In summary, management of chronic illness in late life is an issue for the individual, the family, the health care profession, and the world. Nurses work toward the achievement of the goals of *Healthy People 2010* to prepare individuals for a healthier old age and to enhance health and wellness for those already in late life. Nurses must work with older adults holistically to maximize their assets, minimize their limitations, and make the most of what they have. Nursing roles may include direct caregiver, resource person, advisor, teacher, and facilitator.

This kind of nursing requires a different focus than acute care nursing, where the emphasis is on attention to immediate and life-threatening needs and attempts to cure. Chronic illnesses, on the other hand, are illnesses to live with, and nursing's response is one of long-term caring. Progress is not measured in attempts to achieve cure, but rather in maintenance of a steady state or regression of the condition, all the while remembering that the condition does not define the person. Understanding the meaning of the experience of chronic illness from the person's perspective, a holistic approach, and working collaboratively with the person are of utmost importance.

Living with chronic and disabling conditions often puts a damper on all but the most robust individual. Because an illness limits an older person physically or cognitively, it does not have to limit the person's human potential. Healthy aging does not mean the absence of disease; rather, it means moving toward wellness in spite of disease. Someone once said that a chronic illness is like a grain of sand in an oyster; it irritates and creates a pearl, or the oyster just dies. Part of nursing intervention is aimed at helping create that pearl.

APPLICATION OF MASLOW'S HIERARCHY

Chronic illnesses and the consequences of treatment can affect an older adult's ability to fulfill basic physiological needs without assistance or adaptation. Nursing interventions are directed at enhancing self-care abilities as well as providing care to ensure that basic needs can be met with as much independence as possible. A wellness approach centers on assisting elders to meet as many of Maslow's defined needs as possible. Chronic illnesses and disabilities may impair physical function, but a sense of safety, security, belonging, self-esteem, and self-actualization can still be attained. Maintaining integrity and achieving one's maximal potential despite functional limitations and illness may be one of the greater accomplishments of many older people. Our care must support the potential for wellness at all stages in life.

KEY CONCEPTS

- ▶ Declines in mortality, increasing medical expertise, and sophisticated technological developments have resulted in a great increase in the survival of the very old with multiple chronic disorders.
- ▶ The effects of chronic illness range from mild to life-limiting, with each person responding to unique circumstances in a highly individualized manner.
- ▶ The Chronic Illness Trajectory, Maslow's Hierarchy of Needs, and The Shifting Perspectives Model of Chronic Illness offer useful frameworks to understand chronic illness and design nursing interventions.
- ▶ People with chronic illnesses can achieve wellness, and the role of the nurse is critical in the promotion of wellness.
- ▶ The goals of healthy aging include minimizing risk for disease, encouraging health promotion, and in the presence of disease, alleviating symptoms, delaying or avoiding the development of complications, and maximizing function and quality of life.
- ▶ Loss and grief are common in chronic illness. Nursing interventions include encouraging the person to

Human Needs and Wellness Diagnoses

Self-Actualization and Transcendence
(Seeking, Expanding, Spirituality, Fulfillment)
Seeks meaning in illness and disorders
Surmounts impairments
Maintains values and optimism
Transcends the physical
Seeks knowledge and creative self-expression

Self-Esteem and Self-Efficacy
(Image, Identity, Control, Capability)
Exerts maximum control of self and environment
Maintains strong sense of identity regardless of impairment
Finds ways to express sexuality satisfactorily
Accepts altered body function or appearance
Maintains grooming
Copes effectively with exacerbations of disorders

Belonging and Attachment
(Love, Empathy, Affiliation)
Maintains important network of affiliations
Develops appropriate relationship with
health care providers
Keeps personal commitments
Devises ways to express reciprocity in relationships

Safety and Security
(Caution, Planning, Protections, Sensory Acuity)
Uses adaptive equipment safely
Uses mobility aids to maintain movement
Adheres to medical regimen
Monitors health and performs maintenance as needed
Demonstrates adequate health care

Biological and Physiological Integrity
(Air, Fluids, Comfort, Activity, Nutrition, Elimination, Skin Integrity)
Is attentive to shifts in bodily needs
Maintains intact skin
Has regular schedule of elimination
Has adequate fluid and fiber intake
Recognizes and responds to shifting energy demands

These are not all the possible wellness diagnoses that may be identified. The above
are examples of nursing diagnoses that should be considered when planning care
for the older adult.

talk about his or her losses, providing support through active listening, and recognizing the grief process that may be occurring.

▶ New models of cost-effective care are needed that increase access and improve outcomes and quality of life for persons with chronic illness. Nurses are particularly well prepared to assume major roles in chronic illness care.

▶ The goal of rehabilitation for the older adult is to maintain the highest practicable level of functioning.

ACTIVITIES AND DISCUSSION QUESTIONS

1. What type of education and counseling might the nurse provide to a 40-year-old client to promote health and prevent chronic illness in later life?
2. Discuss ways that one might modify a living situation to accommodate an individual with limited energy resulting from chronic disorders.
3. What do you think would be the most devastating loss in activities of daily living?
4. What are some nursing interventions to assist a person with chronic illness to deal with loss? Practice or role-play various ways that these issues can be addressed.
5. How would you encourage an individual toward maximal participation in self-care?
6. What would be the measures of wellness during chronic illness?

RESOURCES

Organizations
The Center for Aging Services Technologies (CAST)
website: www.agingtech.org/about.aspx

Imagine the Future of Aging
website: www.agingtech.org/imagine_video.aspx

World Health Organization
Chronic diseases and health promotion
website: www.who.int/chp/en/

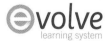

For additional resources, please visit evolve.elsevier.com/Ebersole/gerontological.

REFERENCES

Ahlstrom G: Experiences of losses and chronic sorrow in persons with severe chronic illness, *J Nurs Healthcare Chron Illness* in association with *J Clin Nurs* 16(3a):76-83, 2007.

American Hospital Association: Health for life: focus on wellness, 2007. Accessed 6/17/08 from www.aha.org.

Astin F, Closs SJ: Chronic disease management and self-care support for people living with long-term conditions: is the nursing workforce prepared? *J Nurs Healthcare Chron Illness* in association with *J Clin Nurs 16*(7b):105-106, 2007 (guest editorial).

Berquist S, Neuberger G, Jamison M: Altered mobility and fatigue. In Lubkin I, Larsen P, editors: *Chronic illness: impact and interventions,* ed 6, Sudbury, MA, 2006, Jones & Bartlett.

Brunk D: Robot proves its mettle at LTC facility, *Caring for the Ages* 9(5):12, 2008.

Callahan C, Boustani M, Unverzagt FW et al: Effectiveness of collaborative care for older adults with Alzheimer's disease in primary care, *JAMA* 295(18):2148-2157, 2006.

Centers for Disease Control and Prevention (CDC): *Chronic disease notes and reports: special topic healthy aging* 18(2):1-22, 2007.

Centers for Disease Control and Prevention (CDC) National Center for Health Statistics: U.S. mortality drops sharply in 2006, latest data show, June 11, 2008a. Accessed 6/17/08 from www.ced.gov/nchs/pressroom/08newsreleases/mortalityw006.htm.

Centers for Disease Control and Prevention: Healthy aging for older adults, 2008b. Accessed 6/17/08 from www.cdc.gov/aging/.

Chin P, Papenhausen J, Burgess C: Nurse case management. In Lubkin I, P Larsen P, editors: *Chronic illness: impact and interventions,* ed 6, Sudbury, MA, 2006, Jones & Bartlett.

Corbin JM, Strauss A: *Unending work and care: managing chronic illness at home,* San Francisco, 1988, Jossey-Bass.

Corbin JM, Strauss A: A nursing model for chronic illness management based upon the trajectory framework. In Woog P, editor: *The chronic illness framework: the Corbin and Strauss nursing model,* New York, 1992, Springer.

Curtin M, Lubkin I: What is chronicity? In Lubkin I, Larsen P, editors: *Chronic illness: impact and interventions,* ed 6, Sudbury, Mass, 2006, Jones & Bartlett.

Czaja S, Schulz R: Innovations in technology and aging, *Generations* 30(2):6-8, 2006.

Donnelly G: Chronicity: concepts and reality, *Holis Nurs Prac* 8(1):1-7, 2003.

Dunn HL: *High level wellness,* ed 2, Arlington, VA, 1972, Beatty.

Eliopoulos C: *Gerontological nursing,* ed 6, Philadelphia, 2001, Lippincott Williams & Wilkins.

Espinoza S, Walston JD: Frailty in older adults: insights and interventions, *Cleveland Clinic J Med,* 72(12):1105-1112, 2005.

Fried L, Tangen C, Walston J et al: Frailty in older adults: evidence for a phenotype, *J Gerontol A Biol Sci Med Sci* 56(3):M146-M157, 2001.

Fried L, Ferrucci F, Darer J et al: Untangling the concepts of disability, frailty and co-morbidity: implications for improved targeting and care, *J Gerontol A Biol Sci Med Sci* 59(3)A:255-263, 2004.

Fries JF: Health promotion and the compression of morbidity, *Lancet* 1:1481-483, 1989.

Giddings L, Roy D, Predeger E: Women's experience of ageing with a chronic condition, *J Adv Nurs* 58(6):557-565, 2007.

Hartford Institute for Geriatric Nursing: *Frailty and its implications for care.* Accessed 6/16/08 from www.consultgerirn.org.

Hodges HF, Keeley AC, Grier EC: Masterworks of art and chronic illness experiences in the elderly, *J Adv Nurs* 36(3):389-398, 2001.

Hwang W, Weller W, Ireys H, Anderson G: Out of pocket medical spending for care of chronic conditions, *Health Affairs* 20(6):268-269, 2001.

Jevne R: Enhancing hope in the chronically ill, *Hum Med* 9(2):121-130, 1993.

Larsen P: Chronicity. In Lubkin I, Larsen P, editors: *Chronic illness: impact and interventions,* ed 6, Sudbury, MA, 2006, Jones and Bartlett.

Larsen P, Lewis P, Lubkin I: Illness behavior and roles, In I Lubkin, P Larsen, *Chronic illness: impact and interventions,* ed 6, Sudbury, MA, 2006, Jones & Bartlett.

Lindqvist O, Widmark A, Rasmussen B: Reclaiming wellness—living with bodily problems, as narrated by men with advanced prostate cancer, *Cancer Nurs* 29(4):327-337, 2006.

Lundman B, Jansson L: The meaning of living with a long-term disease: to revalue and be revalued, *J Nurs Chron Illness* in association with *J Clin Nurs* 16(7b):109-115, 2007.

Morley J, Flaherty J: It's never too late: health promotion and illness prevention in older persons, *J Gerontol A Biol Sci Med Sci* 57A(6):M342, 2002.

Morley J, Mitchell P, Miller D: Something about frailty, *J Gerontol A Biol Sci Med Sci* 57A(11): M698-M704, 2002 (editorial).

Orem D: *Nursing: concepts of practice,* ed 2, New York, 1980, McGraw-Hill.

Orem D: *Nursing: concepts of practice, ed 5,* St Louis, 1995, Mosby.

Partnerships for Solutions: Better lives for people with chronic conditions, 2001. Accessed 6/17/08 from www.partnershipsforsolutions.org/problem/index.html.

Partnerships for Solutions: *Care coordination for people with chronic conditions,* Baltimore, MD, 2003, Johns Hopkins University.

Paterson BL: The shifting perspectives model of chronic illness, *J Nurs Scholarsh* 33(1):21-26, 2001.

Roach S: *The human act of caring,* Ottawa, 1992, Canadian Hospital Association.

Strauss A, Glaser B: *Chronic illness and the quality of life,* St Louis, 1975, Mosby.

U.S. Department of Health and Human Services: *Healthy people 2010,* Sudbury, Mass, 2000, Jones & Bartlett.

Warshaw G: Introduction: Advances and challenges in care of older people with chronic illness, *Generations* 30(3): 5-10, 2006.

Williams J: Rehabilitation challenge, *Nurs Times* 18(31):66-70, 1993.

Woog P: *The chronic illness trajectory framework: the Corbin and Strauss nursing model,* New York, 1992, Springer.

World Health Organization: *Preparing a health care workforce for the 21st century: the challenge of chronic conditions,* Geneva, Switzerland, 2005. Accessed 6/19/08 from www.who.int/chp/knowledge/publications/workforce_report.pdf.

Young H: Challenges and solutions for care of frail older adults, *Online J Issues Nurs* 8(2): May 31, 2003. Accessed 1/31/08 from www.nursingworld.org/ojin.

Zauszniewski J, Bekhet A, Lai C et al: Effects of teaching resourcefulness and acceptance on affect, behavior, and cognition of chronically ill elders, *Issues Mental Health Nurs* 28(6):575-592, 2007.

Pain and Comfort

LEARNING OBJECTIVES

Upon completion of this chapter, the reader will be able to:

- Define the concept of pain and how this may be interpreted by the older adult.
- Differentiate acute from persistent pain.
- Identify data to include in a pain assessment.
- Describe pharmacological and non-pharmacological measures to promote comfort for the person in pain.
- Discuss the goals of pain management for the elderly.
- Develop a nursing care plan for an elder in acute pain and chronic pain.

GLOSSARY

Adjuvant A drug that has a primary use other than pain (antidepressant, anticonvulsant) but also is used to enhance the effects of traditional pain medication.

Equianalgesic The dosage and route of administration of one drug that produces approximately the same degree of effect as the dosage of another drug.

Titration The adjustment of the dosage of a given medication until the desired effect is produced with minimal or acceptable side effects.

THE LIVED EXPERIENCE

Ms. S. had cancer of the stomach and was in moderate to severe pain most of the time. She was referred to the local hospice, and the nurse worked with her and her physician to make Ms. S. comfortable. First the nurse assessed potential causes for the pain, the level of pain, the type of pain, and what level of relief was desired. After a careful titration of her medications, it was found that only a long-acting morphine provided her with comfort and an improved quality of life. However, at the dose needed she also hallucinated, seeing several puppies in the room with her. When asked if she wanted to reduce the dosage to eliminate this side effect, she responded, "No—I'll keep the puppies, I know they are not real and they don't hurt anything. I'd rather have them with me than the pain."

Helen, age 93

Comfort is a personal and intrinsic balance of the most basic physiological, emotional, social, and spiritual needs. Without some level of comfort, wellness is beyond reach. Comfort is uniquely defined, experienced, and expressed by each person as members of a family, community, and culture. A person comes to late life with many learned ways of promoting self-comfort and comforting loved ones.

Pain is a sensation of distress, and it occurs at physical, psychological, and spiritual levels and is represented in the foundation level of Maslow's Hierarchy of Needs. Pain is a multidimensional phenomenon, and usually one type is intertwined with another. Physical pain and several chronic diseases (e.g., Parkinson's) can evoke the psychological pain of depression. Any type of pain results in reduced socialization, impaired mobility, and a reconsideration of the meaning of life and self (Jeffery and Lubkin, 2002).

It is not uncommon in the older population to express spiritual and psychological pain in somatic terms of "not feeling well." This is called "somatization" when all possible physical causes have been ruled out. Premature labeling can have disastrous effect or even cause death. How pain is expressed is highly influenced by the unique history of the individual and the meaning ascribed to the pain. It is also important to realize that an individual responds in a way that reflects his or her own cultural expectations and understanding of acceptable behavior. Very simply, pain is whatever a person says it is.

For those with cognitive and expressive impairments (e.g., dementia and aphasia), pain is a particular challenge for the person, the significant others, and the nurse. Expression of pain must be interpreted by others as they attend to subtle cues (Box 16-1). Indicators of discomfort include restless and confusion. Understanding what the person is trying to communicate through his or her behavior is an essential skill in caring for older people with limitations in ability to communicate (Box 16-2). This is discussed in Chapter 21 in more detail.

Other factors affecting the communication of pain include hearing loss, depression, sedating drugs (which do not necessarily ease pain), the personality of the individual, and the way discomfort is acceptably expressed, if at all. The nurse cannot assume that those individuals who cannot or will not verbalize their pain for whatever reason do not have pain or as much pain as others. Instead, the nurse must be alert to the cues that suggest that pain and discomfort are present. A helpful guide to follow is that if the person has a condition that causes pain to those who report it, the condition is also painful to those who are unable to express it for whatever reason. The nurse must initiate assessment and interventions as appropriate and acceptable to the person.

Pain is now considered the fifth vital sign, and assessment of it is expected as part of evidence-based care (Molony et al, 2005). Providing comfort to persons in pain is a quality indicator, that is, a marker of quality care. Patients now have a legislated right to have their pain adequately controlled in the health care context. Yet even in the presence of the directives mandating it, there remains inadequate assessment and undertreatment of

---

Box 16-1   Pain Cues in the Person with Communication Difficulties

Changes in Behavior

Restlessness and/or agitation or reduction in movement
Repetitive movements
Physical tension such as clenching teeth or hands
Unusually cautious movements, guarding

Activities of Daily Living

Sudden resistance to help from others
Decreased appetite
Decreased sleep

Vocalizations

Person groans, moans, or cries for unknown reasons
Person increases or decreases usual vocalizations

Physical Changes

Pleading expression
Grimacing
Pallor or flushing
Diaphoresis (sweating)
Increased pulse, respirations or blood pressure

Box 16-2   "Did My Back Hurt?"

Ms. R., had moderate dementia; she mistook her son for her husband, and did not know that she was in a nursing home. She began moaning from time to time, grimacing and pacing and spending less time "visiting" with the other residents she believed were her guests. She began holding her back and refusing to get out of bed, and when up, to pace with more intensity of motion. An x-ray study of her back showed severe osteoporosis. She was started on calcitonin—a medication for osteoporosis with a side effect of pain relief for some. Over the course of about 6 weeks, Ms. R. began resuming her usual activities and was much cheerier than she had been in a long time. When asked if her back still hurt she responded, "Did my back hurt?" Her back pain was expressed in behavior change. Although she could not express the physical pain, she was nonetheless feeling it: she could only express it in her own way. It was up to the nurse to observe, interpret potential causes, and seek treatment on her behalf.

pain especially when the patient is an older adult, from a minority group or in a nursing home (Smith, 2005).

Nurses have their own definitions and expectations of the expression of pain. As with patients, these are drawn from nurses' personal and professional experiences, culture, and so on. Myths, stereotypes, and generalizations about aging influence the nurse's response, such as that the elderly don't feel as much pain, or that they complain all the time (Box 16-3). These beliefs further the prevalence of undertreatment.

Nurses have a responsibility to let go of their own expectations and promote comfort for those who are suffering, regardless of the cause and manner of expression. They do so with a nonjudgmental approach and with the goal of understanding and developing interventions to relieve, not just lessen, pain of all kinds. In

light of the evidence of undertreatment of pain in the older adult, the gerontological nurses' skill in assessment and intervention is especially important.

ACUTE AND PERSISTENT PAIN

There are two categories of pain, acute and persistent, otherwise known as chronic. Further there are subtypes of each, such as neuropathic and nociceptive. For a more detailed discussion of the sub-types of pain, see Touhy and Jett (2008).

Acute Pain

Acute physical pain is temporary and includes postoperative, procedural, and traumatic pain. Acute physical pain is usually easily controlled by analgesic medications. In the hospital setting an analgesic pump controlled by the patient is used for a restricted period. Acute pain is a universal experience for older adults owing simply to the length of life lived and opportunities for traumatic injury and the development of pain-producing illness. At the same time, the older one is, the more likely one will have an adverse reaction to pain medication (see Chapter 14). For example, most analgesics cause sedation. Although use of the medication may be necessary, this side effect also increases the risk for falls and delirium.

Acute pain may also be psychological or spiritual in nature, such as in early bereavement or in a major depressive episode. Because of the high number of losses in the lives of older adults (see Chapters 23 and 25), the risk for such acute pain is high.

Persistent Pain

Persistent pain results in dramatic changes in lifestyle and the ability to meet personal needs.

The older one is, the higher the risk for developing health problems that are associated with persistent pain and iatrogenic side effects with treatment. Conditions that are degenerative (e.g., arthritis) or pathological (e.g., herpes zoster, stroke, peripheral neuropathy) are common and cause pain at some level. Adverse iatrogenic events include falls and changes in cognitive function; sometimes these are the effect of medications taken at the same time. Loneliness and emotional pain from loss (see Chapter 25) decrease the ability to cope with physical pain. These psychosocial aspects of an elder's pain experience are rarely or superficially assessed by the nurse or included in the plan of care. The current

Box 16-3	Fact and Fiction About Pain in the Elderly

MYTH: Pain is a normal part of aging.
FACT: Pain is not part of the normal changes with aging; however, its occurrence increases with age.
MYTH: Pain sensitivity and perception decrease with aging.
FACT: Not true; however, the older adult may have a greater tolerance for pain owing to adjustment to inadequate relief of long standing.
MYTH: If patients don't complain of pain, they do not have pain.
FACT: Persons may not report pain for a variety of reasons and nonetheless have pain. They may feel that is culturally inappropriate to "complain" of pain or feel that they are burdensome to those around them, including nurses.
MYTH: A person who has no functional impairment, appears occupied, or is otherwise distracted from pain must not have significant pain.
FACT: Patients have a variety of reactions to pain. Many patients are stoic and refuse to "give in" to their pain.
MYTH: Narcotic medications are inappropriate unless used for short periods of time.
FACT: Opioid analgesics are often the best treatment for moderate to severe persistent pain in order to help restore the person's ability to function and have some quality of life.
MYTH: Potential side effects of narcotic medication make them too dangerous to use in the elderly.
FACT: Narcotics may be used safely in the elderly.

cohort of pre–baby boomers in pain may underreport pain and undertreat themselves because of the cost of the medications, belief in an associated stigma, attribution of the pain to normal burdens of "old age," or the fear of addiction.

Persistent pain may be a sequela to an episode of acute pain (e.g., herpes zoster); it is not time-limited and may vary in intensity throughout the day or with changes with activity. For example, persons with dysthymia (chronic lower levels of depression) usually feel the most sadness in the morning with a lifting of mood as the day progresses (Chapter 24). Persons with rheumatoid arthritis also have the most pain in the morning with slow but limited improvement with movement. In most cases pain that occurs with the older adult is superimposed on a preexisting level of persistent pain, primarily because of the very high prevalence of osteoarthritis.

Osteoarthritis

By age 50, the majority of adults have some level of degenerative abnormalities of the lower spine (see Chapter 18). One of the most typical is loss of support of the spinal column from osteoarthritis. Osteoarthritis is the destruction of the inner joint surfaces and the most common form of joint disease. It is also the most common cause of disability in persons over 65 (Touhy, 2008). With osteoarthritis, joint pain and stiffness are initially intermittent and then become persistent. Pain is characterized by aching and stiffness in the joints with inactivity, and discomfort or acute pain with activity

Relief from pain requires the skillful use of both pharmacological and nonpharmacological measures. Acetaminophen (Tylenol) remains the drug of choice for mild osteoarthritic pain. However most people report better relief with the nonsteroidal antiinflammatory drugs (NSAIDs) such as Naproxen or ibuprofen. These are used frequently, and pose a considerable risk for interactions and adverse events (Durrance, 2003). Topical capsaicin may reduce osteoarthritis pain. As it is made from chili peppers, it is necessary to warn patients who use this topical preparation, to wash their hands after application, to keep their hands away from their eyes, and to expect a strong initial sensation of burning. Severe arthritis with unrelieved pain and extensive disability may necessitate the use of local anesthetics such as with corticosteroid injections into affected joints. Hyaluronic acid injections have been found to improve join lubrication in some persons. Both treatments are limited to three to five injections (NIAMS, 2006). In extreme persistent and painful cases surgical intervention is used, such as joint replacement. Long-acting narcotic pain relievers have also been effective.

Nonpharmacological pain management of osteoarthritis includes application of moist heat to relieve pain, spasm, and stiffness, and joint care. Joint care may include orthotic devices such as braces and splints to support joints, weight reduction if necessary, physical therapy, and avoiding overusing the affected joint. Complementary and alternative and cognitive-behavioral measures may also be useful adjuncts (see later discussion).

Herpes Zoster

Nearly 1 million cases of herpes zoster (HZ), or shingles, occur each year, most often in persons between ages 60 and 79. About 1 in 5 people who have had chicken pox will develop shingles at some time in their lives (NIAMS, 2006). HZ is a viral infection of the nerves (see Chapter 11). It is characterized by the sensations of itching, stinging, burning pain along the pathway of the affected nerve (dermatome) finally, erupting into serous vesicles. An acute episode last from days to weeks. When the eye is affected, it is a medical emergency with a high risk of blindness and brain involvement.

Although an outbreak of zoster causes acute pain, it may become chronic with what is diagnosed as postherpetic neuralgia (PHN). PHN is persistent pain from the now damaged nerves following HZ and hard to treat once established. Narcotics may be necessary for pain relief. A combination of antiviral medications, steroids, aspirin, and topical anesthetics may be more effective. Antiviral agents such as acyclovir and famciclovir which may shorten the duration of an acute outbreak and may prevent postherpetic neuralgia when given promptly. Low doses of tricyclic antidepressants (e.g., desipramine, Elavil) have been used for postherpetic neuralgia; however, they are now contraindicated for use in the elderly because of their anticholinergic effects (see Chapter 14). In 2006 the FDA approved the use of a preventive varicella zoster virus (VZV) vaccine for persons of at least age 60 who had chicken pox in the past. (NINDS, 2008).

APPLICATION OF MASLOW'S HIERARCHY

At the lowest level of the hierarchy, pain may result in self-care deficits and prevent one from independently performing ADLs and IADLS (see Chapters 13). The presence of disabling pain or its treatment affects safety needs, for example it can lead to the inability to escape a dangerous situation. Such pain also alters family relationships, limits or restricts one's usual role and social and religious activities, and affects the sense of belonging, self-esteem, and self-actualization (see Chapter 24).

IMPLICATIONS FOR GERONTOLOGICAL NURSING AND HEALTHY AGING

As always, care of the elder in pain begins with assessment and continues through to the evaluation of the interventions. The nurse is usually the person most attuned to the needs of patients and is in a key position to work with the person until their pain is relieved.

Assessment

A comprehensive assessment of pain includes a complete history and physical, as well as a assessment specific to pain (Box 16-4). The Hartford Institute for Geriatric Nursing provides an evidence-based guide in its "Try This" series available on the website (www.hartfordign. org). A number of factors should be considered when caring for older adults (Box 16-5). When the person has

---

Box 16-5   Mnemonics for Pain Assessment

Pain is real (Believe the patient!)
Ask about pain regularly
Isolation (psychological and social problems)
Notice nonverbal pain signs
Evaluate pain characteristics
Does pain impair function?

Onset
Location
Duration

Characteristics
Aggravating factors
Relieving factors
Treatment previously tried

From *Aging Successfully* (newsletter of the Division of Geriatric Medicine, St Louis University School of Medicine; Geriatric Research, Education and Clinical Centers, St Louis Veterans Administration Medical Center; the Gateway Geriatric Education Center of Missouri and Illinois), 11(3):6, 2001.

Box 16-4   Additional Factors to Consider when Assessing Pain in the Elderly

Function: How is the pain affecting the ability to participate in usual activities and perform activities of daily living and instrumental activities of daily living?
Alternative expression of pain: Have there been recent changes in cognitive ability or behavior, such as increased pacing, grimacing, or irritability? Is there an increase in the number of complaints? Are they vague and difficult to respond to? Has there been a change in sleep-wake patterns? Is the person resisting certain activities, movements, or positions?
Social support: What are the resources available to help the person cope and tolerate treatment? How is pain affecting the person's usual role? How is pain affecting the relationship with others?
Pain history: How have previous experiences with pain been managed? What is the perceived meaning of the past and the present pain? What are the cultural factors that affect the belief in the meaning of the pain and the ability to express pain and receive relief?

---

cognitive impairments or difficulties with communication, assessment is particularly challenging.

When possible, assessment begins with a person's self-report of pain. For the person unable to express himself or herself, assessment begins with the nurse's careful observation for any potential indicators of discomfort (see Box 16-1). Many times, older adults will not relate pain complaints unless directly asked specific questions such as, "Do you have pain now?" "Where is your pain?" "Do you have pain every day?" "Does pain keep you from sleeping at night or doing your daily activities?" In some cases the use of alternate words are necessary, such as ache, hurt, or discomfort. The use of written or visual analog scales (Figures 16-1 and 16-2) have also been found useful; most can be used cross-culturally or with a person with limited English proficiency. A person who does not appear to be in pain may be comfortable indicating it on a scale, such as 8 out of 10, or pointing to a grimacing or crying face. Visual analog scales have been clinically tested and meet best-practices guidelines for use with older adults (Taylor et al, 2005). However, their use in persons with dementia has varying results (Taylor et al, 2005).

Assessment includes a history of use and detailed descriptions of pain intensity, frequency, quality, location,

Brief Pain Inventory

Date _____ / _____ / _____   Time: _____

Name: _____ _____ _____
        Last   First   Middle Initial

1) Throughout our lives, most of us have had pain from time to time (such as minor headaches, sprains, and toothaches). Have you had pain other than these everyday kinds of pain today?
1. Yes   2. No

2) On the diagram, shade in the areas where you feel pain. Put an X on the area that hurts the most.

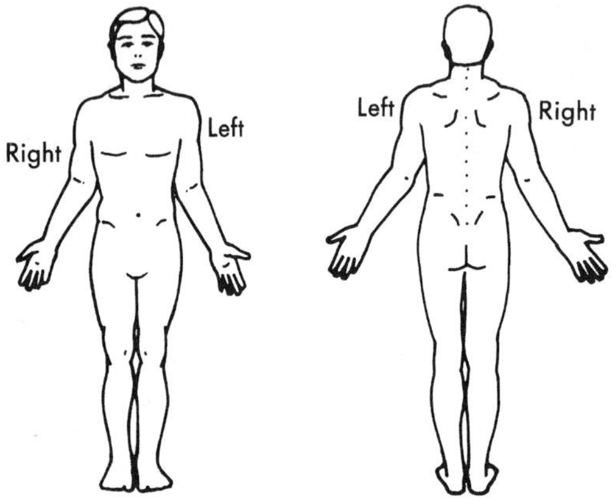

3) Please rate your pain by circling the one number that best describes your pain at its **worst** in the past 24 hours.

0   1   2   3   4   5   6   7   8   9   10
No   Pain as bad as
pain   you can imagine

4) Please rate your pain by circling the one number that best describes your pain at its **least** in the past 24 hours.

0   1   2   3   4   5   6   7   8   9   10
No   Pain as bad as
pain   you can imagine

5) Please rate your pain by circling the one number that best describes your pain on the **average.**

0   1   2   3   4   5   6   7   8   9   10
No   Pain as bad as
pain   you can imagine

6) Please rate your pain by circling the one number that tells how much pain you have **right now.**

0   1   2   3   4   5   6   7   8   9   10
No   Pain as bad as
pain   you can imagine

7) What treatments or medications are you receiving for your pain?

_____

_____

8) In the past 24 hours, how much **relief** have pain treatments or medications provided? Please circle the one percentage that most shows how much relief you have received.

0%   10   20   30   40   50   60   70   80   90   100%
No   Complete
relief   relief

9) Circle the one number that describes how, during the past 24 hours, pain has **interfered** with your:
A. General activity

0   1   2   3   4   5   6   7   8   9   10
Does not   Completely
interfere   interferes

B. Mood

0   1   2   3   4   5   6   7   8   9   10
Does not   Completely
interfere   interferes

C. Walking ability

0   1   2   3   4   5   6   7   8   9   10
Does not   Completely
interfere   interferes

D. Normal work (includes both work outside the home and housework)

0   1   2   3   4   5   6   7   8   9   10
Does not   Completely
interfere   interferes

E. Relations with other people

0   1   2   3   4   5   6   7   8   9   10
Does not   Completely
interfere   interferes

F. Sleep

0   1   2   3   4   5   6   7   8   9   10
Does not   Completely
interfere   interferes

G. Enjoyment of life

0   1   2   3   4   5   6   7   8   9   10
Does not   Completely
interfere   interferes

May be duplicated for use in clinical practice.

Fig. 16-1   Brief pain inventory. (*Copyright Charles S. Cleeland, PhD, Houston.*)

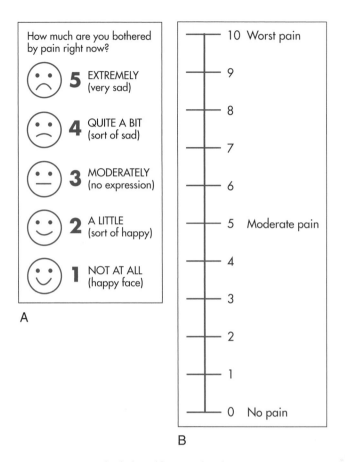

How much are you bothered by pain right now?

😣 5 EXTREMELY (very sad)

🙁 4 QUITE A BIT (sort of sad)

😐 3 MODERATELY (no expression)

🙂 2 A LITTLE (sort of happy)

😊 1 NOT AT ALL (happy face)

A

10 Worst pain
9
8
7
6
5 Moderate pain
4
3
2
1
0 No pain

B

May be duplicated for use in clinical practice.

Fig. 16-2 Examples of visual analog scales. **A,** Example of a visual analog scale (VAS), for example, a series of faces or colors of varying intensities. **B,** Example of a numeric rating scale.

and aggravating and alleviating factors (Box 16-5). Medication history includes prescribed, herbs and supplements, over-the-counter drugs and street drugs. Figure 16-3 presents a standard pain assessment tool. This tool, or a variation of it, is commonly used in hospitals and nursing homes.

Interventions

The goals of pain management in the older adult are to promote comfort and maintain the highest level of functioning and self-care possible. Careful use of pharmacological and nonpharmacological approaches helps to achieve both of these goals. A holistic approach is necessary due to the complex and pervasive nature of pain.

To provide optimal care of the person in pain, attention is given to psychological and social consequences of physical pain. Reducing suffering calls for careful listening, unconditional positive regard, and ongoing support and mobilization of resources. Use of pillows for support or body positioning, appropriate and comfortable seating and mattresses, frequent rest periods, and pacing of activities to balance activity and rest are important aspects of providing comfort.

The nurse encourages elders and their significant others to have an active role in pain management. The patient can keep a personal journal or pain diary of levels of pain; this includes the times, types, and doses of medication taken, its effect, and the duration of its benefit; and which activities increase or decrease the

INITIAL PAIN ASSESSMENT TOOL

Date _____

Patient's name _____ Age _____ Room _____

Diagnosis _____ Physician _____

Nurse _____

I. LOCATION: Patient or nurse mark drawing.

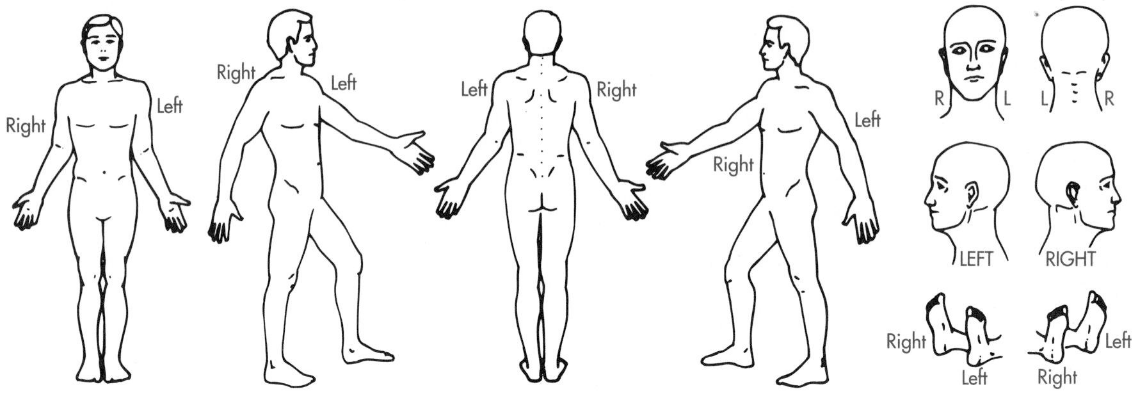

II. INTENSITY: Patient rates the pain. Scale used _____

        Present: _____
        Worst pain gets: _____
        Best pain gets: _____
        Acceptable level of pain: _____
III. QUALITY: (Use patient's own words, e.g., *prick, ache, burn, throb, pull, sharp.*) _____
    _____

IV. ONSET, DURATION VARIATIONS, RHYTHMS: _____
    _____

V. MANNER OF EXPRESSING PAIN: _____
    _____

VI. WHAT RELIEVES THE PAIN? _____
    _____
    _____

VII. WHAT CAUSES OR INCREASES THE PAIN? _____
    _____

VIII. EFFECTS OF PAIN: (Note decreased function, decreased quality of life.) _____
        Accompanying symptoms (e.g., nausea) _____
        Sleep _____
        Appetite _____
        Physical activity _____
        Relationship with others (e.g., irritability) _____
        Emotions (e.g., anger, suicidal, crying) _____
        Concentration _____
        Other _____
IX. OTHER COMMENTS: _____
    _____

X. PLAN: _____

Fig. 16-3   Pain assessment. *(From McCaffery M, Bebee A:* Pain: clinical manual of nursing practice, *St Louis, 1989, Mosby.)*

pain. This type of information helps establish patterns that may be useful in improving pain management by adjusting activity, providing medications at the right times, and helping the patient feel in control of some aspect of care. An example of a pain diary can be found at the website for the American Geriatrics Association (www.americangeriatrics.org). A pain graph provides a visual picture of the highs and lows of the pain. The diary should be reviewed with the care provider and used to adjust dosages or timing for optimal relief (http://www.americangeriatrics.org/education/daily_ pain_diary.pdf).

The nurse also encourages patients to stay as active as is possible within their comfort range. When a person has pain with a needed specific activity (e.g., as in rehabilitation), anticipation anxiety may increase the pain. In this case, the plan of care should include both pharmacological and nonpharmacological interventions such as relaxation before the recommended activity. Administering an effective short-acting medication 20 to 30 minutes before the specific activity may eventually lessen or eliminate the fear of discomfort and can greatly enhance the individual's capacity for that activity. The nurse should learn the patient's ability to cope with pain and work within those parameters.

Pharmacological Interventions

A pharmacologic approach to pain relief is accomplished by medication aimed at altering sensory transmission to the cerebral cortex. This approach is most effective when implementation of the treatment regimen involves teamwork between the patient, the health care providers (nurses included), family members and significant others. In some cultures the patient is not the decision maker regarding treatment. Instead the tribal elders, the oldest son, or others must be consulted first with permission of the patient (see Chapter 4).

A variety of pharmacological interventions are available for pain management. The combination of long-acting drugs and short-acting analgesics has been particularly effective. Nonnarcotic (e.g., acetaminophen, ibuprofen) and narcotic (e.g., morphine) as well as adjuvant medications (antidepressants, anticonvulsants) are currently available for use and may be cautiously prescribed to older adults in physical pain.

The general principles of pain control for older adults are the same as for younger adults; however, older adults may experience more adverse drug reactions related to age-associated changes in drug absorption, distribution, metabolism, and excretion (see Chapter 14). Meperidine (Demerol), which is frequently given for postoperative or posttraumatic injury pain, is absolutely contraindicated for use in older adults. A guideline for the management of pain in older adults was developed by the American Geriatrics Society. This can be found at www.americangeriatrics.org (search Pain).

In gerontological nursing it is essential that pain medications are started at the lowest dose possible. However, it is equally as important for the dosages to be titrated to the point that pain is relieved and the relief is continuous. Too often, while a low dose is started, increases are delayed and suffering is prolonged unnecessarily. The adage "Start low, go slow, but go!" is important to remember. The goal of pain management, particularly for persistent pain, is to prevent the pain, not simply relieve it.

Nonnarcotic Analgesics. Acetaminophen is often adequate for mild to moderate pain, However 4 g (4000 mg) is the maximum for any 24-hour period. Although this may seem like a high dose, with the availability of products such as Extra-Strength Tylenol at 500 or 1000 mg per tablet, the maximum dose is reached quickly. This maximum dose is reduced for persons with renal or hepatic dysfunction or who drink alcohol.

If acetaminophen is not effective or tolerated, nonacetylated salicylates (trisalicylate, choline magnesium) may be tried, or one of the many NSAIDs that are available (e.g., aspirin, ibuprofen) may be used. Over-the-counter NSAIDs are used very commonly. However, they must be used with caution because of the increased risk of adverse effects or death due to acute gastrointestinal bleeding or myocardial infarction (American Gastroenterological Association et al, 2006). NSAIDs may increase or decrease the effect of many prescription medications that older people are likely to be taking such as, anticoagulants, oral hypoglycemics, diuretics, and antihypertensives.

To reduce the risks of bleeding, alternative and adjuvant medications are sometimes used. Although the COX-2 inhibitor celecoxib (Celebrex) has been reported effective for some persons with mild to moderate pain, it cannot be used by someone with sensitivity to sulfa drugs. It should also be noted that more recent research contradicts earlier beliefs about the lowered risk for gastrointestinal effects in COX-2 inhibitors (Stockl et al, 2005).

Narcotic Analgesics. Narcotic medications, especially the opioids, effectively treat both acute and persistent pain. Opiates produce a greater analgesic effect, a higher peak, and a longer duration of effect in older adults when compared to younger adults. This is in part due to prolonged half-lives of the medications (see Chapter 14). The recommendation to start with the lowest anticipated effective dose, monitor response frequently, and titrate slowly to desired effect is especially applicable with the use of narcotic pain relievers. Pain relief should be planned for an "around the clock" approach with a combination of long-acting or sustained-release analgesics and generous use of as-needed (PRN) medications. The dose of the PRN medications are monitored so that the long-acting doses can be adjusted to the point that break-through pain is at a minimum. If breakthrough medication is needed on a regular basis, that is the indication that the long-acting medication dosage needs adjustment. Breakthrough pain may occur occasionally during a stable regimen of long-acting medication, and additional medication should always be available. Opioids used long-term for chronic pain control should be convenient and easy to administer or take. The simplest drug regimen is the one most likely to be effective and to be followed more easily.

Side effects of opioids include gait disturbance, dizziness, sedation, falls, nausea, pruritus and constipation. Several of these will resolve on their own as the body becomes adjusted to the drug. Side effects may be lessened or prevented when the prescribing provider works closely with the patient and the nurse to slowly titrate the dosage of the drug to a point where the best relief can be obtained with the fewest side effects. Sedation and impaired cognition do occur when opioid analgesics are started or dosages increased. This often causes great concern from patients, families, and nurses. Patients and caregivers should be cautioned about the potential for falls, and appropriate safety precautions should be instituted.

The nurse provides close observation of the person's response and works to prevent and promptly treat side effects or adverse drug reactions. Since constipation is almost universal when opioids are used in older patients, the nurse can ensure that an appropriate bowel regimen is begun at the same time as the opioids. A daily dose of a combination stool softener and mild laxative may be very helpful, along with adequate fluid intake.

Although many of the narcotic pain relievers can be used in the older adult, albeit with caution, the use of meperidine (Demerol) is absolutely contraindicated. The metabolites of meperidine can quickly produce confusion, psychotic behavior, and seizure activity. The same can be said for pentazocine (Talwin), and methadone. Propoxyphene (Darvon) has a long half-life and

a metabolite that has been associated with cardiac irregularities and pulmonary edema, and is not recommended (Fick et al, 2003). The nurse can refer to the Agency for Healthcare Research and Quality guidelines for acute and chronic pain management as well as the latest equianalgesic charts if they are needed (www.ahrq.gov).

Nonpharmacological Measures of Pain Relief

Nurses have a long history of comforting patients through nonpharmacological measures. This may be in the form of a caring and supportive relationship or through the use of specific techniques performed either by the nurse or at the recommendation of the nurse.

It has now been shown that a combination of pharmacological and nonpharmacological interventions appears to be most effective in the relief of both acute and chronic pain. In one study it was found that up to 50% of the older adults reported using at least three different strategies at the same time to control their pain (Barry et al, 2005). The basic approach to pain control is to encourage whatever strategies have been effective in the past without causing harm. This is particularly applicable for older adults with a lifetime of experience at managing their own pain and that of others. In some cases, what is now referred to as complementary and alternative medicine (CAM) is actually the formalization of approaches that people have used for years. More and more of what is considered CAM is gaining acceptance by insurers such as Medicare. Several methods that elders use are briefly reviewed here, but it must be acknowledged that this represents only a small sample of what is available (see www.nccam.nih.gov).

Physical Approaches

Cutaneous Nerve Stimulation. Deep and superficial stimulation of nerves for the purpose of pain relief has been practiced for centuries. The Chinese practices of acupuncture, acupressure, and moxibustion are good examples of this approach and are used throughout China. Acupuncture and acupressure are therapies with growing scientific evidence of their effectiveness for chronic pain (NCCAM, 2007a). In some cases Medicare and some private insurance companies will pay for the cost of acupuncture treatment from a licensed acupuncturist.

Nurses have long provided massage, vibration, heat, cold, and ointments. Heat and cold temporarily interrupt the transmission of pain impulses to the cerebral pain center; however, caution must be used in consideration of the cause of the pain. Heat is effective for some things, such as the deep pain of inflammatory musculoskeletal conditions such as rheumatic arthritis. On the other hand, heat will increase the circulation to the area and therefore is contraindicated in occlusive vascular disease and in nonexpansive tissue such as bursae (some joints), where it may increase pain. At the same time, intermittent application of cold packs is helpful in low back pain and some situations of nerve irritation. Care must be taken when applying heat and cold to older skin to prevent skin damage due to normal age-related thinning (see Chapter 6).

Transcutaneous Electrical Nerve Stimulation.
Another method of cutaneous stimulation is transcutaneous electrical nerve stimulation (TENS), low-level laser therapy (LLLT) or percutaneous electrical nerve stimulation (PENS). Electrodes taped to the skin over the pain site or on the spine emit a mild electrical current that is felt as a tingling, buzzing, or vibrating sensation. The electrical impulses are expected to prevent pain signals from reaching the brain. PENS and TENS have been helpful in treating phantom limb pain, PHN, and low back pain (Resnick, 2003). In many cases Medicare will pay for the use of a prescribed TENS unit. The units are available from physical therapists and pain specialists.

Touch.
Touch is a natural form of providing comfort, although its therapeutic properties are still not clearly understood. Touch is now grouped into a category known as "energy medicine" such as reiki. These approaches have been reported to be very effective. Although research is currently under way through the National Center for Complementary and Alternative Medicine, research-based evidence is not yet available (NCCAM, 2007b). When combined with purposeful relaxation, touch may decrease anxiety, reduce muscle tension, and help relieve pain.

Cognitive-Behavioral Approaches

Biofeedback.
Biofeedback is a cognitive behavioral approach that has been applied to pain control. An individual can learn voluntary control over some body processes and alter them by changing the physiological correlates appropriate to them. Training and equipment of some type are needed to learn how to alter one's body response through biofeedback. It requires full cognitive functioning and manual dexterity for self-treatment.

Distraction.
Distraction is a behavioral strategy that lessens the perception of pain by drawing the person's attention away from the pain and relegating it to peripheral awareness. In some instances the individual is completely unaware of the pain; in other instances the intensity of pain is significantly diminished. Pain messages are more slowly transmitted to the pain center in the brain, and therefore less pain is felt.

Mild to moderate pain responds well to distraction. At times, if an individual concentrates intently on another subject, the acute pain may be relieved. The most common forms of distraction include slow rhythmical breathing, slow rhythmical massage, rhythmical singing or tapping, active listening, guided imagery, and humor (Jeffery and Lubkin, 2002). Distraction does not always work, and evaluation of efficacy is important.

Relaxation, Meditation, and Imagery.
As a behavioral strategy, relaxation enables the quieting of the mind and the muscles, providing the release of tension and anxiety. Relaxation should be adjunctive to all pharmacological interventions. Meditation and imagery are two methods of promoting relaxation. Imagery uses the client's imagination to focus on settings full of happiness and relaxation rather than on stressful situations. Several studies using guided imagery have shown that there was a decrease in pain perception in foot pain and abdominal pain. It was suggested that a strong image of a pain-free state effectively alters the autonomic nervous system's responses to pain (NCCAM, 2007b).

Evaluation

Evaluation of pain relief outcomes requires reassessment of the patient's status. Reevaluation of the frequency and intensity of pain, behavioral signs and symptoms that suggest pain, response to pharmacological and nonpharmacological interventions, and the impact of pain on mood, ADLs, sleep, function and other quality of life measures are all included in ongoing reassessment. Adjustments of treatment regimens and interventions are based on reassessment findings. Active involvement of the patient, the family, and all caregivers is essential for comprehensive pain assessment, management, and evaluation.

▶ KEY CONCEPTS

▶ The absence of expressed pain does not necessarily imply comfort. Comfort is a state of ease and satisfaction of body needs, as well as freedom from pain and anxiety.

▶ The experience of pain is not limited to that which is of physical origin. Pain related to psychological or spiritual factors can have the same effect and is often combined with that arising from physical causes.

▶ Assessment of pain is influenced by many misconceptions, myths, and stereotypes about pain. Inadequate treatment of pain is a major concern for older adults in care settings today.

▶ Culture, ethnicity, family, and individual characteristics all influence one's tolerance and expression of pain.

▶ Older people with various degrees of cognitive impairment may demonstrate pain by increased levels of confusion, restlessness, or withdrawal.

▶ Although it is sometimes assumed, it has not been shown that pain sensitivity and perception decrease with age.

▶ The nursing goal is to assist in pain relief. Some pain medications are more appropriate than others for use with elders.

▶ Acute pain and persistent pain necessitate different therapeutic approaches. Persistent pain predominates in the lives of many older adults.

▶ Various combinations of pharmacological and nonpharmacological pain control can be effective but must be individually designed with the elder involved in the decision making.

ACTIVITIES AND DISCUSSION QUESTIONS

1. What is pain?
2. Compare the features of acute and persistent pain.
3. List data necessary for an accurate pain assessment.
4. What are the barriers that interfere with assessment and treatment of pain for all patients? What barriers are associated with pain management in older people?
5. How might pain be expressed in cognitively impaired older people? How does assessment of pain differ in cognitively impaired older people?
6. What pharmacological and nonpharmacological therapy is available, and how can each type work with the other to relieve pain?

RESOURCES

Organizations
American Academy of Pain Management
13947 Mono Way #A
Sonora, CA 95370
(209) 533-9744
website: www.aapainmanage.org

National Center on Complementary and Alternative Medicine
PO Box 7923
Gaithersburg, MD 20898
(888) 644-6226
website: www.mccam.nih.gov

Nurse Healers—Professional Associates International
Alamo Plaza, Suite 111R
4550 W. Oakey Boulevard
Las Vegas, NV 89102
(702) 870-5507
website: www.therapeutic-touch.org

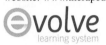

For additional resources, please visit evolve.elsevier.com/Ebersole/gerontological.

REFERENCES

American Gastroenterological Association, Wilcox J, Allison J et al: Consensus development conference on the use of nonsteroidal anti-inflammatory agents, including cyclooxygenase-2 enzyme inhibitors and aspirin. *Clin Gastroenterol Hepatol* 4(9):1082-1089, 2006.

Barry L, Gill T, Kerns R, Reid M: Identification of pain reduction strategies used by community-dwelling older persons. *J Gerontol A Biol Sci Med Sci* 60(12):1569-1575, 2005.

Durrance SA: Older adults and NSAIDs: avoiding adverse reactions, *Geriatr Nurs* 24(6):349-352, 2003.

Fick D, Cooper JW, Wade WE et al: Updating the Beers criteria for potentially inappropriate medications in the elderly: results of a U.S. consensus panel, *Arch Intern Med* 163(22):2716-2724, 2003.

Jeffery JE, Lubkin IM: Chronic pain. In Lubkin IM, Larsen PD, editors: *Chronic illness: impact and interventions*, ed 6, Sudbury, Mass, 2006, Jones & Bartlett.

Molony SL, Kobayashi M, Holleran EA, Mezey M: Assessing pain as a fifth vital sign in long term care facilities: Recommendations from the field, *JGN* 31(3):16-24, 2005.

National Center of Complementary and Alternative Medicine (NCCAM): *An introduction to acupuncture.* 2007a. Available at http://nccam.nih.gov/health/acupuncture. Accessed 7/6/08.

National Center of Complementary and Alternative Medicine (NCCAM): *An introduction to reiki.* June 2007b. Available at http://nccam.nih.gov/health/reiki Accessed 7/6/08.

National Institute of Neurological Disorders and Stroke (NINDS): *NINDS Shingles information page.* Updated July 2008. Available at www.ninhs.nih.gov. Accessed 7/5/08.

National Institute of Arthritis and Musculoskeletal and Skin Diseases (NIAMS): *Osteoporosis.* Updated May 2006. Available at www.naims.nih.gov. Accessed 7/5/08.

Resnick B: Managing chronic pain in the older patient, *Geriatr Nurs* 24(6):373, 2003.

Semla T, Beizer J, Higbee M: *Geriatric dosage handbook: including clinical recommendations and monitoring guidelines,* Cleveland, 2007 Lexi-Comp's Drug Reference Handbooks.

Smith M: Pain assessment in nonverbal older adults with advanced dementia, *Perspect in Psychiatr Care* 41(3):99-113, 2005.

Stockl K, Cyprian L, Chang E: Gastrointestinal bleeding rates among managed care patients newly started on COX-2 inhibitors or nonselective NSAIDs, *J Manag Care Pharm* 11(7):550-558, 2005.

Taylor L, Harris J, Epps C, Herr K: Psychometric evaluation of selected pain-intensity scales for use with cognitively impaired and cognitively intact older adults, *Rehab Nurs* 30:55-61, 2005.

Taylor L, Herr K: Pain intensity assessment: a comparison of selected pain intensity scales for use in cognitively intact and cognitively impaired African American older adults, *Pain Manage Nurs* 4(2):87-95, 2003.

Touhy T: Cognition and caring for persons with cognitive impairment. In Ebersole P et al, editors: *Toward healthy aging: human needs and nursing response*, ed 7, St. Louis, 2008, Mosby.

Touhy T, Jett K: Pain and comfort. In Ebersole P et al, editors: *Toward healthy aging: human needs and nursing response*, ed 7, St. Louis, 2008, Mosby.

World Health Organization (WHO): *Management of cancer pain: adults. Quick Reference Guide for Clinicians no. 9, AHCPR Pub No. 94-0593,* Rockville, Md, 1990 U.S. Department of Health and Human Services, Public Health Service, Agency for Health Care Policy and Research.

Diabetes Mellitus

LEARNING OBJECTIVES

Upon completion of this chapter, the reader will be able to:

- Explain the risks for and complications of diabetes in the older adult.
- Identify the unique aspects of diabetes management in older adults.
- Describe the assessment necessary in the screening and monitoring of persons with diabetes.
- Explain the important components of diabetes management.
- Discuss the nurse's role in diabetes management.
- Develop a nursing care plan for elders with diabetes.
- Propose a reason for the significantly higher rate of diabetes among those over 75 when compared to those over 50.

GLOSSARY

Autoimmune Term applied to the condition where the body sees a part of itself as a foreign object and attempts to destroy it.

Hgb A$_1$c (Glycosylated hemoglobin) A blood test that measures the amount of glucose in the hemoglobin of red blood cells averaged over the 90-day life span of the cell.

Insulin resistance A condition in which body cells are insensitive to the insulin produced by the pancreas, thus impairing glucose metabolism.

THE LIVED EXPERIENCE

I can see that Anna is going to need a lot of help learning to manage her diabetes. I know now that I overwhelmed her with brochures and information right off. She just looked frightened to death, and she really just has a mild elevation in blood sugar; it should be controlled with diet and exercise. I will call her tomorrow and see if she is less anxious.

Anna's gerontological clinical nurse specialist

DIABETES

Diabetes mellitus, now referred to simply as DM (type 1 or 2), is a syndrome of disorders of glucose metabolism resulting in hyperglycemia. Persons with diabetes often have other health problems as well, including problems with the metabolism of lipids and proteins. Diabetes is the leading cause of end-stage renal disease and blindness and is especially prevalent among persons over 65 (Figure 17-1).

The number of persons with diabetes and the risk for diabetes varies by ethnicity, place of residence, and age (Box 17-1). Among Native Americans and Alaskan Natives the rate is 14.2%, with a range of 6% to 29.3% among those living in the American Southwest (NIDDK, 2008a). Persons at least 50 years of age who identify themselves as Hispanic have an overall rate of 25% to 30% with variation by country of origin or residence. Persons from Cuba have the lowest rate (8.2%), persons from Mexico have a rate of 11.9%, and persons

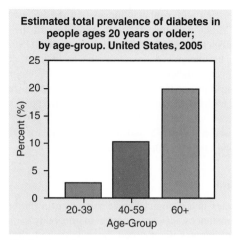

Estimated total prevalence of diabetes in people ages 20 years or older; by age-group. United States, 2005

Fig. 17-1 Prevalence of diabetes among older adults. *(Data from 1999-2002 National Health and Nutrition Examination Survey estimates of total prevalence [both diagnosed and undiagnosed] were projected to year 2005.)*

from Puerto Rico have the highest at 12.6%. Hispanics also have 1.8 times the risk for diabetes of non-Hispanic whites (NIDDK, 2008b)

African Americans are 1.8 times more likely to have DM than their white counterparts. Whereas 14.7% of those over age 20 (5 million) have diabetes, 12.2 million or 23% of persons over age 65 have been diagnosed with diabetes, especially those persons over 74 (NIDDK, 2008c).

The question remains whether diabetes is a primary or secondary event when there is a coexisting illness. Coexisting illnesses, such as hypertension and hyperlipidemia,

---

Box 17-1   Risk Factors for Diabetes Mellitus

- Ethnicity
- Increasing age
- Blood pressure ≥140/90 mm Hg
- First-degree relative (parent, sibling, child) with diabetes mellitus (DM)
- History of impaired glucose tolerance or impaired fasting plasma glucose
- Obesity: >120% of desirable weight or body mass index (BMI) >30 kg/m^2
- Previous gestational DM or having had a child with a birth weight of >9 pounds
- Undesirable lipid levels: high-density lipoproteins (HDLs) <35 mg/dl or triglycerides >250 mg/dl

---

are associated with a decrease in insulin sensitivity. Drugs such as diuretics, glucocorticoids, nonsteroidal antiinflammatory drugs (NSAIDs), and alcohol may also contribute to insulin resistance or the body's failure to utilize the insulin that is present.

Although no direct genetic influence has been found in connection with the development of type 2 DM, genes that are related to the risk for type 1DM have been identified. Among the Pima Indians of the American Southwest, who have the highest rate of diabetes in the world, the *FABP2* gene has been found to be strongly associated with insulin resistance (NIDDK, 2008c).

Type 1 DM (formerly called *insulin-dependent diabetes mellitus [IDDM]* and *juvenile onset*) develops in early life and is a result of autoimmune destruction of the insulin-producing beta cells of the pancreas. The resulting absence of insulin is incompatible with life; without replacement of the insulin, the person will soon die. It has been rare that someone with type 1 DM lives to late life, and it is seen in only 5% to 10% of persons over 18. However this is expected to change dramatically in the very near future due to breakthroughs in treatment options.

The overwhelming number of older persons with DM have type 2 (formerly called *non–insulin dependent diabetes mellitus [NIDDM]* or *adult onset*). In this case, the pancreas is making insulin but not enough to keep up with the needs of the body. This lack of adequate supplies of naturally occurring insulin is combined with the insulin resistance that is characteristic of type 2 DM. The onset is usually insidious, and up to one half of all persons with type 2 DM may be undiagnosed. They may go a number of years without treatment while they are developing serious complications.

Other persons develop conditions that may advance to diabetes if left untreated; these are impaired glucose tolerance (IGT) or impaired fasting glucose (IFG). A fasting plasma glucose value between 110 and 125 is considered IFG, and a glucose level between 141 and 199 mg/dl 2 hours after a glucose challenge is considered IGT. Diabetes is diagnosed after two tests indicating fasting plasma glucose of more than 125 (ADA, 2007). The numbers used to make these decisions do not change with age (Box 17-2).

Complications

Complications occur over the long course of the disease and are microvascular, macrovascular, or both. Macrovascular complications include myocardial infarction,

Box 17-2	Diagnosis of Disorders of Glucose Metabolism

Diagnosis of diabetes mellitus requires either
ONE random plasma glucose ≥200 mg/dl when exhibiting symptoms
or
TWO of any combination of positive tests on different days:
- Fasting plasma glucose (FPG) >126 mg/dl on separate occasions (NOTE: This is not the same as blood glucose levels that are obtained with a fingerstick.)
- Oral glucose tolerance test (OGTT) >200 mg/dl 2 hours after glucose
- Random plasma glucose >200 mg/dl without symptoms

Diagnosis of impaired fasting glucose (IFG) requires
Fasting blood glucose between 110 and 125 mg/dl

Diagnosis of impaired glucose tolerance requires
Glucose between 141 and 199 mg/dl 2 hours after a glucose challenge

stroke, peripheral vascular disease, and neuropathy. The microvascular problems are loss of vision (diabetic retinopathy) and end-stage renal failure from diabetic nephropathy. The advancement of retinopathy also correlates with neuropathy and peripheral neuropathy (ADA, 2007b). There is also delayed wound healing that, when combined with peripheral neuropathy, may lead to amputation.

Combined macrovascular and microvascular damages also lead to male sexual impotence. Impotence in men is a result of reduction in vascular flow, peripheral neuropathy, and uncontrolled circulating blood glucose. Sexual dysfunction is 2 to 5 times greater in this group than in the general population, even though interest and desire are still present.

Persons with diabetes commonly have problems with their feet, which can have a considerable impact on their functional status (see Chapter12). Warning signs of foot problems derive from different body systems and include cold feet and intermittent pain from claudication (vascular); burning, tingling, hypersensitivity, or numbness (neurological); gradual change in shape or sudden, painless change without trauma (musculoskeletal); and infections, skin color and texture changes, and slow-healing, exquisitely painful or painless wounds (dermatological) (ADA, 2007b).

Persons with diabetes most often die of heart disease. Since national efforts to move toward the goals established by *Healthy People 2010* (USDHHS, 2000) there has been a decrease in the number of deaths. However, diabetes-related cardiovascular mortality among those at least 65 years old continues to remain high, with last reports indicating 626 deaths per 100,000 for those between ages 65 and 74, and 2122 per 100,000 for persons aged 75 and above (Centers for Disease Control and Prevention [CDC], 2008).

Goals

Diabetes is a chronic disease that, even in the best of circumstances, causes damage to the body's organs. When diabetes is untreated, or undertreated, the complications develop more quickly and more severely. Therefore, holding back progression of the disease is the major goal. The first step is to maintain glycemic control the majority of the time with target levels for glycosylated hemoglobin (Hgb A_{1c}) as close to 7 as possible, or 8 for those who are medically fragile (ADA, 2007a). Good control of the blood sugar has been found to lead to significant prevention of microvascular complications and slows the progression of the disorder, but clinical trails have not yet included an examination of this effect in older adults (Table 17-1). As might be expected, poor perceptions of one's health, anxiety, and depression are often associated with diabetes, and these may reduce the person's motivation for self-management. Social support, mastery, and self-esteem have been found to have the greatest positive effect on depression and anxiety surrounding the diagnosis of diabetes and living with diabetes. A holistic approach to diabetes and more depth and breadth in nursing practice related to the care of the diabetic patient of any age can facilitate improved health maintenance and adherence to recommended therapies.

IMPLICATIONS FOR GERONTOLOGICAL NURSING AND HEALTHY AGING

Gerontological nurses have great potential for helping individuals and the nation reach the goals set forth in *Healthy People 2010* (USDHHS, 2000), from conducting screenings to patient education and coaching. The nurse can participate in early detection through public screenings or pay attention to the need for screening of persons residing in communal settings such as nursing homes and assistive living centers. The nurse can promote healthy aging by helping people do what they can

Table 17-1 **Maintaining Glycemic Control***			
	PREPRANDIAL	POSTPRANDIAL	3 AM
Blood glucose (mg/dl)	70-120	<180	>65

*Maintaining intensive control has been found to reduce the risk of eye disease (76%), kidney disease (50%), and neuropathic disease (60%).

Data from National Diabetes Education Program: *Diabetes: the science of control,* 2007 (website): *ndep.nih.gov/resources/presentations/diabetescontrol/.* Accessed 6/13/07.

to reduce their risk, such as obtaining or maintaining an ideal body weight, eating a healthy diet that provides for adequate protein without excessive carbohydrates, exercising, and keeping their cholesterol levels and blood pressure under control.

For persons at higher risk for diabetes, especially those with IFG or IGT, attention should be directed at reducing the risk for both diabetes and heart disease. This means education and interventions to help the person reach the following goals:

▶ No smoking
▶ Blood pressure ≤130/80 mm Hg
▶ Cholesterol <200 mg/dl
▶ Low-density lipoprotein (LDL) <100 mg/dl
▶ High-density lipoprotein (HDL) >40 mg/dl
▶ Triglycerides <150 mg/dl
▶ Blood glucose <126 mg/dl

Screening for diabetes by fasting plasma and random blood glucose testing is important for early identification of potential or actual disease. Annual screening of fasting plasma glucose measurements is recommended for all persons in high-risk groups, which includes all persons over 65.

Assessment

The nurse begins with the assessment for risk factors and a subjective report of signs and symptoms, including the evaluation of the presence or absence of hyperglycemia: polydipsia, polyuria, or polyphagia, even though these are rarely seen in older adults. It is more common to find vaguer symptoms, such as fatigue, change in weight, and varied or recurrent infections. When there are symptoms, the duration and character of the these should be described. Family history is important because of the genetic influence. Nutrition, weight, and exercise history are important to identify eating patterns, an active or sedentary lifestyle, and weight control measures, all of which can provide clues for realistic

education and how to encourage better adherence to a therapy regimen, which promotes health and wellness. Assessing economic resources helps establish the person's ability to purchase equipment, materials, and foods that may be needed to maintain diabetes control. This is especially important for older adults, many of whom are on very limited incomes (see Chapter 22). History of the use of alcohol and tobacco provides information related to the risk for complications.

The nursing assessment also includes careful measurement of blood pressure, visual acuity, and gross neurological function. Distant vision can be checked with a Snellen chart and near vision with a newspaper. The skin and feet should be thoroughly inspected for any injury, such as corns, calluses, blisters, cracks, or fungal infections. Use of the Semmes-Weinstein monofilament instrument is recommended to test for peripheral neuropathy. This is available to nurses and easy to use. It is a very helpful measure of the progression of peripheral neuropathy.

Management

Promoting healthy aging in person with diabetes requires an array of interventions and usually involves persons from a number of disciplines working together with the patient and significant others. Management of such a disease requires expertise in medication use, diet, exercise, counseling, and giving support. The persons involved may include the usual care nurses as well as nutritionists, pharmacists, podiatrists, ophthalmologists, physicians or nurse practitioners, certified diabetic educators, and counselors. If the person's disease is hard to control, endocrinologists are involved, and as complications develop, more specialists are called in such as nephrologists, cardiologists, and wound care specialists.

Diabetes self-management (DSM), diabetes self-management education (DSME), and patient empowerment are now the cornerstones of disease management

(Funnell and Anderson, 2004; Mensing et al, 2007) . The skills needed for self-management include knowledge about nutrition, the development of an exercise plan, safe medication use, what to do during periods of other illness, and attention to the psychological aspects of dealing with a chronic illness. Other self-management skills include the use of personal glucose monitors, optimal care of the feet, and knowledge about the disease. The nurse is highly instrumental in the teaching of self-management skills, encouraging patient empowerment and supporting the person while he or she struggles with a complicated and very serious disease. Standards have now been established for DSME, and the cost is covered by many insurance companies including Medicare (Mensing et al, 2007). Medicare will pay 80% of the costs for this education and diabetic supplies after the annual deductible has been met (Centers for Medicare and Medicaid Services [CMS], 2007).

Standards of Care

The American Geriatrics Society, the American Diabetes Association (ADA) and the National Institute of Health have developed a standard for diabetes care (ADA, 2007a). The first and perhaps the most important guideline is that the care of the older adult with diabetes must be individually planned to consider the relative costs and benefits for the frail and very elderly, although the standards of care apply to those who are healthy at any age. Among those recommendations are the following:

▶ When collecting the patient's health history, include smoking history, dietary habits, weight patterns, previous treatment programs, current treatment regimen, exercise and activity levels, infections, illnesses, and complications of diabetes. Information about the approaches that have worked and failed will help the nurse design programs specific to the person.

▶ Annual physical examination includes blood pressure; dilated eye examination; thyroid palpation; palpation of pulses; foot (and repeated at all appointments that are not urgent), periodontal, and skin examination; and neurological examination. Testing fine sensation with a monofilament is recommended.

▶ Laboratory tests should include both a fasting plasma glucose and an Hgb A_1C; fasting lipid profile; serum creatinine if proteinuria is present; urinalysis, including microalbuminuria, and urine culture if indicated; thyroid function (thyroxine [T_4] or thyroid-stimulating hormone [TSH]); and electrocardiogram (ECG).

Nurses must advocate for elders and encourage them to obtain the care we now know can delay or minimize complications.

Demonstrations of techniques for self-monitoring blood glucose (SMBG) include teaching how to obtain a blood sample, use of the glucose monitoring equipment, troubleshooting when there are results indicating an error, and recording the values from the machine. Older adults with arthritis, low vision, or peripheral neuropathy from whatever cause will have difficulties with the mechanics of SMBG and will require creative teaching and perhaps the enlistment of friends or neighbors in the tasks that are necessary; however, new technologies and drug delivery systems are being designed to address management plans (e.g., nasal sprays). The education plan includes helping to determine the timing and frequency of the self-monitoring, the correct adjustment in the schedule when ill, and what to do with the results. Self-care management includes bringing the results to each medical visit and reviewing them with the nurse or other health care provider.

Where appropriate, demonstration and return demonstration should be given for drawing up insulin, selecting the injection site, injecting and storing insulin, and disposing of the used needle and syringes. Again, this is limited by the person's limitations as noted above. Knowing how to safely transport insulin when traveling is also important.

Daily foot care and foot examination should be discussed and demonstrated. Persons who are not particularly flexible will have difficulty reaching and inspecting their feet, and a family member or friend can be asked to do this. As long as vision is adequate, checking can also be done by placing a mirror on the floor to examine the sole. Attention to foot care can reduce the risk of amputation. Awareness of the need for good shoes that fit well is essential (see Chapter 11). Those who have Medicare are eligible for one pair of specially made shoes annually.

Knowledge about the disease and its effects includes knowing what affects the blood sugar and knowing that eating and drinking increases blood sugar. Skipping a meal decreases blood sugar. The elder should have a list of warning signs for high and low blood sugar levels (Box 17-3), and know that extra SMBG should be done any time the person feels clammy or cold, sweaty, shaky, or confused, all signs of low blood sugar. Hypoglycemia is the most common problem for elderly diabetics, especially for those taking sulfonylureas. An identification bracelet is highly recommended especially because of the quick misdiagnosis that can occur is the person is found to be confused and mistakenly believed to have dementia.

Box 17-3	Signs and Symptoms Suggestive of Diabetes in the Elderly

1. General symptoms such as polyphagia, polyuria, polydipsia, and weight loss
2. Recurrent infections, particularly of bacterial or fungal origin, that involve the skin, intertriginous areas, or the genitourinary tract and sores or wounds that tend to heal slowly
3. Neurological dysfunction, including paresthesia, dysesthesia, or hyperesthesia; muscle weakness and pain (amyotrophy); cranial nerve palsies; autonomic dysfunction of the gastrointestinal tract (diarrhea), cardiovascular system (orthostatic hypotension, dysrhythmias), reproductive system (impotence), or bladder (atony, overflow incontinence)
4. Arterial disease (macroangiopathy) involving the cardiovascular, cerebrovascular, or peripheral vasculature structures
5. Small-vessel disease (microangiopathy) involving the kidneys (proteinuria, glomerulopathy, uremia) and eyes (macular disease, exudates, hemorrhages)
6. Lesions of the skin, such as Dupuytren's contractures, facial rubeosis, and diabetic dermopathy
7. Endocrine-metabolic complications, including hyperlipidemia, obesity, and a history of thyroid or adrenal insufficiency (Schmidt's syndrome)
8. A family history of type 1 or type 2 diabetes and a poor obstetrical history (miscarriages, stillbirths, large babies)

Box 17-4	Interaction between Diabetes and the Aging Process

1. A decline in visual acuity can affect the individual's ability to see printed educational material, medication labels, markings on a syringe, and blood glucose monitoring devices.
2. Auditory impairments can lead to difficulty hearing instructions.
3. Altered taste can affect food choices and nutritional status.
4. Poor dentition or changes in the gastrointestinal system can lead to difficulties with food ingestion and digestion.
5. Altered ability to recognize hunger and thirst may lead to weight loss, dehydration, and increased risk for hyperosmolar nonketotic syndrome.
6. Changes in hepatic or renal function can affect ability to self-administer medications.
7. Arthritis or tremors can affect ability to self-administer medications and use monitoring devices.
8. Polypharmacy complicates medication choices.
9. Depression affects motivation for self-management.
10. Cognitive impairment and dementia decrease self-care ability.
11. Inadequate education and poor literacy call for modifications in the method of teaching about diabetes care.
12. The level of income can affect the level of care sought or obtained.
13. Living alone without a resource person for help with management can have a negative effect on the person with diabetes.
14. A sedentary lifestyle and obesity can result in decreased tissue sensitivity to insulin.

We know that the risk of complications is high even with mild hyperglycemia. However, the older we get, the more tolerant we are to hyperglycemia. Therefore an elder may slip into a life-threatening hyperosmolar nonketotic coma as possibly the first and often misdiagnosed sign of hyperglycemia. Experiential teaching, encouragement, and reinforcement of mastery are important factors that promote successful self-management. Some of the factors affecting diabetes control in older adults are identified in Box 17-4.

Nutrition

Adequate and appropriate nutrition is a key factor in the control of diabetes. An initial nutrition assessment with a 24-hour recall will provide some clues to the patient's dietary habits, intake, and style of eating. It is always necessary to know who shops and prepares the food if there is to be any impact on nutritional status. If the person is from an ethnic group different from the nurse, the nurse will need to learn more about the usual ingredients and methods of food preparation to be able to give reasonable instructions. Ideally, all persons with diabetes should have medical nutrition therapy by a registered dietitian who is a certified diabetic educator on an annual basis. At the time of this writing this service is covered by Medicare.

The ADA guidelines (N.D.) focus on a healthful diet with attention to an adequate variety of foods with portion control. Recommended daily caloric intake ranges from 1600 calories for women and a maximum of 2200 calories for men. The goal is to keep the glucose level under control by balancing exercise with eating, weight loss if overweight, and limiting saturated fats in the diet. Carbohydrates are included on the diabetes food pyramid, but these are restricted to those that are full-grain. For details about all aspects of diet and diabetes, see the American Diabetes Association website at www.diabetes.org/nutrition-and-recipes/nutrition/foodpyramid.jsp.

It is part of the nurse's responsibility to learn if there is difficulty with access to food, including food preparation and shopping for food. Working with elders, whose dietary habits have been formed over a lifetime, can be difficult but is not impossible.

Exercise

Exercise is an important aspect of therapy for type 2 DM because it increases insulin production and decreases insulin resistance. Walking is an inexpensive and beneficial way to exercise. Unfortunately, in some communities, crime prevents walking in one's neighborhood. This is most applicable to elders who have lived in their homes many years, since many older neighborhoods have deteriorated over the years. Walking in a local mall, where it is climate controlled, has proved to be a good alternative.

Exercise in conjunction with an appropriate diet may be sufficient to maintain blood glucose levels within normal levels in some cases. A more intensive exercise program should not be started until the older adult has had a physical examination, including a stress test and ECG. A physician or nurse practitioner and a diabetic educator will then have the information necessary to develop safe exercise plans for and with the person. Daily exercise is recommended. Those who have limited mobility can still do chair exercises or if possible use exercise machines that permit sitting and holding on for support. Exercise decreases blood sugar. If the person is using insulin, exercise must be done on a regular rather than an erratic basis, and blood glucose should be tested before and after exercise to avoid hypoglycemia.

Medications

Antihyperglycemics include oral agents and insulin, including the new inhalant insulin. Oral medications are prescribed according to the insulin deficit identified: no secretion of insulin, insulin resistance, or inadequate secretion of insulin. The sulfonylureas (e.g., Glucotrol) and meglitinides (e.g., Starlix) increase insulin secretion. Biguanides (e.g., metformin) or thiazolidinediones (e.g., Actos) have been useful to enhance insulin sensitivity by decreasing insulin resistance.

The mainstay of treatment of type 2 DM in later life is oral medication; however, when the blood sugar is over 200 and difficult to control, insulin may be necessary. It is important to note that the use of insulin by someone with type 2 DM does not "convert" them to a type 1 diabetic, since the diagnosis is made on the type of disorder rather than on the treatment. Diabinase should never be prescribed for the older adult, and metformin (Glucophage) only if the serum creatinine level is at or below 1.5 mg/dl for men and at or below 1.4 mg/dl for women or any time an abnormal creatinine clearance is found (see Chapter 14) (ADA, 2007b).

If other medications are prescribed, they must be carefully reviewed. The effect of drugs on blood glucose must be given serious consideration because a number of medications commonly used for elders adversely affect blood glucose levels (see Box 17-5). Therefore older adults should be advised to ask if a particular drug prescribed affects their therapy and should check with their primary care provider before taking any over-the-counter medications.

Long-Term Care and the Elder with Diabetes

Many of the persons cared for by gerontological nurses in long-term care facilities have diabetes. It is estimated that this number is 24 million, or 50% of long-term care residents (ADA, 2008). In this setting the nurse may be responsible for many of the activities that would otherwise fall to the patient or a home caregiver to carry out. Meals, nutritional status, intake and output, and exercise and activity are monitored. The nurse assesses the person for signs of hypoglycemia and hyperglycemia as well as evidence of complications. The nurse ensures that the standards of care for the person with diabetes are met. The nurse monitors the effect and side effects of diet, exercise, and medication use and encourages self-care whenever possible. The nurse administers or supervises the administration of medications. If the person requires what is called sliding scale insulin, wherein the dosage depends on the current glucose reading, it is the nurse who must make the determination of the dosage under "sliding scale" guidelines.

APPLICATION OF MASLOW'S HIERARCHY

The goals of nursing care are to maintain the older adult with diabetes in the best health that is realistically possible. Maintaining the older adult's health is a team effort. As part of the team, the nurse serves as an educator, care provider, advocate, supporter, and

Box 17-5	Medications Affecting Blood Sugar

Increase Blood Glucose Levels
- Corticosteroids
- Diazoxide
- Estrogens
- Furosemide and thiazide diuretics
- Glucagon
- Lithium
- Phenytoin
- Rifampin
- Sympathomimetics (antihistamines, decongestants, bronchodilators)
- Thyroid replacement preparations

Decrease Blood Glucose Levels
- Alcohol
- Anabolic steroids
- Beta blockers (antihypertensives)
- Salicylates (high doses)

Interactions with Sulfonylureas (Oral Hypoglycemics)
Increased Effects (Lower Blood Glucose Levels Further)
- Allopurinol
- Beta blockers
- Clofibrate
- Histamine antagonists
- Imidazole antifungals
- Low-dose salicylates
- Monamine oxidase inhibitors
- Probenecid
- Tricyclic antidepressants

Drugs Not to Be Taken in Combination with Sulfonylureas
- Azapropazone
- Chloramphenicol
- Dicumarol
- Oxyphenbutazone
- Phenylbutazone
- Salicylates (high dose)
- Sulfonamides

Decreased Effects (Hinder Hypoglycemic Action)
- Barbiturates
- Corticosteroids
- Diuretics
- Estrogens
- Rifampin

Summarized from an unidentified source: handout at workshop, *Chronic disorders of the aged,* sponsored by Arizona State School of Nursing, Phoenix, Sept 1992.

guide for the older person. With a knowledgable nurse, a person's basic needs can be met to facilitate the person's ability to meet higher levels of Maslow's Hierarchy of Needs.

KEY CONCEPTS

▶ Signs and symptoms of diabetes in the older adult may be vague or suggestive of other medical conditions or considered as part of "old age" rather than the usual and expected symptoms of polyuria, polydipsia, and polyphagia.

▶ Close monitoring of blood glucose levels is the most effective way to prevent, delay, or slow the progression of macrovascular, microvascular, and neurological complications of the disease.

▶ Management of diabetes is a comprehensive team effort and should include the elder as much as he or she can realistically participate as part of the team. If this is not possible, the caregiver, if not the nurse, will need to ensure that the medical regimen is effective.

▶ Preventive foot care is essential for prevention of the possibility of future problems.

ACTIVITIES AND DISCUSSION QUESTIONS

1. What are the risks and complications of diabetes for the older adult?
2. State the components of diabetes management, and explain what each component entails.
3. Describe the nurse's role in the management of diabetes.
4. Develop a nursing care plan for an elder in the community, in an acute care hospital, and in long-term care using wellness and North American Nursing Diagnosis Association (NANDA) diagnoses.

RESOURCES

Organizations
American Diabetes Association
National Center
PO Box 25757
1660 Duke Street
Arlington, VA 22314-3427
website: www.diabetes.org

National Diabetes Information Clearing House
1 Information Way
Bethesda, MD 20892-3560
email address: NDIC@info.niddk.nih.gov

Websites
CDC Diabetes Public Health Resource
www.cdc.gov/diabetes

National Institute of Diabetes and Digestive and Kidney Disorders
www.niddk.nih.gov

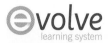
learning system

For additional resources, please visit evolve.elsevier.com/Ebersole/gerontological.

▶ REFERENCES

American Diabetes Association (ADA): Position statement: diagnosis and class of diabetes mellitus, *Diabetes Care* 30(1):S4-S41, 2007a.

American Diabetes Association (ADA): Complications of diabetes, 2007b. Available at www.diabetes.org/diabetes-statistics/complications.jsp. Accessed 7/18/08.

American Diabetes Association(ADA): Economic costs of diabetes in the U.S. in 2007, *Diabetes Care* 31(3):596-615, 2008.

American Diabetes Association (ADA): Using the diabetes food pyramid, N.D. Available at www.diabetes.org/nutrition-and-recipes/nutrition/foodpyramid.jsp. Accessed 7/18/08.

Centers for Disease Control and Prevention (CDC): Death from diabetes, 2008. *Healthy People 2010* Database. Available at http://wonder.cdc.gov/scripts/broker.exe. Accessed 7/13/08.

Centers for Medicare and Medicaid Services (CMS): Diabetes self-management, supplies and other medical services: an introduction, 2007 Available at www.cms.gov. Accessed 7/14/08.

Funnell MM, Anderson R: Empowerment and self-management of diabetes. *Clin Diabetes* 22:123-127, 2004.

Mensing C, Boucher J, Cypress M et al: National standards for diabetes self-management education, *Diabetes Care* 30(Suppl 1):S96-S103, 2007.

NIDDK: American Indians, Alaskan Natives, and Diabetes 2008a. Available at http://diabetes.niddk.nih.gov/dm/pubs/americanindian/index.htm. Accessed 10/19/08

NIDDK: Hispanics / Latinos and Diabetes, 2008b. Available at http://erc.msh.org/mainpage.cfm?file=7.4.3.htm&language=english&module=provider. Accessed 7/14/08.

NIDDK Afrian Americans and Diabetes, 2008c. Available at http://diabetes.niddk.nih.gov/dm/pubs/africanamerican/index.htm. Accessed 10/19/08.

NIDDK: *Genetics of Type 2 Diabetes*. 2008c. Available at http://www2.niddk.nih.gov/Research/ScientificAreas/GeneticsGenomics/GEN1.htm. Accessed 10/19/08.

U.S. Department of Health and Human Services (USDHHS): *Healthy people 2010*, vol 1, ed 2, Washington, DC, 2000, U.S. Government Printing Office. Accessed 10/19/08. Available at www.healthypeople.gov.

Bone and Joint Problems

MUSCULOSKELETAL SYSTEM

A healthy musculoskeletal system not only allows us to be upright but also is necessary to allow us to comfortably carry out the most basic activities of daily living. For some, later life is an opportunity to explore the limits of their ability and become master athletes. For others, later life is a time of significant restriction in movement. However, both athletes and nonathletes may have to deal with the challenges of one or more of the musculoskeletal problems commonly encountered in later life.

The gerontological nurse attends to the needs of older adults with musculoskeletal problems and works to promote healthy bones and joints. In this chapter we discuss osteoporosis and the different forms of arthritis, and their implications for nursing intervention. See

Chapter 10 for a discussion of activity and exercise to maintain musculoskeletal health.

OSTEOPOROSIS

Osteoporosis means *porous bone*. Primary osteoporosis is sometimes thought to be part of the normal aging process, especially for women. Secondary osteoporosis is that which is caused by another disease state, such as Paget's disease, or by medications, such as long-term steroid use. Both are characterized by low bone mineral density (BMD) and subsequent deterioration of the bone structure and changes in posture (Figure 18-1). Osteoporosis affects 10 million people in the U.S., and about 34 million have some degree of bone loss; 68% of these are women (NIAMS, 2007). Osteoporosis is responsible for 1.5 million fractures each year. Of these, 80,000 occur in men, and one third of those with fractures die within 1 year (NIAMS, 2007). Osteoporosis is a silent disorder; a person may never, or not for many years, have symptoms of any kind. With the treatments and interventions now available, some osteoporosis can be prevented or treated and stabilized to some extent. It is always possible to promote healthy aging for the person with osteoporosis.

In the normal process of growth, known as bone turnover, the bones build up mass (formation) and strength while they are at the same time also losing both through resorption. Peak bone mass is reached at about 30 years of age. After that, the loss of BMD is quite minimal at first but speeds up with age. For women, the period of the fastest overall loss of BMD is in the 5 to 7 years immediately following menopause.

A number of other factors increase or decrease a person's risk for both osteopenia and osteoporosis. Some of these cannot be changed (e.g., gender, race, or ethnicity), but others (e.g., calcium intake, exercise) are amenable to change (Box 18-1). African American women have the highest BMD but are still at risk (NAIMS, 2006a).

IMPLICATIONS FOR GERONTOLOGICAL NURSING AND HEALTHY AGING

Osteoporosis is diagnosed through a dual energy X-ray absorptiometry (DEXA) scan but is presumed in older adults with nontraumatic fractures, a loss of 3 inches or more in height, and/or kyphosis (see Figure 18-1). The nurse may be the one to identify the changes that had not yet been medically diagnosed. Without a diagnosis the person cannot be treated.

The U.S. Prevention Services Task Force (USPSTF, 2002) recommends that all persons aged 60 and older

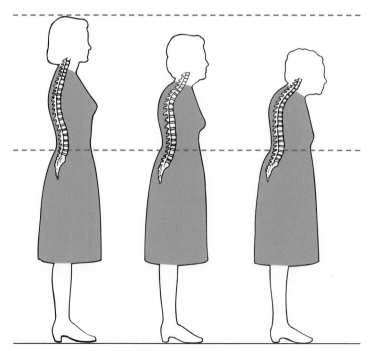

Fig. 18-1   Osteoporosis spine alignment.

Box 18-1	Risk Factors for Osteoporosis

Nonmodifiable Factors
Female sex
Caucasian race
Northern European ancestry
Advanced age
Family history of osteoporosis

Modifiable Factors
Low body weight (underweight)
Low calcium intake
Estrogen deficiency
Low testosterone
Inadequate exercise or activity
Use of steroids or anticonvulsants
Excess coffee or alcohol intake
Current cigarette smoking

and those with more than one risk factor have at least one screening DEXA scan. If the screening is positive the nurse can advocate for the elder to receive appropriate treatment.

Reducing Osteoporosis-Related Risk and Injury

Measures to prevent osteoporosis-related injury or progression of the disease include exercise, nutrition, and lifestyle changes to reduce known risk factors. As with many other diseases, smoking is one risk factor that can be changed. Home safety inspection and education regarding injury prevention strategies are essential (see Chapter 12). An assortment of print and interactive educational materials for both the lay and professional audience can be found at http://www.niams.nih.gov/Health_Info/Bone/Osteoporosis/default.asp.

Weight-bearing physical activity and exercises help to maintain bone mass (Box 18-2). Brisk walking and working with light weights apply mechanical force to the spine and long bones (see Chapter 10). Muscle-building exercises help to maintain skeletal architecture by improving muscle strength and flexibility. The Asian art of tai chi has been used successfully for strengthening of both ambulatory and nonambulatory elders (Wayne et al, 2007). Tai chi and exercise have the added advantage of improving balance and stamina, which may prevent falls or limit the damage if a fall should occur.

Patient teaching includes key aspects of the prevention and treatment of osteoporosis. Information about the sites most vulnerable to injury through accidents, falls, back strain, and poor posture should be provided. Explanation should be given about changes in the upper spine that occur when vertebrae are weakened, and about the pain that results from strain on the lower spine that is caused by the effort to compensate for balance and height changes attributable to alteration of the upper spine. Education also includes the appropriate way to take medications and how to handle their side effects.

Fall prevention is especially important to decrease the morbidity and mortality associated with osteoporosis. Shoes with good support should be worn. Handrails should be used, and walking in poorly lighted areas should be avoided. Basic body mechanics, such as how to lift heavy objects, should be learned. Use of step stools or chairs for reaching things in high places should be discouraged. Attention must be paid to home safety and improvements should include good lighting, railings, and other aids as needed. Walkways should be kept free of obstacles; loose rugs and electrical cords should be arranged so that they do not cause falls (see Chapter 12).

Pharmacological Interventions. Considerable progress has been made in the last decade in the development of pharmacological treatments for both the prevention and the treatment of osteoporosis. Adequate intake of calcium and vitamin D is recommended for persons at all ages and must be taken with all of the prescribed treatments currently available (Kessenich, 2007).

Ideally, optimal nutrition in late life has followed a lifetime of good eating habits (see Chapter 8). The diet during adolescence is probably a key to healthy bones later. A balanced diet that includes food sources of calcium is best (Table 18-1). Persons over 50 should ingest 1200 mg of calcium per day, which can come from combined dietary and supplementary sources (Kessenich, 2007). If using supplements, combination calcium-vitamin D (e.g., Caltrate-D) are recommended. The doses are best spread over the course of the day; for example, 400 mg of calcium is taken in the morning, 400 mg during the day, and another 400 mg before bed. The present recommendation includes the regular use of 400 to 800 international units of supplemental vitamin D (NIAMS, 2007). Patient teaching includes discussion of the factors that inhibit calcium absorption (e.g., excess alcohol, protein, or salt), excretion enhancers (e.g., caffeine; excess fiber; phosphorus in meats, sodas, and preserved foods); and the influence of the body's response to stress (decreased calcium absorption,

Box 18-2	Evidence-Based Practice: "Exercise Plus Program" for Older Women after Hip Fracture

Purpose
This study explores the experiences of older women after hip fracture who were involved in a home-based motivational intervention.

Sample and Setting
The study looked at 70 community-living older women (mean age 80.9) who had some type of surgical repair of a hip fracture and had completed the Exercise Plus Program. The program was implemented by certified exercise trainers and consisted of five exercise sessions (strength training and aerobic) of 30 minutes' duration each. The program was 1 year in duration.

Method
A naturalistic or constructivist inquiry with single open-ended interviews. Basic content analysis was used to analyze data.

Results
The following efficacy enhancement components of the program facilitated motivation:
- Confidence gained from repeatedly exercising and recognizing positive outcomes (e.g., exercise was good for me, exercise builds bone density), importance of a regular schedule
- Verbal encouragement from the trainers (warmth, kindness, and caring from trainers)
- Self-modeling and cues from written materials provided (knowing exactly what exercises to do and how and when to do them; visual cues and the exercise booklet helped)
- Eliminating unpleasant sensations associated with exercise (anxiety, fear of falling, fatigue, pain)

Implications
In setting up exercise programs, specific motivational interventions to encourage continuation of a regular exercise program are important. Focus for exercise programs should be on the benefit of exercise. Simple and clear guidelines for what exercise activity to engage in should be provided, individualized goals established, on-going encouragement and reinforcement of progress toward goals provided in a supportive and caring manner, and ways to overcome barriers to exercise explored. Interventions such as these will help older women to initiate and remain engaged in exercise over time.

Data from Resnick B et al: The Exercise Plus Program for older women post hip fracture: participant perspectives, *Gerontologist* 45(4):539-544, 2005.

increased excretion of calcium in the urine). Constipation, already a problem for many as they age, is worsened by calcium supplements and may reduce the person's willingness to take them. Good nursing care includes developing a preventive plan with the person, including the use of stool softeners and extra fluid intake if not contraindicated. Neither calcium nor calcium-enriched products can be taken at the same time as thyroid preparations.

The highly effective estrogen had been the drug of choice for women. However, the Women's Health Initiative found that although it increased BMD, it also increased the rate of breast cancer, colon cancer, and heart disease, and thus it is no longer recommended for use (Bruckner and Youngkin, 2002).

The currently available medications include bisphosphonates, selective estrogen receptor modulators (SERMs), and parathyroid hormone. All increase bone mass, reduce bone turnover, or both. The bisphosphonates (e.g., Fosamax, Actonel, and Boniva) are often prescribed in daily, weekly, or monthly formulations. However, owing to the seriousness of the risk for esophageal erosion, these must be taken on an empty stomach, with a full glass of water, and with the person completely upright for a half hour after ingestion. They are not appropriate for the person with memory loss or anyone else who cannot comply with the directions.

The SERM Evista is used as a substitute for estrogen and decreases the risk for breast cancer. It is approved for both the prevention and the treatment of

Table 18-1	Calcium Content of Several Common Foods	
FOOD ITEM	SERVING SIZE	CALCIUM (MG)
Plain yogurt, fat-free	8 oz	452
American cheese	2 oz	312
Yogurt with fruit (low fat or fat-free)	8 oz	345
Milk	8 oz	300
Orange juice, calcium-fortified	8 oz	350
Dried figs	10 figs	269
Cheese pizza	1 slice	240
Ricotta cheese, part skim	1/2 cup	334
Ice cream, soft serve	4 oz	103
Spinach	4 oz	139
Cooked soybeans	1 cup	298

Source: National Institutes of Health: *Sources of calcium,* Washington, DC. Available at www.nichd.nih.gov/milk. Accessed 11/1/08.

bone loss, but it can cause hot flashes and coagulation disorders and is contraindicated for use by anyone with a history of a deep venous thrombosis (DVT) or who is taking blood thinners.

The newest treatment for osteoporosis is daily injections of parathyroid hormone in the commercial form of teriparatide (Forteo). It is used for men and women at risk for fractures; however, it has only been approved for 2 years of use at this time (NIAMS, 2007). It is unknown what will happen to people after 2 years. The cost of this treatment can be prohibitive.

Another medication that is quite useful is calcitonin (Miacalcin). It is used to slow bone loss and increase spinal bone mineral density in women who are at least 5 years past menopause. It is not indicated for men. Calcitonin has been found to incidentally reduce back pain in some women. It is given either subcutaneously or as a nasal spray.

ARTHRITIS

Arthritis is the term used to refer to more than 100 diseases that affect 46.4 million individuals of all ages in the United States; this represents an increase in

osteoarthritis and gout but a decrease in rheumatoid arthritis. The overall number is expected to increase to 67 million by 2003 (Lawrence et al, 2008). Arthritis is the number one reason for activity limitations from middle age on. The most common forms of the disease that the gerontological nurse will encounter are osteoarthritis (OA), polymyalgia rheumatica (PMR), rheumatoid arthritis (RA), and gout.

Osteoarthritis

OA, the most common type of arthritis, is a degenerative joint disorder (DJD) that affects at least 20 million Americans. Risk factors include increased age, obesity, family history, and repetitive use of or trauma to the joint. Most persons over 65 will have radiographic evidence of OA even if they are asymptomatic. Native Americans have the highest prevalence of OA, and Asians and Pacific Islanders have the lowest. However, for all, arthritis causes joint stiffening and pain and eventually impairs functioning.

The osteoarthritic joint is one in which the normal soft and resilient cartilaginous lining becomes thin and damaged. This causes the joint space to narrow and the bones of the joint to rub together, causing destruction, pain, swelling, and loss of motion. Bone spurs (osteophytes) may develop in the spaces, causing deformation and deterioration (Figure 18-2). OA results from a complex interplay of many factors, including genetic predisposition, local inflammation, joint integrity, mechanical forces, and cellular and biochemical processes. Treatment is available to lessen pain and increase function (see Chapter 16).

In classic OA there is stiffness with inactivity, which is relieved by activity, and pain with activity, which is relieved by rest. The stiffness is greatest in the morning after the disuse during sleep but should resolve within 30 minutes of arising. As the disease advances, there is pain at rest as well, and more joints become involved. There may be joint instability, and crepitus may be felt or heard and is an indication of the deterioration of the joint. The joint will enlarge, and range of motion is reduced. OA of the cervical spine affects its curvature in a classic fashion (see Figure 18-1). The most common locations for OA are the knees, the hips, the neck (cervical spine), the lower back (lumbar spine), the fingers, and the thumbs (Figure 18-3). Less often it is found in the shoulders. Depression, anxiety, and decreased functional status are all associated with OA.

At this time OA cannot be "cured" without a joint replacement. Many elders elect this procedure for

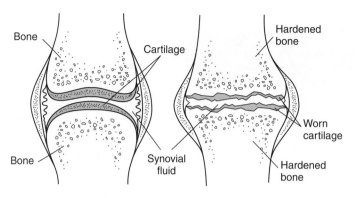

Fig. 18-2   Normal joint and diseased joint.

What Areas Does Osteoarthritis Affect?

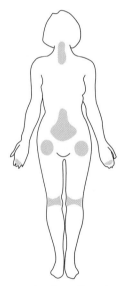

Fig. 18-3   Common locations for osteoarthritis. *(Source: National Institutes of Health: Handout on health osteoarthritis, Washington, DC. Available at http://www.niams.nih.gov/health_info/osteoarthritis/default.asp. Accessed 11/1/08.)*

hips and knees when the pain has become unbearable and the effect on function and quality of life becomes severe. The nurse is involved in the preoperative and perioperative periods and rehabilitation while the person is learning to use the new joint.

Polymyalgia Rheumatica and Giant Cell Arteritis

Polymyalgia rheumatica (PMR) is one of the more common inflammatory diseases seen in older adults. It may occur at the same time as OA, and the two may be difficult to distinguish from each other. The classic presentation of PMR is acute-onset pain beginning in the neck and upper arms and possibly evolving to the pelvic and pectoral girdles. Fatigue and low-grade fever may occur. Pain is usually greatest at night and in the early morning, but usually no joint inflammation is present.

PMR causes stiffness, which occurs especially in the morning and lasts more than 1 hour, as well as severe stiffness and pain in the muscles of the neck, shoulders, lower back, buttocks, and thighs, rather than the joints. The onset may develop very suddenly or slowly. Unlike OA, PMR resolves in 1 to 2 years and necessitates different treatment. Symptoms may be quickly relieved by small does of corticosteroids (Zimmerman-Górska, 2008).

PME rarely occurs in people under age 50 and occurs more often in women than in men; and more in whites in the United States and Europe with a fourfold increase in risk among women (Zimmerman-Górska, 2008). The cause is unknown, but is associated with immune disorders, genetic factors, and a recent infection (NIAMS, 2006b).

Giant cell arteritis (GCA) (also known as *temporal arteritis*) may occur at the same time as PMR. It is an acute inflammation of the arteries of the scalp, especially in the temporal area, which restricts blood flow. Sudden pain in the temporal area or changes in vision are always an emergency. If GCA is not treated early it can result in blindness. Treatment is with high-dose steroids.

Rheumatoid Arthritis

RA is a chronic, systemic, inflammatory joint disorder. It is considered an autoimmune disease in which products from the inflamed lining of the joint invade and destroy the cartilage and bone within the joint. The cause is unknown. RA affects more women then men; about 2.1 million people, or 0.5% to 1% of the U.S. adult population. It most often starts in midlife between the ages of 40 and 60 (Anderson, 2004).

RA is characterized by pain and swelling in multiple joints in a symmetrical pattern; for example, both hands will be affected at the same time. It generally affects the small joints of the wrist, the knee, the ankle, and the hand, although it can affect large joints as well. Whereas morning stiffness in OA lasts less than 30 minutes, in RA it lasts longer than 30 minutes. Since RA is a systemic disease, the person may feel generalized fatigue and malaise and have occasional fevers. The joints are warm and tender. Weight loss is common. The natural course of RA is highly variable, with good and bad days. The disease may last a few months or years or may become a chronic condition with progressive damage to the joints. Risk factors include environmental and genetic factors.

In the past, nonsteroidal antiinflammatory drugs (NSAIDs) were used for treatment early in the disease, and the use of the RA specific drugs was "saved" for later. However, it has been found that prompt efforts may halt or slow the damage (Anderson, 2004). Persons diagnosed with RA usually come under a rheumatologist's care, which involves aggressive therapy using a class of drugs called disease-modifying antirheumatic drugs (DMARDs). All the DMARDs are potentially toxic and are administered with care by a registered nurse, such as the charge nurse in a nursing home.

On-going care of the person with RA includes monitoring the progression of the disease and effectiveness of treatment as well as providing comfort and support. Support groups specific for persons with RA may help to empower, which in turn may improve their quality of life.

Gout

Gout is a common form of inflammatory arthritis in older adults (Ene-Stroescu and Gorbein, 2005). It appears to result from the accumulation of uric acid crystals in a joint. Uric acid is produced when purines found in food break down.

Gout typically starts with an acute attack. The person complains of exquisite pain in the affected joint, often starting in the middle of the night during sleep. The joint is bright purple-red, hot, and too painful to touch. After an acute attack, gout may become chronic with periodic acute "attacks." Risk factors include high blood pressure, a diet high in purines (see Box 18-3), and certain medications: thyazide diuretics, salicylates (e.g., aspirin), niacin, cyclosporines, and levodopa (Synamet) (NIAMS, 2006c).

After the acute attack the medical goal is to prevent another attack, systemic spread of the disease, and the development of chronic gout. This may be done with the avoidance of risk-elevating drugs, or of foods that are high in purine and alcohol, both of which increase uric acid levels; also, medications can be used to either decrease uric acid production (e.g., allopurinol, colchicine) or increase its excretion (e.g., probenecid) (Jett and Lester, 2004). The nurse ensures that the person takes in enough fluids to help flush the uric acid through the kidneys (2 L/day if not contraindicated).

The proximal joint of the great toe is the most typical site, although sometimes the ankle, the knee, the wrist, or the elbow is involved. The development of gout and the body's response to uric acid accumulation is highly individual. It is important to note that some people have elevated levels of uric acid and do not get gout, a clinical picture described as asymptomatic hyperuricemia, and others have gout and low levels of uric acid.

The nurse's roles include teaching the person side effects of medications, how to decrease the likelihood of another attack, and care of the joint. In administering gout-related medications the nurse pays close attention to renal function and notifies the physician or nurse practitioner of any change so that the dosages can be adjusted promptly.

Box 18-3	Examples of Foods High in Purines
Asparagus	Game meat
Beef kidneys	Gravy
Brain	Herring, mackerel, and sardines
Sweetbread	Mushrooms
Dried beans and peas	Scallops

IMPLICATIONS FOR GERONTOLOGICAL NURSING AND HEALTHY AGING

Assessment

When assessing the musculoskeletal system, the nurse examines the joints and muscles for tenderness, swelling, warmth, and redness. In OA, crepitus (a crackling sound) is felt or heard in the affected joints. The hands are examined for the presence or absence of osteophytes. If they appear in the distal joints as deformities of the fingers, they are called Heberden's nodes, and they are called Bouchard's nodes in the proximal joints. In GCA, the temporal arteries enlarge and become tender to touch.

Both passive and active range of motion are evaluated. How far can the person reach and bend all joints without assistance, and what are the reach, flexion, and extension with assistance? The testing of passive range of motion must go only to the point of discomfort and never to that of inducing pain. Test the functional ability of the arms by asking the person to touch the back of the head and the mid-back with both hands.

Interventions

The goals of intervention and management of the different forms of arthritis are to obtain treatment as soon as possible for inflammatory conditions, control pain, and minimize disability. The nurse is very involved in advocacy for adequate and prompt treatment, pain control, medication administration, evaluation, and patient teaching. The reader is referred to Chapter 16 for a discussion of pharmacological treatment of arthritis pain.

Other pharmacological agents used for pain control may include capsaicin cream, made from pepper plants available over the counter. In one study this was found to reduce pain by up to 40% in persons with OA (Grober and Thethi, 2003). It becomes effective after several days of use. Menthol and aspirin creams are also useful and are preferred by many elders.

Pain management and the minimization of disability are interconnected. To minimize disability with OA and RA, the joint must be used, strengthened, and protected.

For severe and disabling pain in the knees and the hips from OA, surgical replacement of the joint (arthroplasty) may be highly successful and restore the person to his or her previous level of functioning. Artificial joints last 10 to 15 years or longer (NIAMS, 2008). Nearly twice as many women as men have joint replacements. Surgical replacements are recommended for even the very old, in select cases.

It cannot be overstated that ongoing therapy from accredited physical therapists is necessary for persons with OA and RA to retain joint use. Weight loss, if necessary, and muscle building are highly recommended. In joint replacement, outcomes depend on the timing of surgery, the number of procedures that the surgeon has performed, the nursing care received, and the patient's medical status before the surgery and ability to participate in rehabilitation.

Exercise has been found to be the cornerstone to maintaining function with OA and RA. Regular exercise can improve flexibility and muscle strength, which in turn help to support the affected joints, reduce pain, and reduce falls. Walking, swimming, and water aerobics are preferred by many, and the latter is often available in senior centers, public pools, and YMCAs in many communities.

Attention should also be given to diet (see Chapter 8). With the decreases in activity associated with pain in all forms of arthritis, it is easy for the person to gain weight. Excess weight significantly increases the pressure and wear and tear on the body, leading to less activity and more weight gain. Weight reduction should be considered for all persons who are overweight. The nurse and the registered dietician will work with the person to identify realistic weight and caloric goals and develop meal plans that are personally and culturally acceptable but still balanced and healthy.

The use of heat and cold is well known in the management of pain in OA and RA. It should not be used in GCA. Patient preference is important, but cold usually works best for an acute process, for example the application of cold packs that decrease muscle spasm, decrease swelling, and relieve inflammatory pain. Heat may be applied superficially or deeply. Ultrasound provides deep heat. Hot packs, hydrotherapy, and radiant heat provide superficial heat. Liquid paraffin baths can be purchased in most drug stores for submerging the hands to provide deep heat and temporary relief (Wright, 2008).

Devices and techniques are available that relieve some of the pressure to the joints and protect the joints and muscles from further stress and, in doing so, to possibly decrease pain and improve balance and function. Canes, crutches, walkers, collars, shoe orthotics, and corsets are such devices in the case of OA and RA. A cane can relieve hip pressure by 60%. A shoe lift can improve lumbar pain. A knee brace is useful, especially if there is lateral instability (the knee "gives out"). If the hands are affected the person can avoid carrying packages by the fingers or can use utensils and household equipment with larger rather than smaller grips. Preventing the exposure of the affected joints to cold temperatures may also help. The person is encouraged to wear leggings, gloves, or scarves as necessary while out-of-doors. Canes may support the person with the muscle weakness which accompanies PMR.

Complementary and Alternative Interventions for OA

A number of complementary and alternative interventions show promise in contributing to pain relief for persons with arthritis. Among the most popular are the dietary supplements glucosamine and chondroitin sulfate, along with acupuncture and massage. While glucosamine and chondroitin have been used for some time as self-treatment, research has now found that their effect on pain is no better than placebos (Swatizke et al, 2008). McCaffrey and Freeman (2003) found a significant reduction in arthritic pain for persons listening to music. Research funded by the National Center for Complementary and Alternative Medicine has confirmed the effectiveness of acupuncture for the treatment of pain with OA (Berman, et al, 2004). Information about these and other techniques can be found at both the Arthritis Foundation and the National Institutes for Health websites (www.nccam.nih.gov).

Acupuncture, a technique used for centuries in China, is increasingly accepted in the United States and is being used in other countries as well. It is a practice of inserting very fine needles along what are called "meridians" on the body in locations specific to the problem. It is now believed that these stimulate the natural, pain-relieving endorphins produced by the nervous system.

APPLICATION OF MASLOW'S HIERARCHY

The acute postsurgical nursing care is designed to restore the physiological functions to address the first level of Maslow's Hierarchy of needs: maintaining fluids, movement, and nutritional adequacy. Effective pain management is critical to ensure that the individual is quickly able to participate in rehabilitation, essential for maximum recovery.

To provide care to the whole person with musculoskeletal disorders the nurse works with a number of approaches and teaches and empowers the person to participate fully in achieving the highest level of wellness possible at all levels of the Hierarchy.

▶ KEY CONCEPTS

- ▶ Most people over the age of 40 will have osteoarthritis at some point in their lives.
- ▶ Osteoporosis is a crippling problem for many elders, especially women. Although it cannot be completely prevented, it can be minimized by early interventions: exercise, weight bearing, and calcium and vitamin D intake.
- ▶ The most serious outcomes of osteoporosis are fractures, which are associated with high mortality.
- ▶ Rheumatoid arthritis produces swelling, inflammation, intense pain, and distortion of the joints.
- ▶ Gout is both an acute and a chronic condition. One of the goals of treatment with gout is to minimize a future attack.
- ▶ Certain types of complementary and alternative interventions have been found to be very helpful to individuals with joint disorders and chronic discomfort.

▶ ACTIVITIES AND DISCUSSION QUESTIONS

1. What are the most effective ways of preventing osteoporosis?
2. What lifestyle issues would you discuss with an individual with advanced osteoporosis?
3. What are the differences in appearance of osteoarthritis and rheumatoid arthritis?
4. What advice would you give someone who is experiencing joint pain and mobility limitations?
5. Discuss your thoughts and experiences relating to alternative methods of dealing with chronic pain.
6. Which of your favorite activities would be difficult if you were afflicted with osteoarthritis?

▶ RESOURCES

Websites
The Arthritis Foundation
www.arthritis.org

National Institute for Arthritis and Musculoskeletal Systems
www.niams.nih.gov

National Institute of Health
Office of Alternative Medicine
www.altmed.od.nih.gov

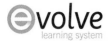

For additional resources, please visit evolve.elsevier.com/Ebersole/gerontological.

REFERENCES

Anderson DL: TNF inhibitors: a new age in rheumatoid arthritis treatment, *Am J Nurs* 104(2):60-68, 2004.

Berman BM, Lao L, Langenberg P et al: Effectiveness of acupuncture as adjunctive therapy in osteoarthritis of the knee: a randomized, controlled trial, *Ann Int Med* 141(12): 901-910, 2004.

Brucker MC, Youngkin EQ: What's a woman to do? Exploring HRT questions raised by the women's health initiative, *AWHONN Lifelines* 6(5):408-417, 2002.

Ene-Stroescu D, Gorbein MJ: Gouty arthritis: A primer in late-onset gout, *Geriatrics* 60(7): 24-31, 2005.

Jett KF, Lester PB: Musculoskeletal disorders. In Youngkin EQ, Sawin K, Israel D, editors: *Pharmcotherapeutics*, ed 2, Upper Saddle River, NJ, 2004, Prentice-Hall.

Kessenich CR: Calcium and vitamin D supplementation for postmenopausal bone health, *JNP* 3(3):155-160, 2007.

Lawrence RC, Felson DT, Hemlick CG et al: Estimates of the prevalence of arthritis and other rheumatic conditions in the United States. Part II, *Arthritis Rheum* 58(1):26-35, 2008.

McCaffrey R, Freeman E: Effects of music on chronic osteoarthritis pain in older people, *J Adv Nurs* 44(5):517-524, 2003.

National Institute of Arthritis and Musculoskeletal and Skin Diseases (NIAMS). *Osteoporosis and ethnic or racial background*, 2006a. Available at http://www.niams.nih.gov/Health_Info/Bone/Osteoporosis/Background/default.asp. Accessed 10/31/08.

National Institute of Arthritis and Musculoskeletal and Skin Diseases (NIAMS): *Polymyalgia rheumatica and giant cell arteritis,* 2006b. Available at www.niams.nih.gov/Health_Info/Polymyalgia/default.asp. Accessed 7/21/08

National Institute of Arthritis and Musculoskeletal and Skin Diseases (NIAMS). *Gout,* 2006c. Available at http://www.niams.nih.gov/Health_Info/Gout/default.asp#cause. Accessed 10/31/08.

National Institute of Arthritis and Musculoskeletal and Skin Diseases (NIAMS). *Osteoporosis,* 2007. Available from http://www.niams.nih.gov/Health_Info/Bone/Osteoporosis/default.asp. Accessed 10/31/08.

National Institute of Arthritis and Musculoskeletal and Skin Diseases (NIAMS). *Once is enough: A guide to prevention fractures,* 2008. Available at http://www.niams.nih.gov/Health_Info/Bone/Osteoporosis/Fracture/preventing_fracture.pdf. Accessed 10/31/08.

U.S. Prevention Services Task Force: *Screening for osteoporosis,* 2002. Available from www.acpr.gov. Accessed 11/1/08.

Sawitzke AD, Shi H, Finco MF et al: The effects of glucosamine and/or chondroitin on the progression of knee osteoarthritis: a report form the glucosamine/chondroitin arthritis intervention trial. *Arthritis Rheum* 58(10): 3183-91, 2008.

Wayne P, Kiel D, Krebs DE et al. The effects of Tai Chi on bone mineral density in postmenopausal women: a systematic review. *Arch Phys Med Rehabil* 88(5):673-80, 2007.

Wright W: Management of mild-to-moderate osteoarthritis: effective intervention by the nurse practitioner, *JNP* 4(1):25-43, 2008.

Zimmerman-Górska I: Polymyalgia rheumatica: clinical picture and principles of treatment, *Pol J Intern Med* 118(6):377-389, 2008.

Diseases Affecting Vision and Hearing

LEARNING OBJECTIVES

Upon completion of this chapter, the reader will be able to:

- Discuss diseases of the eye and ear that may occur in older adults.
- Describe the importance of screening, health education, and treatment of eye diseases to prevent unnecessary vision loss in older adults.
- Increase awareness of the resources available to assist elders with visual and hearing impairments.

GLOSSARY

Drusen Yellow deposits under the retina, often found in people over the age of 60.

Funduscopy Opthalmoscopic examination of the fundus of the eye.

Keratoconjunctivitis sicca Diminished tear production with age.

Lipofuscin Fatty brown pigment found in the tissues related to aging.

Tonometry The procedure used by eye care professionals to determine the intraocular pressure of the eye.

LIVED EXPERIENCE

My Eyes Are Failing

For quite a while now, I've been pretending. That it was just that I was tired. That the light was bad. But my eyes are really getting worse. I'm afraid to go to the doctor because I'm afraid of what he'll say. Which is silly. Either there is something to be done. Or there is not. If it's glasses, hallelujah, and help me find the money. If it's an operation, see me through. If I am going blind, hold me. Help me put down the terror that rises in my gut at the word. Blind. There. I've said it. The ghost word that has been haunting me. Help me remember, if I have to walk in the dark, that I have had a lot of years of seeing clean and clear. I know the slender shape of a birch tree. I have seen thousands and thousands of things in my life. I can conjure them in my mind's eye. No matter what happens, I shall not be without beautiful sights. It is just that I may have to settle for the ones I have already seen.

This chapter discusses diseases that affect vision and hearing in older adults. *Healthy People 2010* (U.S. Department of Health and Human Services [USDHHS], 2001) has set goals for vision and hearing (see Boxes 3-8 and 3-3, respectively). Age-related changes in vision and hearing are discussed in Chapter 6, assessment of vision and hearing in Chapter 13, and communication adaptations for elders with vision and hearing loss in Chapter 3. An extensive resource list related to vision and hearing loss can be found at the end of Chapter 3 and at evolve.elsevier.com/Ebersole/gerontological.

Because visual and hearing impairments affect most daily activities such as driving, reading, maneuvering safely, dressing, cooking, and engaging in social activities, it is very important to assess the effect of these changes on functional abilities, safety, and quality of life. The issues of concern to nurses who care for older adults are appropriate assessment of age-related vision and hearing loss compared to those caused by disease; health teaching for prevention of diseases that affect vision and hearing; referral for appropriate treatment of eye and ear diseases; devising methods to keep the senses functional enough to negotiate the environment safely and effectively; and compensating for sensory losses by supplementing the remaining senses with additional pleasures. The task is to augment and maximize sensory experiences when senses are diminished and to help design a colorful, rewarding environment that fits the needs and abilities of the individual.

DISEASES AFFECTING VISION

For elders with visual impairments, the consequences for functional ability, safety, and quality of life can be profound. Vision loss may be underestimated by health care professionals and it is important to identify elders who have visual impairment. In addition to appropriate assessment, certain signs and behaviors of visual problems that should prompt the nurse to action are noted in Box 19-1.

The major diseases affecting vision are glaucoma, cataracts, macular degeneration, and diabetic retinopathy. To help the student understand more about these diseases, the following website provides a simulation of glaucoma, cataracts, macular degeneration, and diabetic retinopathy: http://visionsimulator.com/.

Vision loss from eye disease is a global concern, particularly in the developing countries, where 90% of the world's blind individuals live. Estimates are that more than 75% of the world's blindness is preventable or treatable. Vision 2020 is a global

---

> **Box 19-1   Signs and Behaviors That May Indicate Vision Problems**
>
> **What Individuals May Report:**
> Pain in eyes
> Difficulty seeing in darkened area
> Double vision and/or distorted vision
> Migraine headaches coupled with blurred vision
> Flashes of light
> Halos surrounding lights
> Difficulty driving at night
> Falls or injuries
>
> **What Health Care Staff May Notice:**
> Getting lost
> Bumping into objects
> Straining to read or not reading
> Stumbling and/or falling
> Spilling food on clothing
> Social withdrawal
> Less eye contact
> Placid facial expression
> TV viewing at close range
> Decreased sense of balance
> Mismatched clothes
>
> Modified from McNeely E, Griffin-Shirley N, Hubbard A: Teaching caregivers to recognize diminished vision among nursing home residents, *Geriatr Nurs* 13(6):332-335, 1992.

initiative for the elimination of avoidable blindness, launched jointly by the World Health Organization (WHO) and the International Agency for the Prevention of Blindness (http://v2020.org/default.asp). A recent survey conducted in the United States reported that among all racial and ethnic groups participating in the survey, Hispanic respondents reported the lowest access to eye health information, knew the least about eye health, and were the least likely to have their eyes examined (National Eye Institute, 2008). Clearly, prevention and treatment of eye diseases is an important priority for nurses and other health care professionals.

Glaucoma

Glaucoma is a major public health problem in the United States. The disease affects about 2.2 million Americans ages 40 and over, half of whom are not aware they have the disease. There are several types of glaucoma: primary open-angle glaucoma, low tension or normal tension glaucoma, and acute angle-closure glaucoma, which is an emergency. The etiology of glaucoma is variable and often unknown; however, when the natural fluids of the eye are blocked by ciliary muscle rigidity and the buildup of pressure, damage to the optic nerve occurs. Glaucoma can be bilateral, but it more commonly occurs in one eye.

Open-angle glaucoma accounts for about 80% of cases and is asymptomatic until very late in the disease, when there is a noticeable loss in visual fields. Glaucoma has been described as the "silent thief" because it will steal vision with no forewarning (Higginbotham et al, 2004). When glaucoma is diagnosed in elders, many of whom have undiagnosed glaucoma that has not been screened or evaluated, about 20% of loss of visual fields is found to have already occurred (Luggen, 2001). However, if detected early, glaucoma can usually be controlled and serious vision loss prevented. Signs of glaucoma include headaches, poor vision in dim lighting, increased sensitivity to glare, "tired eyes," impaired peripheral vision, a fixed and dilated pupil, and frequent changes in prescriptions for corrective lenses (Miller, 2008). Figure 19-1 illustrates the effects of glaucoma on vision.

An acute attack of angle-closure glaucoma is characterized by a rapid rise in intraocular pressure (IOP) accompanied by redness and pain in and around the eye, severe headache, nausea and vomiting, and blurring of vision. It occurs when the path of the aqueous humor is blocked and intraocular pressure builds up to more than 50 mm Hg. If untreated, blindness can occur in 2 days. An iridectomy, however, can ease pressure. Many drugs with anticholinergic properties including antihistamines, stimulants, vasodilators, clonidine, and sympathomimetics, are particularly dangerous for patients predisposed to angle-closure glaucoma. Older people with glaucoma should be counseled to review all medications, both over-the-counter and prescribed, with their primary care provider.

Low tension or normal tension glaucoma is a type of glaucoma that also occurs in older adults. In this type, intraocular pressure is within normal range but there is damage to the optic nerve and narrowing of the visual fields. The cause is unknown, but risk factors include a family history of any kind of glaucoma, Japanese ancestry, and cardiovascular disease. Management consists of the same medications and surgical interventions that are used for chronic glaucoma (Glaucoma Research Foundation, 2008).

A family history of glaucoma, as well as diabetes, steroid use, and past eye injuries have been noted as risk factors for the development of glaucoma. Age is the single most important predictor of glaucoma, and older women are affected twice as frequently as older men. Among African Americans, glaucoma is the leading cause of blindness. African Americans develop glaucoma at younger ages, and the incidence of the disease is 6 to 8 times more common in African Americans than in whites. Mexican Americans are also at higher risk for glaucoma (National Eye Institute, 2006a). Among African Americans, other factors that may contribute to the high incidence of the disease include earlier onset of the disease as compared with other races, later detection

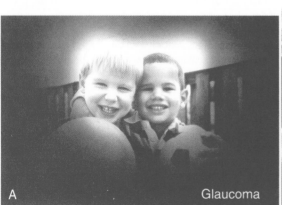
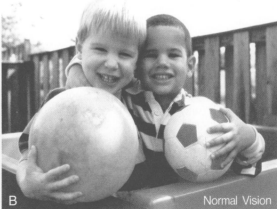

Fig. 19-1   A, Simulated vision with glaucoma. B, Normal vision. *(From National Eye Institute, National Institutes of Health, 2004).*

of the disease, and economic and social barriers to treatment (Boyd-Monk, 2005).

Management of glaucoma involves medications (oral or topical eye drops) to decrease IOP and/or laser surgery. Medications lower eye pressure either by decreasing the amount of aqueous fluid produced within the eye or by improving the flow through the drainage angle. Beta blockers are the first-line therapy for glaucoma, and the patient may need combinations of several types of eye drops. When caring for older adults in the hospital or long-term care settings, it is important to obtain a past medical history to determine if the person has glaucoma and to ensure that eye drops are given according to the person's treatment regimen. Without the eye drops, eye pressure can rise and cause an acute exacerbation of glaucoma (Capezuti et al, 2008). Usually medications can control glaucoma, but laser surgery treatments (trabeculoplasty) may be recommended for some types of glaucoma. Surgery is usually recommended only if necessary to prevent further damage to the optic nerve.

Screening

Adults over the age of 65 should have annual eye examinations, and those with medication-controlled glaucoma should be examined at least every 6 months. Annual screening is also recommended for African Americans and other individuals with a family history of glaucoma who are older than 40. A dilated eye examination and tonometry are necessary to diagnose glaucoma. These procedures can be performed by a primary care provider, optometrist, or a nurse practitioner, who will then refer the person to an ophthalmologist is glaucoma is suspected. Medicare pays for annual screening for glaucoma but only in high-risk patients.

Cataracts

Cataracts are a prevalent disorder among older adults caused by oxidative damage to lens protein and fatty deposits (lipofuscin) in the ocular lens. By age 80, more than half of all Americans either have a cataract or have had cataract surgery. When lens opacity reduces visual acuity to 20/30 or less in the central axis of vision, it is considered a cataract. Cataracts are categorized according to their location within the lens and are usually bilateral. They are virtually universal in the very old but may be only minimally visible, particularly in individuals with pale irises.

Cataracts are recognized by the clouding of the ordinarily clear ocular lens; the red reflex may be absent or may appear as a black area. The cardinal sign of cataracts is the appearance of halos around objects as light is diffused. Other common symptoms include blurring, decreased perception of light and color (giving a yellow tint to most things), and sensitivity to glare. Figure 19-2 illustrates the effects of a cataract on vision.

The most common causes of cataracts are heredity and advancing age. They may occur more frequently and at earlier ages in individuals who have been exposed to excessive sunlight, have poor dietary habits, diabetes, hypertension, kidney disease, eye trauma, or history of alcohol intake and tobacco use. Cataracts are more likely to occur after glaucoma surgery or other types of eye surgery. There is some evidence that a high dietary intake of lutein and zeaxanthin, compounds found in yellow or dark leafy vegetables, as well as intake of vitamin E from food and supplements, appears to lower the risk of cataracts in women. Further research is indicated (Moeller et al, 2008).

When visual acuity decreases to 20/50 and the cataract affects safety or quality of life, surgery is recommended (Miller, 2008). Cataract surgery is the most common surgical procedure performed in the United States. Most often, cataract surgery involves only local anesthesia and is one of the most successful surgical procedures, with 95% of patients reporting excellent vision after surgery. The surgery involves removal of the lens and placement of a plastic intraocular lens (IOL). If the plastic lens is not inserted, the patient may wear a contact lens or glasses. This is not commonly done because the older adult may have difficulty placing and removing the contact lens, and the glasses would be very thick. Cataract surgery is performed with local anesthesia on an outpatient basis, and the procedure has greatly improved with advances in surgical techniques.

Nursing interventions when caring for the person experiencing cataract surgery include preparing the individual for significant changes in vision and adaptation to light and insuring that the individual has received adequate counseling regarding realistic postsurgical expectations. Postsurgical teaching includes covering the need to avoid heavy lifting, straining, and bending at the waist. Eye drops may be prescribed to aid healing and prevent infection. If the person has bilateral cataracts, surgery is performed first on one eye with the second surgery on the other eye a month or so later to ensure healing (Tabloski, 2006).

Although race is not a factor in cataract formation, racial disparities exist in cataract surgery in the

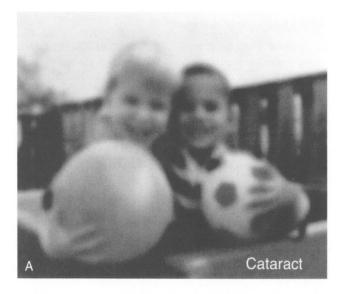

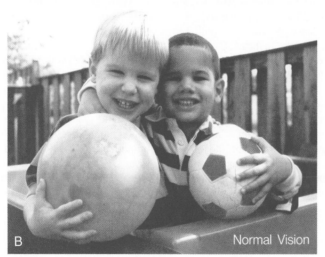

Fig. 19-2 A, Simulated vision with cataracts. B, Normal vision. *(From National Eye Institute, National Institutes of Health, 2004).*

United States, with African American Medicare recipients only 60% as likely as whites to undergo cataract surgery (Miller, 2008; Wilson and Eezzuduemhoi, 2005). Cataracts are of even greater concern in Africa and Asia and account for at least half of the blindness in those countries despite the well known technology that can restore vision at an extremely low cost. Recommendations from Vision 2020 include reducing the backlog of the cataract-blind by increased training of ophthalmic personnel, strength-

ening of the health care infrastructure, and provision of needed surgical supplies in these countries (www. who.int/ncd/vision2020_actionplan/documents/ V2020priorities.pdf2004).

Unfortunately, cataracts and other related eye diseases such as maculopathy, diabetic retinopathy, or glaucoma often occur simultaneously, which complicates the management of each. Individuals who have had cataract surgery are less likely to be effectively treated with surgery for glaucoma.

Diabetic Retinopathy

Some visual disabilities are acquired through the deleterious effects of elevated blood sugar due to diabetes. "Diabetic retinopathy is considered a disease of the retinal microvasculature and is characterized by increased vessel permeability. Blood and lipid leakage leads to macular edema and hard exudates (composed of lipids). In advanced disease, new fragile blood vessels form that hemorrhage easily" (Whiteside et al, 2006, p. 55). Because of the vascular and cellular changes accompanying diabetes, there is often rapid worsening of other pathologic vision conditions as well.

Diabetic retinopathy is the third leading cause of blindness in the United States, and the incidence curves abruptly with increasing age. Approximately 4.1 million U.S. adults 40 and older have diabetic retinopathy; 1 of every 12 persons with diabetes in this age group has advanced, vision-threatening retinopathy (National Eye Institute, 2006b). Most diabetic patients will develop diabetic retinopathy within 20 years of diagnosis.

There is little to no evidence of retinopathy until 3 to 5 years or more after the onset of diabetes. Early signs are seen in the funduscopic examination and include microaneurysms, flame-shaped hemorrhages, cotton wool spots, hard exudates, and dilated capillaries. Constant, strict control of blood glucose, cholesterol, and blood pressure and laser photocoagulation treatments can halt progression of the disease (Ham et al, 2007). Laser treatment can reduce vision loss in 50% of patients. Annual dilated funduscopic examination of the eye is recommended beginning 5 years after diagnosis of diabetes type 1 and at the time of diagnosis of diabetes type 2.

Macular Degeneration

Age-related macular degeneration (AMD) is the most common cause of legal blindness and the most common visual impairment of individuals over the age of 50. The prevalence of AMD increases drastically with age, with more than 15% of white women over the age of 80 having the disease. Whites and Asian Americans seem to be more vulnerable to AMD than African Americans or Mexican Americans (Feret et al, 2007). With the number of older adults affected projected to increase over the next 20 years, AMD has been called a growing epidemic (Bressler et al, 2004).

AMD is a degenerative eye disease that affects the macula, the central part of the eye responsible for clear central vision. The disease causes the progressive loss of central vision, leaving only peripheral vision intact. It usually starts in one eye, but there is a high risk (greater than 40%) that the disease will affect the other eye within 5 years (Bressler et al, 2003). Early signs of AMD include difficulty reading and driving, increased need for bright light, colors that appear dim or gray, and an awareness of a blurry spot in the middle of vision (Feret et al, 2007). Figure 19-3 illustrates the effects of AMD on vision.

AMD results from systemic changes in circulation, accumulation of cellular waste products, tissue atrophy, and growth of abnormal blood vessels in the choroid layer beneath the retina. Fibrous scarring disrupts nourishment of photoreceptor cells, causing their death and loss of central vision. The greatest risk factor for AMD is age. Although etiology is unknown, risk factors are thought to include genetic predisposition, smoking, obesity, family history, and excessive sunlight exposure.

There are two forms of macular degeneration, the "dry" form and the "wet" form. Dry AMD accounts for the majority of cases and rarely causes severe visual impairment, but can lead to the more aggressive wet AMD. Dry AMD has three stages, which may occur in one or both eyes (Box 19-2). One in 10 persons with early AMD will develop the advanced form (Feret et al, 2007). Dry AMD occurs when the light-sensitive cells in the macula slowly break down, blurring central vision in the affected eye. As dry AMD gets worse, the individual may see a blurred spot in the center of vision. One of the most common early signs is drusen. Drusen are yellow deposits under the retina and are often found in people over the age of 60. The relationship between drusen and AMD is not clear, but an increase in the size or number of drusen increases the risk of developing either advanced AMD or wet AMD (National Eye Institute, 2006c).

Wet AMD occurs when abnormal blood vessels behind the retina start to grow under the macula. These new blood vessels are fragile and often leak blood and fluid, which raise the macula from its normal place at the back of the eye. With wet AMD, the severe loss of central vision can be rapid, and many people will be legally blind within 2 years of diagnosis. Peripheral vision usually remains normal, but the person will have difficulty seeing at a distance or doing detailed work such as sewing or reading. Faces may begin to blur, and it become harder to distinguish colors. An early sign may be distortion that causes edges or lines to appear wavy. An Amsler grid is used to determine clarity of central vision (Figure 19-4). A perception of wavy lines

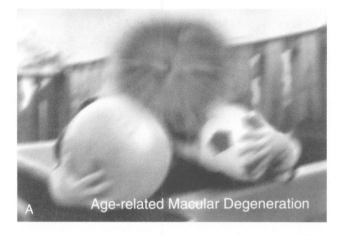

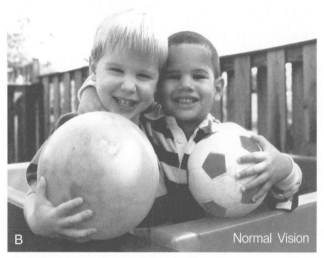

Fig. 19-3   A, Simulated vision with age-related macular degeneration (AMD). B, Normal vision. *(From National Eye Institute, National Institutes of Health, 2004).*

is diagnostic of beginning macular degeneration, and vision loss can occur in days. In the advanced forms, the person may begin to see dark or empty spaces that block the center of vision. According to Miller (2008, p. 345), "People with AMD are usually taught to test their eyes daily using the Amsler grid so that they will be aware of sudden changes."

Patients in the early stage of the disease may attribute their vision problems to normal aging or cataracts. Early diagnosis is the key, and individuals over the age of 40 should have an eye examination at least every 2 years. The National Eye Institute's Age-Related Eye Disease Study (AREDS) (www.nei.nih.gov/) found that a high-dose formulation of antioxidants and zinc significantly

reduces the risk of advanced AMD and associated vision loss. Individuals with intermediate AMD in one or both eyes or advanced AMD (wet form) in one eye but not the other should consider taking the formulation (Box 19-3) (National Eye Institute, 2006c).

Treatment of wet AMD includes photodynamic therapy (PDT) and laser photocoagulation (LPC). Lucentis and Avastin (anti–vascular endothelial growth factor (VEGF) therapy), are biological drugs that are the most common form of treatment in advanced AMD. Abnormally high levels of a specific growth factor occur in eyes with wet AMD, which promote the growth of abnormal blood vessels. Anti-VEGF therapy blocks the effect of the growth factor. These drugs are injected

---

Box 19-2 | Stages of Dry Age-related Macular Degeneration (AMD)

1. Early AMD: People in this stage may have several small drusen or a few medium-sized drusen. At this stage, there are no symptoms and no vision loss.
2. Intermediate AMD: People at this stage have either many medium-sized drusen or one or more large drusen. Some people see a blurred spot in the center of their vision. More light may be required for reading and other tasks.
3. Advanced AMD: In addition to drusen, there is a breakdown of light-sensitive cells and supporting tissues in the central retinal area. This may cause a blurred spot in the center of vision, which may get bigger and bigger. There may be difficulty reading or recognizing faces until they are very close.

From: National Eye Institute: Facts about age-related macular degeneration, 2006. Accessed 3/13/08 from www.nei.nih.gov/health/maculardegen/armd_facts.asp.

Box 19-3 | AREDS Formulation Recommendations

- Vitamin C 500 milligrams
- Vitamin E 400 international units
- Beta carotene 15 milligrams (often labeled as equivalent to 25,000 international units of vitamin A
- Zinc oxide 80 milligrams
- Copper (cubric oxide) 2 milligrams

AREDS, Age-Related Eye Disease Study.

Source: National Eye Institute: *Age-related macular degeneration,* 2006. Accessed 11/5/08 from www.nei.nih.gov/amd/summary.asp; The Age-Related Eye Disease Study Research Group: A randomized placebo-controlled, clinical trial of high-dose supplementation with vitamins C and E, beta carotene, and zinc for age-related macular degeneration and vision loss, *Arch Opthalmol* 119(10):1417-1436.

---

into the eye as often as once a month and can help slow vision loss from AMD, and in some cases can improve sight. Other treatments being researched include gene therapy, human retinal transplantation, antiinflammatory treatment, artificial vision, retinal prosthesis, and neuroprotection (Feret et al, 2007).

Giant Cell (Temporal) Arteritis

Although not a disease of the eye, giant cell arteritis (GCA) can cause vision loss. GCA is an autoimmune disease that causes inflammation of the temporal artery. It primarily affects persons older than 50 years (Hellmann and Stone, 2006). Symptoms include malaise, scalp tenderness, unilateral temporal headache, jaw claudication, throat pain, and sudden vision loss (usually unilateral). The vision loss is considered a medical

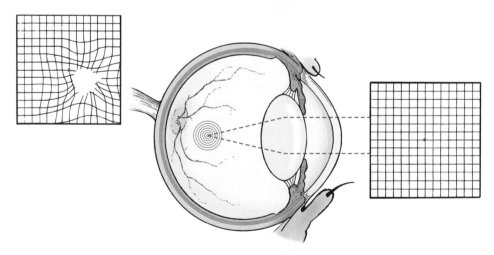

Fig. 19-4   Macular degeneration: distortion of center vision; normal peripheral vision. *(Illustration by Harried R. Greenfield, Newton, MA).*

emergency because of the possibility of ensuing blindness. It is potentially reversible if identified immediately. If the symptom develops, the individual needs to see an ophthalmologist or go to an emergency room immediately

Detached Retina

This condition can develop in persons with cataracts or recent cataract surgery or trauma, or can occur spontaneously. It manifests as a curtain coming down over the person's line of vision. It necessitates immediate emergency treatment.

Dry Eye

Dry eye is not a disease of the eye but is a frequent complaint among older people. Tear production normally diminishes as we age. The condition is termed keratoconjunctivitis sicca. It occurs most commonly in women after menopause. There may be age-related changes in the mucin-secreting cells necessary for surface wetting, in the lacrimal glands, or in the meibomian glands that secrete surface oil, and all of these may occur at the same time (Beers and Berkow, 2000). The older person will describe a dry, scratchy feeling in mild cases (xerophthalmia). There may be marked discomfort and decreased mucus production in severe situations.

Medications can cause dry eye, especially antihistamines, diuretics, beta blockers, and some sleeping pills. The problem is diagnosed by an ophthalmologist using a Schirmer tear test, in which filter paper strips are placed under the lower eyelid to measure the rate of tear production. A common treatment is artificial tears, but dry eyes may be sensitive to them because of preservatives, which can be irritating. The ophthalmologist may close the tear duct channel either temporarily or permanently. Other management methods include keeping the house air moist with humidifiers, avoiding wind and hair dryers, and the use of artificial tear ointments at bedtime. Vitamin A deficiency can be a cause of dry eye, and vitamin A ointments are available for treatment. Sjögren's syndrome, which can occur in elderly people, is a cell-mediated autoimmune disease whose manifestations include decreased lacrimal gland activity. Systemic manifestations of the autoimmune disease include Raynaud's phenomenon, polyarthritis, interstitial pneumonitis, vasculitis, psychiatric manifestations, and loss of exocrine functions (Beers and Berkow, 2000).

DISEASES OF THE EAR

Tinnitus

Tinnitus is defined as the perception of sound in the absence of acoustic stimulus. It is characterized by ringing in the ear and may also manifest as buzzing, hissing, whistling, cricket chirping, bells, roaring, clicking, pulsating, humming, or swishing sounds. The most common type is high-pitched tinnitus with sensorineural loss; less common is low-pitched tinnitus with conduction loss such as is seen in Meniere's disease. The sounds may be constant or intermittent and are more acute at night or in quiet surroundings.

Tinnitus generally increases over time. It is a condition that afflicts many older people and can interfere with hearing, as well as become extremely irritating. It is estimated to occur in nearly 11% of elders with presbycusis. Approximately 50 million people in the United States have tinnitus, and 12 million people are estimated to have tinnitus to a distressing degree (American Tinnitus Association, 2007). The incidence of tinnitus peaks between ages 65 and 74 and is higher in men than in women; in men, the incidence seems to decrease after this age. Tinnitus is the most commonly referred otological problem (American Tinnitus Association, 2007).

Tinnitus can be caused by loud noises, excessive cerumen or auditory canal obstruction, disorders of the cervical vertebrae or the temporomandibular joint, allergies, an underactive thyroid, cardiovascular disease, tumors, conductive hearing loss, anxiety, depression, degeneration of the bones in the middle ear, infections, or trauma to the head or ear. In addition, more than 200 prescription and nonprescription medications list tinnitus as a potential side effect, aspirin being the most common.

Assessment

Tinnitus may be described as pulsatile (matching the beating of the heart) or nonpulsatile (unilateral, asymmetric, or symmetric). Tinnitus may be subjective (audible only to the person) or objective (audible to the examiner). Subjective tinnitus is more common. Objective tinnitus is rare and is frequently due to a vascular or neuromuscular condition. The mechanisms of tinnitus are unknown but have been thought to be analogous to cross-talk on telephone wires, phantom limb pain, or transmission of vascular sounds such as bruits. A simulation of the sounds of tinnitus can be found on the American Tinnitus Foundation website: www.ata.org.

A Tinnitus Handicap Questionnaire developed by Newman et al (1995) measures physical, emotional, and social consequences of tinnitus. It also can be used to assess the changes the individual experiences with treatment. Some persons with tinnitus will never find the cause; for others the problem may arbitrarily disappear. Hearing aids can be prescribed to amplify environmental sounds to obscure tinnitus, and there is a device that combines the features of a masker and a hearing aid, which emits a competitive but pleasant sound that distracts from head noise. Therapeutic modes of treating tinnitus include transtympanal electrostimulation, iontophoresis, biofeedback, tinnitus masking with alternative sound production (white noise), dental treatment, cochlear implants, and hearing aids. Some have found hypnosis, acupuncture, chiropractic, naturopathic, allergy, or drug treatment to be effective.

Interventions

Nursing actions include discussions with the client regarding times when the noises are most irritating and having the person keep a diary to identify patterns. There is some evidence that caffeine, alcohol, cigarettes, stress, and fatigue may exacerbate the problem. Assess medications for possibly contributing to the problem. Discuss lifestyle changes and alternative methods that some have found effective. Also, refer clients to the American Tinnitus Association for research updates, education, and support groups.

Prelingual Deafness

Prelingual deafness in older adults is rarely addressed because it is assumed that individuals deaf since childhood have learned to communicate early in life through the use of sign language. Until 50 years ago, it was common for deaf children to be placed in a state school for the deaf to develop within a culture of their own; therefore many elders with prelingual deafness will have had an entirely different childhood than those with hearing. The prelingual deaf often learn audible speech and/or sign language and lip reading very well. However, their reading and writing skills may be impaired even though their intelligence is normal. For those dependent on visual cues, communication can also be compromised when vision changes occur. For these individuals, signing is their first language and English their second. Subtleties of verbal communication may be lost to them, although they often compensate and become extremely alert to nonverbal cues and feelings. At times a certified interpreter, who is well established in the network of the deaf world, will be needed.

IMPLICATIONS FOR GERONTOLOGICAL NURSING AND HEALTHY AGING

When vision and hearing are impaired, the elder is deprived of major sensory input, which has a direct effect on his or her everyday life. Such sensory losses can potentiate isolation, depression, withdrawal, and loss of self-esteem; raise personal safety issues; and affect health. Nurses can take a leadership role in education about diseases of the eye and the ear, particularly for racially and culturally diverse elders. To promote healthy aging and quality of life, gerontological nurses in all settings must be knowledgeable about the impact of hearing and vision changes on the functional abilities and quality of life of older adults, vision and hearing assessment, prevention and treatment of diseases affecting vision and hearing, effective communication techniques, and ways to assist the individual in adapting to and compensating for these losses.

In assessment of vision and hearing losses, it is important to include the impact of losses on functional ability, mood, and quality of life. A recent study found that depression frequently develops within a few months after AMD is diagnosed in both eyes. Problem-solving training sessions in conjunction with usual medical care were found to correlate with less depression than in those receiving usual care (Rovner et al, 2007). The problem-solving sessions, led by a nurse or counselor in the patient's homes, focused on identifying problems caused by loss of eyesight and finding ways to compensate.

APPLICATION OF MASLOW'S HIERARCHY

Hearing and vision impairments can contribute to challenges at all levels of the hierarchy from meeting biological integrity needs, such as activity, safety, and security needs to the higher-level needs such as a sense of belonging, feeling of self-esteem, and self-actualization. The consequences of these impairments severely affect quality of life and predispose the individual to potential negative health and quality of life outcomes. Whatever the age or the impairments experienced, continued growth and development toward self-actualization, the task of aging, requires interactions and environments in which the older adult is assured that basic needs are met, compensations are made for losses, and meaningful and satisfying experiences continue to be a part of life.

KEY CONCEPTS

▶ Vision and hearing impairment can significantly affect functional ability, safety, and quality of life among older adults.

▶ Vision loss from eye disease is a global concern and prevention of treatment of eye diseases is an important priority for nurses and other health care professionals.

▶ The major diseases affecting vision are glaucoma, cataracts, macular degeneration, and diabetic retinopathy. Many of these diseases can be identified and appropriately treated through proper screening. All adults over the age of 65 should have annual eye examinations.

▶ Tinnitus is a common condition among older people and can interfere with hearing, as well as become extremely irritating. It is characterized by ringing in the ear and may also manifest as buzzing, hissing, whistling, clicking, pulsating, or swishing sounds.

▶ To promote healthy aging and quality of life, nurses in all settings must be knowledgeable about the impact of hearing and vision changes on the functional abilities and quality of life of older adults, vision and hearing assessment, prevention and treatment of diseases affecting vision and hearing, effective communication techniques, and ways to assist the individual in adapting to and compensating for these losses

ACTIVITIES AND DISCUSSION QUESTIONS

1. How can nurses enhance awareness and education about vision and hearing disorders?
2. What is the role of a nurse in the acute care setting in screening and assessment for eye and ear diseases?
3. Develop a teaching plan for an older adult with glaucoma.
4. What type of resources could a nurse in any setting offer to an older adult who has vision and hearing loss?
5. Develop a plan of care for an older adult with diabetic retinopathy.

RESOURCES

See Chapter 3 and evolve.elsevier.com/Ebersole/gerontological for a complete listing of resources for vision and hearing impairment.

REFERENCES

American Tinnitus Association: *About tinnitus,* 2007. Accessed 3/13/08 from www.ata.org.

Beers MH, Berkow R: *The Merck manual of geriatrics,* ed 3, Whitehouse Station, NJ, 2000, Merck Research Laboratories.

Boyd-Monk H: The eyes have it: understanding problems of the aging eye, *Am J Nurs* 3(5):34-45, 2005.

Bressler NM, Bressler SB, Congdon NG et al: Age-related macular degeneration is the leading cause of blindness, *JAMA* 291(15):1900-1901, 2004.

Bressler NM, Bressler S, Congdon N, Ferris F: Potential public health impact of Age-Related Eye Disease Study results: AREDS Report no. 11, *Arch Ophthalmol* 121(11): 1621-1624, 2003.

Capezuti J, Swicker D, Mezey M, Fulmer T, editors: *Evidence-based geriatric nursing protocols for best practice,* New York, 2008, Springer.

Feret A, Steinweg S, Griffin H, Glover S: Macular degeneration: types, causes, and possible interventions, *Geriatr Nurs* 28(6):387-392, 2007.

Glaucoma Research Foundation: *Are you at risk for glaucoma?* Accessed 3/10/08 from www.glaucoma.org.

Ham R, Sloane P, Warshaw G: *Primary care geriatrics,* ed 5, St Louis, 2007, Mosby.

Hellmann DR, Stone JH: Arthritis and musculoskeletal disorders. In Tierney LM, McPhee S, Papadakis M, editors: *Current medical diagnosis and treatment,* New York, 2006, McGraw-Hill.

Higginbotham EJ, Gordon MO, Beisner JA et al: The Ocular Hypertension Treatment Study: topical medication delays or prevents primary open-angle glaucoma in African American individuals, *Arch Ophthalmol* 122(6):813-820, 2004.

Luggen AS: Sensory problems. In Luggen A, Meiner S, editors: *NGNA core curriculum for gerontological nursing,* ed 2, St Louis, 2001, Mosby.

Maclay E: *Green winter: celebrations of old age,* New York, 1977, Thomas W. Crowell.

Miller C: *Nursing for wellness in older adults,* ed 5, Philadelphia, 2008, Wolters Kluwer/Lippincott Williams & Wilkins.

Moeller S, Taylor A, Tucker K et al: Associations between age-related nuclear cataract and lutein and zeaxanthin in the diet and serum in the carotenoids in the Age-Related Eye Disease Study (CAREDS), an ancillary study of the Women's Health Initiative, *Arch Opthalmol* 126(3):354-364, 2008.

National Eye Institute: *Glaucoma,* 2006a. Accessed 3/13/08 from: www.nei.nih.gov/glaucoma/.

National Eye Institute, *Diabetic Retinopathy,* 2006b. Accessed 313/08 from http://www.nei.nih.gov/health/diabetic/retinopathy.asp.

National Eye Institute: *Age-Related Macular Degeneration,* 2006c. Accessed 3/10/08 from www.nei.nih.gov/health/maculardegen/armd_facts.asp.

National Eye Institute: *Survey of public knowledge, attitudes, and practices related to eye health and disease,*

2008. Accessed 3/13/08 from: www.nei.nih.gov/news/pressreleases/031308.asp.

Newman CW, Wharton JA, Jacobsen GP: Retest stability of the tinnitus handicap questionnaire, *Ann Otol Rhinol Laryngol* 104(9 pt 1):718-723, 1995.

Rovner BW, Casten RJ, Hegel MT et al: Preventing depression in age-related macular degeneration, *Arch Gen Psychiatry* 64(8):886-92, 2007.

Tabloski P: *Gerontological nursing*, Upper Saddle River, NJ, 2006, Pearson Prentice Hall.

The Age-Related Eye Disease Study Research Group: A randomized placebo-controlled, clinical trial of high-dose supplementation with vitamins C and E, beta carotene, and zinc for age-related macular degeneration and vision loss, *Arch Opthalmol* 119(10):1417-1436.

U.S. Department of Health and Human Services: *Healthy People 2010. understanding and improving health,* Washington, DC, 2001, The Department.

Whiteside M, Wallhagen M, Pettengill E: Sensory impairment in older adults. Part 2: Vision loss, *Am J Nurs* 106(11):52-61, 2006. Available at www.nursingcenter.com/ajnolderadults. Accessed 6/16/2008.

Wilson MR, Eezzuduemhoi DR: Opthalmologic disorders in minority populations, *Med Clin North Am* 89(4):795-804, 2005.

Cardiovascular and Respiratory Disorders

20

LEARNING OBJECTIVES

Upon completion of this chapter, the reader will be able to:

- Identify most common types of cardiovascular and respiratory diseases occurring in late life.
- Discuss assessment of and intervention for cardiovascular and respiratory disease in the elder.
- Suggest ways to prevent cardiovascular and respiratory disease to the extent possible.
- Differentiate infectious, obstructive, and restrictive lung disease.
- Discuss the signs and symptoms of pneumonia in which rapid hospitalization is recommended if this is consistent with the wishes of the patient or health care surrogate.
- Develop a tuberculosis surveillance plan for a long-term care facility.

GLOSSARY

Comorbidity More than one disease or health condition existing at the same time.

Dyspnea The subjective report of shortness of breath.

Morbidity Disability as the result of a health condition.

Mortality Death as a result of a health condition or event.

Nosocomial Pertaining to the institutional setting or treatment as the source (as in nosocomial infection).

THE LIVED EXPERIENCE

When I first had that heart attack, I was so frightened it seemed I would die just from the fear. It was the first time I realized how comforting calm and efficient nurses could be. There was the one who came into the room a few days later and talked to me about the cardiac rehab program and that I could continue doing the things I had always done, except for changes in diet and more exercise. Even sex! I would never have asked that young thing, but she just told me it was OK.

Jerry, age 63

When Dad had that heart attack, it really scared us all, and I know we were afraid we would say or do something that would bring on another. I think he was also afraid of everything. I'm so grateful for the nurses at the hospital. They seem to give him lots of attention and information about the things he needs to know. He seems quite relaxed with himself now.

Ruth, Jerry's youngest daughter

Caring for older adults means caring for persons with cardiovascular disease (CVD), respiratory problems, or both. These two systems are interconnected. A problem in one is likely to cause or complicate a problem in the other. When the nurse is addressing a cardiac problem, such as heart failure, the respiratory system must be assessed as well. For example, pneumonia may trigger heart failure. Nursing interventions frequently overlap. One carefully planned action can address several systems at the same time and achieve goals of homeostasis and energy conservation, meeting basic physiological needs, and therefore reducing mortality and morbidity and promoting health as much as possible.

CARDIOVASCULAR DISORDERS

Although the numbers of deaths from heart disease have decreased, it remains the leading cause of death, the second most common cause of disability, and the primary diagnosis of persons admitted to long-term care facilities in the United States (U.S. Department of Health and Human Services [USDHHS], 2007) (Figures 20-1 and 20-2) The rate of deaths per 100,000 increases dramatically with age from a combination of normal changes with aging (see Chapter 6) and the presence of risk factors (Box 20-1). Older adults also undergo the majority of CVD-related procedures, but treatment approaches are highly variable by ethnicity and sex (Box 20-2). The American Heart Association identifies the major cardiovascular diseases as hypertension

(HTN); coronary heart disease (CHD), including myocardial infarction (MI) and angina; and heart failure (HF) (Figure 20-3).

Hypertension

Hypertension (HTN) is the most common chronic cardiovascular disease encountered by the gerontological nurse. Both the definition of and the guidelines for treatment of HTN are provided by the Joint National Committee of the Detection, Evaluation, and Treatment of High Blood Pressure (JNC) (Box 20-3). HTN is diagnosed any time the diastolic blood pressure reading is 90 mm Hg or higher or the systolic reading is 140 mm Hg or higher on two separate occasions (JNC 7, 2003) (Table 20-1). Blood pressure increases slightly with age, with a leveling off or decrease of the diastolic pressure for persons about 60 years of age and older. Older adults most often have isolated systolic hypertension, which is an elevation in only the systolic reading. This is quite different from the younger person, who is more likely to have an elevation in just the diastolic or in both. During the Joint National Committee of the Detection, Evaluation, and Treatment of High Blood Pressure's (JNC's) last review (#7) in 2003, it was noted that the definition for HTN does not change regardless of age. The current blood pressure goal for all persons is 120/60 mm Hg (Joint National Committee of the Detection, Evaluation, and Treatment of High Blood Pressure, 2003).

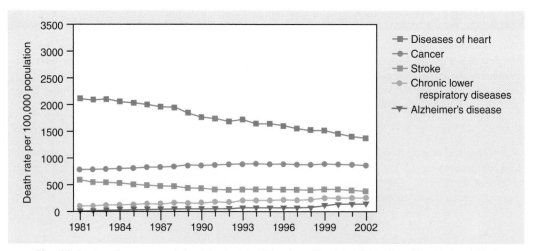

Fig. 20-1   Leading causes of death in women older than 65 years. *(Data from The National Vital Statistics System. The Data Warehouse on Trends in Health and Aging [website]: www.cdc.gov/nchs/ agingact.htm. Accessed 7/1/06.)*

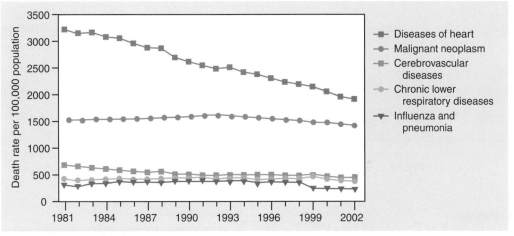

Fig. 20-2 Leading causes of death in men older than 65 years. *(Data from The National Vital Statistics System. Redrawn from the Data Warehouse on Trends in Health and Aging. Available at www.cdc.gov/nchs/agingact.htm. Accessed 7/1/06.)*

Box 20-1	Risk Factors for Heart Disease

- Age (>55 years for men; >65 years for women)
- Family history of premature CHD (<55 years for men; <65 years for women)
- Microalbuminuria or estimated GFR <60 ml/min
- Hypertension*
- Cigarette smoking
- Central obesity
- Physical inactivity
- Dyslipidemia*
- Diabetes, IGT, or IFG*

*Components of metabolic syndrome.

BMI, Body mass index; *CHD,* coronary heart disease; *GFR,* glomerular filtration rate; *IFG,* impaired fasting glucose; *IGT,* impaired glucose tolerance.

Box 20-2	Treatment of Chest Pain Differs by Sex and Ethnicity

The complaint of chest pain is often expressed by adult patients, especially in late life. When this chest pain is attributed to a cardiac origin, men are more likely than women to be diagnosed with angina (18% vs 4%) and intermediate coronary syndrome (ICS) (21% vs 10%), and women are more likely than men to be diagnosed with vague chest pain only (86% vs 61%). Blacks received more chest pain diagnoses than whites (71% vs 62%) with similar angina and ICS diagnoses. However, both blacks and women received fewer cardiovascular medications than white men.

Data from Hendrix KH, Mayhan S, Lackland DT, Egan BM: Prevalence, treatment, and control of chest pain syndromes and associated risk factors in hypertensive patients, *Am J Hypertens* 18(8):1026-1032, 2005.

It is anticipated that the updated JNC 8 guidelines will be prepared in the next several years.

Although often treatable, and in some cases preventable, the rates of HTN changed little during the last 10 years of the 1900s, and significant disparities exist among ethnic groups. If one does not have hypertension at 55, there is still a 90% chance of developing it later in life (USDHHS, 2007). Although race, ethnicity, and a family history of hypertension cannot be changed, a number of other factors are within control of the individual to reduce his or her risk for hypertension (Box 20-4).

Most HTN is discovered during health screening or examination for another problem, when related complications may have already developed. The most important complication of HTN is the long-term effects resulting in end-organ damage, especially to the heart. Older persons with HTN have an absolute higher risk

Hypertension (HTN)	Coronary heart disease (CHD)	Heart failure (HF)	Cerebrovascular disease (CVD)	Atrial fibrillation (AF)
50 million	12 million 85% of CHD deaths occur in those over age 65	5 million 75% over age 65	4 million 600,000 strokes annually 158,000 deaths annually Silent infarcts may increase the risk of dementia	2 million 70% between ages 65 and 85 Responsible for 15% of strokes

Fig. 20-3   Cardiovascular disease statistics. *(Modified from U.S. Department of Health and Human Services [USDHHS]. Available at www.healthypeople.gov/document/tableofcontents.htm. Accessed 11/6/08.)*

Box 20-3   Key Points of the JNC 7

- For persons older than 50 years, SBP is more important than DBP as a CVD risk factor.
- Starting at 115/75 mm Hg, CVD risk doubles with each increment of 20/10 mm Hg throughout the BP range.
- Persons who are normotensive at age 55 years have a 90% lifetime risk for developing HTN.
- Those with SBP 120-139 mm Hg or DBP 80-89 mm Hg should be considered prehypertensive, and they require health-promoting lifestyle modifications to prevent CVD.
- Thiazide type of diuretics should be the initial drug therapy either alone or combined with other drug classes unless compelling reasons are present.
- Certain high-risk conditions are compelling indications for other drug classes.
- Most patients will require two or more antihypertensive drugs to achieve goal BP.
- If BP is >20/10 mm Hg above goal, initiate therapy with two agents; one usually should be a diuretic of the thiazide type.

BP, Blood pressure; *CVD,* cardiovascular disease; *DBP,* diastolic blood pressure; *HTN,* hypertension; *JNC,* Joint National Committee of the Detection, Evaluation, and Treatment of High Blood Pressure; *SBP,* systolic blood pressure.

Adapted from JNC 7: *JNC 7 Express: the seventh report of the Joint National Commission of the Prevention, Detection, Evaluation and Treatment of High Blood Pressure, USDHHS Pub No 03-5233,* 2003. Available at http://www.nhlbi.nih.gov/guidelines/hypertension/. Accessed 11/8/08.

Table 20-1   Blood Pressure Classification

CLASSIFICATION	BLOOD PRESSURE
Normal	<120 systolic and <80 diastolic
Prehypertension	120-139 systolic or 80-89 diastolic
Stage 1 HTN	140-159 systolic or 90-99 diastolic
Stage 2 HTN	>160 systolic or >100 diastolic

HTN, Hypertension.

Box 20-4   Modifiable Factors That Increase the Risk for Essential Hypertension

- Cigarette smoking or tobacco use
- Excessive alcohol intake
- Sedentary lifestyle
- Inadequate stress and/or anger management
- High-sodium diet
- High-fat diet

for cardiac disease such as CHD, atrial fibrillation, and heart failure, as well as acute cardiovascular and cerebrovascular events such as myocardial infarction, stroke, and sudden death. Poorly controlled HTN is also implicated in chronic renal insufficiency, end-stage renal disease, and peripheral vascular disease (Langford and Thompson, 2005).

Coronary Heart Disease

The beating heart, like other muscles, needs oxygen and other nutrients to provide energy for its work. However, the blood passing through the heart with each beat is not available to provide oxygen or nutrients to the organ itself. Instead, like all other muscles, the heart receives its oxygen from arteries within it. CHD is caused from a blockage of these vessels and may be referred to as *arteriosclerosis*, or "hardening of the arteries." Coronary artery disease (CAD) develops when cholesterol and other fats are deposited in the layers of the arteries, narrowing the channel through which blood flows and therefore limiting the amount of oxygen reaching the tissue, which is known as ischemia. CAD is in part a direct consequence of chronic, untreated or inadequately treated hypertension (Cooper, 2007). Seventy-five percent of all cardiac-related deaths each year is attributed to CHD (USDHHS, 2007).

The symptoms of gripping chest pain, radiation to the shoulder, etc., that are usually thought to indicate acute ischemia (an acute myocardial infarction [AMI]) are not usually seen in older adults. Instead the person is more likely to have what is called a *silent MI*. His or her discomfort may be mild and may be localized to the back, the abdomen, the shoulders, or either or both arms. Nausea and vomiting, or merely a sensation like heartburn, may be the only symptoms. More often there are no noticeable signs or symptoms as all, and the event is only noticed at the time of death or when an electrocardiogram (ECG) is performed for some other purpose. These vague symptoms are often not brought to the attention of a medical provider.

Heart Failure

The damage to the heart from CHD may lead to heart failure (HF), which is the most frequent cause for hospitalization of an older adult. Sixty-five to seventy percent of all hospitalizations in 2004 included a diagnosis of HF. Those 65 and older represented 80% of those hospitalized. Often this resulted in a transfer to a long-term care facility (Fang et al, 2008).

HF is a disease of the heart muscle in which the muscle is damaged, malfunctions, and can no longer pump enough blood to meet the needs of the body. The severity of malfunctioning depends on whether it is a mechanical or functional abnormality. Causes of HF include hypertension, fever, hypoxia, anemia, metabolic disease, and infection (Langford and Thompson, 2005). Over time the heart is further damaged because of poor control of the underlying problem (e.g., hypertension or CHD) leading to more and more severe HF, known as CHF or congestive heart failure. An unhealthy diet, smoking, and lack of exercise aggravate the development of heart disease and the extent of damage, especially for those who have a family (genetic) history of heart disease. There is no cure for HF, only the management of symptoms and the attempt to prevent worsening. About 50% of persons with HF die within 1 year; the vast majority of these persons are over 65 (Hudspeth, 2006).

Clinical HF is categorized as left-sided, right-sided, or both-sided (biventricular) failure. It can also be described as either systolic or diastolic dysfunction (Baker and Carey, 2007). Left-sided and diastolic failure are the most common types found in the elderly. The New York Heart Association and the American College of Cardiology–American Heart Association provide us with convenient ways to classify the symptomatic experience of the HF, from symptom-free to severely disabled (Box 20-5).

Common signs and symptoms of heart failure in the elderly include fatigue or shortness of breath (dyspnea) with exertion, inability to lie flat without getting short of breath (orthopnea), waking up at night gasping for air, weight gain, and swelling in the lower extremities. Dyspnea may occur at rest or on exertion, or it may appear intermittently at night (paroxysmal nocturnal dyspnea). The dyspnea may be relieved by sitting up or sleeping on multiple pillows or with the head of the bed elevated. If a cough is present, it is worse at night.

In addition, the nurse should be alert for the atypical clinical presentation of exacerbations of HF in the elderly. The person may appear confused, or delirious; begin falling; or complain of insomnia or urinary frequency at night (nocturia). He or she may complain of dizziness or may have syncope (fainting). Or more often, the nurse will notice that the person has the "droops," or malaise and a subtle decline in activity tolerance or functional or cognitive abilities.

One of the major ways that cardiac conditions differ from other chronic problems is that when they become acute problems, they can do so very rapidly, and often necessitate acute hospitalization and intensive treatment followed by rehabilitation. Many other chronic disorders are managed at home.

Box 20-5	Classification of Heart Failure

Class I: Asymptomatic
Cardiac disease without resulting limitations of physical activity

Class II: Mild Heart Failure
Slight limitation of physical activity
Comfortable at rest
An increase in activity may cause fatigue, palpitations, dyspnea, or anginal pain

Class III: Moderate Heart Failure
Marked limitation in physical activity
Comfortable at rest
Ordinary walking or climbing of stairs can quickly bring on symptoms of fatigue, palpitations, dyspnea, or anginal pain
Substantial periods of bed rest required

Class IV: Severe Heart Failure
Almost permanently confined to bed
Inability to carry out any physical activity without discomfort or severe symptoms
Some symptoms occur at rest
Chronic shortness of breath is common

Developed by the NY Heart Association in 1928. Disseminated broadly. See http://www.abouthf.org/questions_stages.htm and http://www.americanheart.org/presenter.jhtml?identifier=4569. Accessed 11/8/08.

IMPLICATIONS FOR GERONTOLOGICAL NURSING AND HEALTHY AGING

Assessment

As with any assessment, obtaining a pertinent history of the events leading up to and including the presentation of cardiovascular problems is essential, whether the history is from the patient or a friend or family member. Monitoring of vital signs, laboratory results, and kidney function, and assessing the cardiac and respiratory function and conducting a mental status exam level are essential (see Chapters 13 and 21). Members of the University of Iowa Gerontological Nursing Intervention Center offer an evidence-based assessment tool that can be used as a basic assessment measure as well as one that indicates change in long-term care patients with heart failure (Harrington, 2008). The tool can be used to document status in three categories: activities of daily living, quality of sleep, and dyspnea. It is available for free (acknowledged) use from www.nursing.uiowa.edu/excellence/nursing_interventions/index.htm.

Interventions

For the person with CVD, the goals of therapy are to provide relief of symptoms, improve the quality of life, reduce mortality and morbidity, and slow or stop progression of dysfunction through the use of aggressive drug therapy. Additional goals are to maximize the function and quality of life for the person with CVD and, when appropriate, provide expert palliative care. Concurrent and supportive therapies include modifying the diet by decreasing fat, cholesterol, and sodium; exercise; education; and family and social supports (Hudspeth, 2006).

Nursing interventions assist the person to accomplish these goals and have been found to be highly effective (Sisk et al, 2006). What specific interventions are used will depend on the severity of the disease, the person, and the desire for either palliative or aggressive care. Nursing actions range from teaching the older adult about lifestyle changes in diet, activity, and rest (see Chapter 10), to acute measures, such as the administration of oxygen. In general, interventions about which the nurse should be knowledgeable are related to those assessed:

▶ Response to prescribed exercise
▶ Medication administration and the evaluation of medication effects
▶ Monitoring for signs and symptoms of CHF
▶ Monitoring fluid intake and output and diet
▶ Monitoring weight (either daily, biweekly, or weekly)
▶ Auscultating heart and lung sounds
▶ Monitoring laboratory values
▶ Education related to all of the above
▶ Providing comfort (see Chapter 25)

The goal of the management of HTN is to minimize the risk of complications and reduce or eliminate modifiable risk factors. This means keeping the blood pressure less than 140/90 mm Hg for otherwise healthy adults and less than 130/80 mm Hg for persons with diabetes. By doing so, many of the long-term complications (e.g., heart disease) can be avoided, minimized, or delayed (Box 20-6 and 20-7). To accomplish this, the nurse has a responsibility to work with the elder and his or her family comprehensively to promote healthy aging. Fortunately, the work of the American Heart Association and the JNC provides detailed evidence-based treatment guidelines for most children and adults. Unfortunately, less is known about the

Box 20-6	Minimizing Risk for Heart Disease

Maintain:
  Blood pressure ≤130/80
  Total cholesterol <200
  LDL <100
  HDL >40
  Triglycerides <150

HDL, High-density lipoprotein; *LDL,* low-density lipoprotein.

Box 20-7	Benefits of Controlling Blood Pressure

	Average percent reduction in risk for new events
Stroke decreases	35%-40%
Myocardial infarction decreases	20%-25%
Heart failure decreases	50%

appropriate treatment of fragile older adults with CVD who are residing in long-term care facilities. A more careful risk-benefit analysis must be done related to treatment and outcomes in this setting. For someone with a limited life expectancy, the significant side effects of some medications and limitations in food choices may result in an unnecessary decrease in quality of life. When aggressive treatment is no longer affective, a referral to hospice may be a possibility (see Chapter 25).

The potential for wellness after a major cardiac event or procedure is increased when elders participate fully in a cardiac rehabilitation program, if available. Otherwise disability can progress rapidly, especially if the person believes that any exertion overtaxes the heart and will cause acute CHF, another heart attack, or death. To prevent this, cardiac exercise rehabilitation programs are designed to address the physical, mental, and spiritual needs and overall health of the person and his or her family. Reductions in mortality are reported from 18% to 45% (Franklin and Vanhecke, 2007). Typical programs are prescribed by the physician or nurse practitioner and begin with self-management education and light activity

progressing to moderate activity under the supervision of a rehabilitation nurse and physical therapist. For those who are more physically compromised, it is necessary to identify energy-conserving measures applicable to their daily tasks.

The nurse and the person with CVD must be cautious about exercise. For those who have had an AMI, exercise-related orthostatic hypotension is more likely to occur as a result of age-related decreases in baroreceptor responsiveness, which controls the body's ability to respond to the need for changes in blood pressure (see Chapter 6). Because thermoregulation is also impaired, exercise intensity must be reduced in hot, humid climates (see Chapter 12). A healthy alternative is to encourage "mall walking" in local covered and climate-controlled shopping centers. In some locations this has become a social event as well as a safe way to exercise.

Risk reduction programs should be instituted with a clear understanding of the difficulties involved in attempts to alter harmful lifestyle practices such as smoking, overeating, habitual anger or irritation, and a sedentary lifestyle. These practices may have been going on for a lifetime and are not easily changed by "education." The nurse's role in these instances is to discuss these practices in a nonjudgmental manner, providing acceptance, encouragement, resources, knowledge, and affirmation of both the difficulty of making lifestyle changes and the person's right to choose.

RESPIRATORY DISORDERS

The normal physical changes with aging (see Chapter 6) result in a greater risk for respiratory problems, and when they occur, there is a higher risk for death than in younger persons. Diseases of the respiratory system are identified as infectious, as acute or chronic, and as involving the upper or lower respiratory tract. They are further defined as either *obstructive*—preventing airflow out as a result of obstruction or narrowing of the respiratory structures; or *restrictive*—causing a decrease in total lung capacity as a result of limited expansion. Almost all chronic obstructive pulmonary disease in late life arises from tobacco use or exposure to tobacco and other pollutants earlier in life. Although asthma may be triggered by environmental factors, there are strong genetic and allergic factors which contribute to its occurrence. The nurse's focus is on helping the person maintain function and quality of life, while being vigilant for signs of infection.

Chronic Obstructive Pulmonary Disease

Chronic obstructive pulmonary disease (COPD) is a catch-all term used to encompass those conditions that affect airflow. It includes asthma, bronchitis, and emphysema and as a group, is the fourth leading cause of death for both older men and women; however, it is expected to be the third leading cause of death by 2020. While overall the death rate from COPD has decreased, the age-adjusted death rate for women over 45 years increased from 100.8 per 100,000 persons in 1999 to 103.4 in 2005; the rate for men during this same time period decreased from 123.9 to 118.8. For persons from racial and ethnic groups other than non-Hispanic whites, the rate is considerably lower. The reduction is attributed to a decrease in the cigarette smoking rate (USDHHS, 2008).

COPD also contributes to activity limitations. For all persons older than 45 years, the activity limitation rate was 2.5% in 1997, as it was in 2002. This varies by ethnicity, with Hispanics with the lowest rate of activity limitation (1.4%) and the highest in non-Hispanic whites (2.6%) (Figure 20-4).

The type of signs and symptoms seen varies with the type of COPD. For example, persons with emphysema have little sputum production and appear pink since they are receiving adequate oxygen. On the other hand, persons with bronchitis have chronic sputum production, frequent cough, and are pale and somewhat cyanotic. Thorough discussions of these symptoms can be found in medical-surgical nursing and pathophysiology texts. What is crucial to gerontological nursing is the need to watch the person with COPD very closely for signs of worsening infection and of aggravation of any underlying heart disease.

When respirations exceed 30/min, the person with COPD is having a worsening of his or her illness and prompt response by the nurse is necessary. An acute episode of COPD is characterized by significantly worsened dyspnea and increased volume and purulence of sputum (Langford and Thompson, 2005). A number of factors including viral or bacterial infections, air pollution or other environmental exposures, or changes in the weather may trigger a change in the person's respiratory health.

Persons with advanced COPD, as seen in most of the older adults with the disease, can expect to have periods of worsening of symptoms and functioning between periods of control. During periods of illness, medication changes are usually needed. Persons who have well-developed skills in self-management often

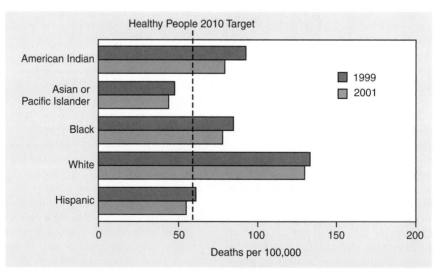

Fig. 20-4 Activity limitation because of chronic respiratory problems. *NOTE:* Data are for ages 45 years and older and age adjusted to the 2000 standard population. Black and white exclude persons of Hispanic origin. Persons of Hispanic origin may be any race. Persons reported one or more races. Data by single race category are for persons who reported only one racial group. *(Data from National Health Interview Survey, NCHS, CDC. Redrawn from Respiratory Disease http://www. healthypeople.gov/document/html/volume2/24respiratory.htm. Accessed 11/7/08.)*

will begin to deal with the changes before consulting a health care provider. Hospitalization is always a possibility with COPD exacerbations, especially when one has or is suspected of having an infection.

Pneumonia

Pneumonia is a bacterial or viral lower respiratory tract infection that causes inflammation of the lung tissue. Pneumonia and influenza are between the fourth and the eighth leading causes of death for persons over the age of 65, depending on age and ethnicity (Centers for Disease Control and Prevention [CDC], 2006). Particularly susceptible are elders with comorbid conditions such as alcoholism, asthma, COPD, or heart disease, or those who live in institutional settings. Elders residing in nursing homes, regardless of the reason, have a 10-fold greater incidence of pneumonia. Other factors that increase the risk of acquiring pneumonia relate to normal changes of aging of the respiratory system, such as a diminished cough reflex, increased residual volume, and decreased chest compliance (see Chapter 6). Many cases of pneumonia can be either prevented by immunization or treated effectively.

Pneumonia is classified as either community-acquired or nosocomial. That is, it is either acquired as a consequence of living in the community or as a result of medical treatment or institutionalization. In the nursing home the most frequent causes of aspiration pneumonia are reflux of colonized oral secretions, from a feeding tube or simply eating.

The usual signs and symptoms of pneumonia such as cough, fatigue, and dyspnea may easily be attributed initially to something else, such as the underlying COPD or medications. In older adults, other signs may be seen such as falling, mental status changes or signs of confusion, general deterioration, weakness, anorexia, rapid pulse, and rapid respirations. When one appears to have pneumonia, an abnormal chest x-ray, fever, and elevated white blood count are expected. However, these signs may be delayed in an older adult, and if treatment is not started until these are present, it may be too late and the result may be death. For the best possibility of survival of a frail elder with pneumonia, very prompt interventions are necessary. For the frail and medically compromised, interventions may be necessary as soon as an infection is determined to be a reasonable explanation for a sudden change (Jett, 2006).

One of the most important questions a nurse needs to consider is if a recommendation and advocacy for hospitalization is appropriate. Fortunately there are several evidence-based guidelines to help the nurse make this decision. The indicators of an increased likelihood of pneumonia-related death for persons in the community are as follows: (1) aggravation of another health condition at the same time, (2) respiratory rate >25, and (3) elevated C-reactive protein, if known. The indicators for an increased risk for death within 30 days for those in nursing homes are respiratory rate >30, pulse >125, altered mental status, and history of dementia. Studies have found that the death rate increases with even one risk factor, with greater risk for each additional factor (Ladenfeld et al, 2004). However, the ultimate decision regarding hospitalization is always up to the patient or the health care surrogate (see Chapter 22). For the elder, especially one who is frail or decompensated, the decision to hospitalize or not will be determined by the patient's wishes regarding aggressive treatment. It is always imperative to make sure that the patient and the significant others realize the severity of the situation and that there are always options. In this case, the options are "as aggressive as possible" care in the facility (e.g., intravenous [IV] antibiotics, oxygen per cannula), "comfort measures," or "acute treatment," which will most likely include an emergency room visit and artificial ventilation in an intensive care unit (Gulick and Jett, 2006). The decision will always be a personal one.

IMPLICATIONS FOR GERONTOLOGICAL NURSING AND HEALTHY AGING

Assessment

The nursing assessment of the person with respiratory problems focuses on the objective observations of oxygen saturation, sputum production, and coughing and the subjective reports of dyspnea, its affect on functional status, and quality of life. Only persons experiencing a problem can really tell us what it is like for them. Visual analog scales and numeric rating scales, similar to those used to assess pain, may be helpful (see Chapter 16). Persons can be asked how they would rate their breathing, from 1 (no dyspnea) to 10 (the worst dyspnea possible), and so on.

When an infection is suspected, it is never appropriate to use a "wait and see" approach; elevations in temperature or in white blood cell count may not occur until the person is in a septic state, and chest x-ray exams in debilitated persons are often falsely negative at the beginning of the infection or with dehydration. Patients and their families should be told the seriousness of this or any infection in older adults. More timely diagnosis calls for sensitive clinical assessments by both the nurse and the other health care providers.

Assessment includes detailed information about cough. When did it start? How long are the episodes of coughing? Is there any associated pain? What seems to make it better, and what makes it worse? Is the person using anything to treat the cough? Is the person smoking (and how much) or exposed to smoke or other respiratory irritants? If the cough is productive, what is the color, texture, and odor of the mucus? Does the color change according to the time of the day?

The remaining physical examination is the same as that used for persons with cardiac disease, since it is not always clear whether symptoms such as fatigue and shortness of breath are cardiac or respiratory in nature. Observation of airway clearance, breathing patterns, and mobility; the measurement of pulse oximetry; a mental status examination; and a functional assessment provides a clearer picture of the person's health status. Pulmonary function testing is most definitive in terms of lung capacity, and along with a chest x-ray examination, can show the extent of respiratory damage from acute or chronic conditions. Box 20-8 presents the key aspects of a respiratory assessment.

Box 20-8   Respiratory Assessment

Obtain Following History:
Family
Past medical
Symptoms

Perform Assessment of the Following:
Overall body configuration (e.g., posture, chest symmetry, shape, etc.)
Respirations, including ease of ventilation, use of accessory muscles, etc.
Detailed description of level of dyspnea per activity
Oxygenation (pulse oximetry, skin color, capillary refill, pallor)
Sputum (color, amount, consistency)
Palpation, percussion, and auscultation
Functional status
Cognitive status if indicated
Mood if indicated
Discussion of wishes for treatment and advance planning
Presence or absence of a living will and designated health care surrogate

---

Interventions

As with heart failure, many respiratory diseases in late life cannot be cured. Nursing interventions are based on palliative goals, namely, stabilizing the disease, reducing the risk of exacerbations and hospitalizations, promoting maximal functional capacity, and preventing premature disability. Education always includes smoking cessation, secretion clearance techniques, identification and management of exacerbations, breathing retraining, management of depression and anxiety, nutritional support, the proper use and administration of medications, and dealing with supplemental oxygen therapy if and when it is necessary (Langford and Thompson, 2005). Except in severe cases, treatment can occur in a skilled nursing facility if the person is already there, as long as oxygen therapy, parenteral fluids, and antibiotics can be administered by the nursing staff.

If there is a person available to assume a caregiver role, care and treatment can occur in the elder's home with temporary home health service support. If the elder fails to improve or deteriorates in either setting, then hospitalization is often necessary, unless this is against the wishes of the patient. A change to active palliative care may be appropriate at any time (see Chapter 25). If the person is hospitalized, a prolonged rehabilitation may be necessary, either at home or in a skilled nursing facility or both (see Chapter 26). Pharmacological and mechanical interventions for the treatment of infection are individually tailored based on the health status of the person before the infection, expected outcomes of treatment, where treatment will be provided, and wishes of the patient as noted above.

Interdisciplinary Care

Education is a part of every aspect of pulmonary care (Box 20-9). The person is taught to recognize the signs and symptoms of respiratory infection; how to maintain adequate nutrition; how to use an inhaler, nebulizer, and a peak flow meter, and how to clean them; the safe use of oxygen; the type of exercise that is beneficial; how to pace activities; coping strategies; and about other issues, such as sexual function. Each of these areas calls for teaching and indicates specific interventions that will help older adults and their families to participate in self-management.

Diet education should address the reason for monitoring weight and the signs of malnutrition. Weight loss can occur rapidly because of the energy expenditure needed to breathe while eating. A sense of being full early in the meal is caused by congestion

Box 20-9	Instructions for Persons with Chronic Obstructive Pulmonary Disease

Nutrition

Eat small, frequent meals with high protein and caloric content.*

Select foods that do not require a lot of chewing or cut in bite-size pieces to conserve energy.

Drink 2 to 3 L of fluid daily.*

Weigh self at least twice each week.

Activity Pacing to Conserve Energy

Plan exertion during the best periods of the day.

Arrange regular rest periods.

Allow plenty of time to complete activities.

Schedule sex around best-breathing time of day.

Use prescribed bronchodilators 20 to 30 minutes before.

Use a position that does not call for pressure on the chest or support of the arms.

General Instructions

Participate in regular exercise.*

Select and wear clothing and shoes that are easy to put on and remove.

Avoid indoor and outdoor pollutants.

Avoid exposure to others with illness.

Obtain an annual flu shot if not allergic.

Obtain pneumococcal immunization as appropriate.

Notify health care provider of changes:

  Temperature elevation

  Sputum color or amount produced

  Increased shortness of breath

*As prescribed.

---

in the abdomen due to a flattened diaphragm. Anorexia or decreased appetite occurs as a result of sputum production and gastric irritation from the use of bronchodilators and steroids.

Activity and exercise tolerance should be assessed by the occupational and respiratory therapist, and activities should be prescribed to increase endurance and improve respiratory status. Exercise may be done with or without oxygen as a supplement to control symptoms so that the older adult can spend enough time in exercise to benefit from it. The person should be informed that sexual activity is still possible, and education and counseling information should be provided, either by the rehabilitation nurse or a professional medical counselor.

Medications are used to treat infection and control dyspnea, cough, and sputum production. As with any medication teaching, the nurse can make sure that the person knows the purpose and the correct dosage and regimen of any medication he or she is taking, its side effects, and what to do if side effects occur (see Chapter 14). Inhalers are difficult for those with limited manual dexterity and/or strength, as with arthritis in the hands. If needed, special adaptive devices are available.

Rehabilitation is an important aspect of maximizing quality of life for the person with respiratory problems, as it is for those with cardiovascular problems. An older adult with COPD would be considered a candidate for pulmonary rehabilitation as long as he or she has pulmonary reserve and stable heart disease. Rehabilitation programs for the older adult with COPD consist of drug therapy, reconditioning exercises, and counseling. A multidisciplinary team of health professionals works collectively to help the older adult achieve the following goals:

▶ Increase the level of independence

▶ Maintain individuality and autonomy

▶ Improve function in his or her environment

▶ Decrease the number of hospitalizations and need for hospitalization

▶ Increase exercise tolerance

▶ Increase self-esteem and self-care skills

▶ Improve the quality of life and comfort

The number of goals achieved depends on many factors, including extent of illness and of coexisting conditions. For those recovering from pneumonia, the rehabilitative period may be prolonged.

Economic issues are always a concern for persons with chronic disease (see Chapter 15). A number of medications are used and can be very expensive, especially when needed for an indefinite period of time. The expense of oxygen therapy for persons with a limited income may also interfere with the adequacy of therapy and create feelings of anxiety. Medicare coverage for oxygen is limited to those persons with a moderate to severe level of disease as determined by their oxygen saturation rates, and oxygen is never covered by insurance for comfort only.

Mouth care is very important, especially for the person receiving supplemental oxygen and all who are medically or physically debilitated. Inadequate mouth care leads to the propagation of bacteria, which compounds an already serious situation. Inadequate oral care may lead to aspiration pneumonia. Sputum is considered potentially infectious and must be handled appropriately.

Monitoring nutrition and obtaining nutritional consultation as necessary is the responsibility of the nurse in all settings. The nurse will also ensure that the person recovering from pneumonia is adequately nourished and hydrated while monitoring fluid volume. Overload is a risk for persons with coexisting heart disease. Mobilizing the older person and referring him or her for physical and occupational therapy to prevent or stop functional decline should occur as soon as the person's condition allows.

APPLICATON OF MASLOW'S HIERARCHY

For persons with cardiovascular or respiratory disorders, all efforts of professionals, family caregivers, and the older adult are directed toward creating a safe and comfortable environment that will maximize function and attainment of the highest level of functioning and wellness, with or without direct assistance. While Maslow's lowest level of basic needs is often the priority, efforts can be made for the person to be able to reach for satisfaction of higher level needs as well.

The nurse also has a role in the prevention of complications. Adults older than 65 years of age and those with chronic conditions should be encouraged to receive the 1-time pneumococcal vaccine (Pneumovax) unless they are at high risk. In that case, their health care providers may recommend a second immunization after about 5 years. Influenza-related pneumonias may be avoided or ameliorated with yearly (October to December) flu vaccinations. Finally, yearly dental cleanings and examinations should be encouraged as well, since dental caries and periodontal disease predispose one to develop pneumonia as a secondary infection (Karnath et al, 2003).

Tuberculosis

Tuberculosis (TB) is a communicable and infectious disease caused by the bacteria *Mycobacterium tuberculosis*. The term *tuberculosis infection* refers to a positive TB skin test with no evidence of active disease. *Tuberculosis disease* refers to cases that have positive acid-fast smear or culture for *M. tuberculosis* or radiographical and clinical presentation of TB.

It is estimated that one third of the world's population is infected with *M. tuberculosis* (Cohen, 2006). *M. tuberculosis* was considered to be conquered in the 1950s with the development of the drug isoniazid (INH). Many of our present elders were treated following infections during World War II. Many others were infected as children. As they become immunocompromised as a result of chemotherapy, extreme old age, or

human immunodeficiency virus (HIV) infection, the bacterium could be reactivated.

The number of cases of TB in the United States has steadily decreased, with a drop from 4.4 per 100,000 in 2006 to 4.2 in 2007, the lowest in recorded history. However, this low rate is because of the very low rate in white, natural citizens. The rate of persons born outside of the United States is 9.7 times higher. Furthermore, though highly variable, the rate is higher in minority populations (CDC, 2008).

Although the numbers of cases in the U.S. in 2006 were low, TB continues to be found in at least one long-term care facility in 41 of 52 reporting areas (50 states, District of Columbia, and New York City). Out of a total of 312 cases in 2006, the highest incidence in long-term care facilities in 2006 was in California (62) and Texas (24) (CDC, 2007). Gerontological nurses working in these areas must be particularly knowledgeable about this potentially life-threatening disease and protect themselves and others. Persons who are immunosuppressed, who are from areas with high infection rates, or who live in group settings are at particular risk. Older residents of congregate living settings are between 2 and 7 times more likely to acquire the disease than those who live in the community (Ferebee, 2006).

Symptoms include unexplained weight loss or fever and a cough lasting more than 3 weeks, regardless of age-group. Night sweats and generalized anxiety may be present. In more advanced stages, the person will also have dyspnea, chest pain, and hemoptysis. Laboratory results in the elderly may show an increased sedimentation rate and lymphocytopenia. Because these signs and symptoms are associated with many disorders common in older adults, diagnosis often is made during a health screening (Libow, 2005). For persons with positive skin tests, it is necessary to confirm a diagnosis with a chest x-ray and sputum culture.

Implications for Gerontological Nursing in Long-Term Care Settings

In promoting healthy aging in the context of TB, the nurse has a responsibility to both the public and the individual. The nurse must be proactive in the prevention of contagious disease and in the prompt treatment of those who become or are ill. This is especially important in the long-term care setting. Elders in these settings are at higher risk because of communal living situations and the high rate of medical frailty. In 1990 the Centers for Disease Control and Prevention (CDC) recommended that every person entering a long-term care facility as a resident or an employee undergo annual testing for TB

(CDC, 2008). In 2005 the guidelines were updated considerably to reflect the changes in both incidence and prevalence in different geographic areas. To ensure prompt identification of persons with TB and limit its spread, especially in the long-term or extended-care facility, nurses should develop and implement an appropriate surveillance plan (Box 20-10). If such a plan is not already in place, the CDC and the state health departments are excellent sources of guidance and assistance.

TB is a reportable condition, which means that all suspected and confirmed cases are reported to the local or state health authorities (Chesnutt et al, 2009). The local public health nurses usually conduct investigations to ensure that all potentially infected people have been tested and that all persons with the disease receive treatment. The nurse actively participates in health screenings that may include TB testing. As a health care provider, the nurse is also at risk for acquiring the infection and needs to be screened regularly to prevent becoming a carrier (Box 20-11).

Nurses have a role in monitoring laboratory values, assessing for adverse drug reactions, and monitoring drug compliance in persons with TB, all of which are crucial to treatment effectiveness and the patient's well-being. The gerontological nurse participates in screening, educating regarding the seriousness of the infection,

---

Box 20-10   Surveillance Guidelines for Tuberculosis in the Long-Term Care Setting*

- Each facility should have an individual responsible for tuberculosis (TB) infection control and an infection prevention and control plan.
- Each facility should conduct a TB risk assessment on a regularly scheduled basis that considers both patients and residents and health care workers (low–moderate and high risk).
- Determine the need for TB screening based on the results of the risk assessments.†
  For low risk settings:
  - Screen all new residents on admission and employees on hire for symptoms, and consider using the two-step tuberculin skin test (TST) or the blood assay for *Mycobacterium tuberculosis* (BAMT).
  - Repeat annually.
  - For those who test positive or have had a positive test in the past, perform one chest radiograph and then an annual review of symptoms rather than repeat of film.
- No persons with a diagnosis of TB should remain in a long-term care facility unless adequate administrative and environmental controls and a respiratory protection program is in place.

*For more details, see the Centers for Disease Control and Prevention (CDC): Guidelines for preventing the transmission of *Mycobacterium tuberculosis* in health-care settings, 2005. *MMWR Morb Mortal Wkly Rep* 54(RR17):1-141, 2005; http://www.cdc.gov/tb/pubs/slidesets/InfectionGuidelines/default.htm. Accessed 11/6/08.

†Each state public health unit provides guidelines and directions specific to the geographic area and the known risk estimates.

Box 20-11   First-Person Clinical Note: Community Nursing and Persons with Tuberculosis

As a young public health nurse, it was my responsibility to periodically check on all persons in my assigned district who were undergoing treatment for tuberculosis (TB). A new person had moved into one of the many boarding houses of this inner-city neighborhood. Mr. Jones was a pleasant, robust 60-year-old who expressed pleasure in the visit and reported that he was doing well, that he had plenty of medications, and that they were not causing him any problems. He dashed out of the room, returned with a small suitcase, and opened it for me to assure me of his supply, and there before me were dozens of unopened bottles of isoniazid (INH), one of the staples of TB treatment. I called the medical director, who recommended that Mr. Jones be sent to the local hospital and, to make sure he got there, to deliver him forthwith. So I loaded him and his suitcase into my car and away we went; thinking of what Florence Nightingale would say, I left the windows open wide. When I returned to the health department, my first stop was for a TB test for myself and the plans for a follow-up after the incubation period. All for the sake of community well-being!

Kathleen Jett

and helping persons obtain the appropriate treatment as needed.

KEY CONCEPTS

▶ Heart disease is the most common cause of death for persons in the United States.

▶ The underlying cause for the majority of cardiovascular and pulmonary disease is smoking, therefore assisting persons in smoking cessation can have a significant impact on improving their health.

▶ Pneumonia and influenza are particularly important health problems for those over 65 and significantly more so for those who are frail, immunocompromised, have HIV, or are otherwise decompensated.

▶ The mortality associated with pneumonia can be minimized through the use of pneumonia and influenza vaccinations and excellent oral hygiene.

▶ The goal of therapy for cardiac and respiratory disorders is to relieve symptoms, improve the quality of life, reduce mortality, stabilize and slow the progression of the disease, reduce the risk of exacerbation, and maximize functional capacity.

▶ Careful attention to the early detection and prompt treatment of tuberculosis is necessary to continue in the attempt to completely eradicate this communicable disease.

ACTIVITIES AND DISCUSSION QUESTIONS

1. What is congestive heart failure?
2. Discuss assessment and intervention for elders with a diagnosis of congestive heart failure, chronic obstructive pulmonary disease, or pneumonia.
3. Why is pneumonia so dangerous to the older adult?
4. What preventive measures can be instituted to prevent or lessen the severity of pneumonia and tuberculosis among the elder population?
5. Develop a nursing care plan for an elder with congestive heart failure or a respiratory condition using wellness and North American Nursing Diagnosis Association (NANDA) diagnoses.

REFERENCES

Baker MD, Carey L: Heart failure: Ambulatory management, *Clin Rev* 17(6):36-42, 2007.

Centers for Disease Control and Prevention (CDC): *Death rate for 113 select causes by age, U.S., 2005.* 2006. Available at www.nchs.cdc.gov. Accessed 7/21/08.

Centers for Disease Control and Prevention (CDC): Table 31. *Tuberculosis cases and percentages by residence in long term care facilities, age >15: Reporting areas, 2006.* 2007. Available at www.cdc.gov/tb/surv/surv2006/pdf/table31.pdf. Accessed 7/21/08.

Centers for Disease Control and Prevention (CDC): *Trends in Tuberculosis—United States 2007.* 2008. *MMWR Morb Mortal Wkly Rep* 57(11):281-285, 2008. Available at www.cdc.gov/mmwr/preview/mmwrhtml/mm5711a2.htm. Accessed 7/21/08.

Chesnutt MS, Murray JA, Prendergast TJ: Pulmonary disorders. In McPhee SJ & Papadakis MA (editors*), 2009 Current medical diagnosis and treatment*, New York, 2009, McGraw-Hill.

Cohen SM: Diagnosis and treatment of tuberculosis, *JNP* 2(6):390-396, 2006.

Fang J, Mensah GA, Croft JB, Keenan NL: Heart failure-related hospitalization in the U.S., 1979-2004. *J Am Coll Cardiol,* 52(6):428-434, 2008.

Ferebee L: Respiratory function. In Meiner SE, Luecknotte AG, editors: *Gerontologic nursing,* ed 3, St Louis, 2006, Mosby.

Franklin BA, Vanhecke TE: Preventing reinfarction: changing behavior after the MI. Part 1, *Consultant* 47(6):517-522, 2007.

Gulick G, Jett KF: Applying evidence-based findings to practice: caring for older adults in subacute units, *Geriatr Nurs* 27(5):280-283, 2006.

Harrington CC: Evidence-based guideline: assessing heart failure in long-term care facilities, *J Gerontol Nurs* 34(2):9-14, 2008.

Hudspeth T: Heart failure: lost in translation, *ADVANCE Nurs Pract* 14(7):55-58, 2006.

Jett KF: Examining the evidence: knowing if and when to transfer a resident with pneumonia from the nursing home to the hospital or subacute unit, *Geriatr Nurs* 27(5):280, 2006.

Joint National Committee of the Detection, Evaluation, and Treatment of High Blood Pressure (JNC): *JNC 7 Express: the seventh report of the Joint National Commission of the prevention, detection, evaluation and treatment of high blood pressure,* USDHHS Pub No 03-5233, 2003. Available at www.nhlbi.nih.gov. Accessed 7/22/08.

Karnath B, Agyeman A, Lai A: Pneumococcal pneumonia: update on therapy in the era of antibiotic resistance, *Consultant* 42(3):321-326, 2003.

Landefeld CS, Palmer RM, Johnson MA et al: *Current geriatric diagnosis and treatment.* New York, 2004, McGraw Hill.

Langford R, Thompson J: *Mosby's handbook of diseases,* ed 3, St. Louis, 2005, Mosby.

Libow LS: Preventing the spread of tuberculosis in the nursing home, *Long-Term Care Interface* (March):8-10, 2005.

Sisk J, Herbert P, Horowitz C et al: Effects of nurse management on the quality of heart failure care in minority communities: a randomized clinical trial, 2006, *Ann Intern Med* 145(4):273-283, 2006.

U.S. Department of Health and Human Services (USDHHS): *Progress review: Respiratory diseases.* 2008. Available at http://www.healthypeople.gov/Data/2010prog/focus24/default.htm. Accessed 11/6/08.

U.S. Department of Health and Human Services (USDHHS): *Progress review: Heart disease and stroke.* 2007. Available at http://www.healthypeople.gov/Data/2010prog/focus12. Accessed 11/8/08.

Cognitive Impairment

LEARNING OBJECTIVES

Upon completion of this chapter, the reader will be able to:

- Differentiate between dementia, delirium, and depression.
- Discuss the different types of dementia and appropriate diagnosis.
- Explain the differences between hemorrhagic and ischemic stroke.
- Describe the effects of Parkinson's disease and appropriate nursing interventions.
- Describe nursing models of care for persons with dementia.
- Discuss common concerns in care of persons with dementia and nursing responses.
- Develop a nursing care plan for an individual with delirium.
- Develop a nursing care plan for an individual with dementia.

GLOSSARY

Ataxia An impaired ability to coordinate movement, typified especially by a staggering gait.

Computed tomography An x-ray technique that produces a film representing a detailed cross-section of tissue. Used primarily to diagnose space-occupying lesions

Embolus A quantity of air, gas, or tissue that circulates and becomes lodged in a blood vessel.

Excess disability A reversible deficit that is more disabling than the primary disability. Examples would be a patient with dementia who is kept in a wheelchair and therefore loses the ability to walk or a patient with a stroke who experiences a contracture or pressure ulcer on the affected side as a result of poor positioning or pressure relief.

Intracerebral Within the tissue of the brain.

Milieu The environment or setting.

Subarachnoid The space under the arachnoid membrane and above the pia mater, which may fill with blood during cerebral hemorrhage.

Thrombus A lump of platelets, fibrins, and cellular elements attached to the inner wall of an artery or vein, sometimes blocking the flow of blood.

THE LIVED EXPERIENCE

"The Alzheimer's patient asks nothing more than a hand to hold, a heart to care, and a mind to think for them when they cannot; someone to protect them as they travel through the dangerous twists and turns of the labyrinth. These thoughts must be put on paper now. Tomorrow they may be gone, as fleeting as the bloom of night jasmine beside my front door."

Diana Friel McGowin, who was diagnosed with Alzheimer's disease when she was 45 years old (McGowin, 1993, p. viii).

This chapter focuses on cognitive impairment and the diseases that affect cognition. Included in the chapter is a discussion of delirium and Alzheimer's disease and other dementias. Stroke and Parkinson's disease are also included, since both can affect cognitive functioning. The chapter also presents nursing interventions for people experiencing delirium and dementia as well as caregiving for persons with dementia. Cognitive function in aging is discussed in Chapter 7; instruments for cognitive assessment in Chapter 13; and communication with persons experiencing cognitive impairment in Chapter 3.

We have artificially separated cognitive function from mental health, though they are in most ways interdependent. The mind is in some ways limited by the capacities of the brain, yet just as in medicine, there is a danger of evaluating the person by the measured and tested efficiency of cells and organs. Nowhere is this more important than in examining the cognition of older people. Citing John Morris, professor of neurology at Washington University in St. Louis, Crowley (1996) says that if brain function becomes impaired in old age, it is a result of disease, not aging.

OVERVIEW OF COGNITIVE IMPAIRMENT

Cognitive impairment (CI) is a term that describes a range of disturbances in cognitive functioning, including disturbances in memory, orientation, attention, and concentration. Other disturbances of cognition may affect intelligence, judgment, learning ability, perception, problem solving, psychomotor ability, reaction time, and social intactness.

Cognitive Assessment

An older person with a change in cognitive function needs a thorough assessment to identify the presence of specific pathological conditions (Box 21-1). Pathological conditions causing impairment of cognition include delirium, dementia, and depression. The literature reveals that both physicians and nurses routinely fail to appropriately assess an individual's cognitive functioning in all settings. Pathological conditions are often undiagnosed, reversible causes not identified, and opportunities for

---

Box 21-1	**Overview of Cognitive Assessment**

A. Concepts and Categories
1. Definition: *cognitive function:* the processes by which an individual perceives, registers, stores, retrieves, and uses information
2. Categories of cognitive change and/or decline
   a. The dementias (e.g., Alzheimer's, vascular) are chronic, progressive, insidious, and permanent states of cognitive impairment
   b. Delirium and/or acute confusion: an acute and sudden impairment of cognition that is considered temporary, generally an identifiable, biophysical cause
   c. Impairment in thought processes

B. Assessment
1. Methods of assessment
   a. Formal—cognitive testing using standardized instruments
      i. Advantages: standardized; enables comparison across individuals and nurses
      ii. Disadvantages: individual performance influenced by pain, education, fatigue, cultural background, and perceptual and physical abilities
   b. Informal—through structured observations of nurse-individual interactions
      i. Advantages: may have greater meaning about individual's actual cognitive ability-performance
      ii. Disadvantages: difficult to make judgments regarding change in individual condition; variability in interpretation
2. Other considerations for assessment
   a. Characteristics of the environment for assessment
      i. Physical environment
         —Comfortable ambient temperature
         —Lighting adequate but not glaring

Box 21-1   Overview of Cognitive Assessment—cont'd

        —Free of distractions (e.g., should be conducted in the absence of others and other activities)
        —Position self to maximize individual's sensory abilities
    ii. Interpersonal environment
        —Use individual's self-paced rate for assessment
        —Emotionally nonthreatening
  b. Timing considerations
    i. Timing should reflect the actual cognitive abilities of the individual and not extraneous factors
    ii. Times of the day to generally avoid:
        —Immediately on awakening from sleep; wait at least 30 minutes
        —Immediately before or after meals
        —Immediately before or after medical diagnostic or therapeutic procedures
        —When patient has pain or discomfort
3. Parameters of assessment
  a. Alertness and/or level of consciousness: the most rudimentary cognitive function and level of arousal, or responsiveness to stimuli determined by interaction with individual, and determination of level made on the basis of the individual's best eye, verbal, and motor response to stimuli
    i. Alertness—able to interact in a meaningful way with the examiner
    ii. Lethargy or somnolence—not fully alert; individual tends to drift to sleep when not stimulated, diminished spontaneous physical movement, loses train of thought, ideas wander
    iii. Obtundation—transitional stage between lethargy and stupor; difficult to arouse, meaningful testing futile, requires constant stimulation to elicit response
    iv. Stupor or semicoma—individual mumbles and/or groans in response to persistent and vigorous physical stimulation
    v. Coma—completely unable to be aroused, no behavioral response to stimuli
  b. Attention: ability to attend and/or concentrate on stimuli: can follow through with directions, especially a three-stage command; is easily distracted
  c. Memory: ability to register, retain, and recall information both new and old. Does individual remember your name? Is individual able to learn and remember new information?
  d. Orientation: to time, place, and person
  e. Thinking: ability to organize and communicate ideas; thoughts should be organized, coherent, and appropriate perception: presence or absence of illusions, delusions, or visual or auditory hallucinations
  f. Psychomotor behavior: ability to comprehend and perform simple motor skills; execution ability: ask the individual to perform certain ADLs and IADLs, or to perform a three-step command, and to copy a figure
  g. Insight: ability to understand oneself and the situation in which one finds oneself
  h. Judgment: ability to evaluate a situation (real or hypothetical) and determine an appropriate action

C. Outcomes of Assessment
1. Individual
  a. Detection of deviations will be prompt and early, with appropriate care and treatment instituted in a timely manner
  b. Plans of care will appropriately address cognitive functioning, with corrective and supportive components
2. Health care provider
  a. Assessment and documentation of cognitive function
  b. Appropriate strategies to address any deviation in cognitive function
  c. Competence in cognitive assessment
  d. Evidence of ability to differentiate among the different types of cognitive change and/or decline
3. Institution
  a. Documentation of cognitive function will increase
  b. Referral to appropriate advanced practitioners (e.g., geriatrician, geriatric or gerontologic or psychiatric clinical nurse specialist or nurse practitioner, consultation-liaison service) will increase

ADLs, Activities of daily living; *IADLs,* instrumental activities of daily living.

From Foreman MD, Fletcher K, Mion L et al: Assessing cognitive function, *Geriatr Nurs* 17(5):228, 1996.

early intervention missed. As a result, the person experiences greater impairment and functional decline (Braes et al, 2008).

Some of the reasons for this include the complexity of cognitive assessment and the existence of several conditions with similar symptoms (dementia, depression, delirium) (Table 21-1), the often atypical symptom presentation in older adults, and the belief that alterations in cognitive functioning are "normal" in older people (Braes et al, 2008; Fletcher, 2008) (see Chapter 7 and Box 7-6). It is important for nurses to have the skills to recognize cognitive impairment and monitor cognitive functioning. "Assessment of cognitive function is the first and most critical step in a cascade of strategies to prevent, reverse, halt, or minimize cognitive decline" (Braes et al, 2008, p. 42). There are a number of excellent resources

to assist nurses in assessing cognition (Box 21-2). Many of these resources are available in both print and video formats.

Screening for Cognitive Impairment

Screening is used to determine if cognitive impairment exists, but basic screening methods do not diagnose specific pathological conditions. If impairment is identified through screening, the person should be referred for a more comprehensive evaluation to confirm a diagnosis of dementia, delirium, or depression, or some other health problem (Braes et al, 2008). A comprehensive evaluation includes a complete assessment, including laboratory workup, to rule out any medical causes of cognitive impairment. Screening for depression using instruments such as the Geriatric Depression Scale

Table 21-1   Differentiating Delirium, Depression, and Dementia

CHARACTERISTIC	DELIRIUM	DEPRESSION	DEMENTIA
Onset	Sudden, abrupt	Recent, may relate to life change	Insidious, slow, over years and often unrecognized until deficits obvious
Course over 24 hr	Fluctuating, often worse at night	Fairly stable, may be worse in the morning	Fairly stable, may see changes with stress
Consciousness	Reduced	Clear	Clear
Alertness	Increased, decreased, or variable	Normal	Generally normal
Psychomotor activity	Increased, decreased, or mixed Sometimes increased, other times decreased	Variable, agitation or retardation	Normal, may have apraxia or agnosia
Duration	Hours to weeks	Variable and may be chronic	Years
Attention	Disordered, fluctuates	Little impairment	Generally normal but may have trouble focusing
Orientation	Usually impaired, fluctuates	Usually normal, may answer "I don't know" to questions or may not try to answer	Often impaired, may make up answers or answer close to the right thing, or may confabulate, but tries to answer
Speech	Often incoherent, slow or rapid, may call out repeatedly or repeat the same phrase	May be slow	Difficulty finding word, perseveration
Affect	Variable but may look disturbed, frightened	Flat	Slowed response, may be labile

Adapted from Rapp CG, Mentes J, Titler M: Acute confusion/delirium protocol, *J Gerontol Nurse* 27(4):21-33, 2001. Reprinted with permission from SLACK, Inc, Thorofare, NJ.

Box 21-2   Resources for Assessment of Cognition

Try This Series (ConsultGeriRN.org) Resources:
Issue 3: Mental status assessment of older adults: The Mini-Cog (article and video)
Issue 13: Confusion Assessment Method (CAM) (article and video)
Issue 25: The Confusion Assessment Method for the Intensive Care Unit (CAM-ICU)
Issue D3: Brief evaluation of executive dysfunction—an essential refinement in the assessment of cognitive impairment
Issue D8: Assessing and managing delirium in persons with dementia (article and video)

Other Resources:
American Association of Neuroscience Nurses: *Neurological assessment of the older adult: a guide for nurses*, 2007. Available at www.aann.org. Accessed 7/8/08.
Braes T, Millisen K, Foreman M et al: *Nuring standard of practice protocol: assessing cognitive functioning*, In Capezuti E, Swicker D, Mezey M et al, editors: *Evidence-based geriatric nursing protocols for best practice*, ed 3, New York, 2008, Springer.
Hospital Elder Life Program (HELP): http://elderlife.med.yale.edu/public/public-main.php.
Malone M: ACE cards for assessing delirium. Complete series of ACE cards to help manage common geriatric conditions. Available at Michael.Malone.md@aurora.org.
Management related to management of brain dysfunction in critically ill patients: www.icudelirium.org. Accessed 7/8/08.
Mini-Mental State Examination: www.minimental.com. Accessed 7/8/08.
Rapp C, Mentes J, Titler M et al: Acute confusion/delirium protocol, *J Gerontol Nurs* 27(4):21-33, 2001.
Registered Nurses Association on Ontario (RNAO): *Caregiving strategies for older adults with delirium, dementia, and depression* (www.guidelines.gov). Accessed 7/8/08.
Tullmann D, Mion LC, Fletcher K et al: *Nursing standard of practice protocol: delirium: prevention, early recognition, and treatment*, In Capezuti E, Swicker D, Mezey M et al, editors: *Evidence-based geriatric nursing protocols for best practice,* ed 3, New York, 2008, Springer. Available at www.consultgerirn.org.

Source: The Hartford Institute for Geriatric Nursing (www.hartfordign.org/TryThis)

(GDS) should be conducted. Formal cognitive testing, neuropsychological examination, interview (family and patient), observation, and functional assessment are additional components of a comprehensive assessment. Computerized tomography (CT), magnetic resonance imaging (MRI), and an electroencephalogram (EEG) may be indicated in the diagnostic process. Several evidence-based guidelines are available for assessment of changes in mental status and diagnosis of dementia (www.guidelines.gov), and Fletcher (2008) presents a "Nursing Standard of Practice Protocol: Recognition and Management of Dementia."

The Minimental State Examination (MMSE), the Short Portable Mental Status Questionnaire (SPMSQ), Clock Drawing Test (CDT), the Mini-Cognition (Mini-Cog), the Confusion Assessment Method (CAM), and the NEECHAM (Neecham-Champagne) Confusion Scale, are examples of screening instruments. These instruments may also be used to monitor and evaluate cognitive status in the hospital or during treatment.

Box 21-2 presents other suggestions for assessment and screening of cognitive impairment.

The MMSE is generally considered the best available method for screening for cognitive impairment and is commonly used. However, there are concerns related to the time needed for administration and its lack of sensitivity in detecting early or mild dementia (Fletcher, 2008). In addition, performance on the MMSE is strongly related to education (individuals with less than an eighth-grade education commit more errors), language (individuals for whom English is not their primary language commit more errors), verbal ability (can only be used with individuals who can respond verbally to questions), and culture (culture bias) (Braes et al, 2008; Fletcher, 2008).

Considerations in Cognitive Assessment

Assessment of cognitive functioning is often perceived as a very stressful experience for older adults. Too often, assessments are done when a person is not wearing hearing aids or glasses, or he or she is rushed through a series of questions in a noisy, distracting environment without any preparation or explanation. Most older adults worry about developing memory problems or getting Alzheimer's disease. Cognitive testing or poor performance on tests of memory is often the cause of great anxiety. Assessment of cognitive functioning can be perceived as "intrusive, intimidating, fatiguing, and offensive—characteristics that can seriously and negatively affect performance" (Braes et al, 2008, p. 48).

It is important to attend to these concerns by establishing rapport and developing a therapeutic relationship, ensuring comfort (pain relief), accommodating for physical impairments such as hearing and vision loss, creating an environment free of distractions, and putting the person in the best environment to ensure that performance is truly reflective of ability. The challenge is to stress the importance of the assessment without creating undue anxiety. Braes and colleagues (2008) warn that "It can be counterproductive to describe the assessment as consisting of 'simple,' 'silly,' or 'stupid' questions in an attempt to alleviate anxiety. Such explanations tend to diminish motivation to perform and only heighten anxiety when errors are committed. Anxiety also is heightened following a series of failures on assessment" (p. 48).

Timing is also important, and cognitive assessments should not be conducted immediately upon awakening from sleep, or immediately before and after meals or medical diagnostic and therapeutic procedures (Braes et al, 2008). It is wise to remember that what seems to be a routine procedure to health professionals can be very intimidating for an older person, especially one who is ill or frail.

Delirium

Dementia, delirium, and depression have been called the *three D's of cognitive impairment* because they occur frequently in older adults. These conditions are not a normal consequence of aging, although incidence increases with age. Older people, particularly those with dementia and acute illnesses and stressors, are especially prone to delirium. Because cognitive and behavioral changes characterize all three D's, it can be difficult to diagnose delirium, delirium superimposed on dementia (DSD), or depression. Inability to concentrate, with resulting memory impairment and other cognitive dysfunction, is common in late-life depression. The term *pseudodementia* has been used to describe the cognitive impairment that may accompany

depression in older adults (see Chapter 24 for discussion of depression).

Delirium is characterized by a rapid onset and fluctuating course. Symptoms include disturbances in consciousness and attention and changes in cognition (memory deficits, perceptual disturbances). In contrast, dementia typically has a gradual onset and a slow, steady pattern of decline without alterations in consciousness (Sweeny et al, 2008). Knowledge about cognitive function in aging and appropriate assessment and evaluation are keys to differentiating these three syndromes. Table 21-1 presents the clinical features and the differences in cognitive and behavioral characteristics in delirium, dementia, and depression. The accepted criteria for a diagnosis of delirium are presented in the *Diagnostic and Statistical Manual of Mental Disorders* (APA, 2000).

Etiology

The development of delirium is a result of complex interactions among multiple causes (Inouye, 2006). The exact pathophysiological mechanisms involved in the development and progression of delirium remain uncertain, and further research is needed to understand its neuropathogenesis. Delirium is thought to be related to disturbances in the neurotransmitters in the brain that modulate the control of cognitive function, behavior, and mood. Irving and Foreman (2006) note that "there is growing evidence of cholinergic failure as a common pathway in delirium" (p. 122). Poor cerebral blood flow is also a factor in the development of delirium (Flaherty and Morley, 2004). The causes of delirium are potentially reversible; therefore accurate assessment and diagnosis are critical. Delirium is usually a complication of a medical illness, a drug's or substance's effect on the brain, or a surgical procedure involving general anesthesia. Delirium is given many labels: *acute confusional state, acute brain syndrome, confusion, reversible dementia, metabolic encephalopathy,* and *toxic psychosis.*

Incidence and Prevalence

Delirium is a prevalent and serious disorder that occurs in elders across the continuum of care. Estimates are that delirium may affect more than half of hospitalized older adults and as many as 87% of older adults in intensive care units (ICUs) (Dahlke and Phinney, 2008; Sweeny et al, 2008). Older people who have undergone surgery and those with dementia are particularly vulnerable to delirium. The prevalence of delirium is as high as 65% after orthopedic surgery, particularly hip fracture repair (Rigney, 2006). At the time of discharge from the hospital, approximately 30% to 90% of patients who experienced delirium continue to manifest symptoms. In a study of older patients admitted to a home care agency after hospital discharge, 46% were delirious upon admission. Of even greater significance, 50% of that group lived alone. Delirium also occurs in long-term care facilities and can significantly affect functional outcomes (Marcantonio et al, 2003).

The incidence of delirium superimposed on dementia (DSD) ranges from 22% to 89% (Tullmann et al, 2008). Older patients with dementia are 3 to 5 times more likely to develop delirium, and it is less likely to be recognized and treated than is delirium without dementia (Fick and Mion, 2005). DSD is associated with high mortality among hospitalized older people (Bellelli et al, 2008). Changes in the mental status of older people with dementia are often attributed to underlying dementia, or "sundowning," and not investigated. This is particularly significant since about 25% of all older hospitalized patients may have Alzheimer's disease or another dementia (Voelker, 2008). Despite its prevalence, DSD has not been well investigated, and there are only a few relevant studies in either the hospital or community setting.

Recognition of Delirium

Delirium is a medical emergency and one of the most significant geriatric syndromes (Waszynski and Petrovic, 2008). However, it is often not recognized by physicians or nurses. Studies indicate that delirium is unrecognized in 66% to 84% of patients (Hustey and Meldon, 2002; Sanders, 2002; Pisani et al, 2006; Balas et al, 2007). A comprehensive review of the literature suggested that "nurses are missing key symptoms of delirium and appear to be doing superficial mental status assessments" (Steis and Fick, 2008, p. 47). Failure to recognize delirium, identify the underlying causes, and implement timely interventions contributes to the negative sequelae associated with the condition (Tullmann et al, 2008).

The literature suggests that factors contributing to the lack of recognition of delirium among health care professionals include inadequate education about delirium, a lack of formal assessment methods, and ageist attitudes (Waszynski and Petrovic, 2008). A recent qualitative study (Dahlke and Phinney, 2008) investigated interventions nurses use to assess, prevent, and treat delirium, as well as the challenges and barriers nurses face in this work. The authors concluded that cognitive changes in older people are often labeled *confusion* by nurses and physicians, are frequently accepted as part of normal aging, and are rarely questioned. If the nurse believed that confusion was normal

in older adults, he or she would be less likely to recognize symptoms of delirium as a medical emergency necessitating their attention and intervention. Confusion in a child or younger adult would be recognized as a medical emergency, but confusion in older adults may be accepted as a natural occurrence, "part of the older person's personality" (p. 46).

In the Dahlke and Phinney study, nurses reported that caring for patients with delirium was seen as "annoying, frustrating and not interesting" (2008, p. 45). Nurses expressed that the care of older patients with delirium interfered with what was perceived as the "real work" of caring for a medical or surgical patient. Insufficient knowledge and inadequate time and resources also influenced appropriate care. The authors conclude that nurses are faced with the predicament of fitting care for older adults into a system that does not recognize the unique needs of this population. Clearly, education and attitudes about older people must be addressed if we want to improve care outcomes for the growing number of older adults who will need care.

Risk Factors for Delirium

Identification of risk factors, prompt and appropriate assessment, and continued surveillance are the cornerstones of delirium prevention. More than 35 potential risk factors have been identified for delirium; among the most common are acute illness, infections, metabolic disturbances, alcohol or drug abuse, sensory impairments, surgery, hip fracture, and cognitive impairment. Unrelieved or inadequately treated pain significantly increases the risk of delirium (Irving and Foreman, 2006). Medications account for 22% to 39% of all deliriums, and all medications, particularly those with anticholinergic effects and any new medications, should be considered suspect. Invasive equipment such as nasogastric tubes, intravenous (IV) lines, catheters, and restraints also contribute to delirium by interfering with normal feedback mechanisms of the body (Box 21-3).

Clinical Subtypes of Delirium

Delirium is categorized according to the level of alertness and psychomotor activity. The clinical subtypes are hyperactive, hypoactive, and mixed. Box 21-4 presents the characteristics of each of these clinical subtypes. In non-ICU settings, approximately 30% of delirium is hyperactive, 24% hypoactive, and 46% mixed. Because of the increased severity of illness and the use of psychoactive medications, hypoactive delirium may be more prevalent in the ICU. Although the negative

Box 21-3	Diseases and Disorders Placing Older People at Risk for Delirium

- Age
- Male sex
- Dementia
- Pharmacological agents, especially anticholinergics, hypnotics, anxiolytics, antipsychotics, nonsteroidal antiinflammatory drugs (NSAIDs), antidepressants, narcotics, H_2 receptor antagonists, corticosteroids
- Hypoxemia and metabolic disturbances
- Dehydration, with and without electrolyte disturbances
- Electrolyte imbalances
- Withdrawal symptoms (alcohol and sedative-hypnotic agents)
- Major medical and surgical treatments (especially hip fracture surgery)
- Nutritional deficiencies
- Circulatory disturbances (congestive heart failure, myocardial infarction, cerebrovascular accident)
- Anemia
- Pain (either unrelieved or inadequately treated)
- Sensory deficits
- Social isolation, lack of family contact
- Retention of urine and feces
- Emergency admission or admission from a long-term care facility
- Restraint use
- Use of invasive equipment (including indwelling catheters)
- Abrupt loss of significant person
- Multiple losses in short span of time
- Move to radically different environment (hospitalization, nursing home)

Box 21-4	Clinical Subtypes of Delirium

Hypoactive Delirium
"Quiet or pleasantly confused"
Reduced activity
Lack of facial expression
Passive demeanor
Lethargy
Inactivity
Withdrawn and sluggish state
Limited, slow, and wavering vocalizations

Hyperactive Delirium
Excessive alertness
Easy distractibility
Increased psychomotor activity
Hallucinations, delusions
Agitation and aggressive actions
Fast or loud speech
Wandering; nonpurposeful, repetitive movement
Verbal behaviors (yelling, calling out)
Removing tubes
Attempting to get out of bed

Mixed
Unpredictable fluctuations between hypoactivity and hyperactivity

consequences of hyperactive delirium are serious, the hypoactive subtype may be missed more often and is associated with a worse prognosis because of the development of complications such as aspiration, pulmonary embolism, pressure ulcers, and pneumonia. Increased hospital stays, longer duration of delirium, and higher mortality have been associated with hypoactive delirium (Truman and Ely, 2003).

Consequences of Delirium

Delirium has serious consequences and is a "high priority nursing challenge for all nurses who care for older adults" (Tullmann et al, 2008, p. 113). Delirium results in significant distress for the patient, his or her family and significant others, and nurses. Delirium during hospitalization is associated with high morbidity and mortality, functional decline, increased postoperative complications, increased length of hospital stay and hospital readmissions, increased services after discharge, long-term cognitive decline, and high rates of institutionalization (Rigney, 2006; Sweeny et al, 2008; Tullmann et al, 2008).

Although delirium is considered a reversible cause of altered mental status, a significant number of older adults with delirium never return to their baseline cognitive status, especially in the presence of preexisting dementia (McCusker et al, 2001; Marcantonio et al, 2003; Rigney, 2006). Several studies reported that patients with delirium continue to manifest symptoms up to 6 months after discharge, with persistent memory deficits of particular significance (Foreman et al, 2001).

IMPLICATIONS FOR GERONTOLOGICAL NURSING AND HEALTHY AGING

Assessment

Several instruments can be used to assess the presence and severity of delirium. To detect changes, it is very important to determine the person's usual mental status. If the person cannot tell you this, family members or other caregivers who are with the patient can be asked to provide this information. If the patient is alone, the responsible party or the institution transferring the patient can provide this information by phone. Do not assume the person's current mental status represents his or her usual state, and do not attribute altered mental status to age alone or assume that dementia is present. All older patients, regardless of their current cognitive function, should have formal assessment to identify possible delirium when admitted to the hospital (see Box 21-2).

The MMSE is considered a general test of cognitive status that helps identify mental status impairment. Although the MMSE alone is not adequate for diagnosing delirium, it represents a brief, standardized method to assess mental status and can provide a baseline from which to track changes. Several delirium-specific assessment instruments are available, such as the CAM (Inouye et al, 1990) and the NEECHAM Confusion Scale (Neelon et al, 1996). The CAM-ICU is another instrument specifically designed to assess delirium in an intensive care population and has recently been validated for use in critically ill, nonverbal patients who are on mechanical ventilation (Ely et al, 2001; Rigney, 2006).

The CAM is designed to detect delirium in hospitalized patients and may not adequately identify delirium in nursing home residents (Galik and Resnick, 2007). In this setting, the Delirium-O-Meter (deJonghe et al, 2005), a 12-item behavioral rating scale that determines delirium severity, may be more useful. Psychometric properties are comparable with the CAM. Because nursing assistants often work with residents over time, they are often the ones to first identify subtle changes that may indicate delirium, so nurses in this setting must investigate any report of changes in behavior by the nursing assistant (Galik and Resnick, 2007). Dosa and colleagues (2007) reported on the development of a Nursing Home Confusion Method (NH-CAM).

Assessment using the MMSE, CAM, and NEECHAM should be conducted on admission to the hospital, throughout the hospitalization for all patients identified at risk for delirium, and for all patients who exhibit signs and symptoms of delirium or develop additional risk factors (Steis and Fick, 2008). Results of a study (Waszynski and Petrovic, 2008) suggested that the CAM was useful in identifying delirium in hospitalized adults, and nurses found it very helpful in identifying changes in cognitive functioning. As a result of these findings, the CAM was made a customary part of the daily flow sheet.

Once a patient is identified as having delirium, reassessment should be conducted every shift. Documenting specific objective indicators of alterations in mental status rather than using the global, nonspecific term *confusion* will lead to more appropriate prevention, detection, and management of delirium and its negative consequences. Findings from assessment using a validated instrument are combined with nursing observation, chart review, and physiological findings. Delirium often has a fluctuating course and can be difficult to recognize, so assessment must be ongoing and include multiple data sources.

Interventions

Nonpharmacological

Intervention begins with prevention. An awareness and identification of the risk factors for delirium and a formal assessment of mental status are the first-line interventions for prevention. Balas and colleagues (2007) suggest that "nurses make multiple decisions throughout the day that can potentially enhance or diminish the likelihood that their patients will experience delirium" (p. 152). Nurses play a pivotal role in the identification of delirium, and it is imperative that they accurately report patients' mental status to the medical team so that causative factors can be identified and treated (Irving and Foreman, 2006). Multidisciplinary approaches, including education, to delirium prevention seem to show the most promising results, but continued research is needed to evaluate what type of approach has the most beneficial effect in specific clinical settings. The current disease model of delirium care is not effective (Dahlke and Phinney, 2008).

Borrowing the concept of a "doula" from maternity care, the delirium doula is an innovative approach mentioned in the literature (Balas et al, 2004; Balas et al, 2007; Irving and Foreman, 2006; Sweeny et al, 2008). Of interest, this concept was designed by student nurses who had completed a maternity placement where doulas were used. The proposed role of the delirium doula would include providing support, adjusting the environment to meet the patient's behavior or needs, and assisting the patient to get help when required. A 40% reduction in delirium development among high-risk patients was reported in a specialized delirium unit using a multidisciplinary team approach, behavioral interventions as first-line treatment, and higher nurse-patient staffing ratios (Flaherty et al, 2003).

A well-researched multidisciplinary program of delirium prevention in the acute care setting, the Elder Life Program (Inouye et al, 1999; Bradley et al, 2005; Rubin et al, 2006) focuses on managing six risk factors for delirium: cognitive impairment, sleep deprivation, immobility, visual impairments, hearing impairments, and dehydration. Patient outcomes with the use of this model include a 40% reduction in the incidence of delirium and a decrease in the number of days and episodes of delirium. Most of the interventions can be considered quite simple and part of good nursing care.

Examples of interventions in the Elder Life Program include the following: offering herbal tea or warm milk instead of sleeping medications, keeping the ward quiet at night by using vibrating beepers instead of paging systems, using silent pill crushers, removing catheters and other devices that hamper movement as soon as possible, encouraging mobilization, assessing and managing pain, and correcting hearing and vision deficits. Fall risk reduction interventions such as bed and chair alarms, low beds, reclining chairs, volunteers to sit with restless patients, and keeping routines as normal as possible with consistent caregivers are other examples of interventions. Further information on the Elder Life Program can be found at http://elderlife.med.yale.edu/public/public-main.php. Other programs in acute care are described by Sweeny and colleagues (2008) and Voelker (2008). Box 21-5 presents suggested interventions for delirium.

A commonly used intervention for patients with delirium in acute care is the use of "sitters" or "constant observers (COs)." Costs associated with this practice can be very high, and data indicate that the use of sitters or COs does not consistently decrease the incidence of unsafe patient behavior in the patient with delirium. Nor do they assist in identifying causes and delirium or identifying appropriate interventions. Sweeny and colleagues (2008) report on the implementation of a multicomponent, evidence-based alternative to COs for care of patients with delirium in an acute care hospital. The program focused on fall risk–reduction strategies, as well as assessment of delirium using the CAM, and a protocol for intervention. Results suggest that costs associated with COs decreased from $1.5 million to $250,000 in 2 years with no change in the use of restraints or the incidence of falls.

Pharmacological

Pharmacological interventions to treat the symptoms of delirium may be necessary if patients are in danger of harming themselves or others, or if nonpharmacological interventions are not effective. However, pharmacological interventions should not replace thoughtful and careful evaluation and management of the underlying causes of delirium. Pharmacological treatment should be one approach in a multicomponent program of prevention and treatment. Research on the pharmacological management of delirium is limited, but it has been suggested that "with increased understanding of the neuropathogenesis of delirium, drug therapy could become primary to the treatment of delirium" (Irving and Foreman, 2006, p. 122).

In a recent study, low-dose haloperidol prophylactic treatment reduced the severity and duration of postoperative delirium in high-risk elderly patients who had hip surgery, but had no effect on reducing the incidence of delirium. The study protocol also included consultation by experienced geriatric nurses and geriatricians and a comprehensive delirium protocol that included many of the nonpharmacological interventions discussed previously (Kalisvaart et al, 2005). Ozbolt et al (2008) conducted a literature review of the use of antipsychotics for treatment of delirious elders and concluded that the atypical antipsychotics demonstrate similar rates of efficacy to haloperidol for the treatment of delirium and have a lower rate of extrapyramidal side effects. Further research is needed since no double-blind placebo trials exist. Short-acting benzodiazepines are often used to control agitation but may worsen mental status. In ICU patients with delirium, lorazepam has been identified as an independent risk factor for developing delirium (Pandharipande et al, 2006). Psychoactive medications, if used, should be given at the lowest effective dose, monitored closely, and reduced or eliminated as soon as possible so that recovery can be assessed (Rigney, 2006).

Caring for patients with delirium can be a challenging experience. Patients with delirium can be difficult to communicate with, and disturbing behaviors such as pulling out IV lines or attempting to get out of bed disrupt medical treatment and compromise safety. It is important for nurses to realize that behavior is an attempt to communicate something and express needs. The patient with delirium feels frightened and out of control. The more calm and reassuring the nurse is, the safer the patient will feel. Box 21-6 presents some communication strategies that are helpful in caring for people experiencing delirium.

Box 21-5	Suggested Interventions to Prevent Delirium

Appropriate Assessment
- Know baseline mental status, functional abilities, living conditions, medications taken, alcohol use
- Assess mental status using Minimental State Examination (MMSE), Confusion Assessment Method (CAM), or NEECHAM Confusion Scale (Neelon et al, 1996), and document findings
- Assess for and correct underlying physiological alterations
- Assess for sensory deficits and compensate for sensory deficits (hearing aids, glasses, dentures)

Attention to Basic Needs
- Encourage fluid intake and make sure fluids are accessible
- Avoid long periods of giving nothing orally
- Explain all actions with clear and consistent communication
- Avoid excessive bed rest; institute early mobilization
- Establish a toileting schedule
- Encourage participation in care for activities of daily living (ADLs)
- Assess and treat pain
- Allow for periods of interrupted rest and sleep

Medication Review
- Avoid multiple medications and avoid problematic medications (see Beers List of Inappropriate Medications for Older People at www. hartfordign.org)
- Be vigilant for drug reactions or interactions; consider onset of new symptoms as an adverse reaction to medications
- Avoid the use of sleeping medications—use music, warm milk, decaffeinated herbal tea, attention to sleep hygiene, adequate periods of rest and sleep

Understand Behavior
- Attempt to find out why behavior is occurring rather than simply medicating it (e.g., toileting needs, fear, hunger, thirst)

Maintain Safety without the Use of Restraints
- Keep bed in low position or use a low bed—consider mats on the floor
- Activate bed and chair alarms
- Assess fall risk
- Institute fall risk reduction strategies
- Consult with physical therapy for ambulation training, assistive devices
- Encourage use of assistive devices if patient is accustomed to them
- Place the person near the nursing station for close observation
- Have family, volunteers, or paid caregiver stay with the patient

Minimize Use of Invasive Equipment
- Minimize the use of catheters, restraints, or immobilizing devices
- Use least restrictive devices (mitts instead of wrist restraints, reclining gerichairs instead of vest restraints)
- Hide tubes (stockinette over intravenous [IV] line) or use intermittent fluid administration

Environmental Modifications
- Pay attention to environmental noise
- Normalize the environment (provide familiar items, routines, clocks, calendars)
- Minimize the number of room changes and interfacility transfers
- Do not place a delirious patient with another delirious patient

Box 21-6	Communicating with a Person Experiencing Delirium

- Know the person's past patterns
- Look at nonverbal signs, such as tone of voice, facial expressions, gestures
- Speak slowly
- Be calm and patient
- Face the person and maintain eye contact—get to the level of the person rather than standing over him or her
- Explain all actions
- Smile
- Use simple, familiar words
- Provide frequent reassurance and help the patient to interpret the environment and what is happening to him or her. If patient becomes upset, modify approach to one that is more reassuring and validates the patient's experience rather than reorienting—respond to the emotions expressed (Tullman et al, 2008).
- Allow adequate time for response
- Repeat if needed
- Tell the person what you want him or her to do rather than what you don't want him or her to do
- Give one-step directions, use gestures and demonstration to augment words
- Reassure person of safety
- Keep caregivers consistent
- Assume that communication and behavior are meaningful and an attempt to tell us something or express needs
- Do not assume the person is unable to understand or is demented

OVERVIEW OF DEMENTIA

In contrast to delirium, which is usually a reflection of an acute physiological disturbance, dementia is an irreversible state that progresses over years. Ham (2002) defines dementia as "a clinical state in which a persistent change in cognitive function occurs, with memory loss, and at least one other type of cognitive deficit. These losses are severe enough to impair social and occupational function and to be a clear change from a prior level of function, not occurring during the course of a delirium" (p. 253).

Other clinical features of the syndrome of dementia include at least one of the following:

▶ *Aphasia*—loss of ability to speak with relevance and fluency

▶ *Apraxia*—inability to carry out purposeful movements although motor and sensory abilities are intact
▶ *Agnosia*—inability to recognize common objects or faces of familiar people despite intact sensory abilities
▶ Disturbances in executive functioning (planning, organizing, sequencing, abstracting)

Types of Dementia

Dementia has more than 70 causes, and any person with symptoms of dementia should have a thorough workup to determine the etiology. Dementia can be categorized as primary or secondary. Primary dementias are progressive disorders caused by pathological conditions of the brain (e.g., Alzheimer's disease [AD]); secondary dementias produce pathological conditions of the brain as a result of other conditions (e.g., dementia related to the effects of alcohol). Many dementias in old age can be described as mixed dementia, produced by a number of primary and secondary causes. For example, dementia can be caused by a combination of AD, vascular brain changes, and prior alcoholism (two primary causes and one secondary cause).

Incidence and Prevalence

Dementia of the AD type is the most common, accounting for 50% to 60% of all dementias. AD affects an estimated 5.2 million Americans and more than 16 million individuals worldwide. The prevalence, incidence, and cumulative risk of AD appear to be much higher in African Americans than in non-Hispanic whites. The actual proportion of people with pure AD is probably smaller, and recent studies indicate that half of all people with AD have concomitant vascular disease or cortical Lewy bodies (Bhidayasiri, 2006).

The prevalence of AD increases with age, doubling approximately every 5 years in individuals between the ages of 60 and 95 years. An estimated 50% of individuals older than 85 years have AD. If current trends continue, by the year, 2050, the prevalence of AD is expected to quadruple, affecting almost 107 million people. One in four individuals will either have AD or be caring for someone who does. Ten million baby boomers will develop Alzheimer's disease (Alzheimer's Association, 2008). It is the sixth leading cause of death and the nation's third most expensive medical condition, carrying an annual cost of $110 billion (Ham, 2002; Solomon and Murphy, 2006; Sullivan, 2007). These costs do not take into account the financial impact on families caring for people with Alzheimer's in their own homes.

Dementia has a number of other causes. These include vascular dementia (VaD) (about 10% of dementias); Lewy body dementia (LBD) (about 15% to 25% of dementias); and mixed dementias (usually AD and vascular). Other less commonly occurring dementias are frontotemporal dementia (FTD); Creutzfeldt-Jakob disease (CJD) (subacute spongiform encephalopathy); and human immunodeficiency virus (HIV)–related dementia.

Normal pressure hydrocephalus (NPH) causes a dementia characterized by ataxic gait, incontinence, and memory impairment. This disease is reversible and treated with a shunt that diverts cerebrospinal fluid away from the brain. Many dementias manifest symptoms of cognitive impairment, but associated features, as well as age of onset, vary among the different types of dementing syndromes (Table 21-2).

Accurate diagnosis is important, since treatment and prognosis vary. The rate of diagnosis of dementia

Table 21-2   Classification of Dementing Disorders

DEMENTING DISORDER	SUGGESTIVE FEATURES
Vascular dementia (VaD) Also called multi-infarct dementia	Stepwise deterioration (50%) Focal neurological signs Neuroimaging evidence of cerebrovascular insufficiency
Dementia with Lewy bodies (DLB)	Fluctuations in performance Visual hallucinations, delusions Bilateral symmetric parkinsonism Neuroleptic hypersensitivity
Frontotemporal lobe dementia (FTD)	Early personality changes Early age of onset (before 60) Cortical atrophy selective to frontal and temporal lobes Early language dysfunction Relatively preserved memory and visuospatial function
Parkinson disease dementia (PDD)	Asymmetric parkinsonian features Later onset of dementia, at least 1 year after onset of parkinsonian features Subcortical dementia with impairment of frontal-executive functions
Creutzfeldt-Jakob disease (CJD) and nvCJD (transmissible spongiform encephalopathy)	*CJD:* Rare form of dementia characterized by tiny holes that give the brain a "spongy" appearance under microscope May be hereditary or occur sporadically or through transmission from infected individuals Onset of symptoms at about age 60 90% of patients die within 1 year Failing memory, behavioral changes, lack of coordination, visual disturbances *nvCJD (bovine spongiform encephalopathy or mad cow disease):* Occurs in younger patients and may be caused by contaminated feed

Data from National Institute of Neurological Disorders and Stroke: *Dementia: hope through research,* 2008. Available at www.ninds.nih.gov/disorders. Accessed 11/7/08; Bhidayasiri R: When it's not AD: atypical dementing illnesses. Part 1. *CNS Senior Care* 5(2):17, 2006.

is quite low despite advances in technology and knowledge about the different types and causes of dementia. In some studies, as many as 75% of patients with moderate to severe dementia and more than 95% of those with mild impairment escape diagnosis in the primary care setting. Clearly, education of both professionals and the community is needed so that more timely diagnosis and treatment can be initiated (Stefanacci, 2008).

Alzheimer's Disease

AD was first described by Dr. Alois Alzheimer in 1906 and is a cerebral degenerative disorder of unknown origin. AD destroys proteins of nerve cells of the cerebral cortex by diffuse infiltration with nonfunctional tissue called neurofibrillary tangles and plaques. The tangles and plaques represent the death of nerve cells throughout the brain. The brain shrinks to about one third of its normal weight. The tangles consist of a protein called *tau* that "clogs" the insides of brain cells and their connections. Deposits of beta amyloid accumulate abnormally in the brains of patients with AD. The disease is progressive and is accompanied by increasing memory loss, inability to concentrate, personality deterioration, and impaired judgment.

The course of AD ranges from 1 to 15 years; typical life expectancy is 8 to 9 years after symptom onset, with death usually occurring as a result of pulmonary infections, urinary tract infections, pressure ulcers, or iatrogenic disorders. Risk factors include increasing age, family history and genetics, Down syndrome, female sex, environmental toxins, low formal education and occupational attainment, previous head trauma, and cerebrovascular disease. Diabetes is also associated with increased risk of AD.

The cause of the disorder is still unknown, and research is ongoing. Current research focuses on many aspects of AD: anatomy, biochemistry, diagnosis, genetics, language, memory, nutrition, perception, pharmacology, physiology, psychosocial issues, and virology. Some research indicates that flaws in processes governing production, accumulation, or disposal of beta amyloid are the primary causes of AD. Although the "amyloid hypothesis" remains the most widely accepted theory, other active areas of research include tau, inflammation, disruptions of cell-signaling pathways, and cardiovascular risk factors. Other clinical research trials have begun looking at homocysteine, which is linked to an increased risk of developing AD over time. This amino acid is known to be linked to an increase in heart disease risk,

and higher homocysteine levels may increase the risk for AD (Alzheimer's Association, 2008).

The two recognized forms of AD are familial and sporadic. Familial AD is quite rare and usually occurs before the age of 60 years. In familial AD, the person has inherited an abnormal variation (mutation) in one of three genes that are known causes of the disease: *PS1*, *PS2*, and *APP*. The gene mutations influence the production of beta amyloid. Sporadic AD is not inherited in any direct pattern, but genetic variations may influence susceptibility to AD. Gene research is an area of active investigation. For more information on current research, see www.alz.org.

Diagnosis of Alzheimer's Disease

The only method of confirming the diagnosis of AD is to perform a brain biopsy or autopsy. Clinically, AD is diagnosed most thoroughly based on the history from the family and testing to rule out other disorders that may mimic the disease. Probable AD can be clinically diagnosed if the onset is typically insidious with progression and if no other systemic or brain diseases could account for the progressive cognitive deficits. Earlier diagnosis and better diagnostic testing has led to an increase in the diagnosis of mild cognitive impairment (MCI). MCI is defined as cognitive decline greater than expected for an individual's age that minimally interferes with activities of daily living (ADLs). MCI may be a precursor of dementia, and individuals diagnosed with MCI are more than 3 times as likely to develop AD than a cohort of individuals without MCI (Fletcher, 2008) (see Chapter 7).

Symptoms of AD are usually present several years before a diagnosis is made. Symptoms of apathy and depression may be the first and earliest signs of AD, occurring up to 3 years before the disease is diagnosed. The history given by the family is another important part of assessing and diagnosing probable AD. A 2006 survey by the Alzheimer's Foundation of America found that the stigma associated with Alzheimer's disease among patients and families can delay the diagnosis for up to 6 years after symptoms first appear. A delayed diagnosis means that patients and families are without critical support, resources, and treatment (see www.alzfdn.org). *The Diagnostic and Statistical Manual of Mental Disorders* (DSM-IV-TR) presents the criteria for dementia of the Alzheimer's type (APA, 2000).

Cultural Differences

Research is limited regarding the influence of culture and ethnicity on the recognition and interpretation of cognitive changes and the assessment, diagnosis, and treatment of AD and other dementias. Further research is needed to understand how individuals from racially and culturally diverse groups view dementia and how cultural beliefs about disease etiology and symptoms influence diagnosis, treatment, and help-seeking behaviors (Neary and Mahoney, 2005; Hargrave, 2006). Studies have shown that African Americans may view dementia as a "normal consequence of aging, a form of mental illness, or manifestation of culture-specific physical syndromes" (e.g., "worriation" or "spells"). These health beliefs may lead to normalizing or minimizing symptoms, promote denial, and delay help-seeking behaviors (Hargrave, 2006, p. 37).

Hispanics may attribute the etiology of dementia to a "lack of balance in one's lifestyle, punishment for bad behavior, or mental illness (*locos*) or a temporary state of *nervious*, or nervousness" (Neary and Mahoney, 2005, p. 169). However, recent studies suggest that limited knowledge about dementia is a more significant deterrent to recognizing its symptoms and seeking assessment and treatment (Hargrave, 2006; Neary and Mahoney, 2005). Development of culturally and linguistically appropriate sources of information about dementia is important (Neary and Mahoney, 2005). The Diversity Toolbox, prepared by the Alzheimer's Association (www.alz.org/professionals_and_researchers_caring_for_diverse_populations.asp) is an important resource for nurses and other health professionals working with culturally and racially diverse older adults.

Pharmacological Treatment

Drug therapy with cholinesterase inhibitors (CIs) has transformed the treatment of AD, offering hope for enhanced function and reduction of the speed of decline. CIs approved to treat AD include donepezil (Aricept), rivastigmine (Exelon), and galantamine (Razadyne). The most recently approved drug, memantine (Namenda), is a new class of medication (N-methyl-D-aspartate [NMDA] antagonist) indicated for the treatment of moderate to severe AD. Unlike the CIs, which increase the amount of acetylcholine in the brain, memantine blocks the effect of abnormal glutamate activity that may lead to neuronal cell death and cognitive dysfunction. Memantine may be used alone or in combination with the CIs. The use of CIs are associated with a decreased risk of rapid cognitive deterioration, institutionalization, and weight loss (Gilette-Guyonnet et al, 2006). Therapy with a CI plus memantine may slow cognitive and functional decline more than therapy with a CI alone (Atri et al, 2008).

Current treatment guidelines recommend CI therapy as first-line treatment in patients with mild to moderate AD, and these medications may also be prescribed for MCI. Duration of therapy should be long-term, even if the patient shows slight decline, provided that function is better than it would have been without treatment. These medications are usually well tolerated, but side effects include gastrointestinal disturbances (nausea, vomiting, diarrhea, anorexia), sleep disturbances, and sedation (Fletcher, 2008). Starting at a low dose with slow titration is recommended to minimize side effects. Rivastigmine (Exelon) is now available in a patch that may be more convenient to use, have fewer side effects, and provide a consistent day-long dose. No published study directly compares these drugs. Because they work in a similar way, it is not expected that switching from one of these drugs to another will produce significantly different results. However, a person may respond better to one drug than another (National Institute on Aging, 2008).

Medication therapy is directed toward the symptoms of AD and does not affect the neuronal decline that will eventually produce severe disability. However, medications are likely to produce a plateau of brain function and functional abilities and delay the progression of AD. Delaying both disease onset and progression would significantly reduce the burden of AD, particularly in the late stages of the disease (Sullivan, 2007). Positive effects on the behavioral manifestations of AD have also been shown with CI therapy, suggesting that cholinergic mechanisms, among other neurotransmitters, are involved in the manifestation of some behavioral and psychological symptoms of dementia (Figiel and Sadowsky, 2008).

Vascular Dementia

Vascular dementia (VaD) (also known as multi-infarct or post-stroke dementia or vascular cognitive impairment) refers to a group of heterogeneous disorders arising from cerebrovascular insufficiency or ischemic or hemorrhagic brain damage. VaD often coexists with AD, is more common among African Americans and Japanese Americans, and is associated with advancing age, male sex, and stroke (Fladd, 2005; Bhidayasiri, 2006). The ratio of VaD to AD is generally 1:5, and dementia after stroke is thought to occur in one quarter to one third of stroke cases. Hypertension, cardiac disease, diabetes, smoking, alcoholism, and hyperlipidemia are additional risk factors for VaD (Box 21-7).

Diagnostic criteria for VAD include the DSM-IV criteria, the Hachinski Ischemic Score, and the National

Box 21-7	Vascular Brain Disease

Vascular brain disease may result from any of the following:

- Arteriosclerotic plaques blocking circulation to cerebral cells
- Blood dyscrasias interfering with platelet and clot formation
- Cardiac decompensation resulting in insufficient perfusion to the brain
- Cerebrovascular hemorrhage (strokes) of small or large magnitude
- Diabetic deterioration of blood vessels
- Primary hypertension causing deterioration of capillary walls because of sustained pressure (Cerebral cells dependent on the deteriorated capillaries no longer function. Over time, hypertensive persons show greater decrements in cognitive performance than persons with normal blood pressure.)
- Rupture of cerebrovascular or aortic aneurysms
- Sustained severe anemia
- Systemic emboli lodging in cerebrovascular pathway
- Transient ischemic attacks (TIAs) lasting up to 24 hours, resulting from spasms of blood vessels in certain segments of the brain, which produce temporary disturbances in sensation, cognition, and motor activity and are often a warning sign of impending stroke

Institute of Neurological Disorders and Stroke-Association Internationale pour le Recherche et l'Enseignement en Neurosciences (NINDS-AIREN) criteria (Bhidayasiri, 2006). Management of diabetes, hypertension, and hyperlipidemia is important in the primary prevention of VaD. Secondary prevention includes treatments to prevent the recurrence of a vascular accident (use of antihypertensives and antiplatelet medications) or minimize further cognitive damage (use of CIs).

Stroke

Cerebrovascular disease is the most commonly occurring neurological disorder. It is a group of pathological processes in cerebral blood vessels resulting in brain injury. The injury may be the result of an occlusion of the vessel lumen from a thrombus or embolus; rupture of the vessel; or an alteration in vessel permeability, such as changes in blood viscosity

(Boss, 2006). Cerebrovascular disease is manifested as either a stroke or a transient ischemic attack (TIA). Because the immediate effects of the events are similar, diagnosis is geared toward identifying the specific cause of the symptoms seen and the location of the brain injury. Only when the cause is known can appropriate therapy be implemented.

In the United States each year, about 500,000 people have a stroke, 150,000 of whom die (Boss, 2006). More than 70% of all strokes occur in persons older than 65 years, and they are more common in African Americans and less common in Hispanics. The rate among African Americans is 2.5 times higher than among their white counterparts. They also suffer more disability from the stroke and are 200% more likely to die (Boss, 2006). The age-adjusted death rate is about equal in men and women.

Etiology of Ischemic Stroke

The four main types and causes of ischemic strokes are arterial disease, cardioembolism, hematological disorders, and systemic hypoperfusion. Arterial disease in the form of the inflammatory arteriosclerosis is probably most common. Cardioembolism includes those caused by a dysrhythmia such as atrial fibrillation, which is frequently seen in coronary heart disease. The use of antithrombotics (e.g., aspirin, warfarin) in persons with heart disease is an attempt to reduce the risk for stroke. Hematological disorders include coagulation disorders and hyperviscosity syndromes. Hypoperfusion can occur from dehydration, hypotension (including overtreatment of hypertension), cardiac arrest, or syncope (Leira and Adams, 2004). As a result of better preventive treatment and emergency care, hospitalizations for ischemic stroke fell by one-third between 1997 and 2005. Hospitalizations for hemorrhagic stroke remained relatively stable during the same period (Russo and Andrews, 2008).

Transient Ischemic Attack

Transient ischemic attacks (TIAs) are considered transient strokes that last only a few minutes, usually when the blood supply to part of the brain is briefly interrupted. TIA symptoms usually occur suddenly and are similar to those of stroke but do not last as long. Most symptoms of a TIA disappear within an hour but may persist for up to 24 hours (Box 21-8). TIAs are often warning signs that a person may be at risk for a more serious and debilitating stroke. About one-third of those who have a TIA will have an acute stroke some time in the future. Because the symptoms of a TIA and an acute stroke are similar, patients should assume that all stroke-like symptoms are an emergency and should seek immediate evaluation. Often people ignore the symptoms and attribute them to something else since they generally subside after 10 to 15 minutes. Depending on the evaluation, drug therapy or surgery may be recommended to reduce the risk of stroke in people who have had a TIA (National Institute of Neurological Disorders and Stroke, 2008b).

Etiology of Hemorrhagic Stroke

Hemorrhagic strokes are caused primarily by uncontrolled hypertension and less often by malformations of the blood vessels (e.g., aneurysms). Although the exact mechanism is not fully understood, it appears that the chronic hypertension causes thickening of the vessel wall, microaneurysms, and necrosis. When enough damage to the vessel accumulates, it is at risk for rupture. The rupture may be large and acute or small with a slow leaking of blood into the adjacent brain tissue. In many cases, there is a rupture or seepage of blood into the ventricular system of the brain with damage to the affected tissue through necrosis (Boss, 2006). Resolution of the event can occur only with the resorption of excess blood and damaged tissue. Hemorrhagic strokes are more life threatening but much less frequent than thrombotic strokes.

Signs and Symptoms

Both strokes and transient ischemic attacks manifest with acute neurological deficits that are reflective of the part of the brain affected. They are often heralded by a severe headache. In subarachnoid hemorrhages, the headache is not only sudden but also explosive, very severe, and without other neurological manifestations (Leira and Adams, 2004).

Some of the clinical signs and symptoms are suggestive of either ischemia or hemorrhage (see Box 21-8). Persons with hemorrhage have more focal neurological changes and a more depressed level of consciousness than those with an ischemic stroke. If a deep unresponsive state occurs, the person is unlikely to survive (Boss, 2006). Seizures are more common in intracerebral hemorrhage. Nausea and vomiting are suggestions of increased cerebral edema in response to the event. Focal neurological deficits include alternations in motor, sensory, and visual function, coordination, cognition, and language. The deficits are specific to the area of damage. Diagnostic methods include determination of extracerebral causes, if any (e.g., infection or hypoglycemia), as well as localization of the brain damage by an unenhanced CT or MRI Scan.

Box 21-8	Symptoms of TIA or Stroke

- Sudden weakness or numbness on one side of the body (face, arm, or leg)
- Dimness or loss of vision in one eye
- Slurred speech, loss of speech, difficulty comprehending speech
- Dizziness, difficulty walking, loss of coordination, loss of balance, a fall
- Sudden severe headache
- Difficulty swallowing
- Sudden confusion
- Nausea and vomiting

FAST Acronym to Detect Stroke Signs:
Face: Is it droopy?
Arms: Is one side of the body weak or numb?
Speech: Is it slurred?
Time: The window for the clot-busting drug tPA to be effective is 3 hours. To be a candidate you need to get to the hospital within 2 hours of these symptoms.

TIA, Transient ischemic attack.

Complications

The long-term effects of a stroke can include paralysis and hemiparesis, dysarthria, dysphagia, and aphasia, depending on type, extent, and area affected, as well as depression. There is a high incidence of major depression following a stroke (see Chapter 24). Aphasia is discussed in Chapter 3 and dysphagia in Chapter 8. Whenever paralysis results from a stroke, the development of spasticity in the affected limb(s) is a risk. Spasticity can lead to contractures if it is not managed. Iatrogenic types of complications include deep venous thrombosis (DVT) in a flaccid lower limb, aspiration pneumonia, and urinary tract infections. VaD, discussed earlier, is more common in people who have a history of hypertension, TIAs, or stroke.

Management

All actual or potential cerebrovascular events are considered emergencies and should be treated as such. Acute management is usually accomplished in emergency departments and intensive care units. The acute management of the stroke requires careful attention to the accuracy of the diagnosis. Reperfusion therapy (recombinant tissue-type plasminogen activator [rt-PA]) is used for occlusive strokes only if a CT scan confirms the absence of hemorrhage. The sooner rt-PA or other appropriate treatment is begun, the better the chances for recovery. Most occlusive strokes are embolic. If the person actually has a hemorrhagic event and is misdiagnosed, the bleeding will be rapidly accelerated by the rt-PA, and the person will die. The initial response to the hemorrhagic stroke is to find a means to stop the bleeding rather than dissolve an occlusion.

Post–ischemic stroke management begins immediately with anticoagulants or antiplatelets. Aspiration and sepsis precautions, pneumatic stocking devices, attention to bowel function, physical, speech, and occupational therapy, and early mobilization are necessary following all cerebrovascular accidents (CVAs). A period of intense rehabilitation often takes place in a rehabilitation or skilled nursing facility setting and continues long after the person returns home or to an assisted living setting. An important role for the nurse is documenting clearly and in detail the functional capacities that are retained and those that are impaired. The assessment must be redone routinely to carefully evaluate and document areas of progress, areas of need, and signs of depression, a common sequela.

New support services are primary stroke centers. The major elements of a stroke center are patient care areas, acute stroke teams, written care protocols, emergency medical services, stroke unit, neurology service, support services, a stroke center director with support from the medical organization, neuroimaging services, laboratory services, outcome and quality improvement activities, and continuing education. Specialized stroke units have been found to improve outcomes in persons after ischemic strokes.

Nowhere in the care of elders is the multidisciplinary team more essential than in the care of persons after a stroke. The assessment of needs after stroke is extremely complex; it calls for evaluation by a team coordinated by a nurse and includes a neurologist; a physiatrist; speech, occupational, and physical therapists; an ophthalmologist; a rehabilitation specialist; and a psychologist. It also may include a spiritual advisor. It always includes the person's significant other, who may be involved with the day-to-day life and needs of the elder after a stroke. The American Heart Association and the American Stroke Association (see Resources at end of chapter and at evolve.elsevier.com/ Ebersole/gerontological) provide excellent educational resources, as well as support groups, for patients and their families.

Lewy Body Dementia

Lewy body dementias (LBDs) are the second most common form of degenerative dementia and are widely underdiagnosed. LBD is not a single disorder but a spectrum of disorders including dementia with Lewy bodies (DLB), and Parkinson's disease dementia (PDD). Many individuals with LBD are erroneously diagnosed as having other types of dementia, most commonly AD, or Parkinson's disease if they present with movement problems. The presence of Lewy bodies (protein deposits in the nerve cells) characterizes LBD, and presentation is different from AD. Symptoms include cognitive fluctuations, unpredictable changes in concentration and attention, hallucinations, parkinsonian symptoms (discussed later in the chapter), and REM (rapid eye movement) sleep behavior disorder (see Chapter 10), and severe sensitivity to neuroleptics (Galvin et al, 2007).

There are no medications approved specifically for the treatment of LBD, but CIs are used and can offer symptomatic benefits. Early and accurate diagnosis of LBD is essential because a variety of drugs, including typical neuroleptics (e.g., haldoperidol) and atypical neuroleptics (e.g., olanzapine and risperidone), can cause a severe worsening of movement and a fatal condition known as neuroleptic malignant syndrome (NMS). NMS causes severe fever, muscle rigidity, and breakdown that can lead to kidney failure (Lewy Body Dementia Association, 2008). Quietapine and clozapine may be preferred if psychosis warrants treatment. Anticholinergics and some antiparkinsonian medications can worsen the symptoms. Agranulocytosis that may be fatal is a side effect of clozapine, and close monitoring of the neutrophil count is essential. For more information on LBD, see www.lbda.org/.

Parkinson's Disease

Parkinson's disease (PD) is a progressive disease of the basal ganglia (corpus striatum) and involves the dopaminergic nigrostriatal pathway. This type of disorder produces a syndrome of abnormal movement called parkinsonism that leads to difficulty with mobility.

Epidemiology. PD is the second most common neurodegenerative disease after Alzheimer's disease. PD appears to be slightly more common in men than in women, and the average age of onset is about 60 years. Prevalence and incidence increase with age, but 15% of those diagnosed are younger than 50 years. All races and ethnicities throughout the world appear to be affected; however, a number of studies have found a higher incidence in developed countries. PD was first described in 1817 in a paper by Dr. James Parkinson, a British physician, who described "the shaking palsy" and presented the major symptoms of the disease.

PD is a clinical syndrome characterized by the following: bradykinesia (slow movement); resting tremor; rigidity; abnormalities of posture, balance, and gait; and deficiency of the neurotransmitter dopamine. Parkinson's disease is called either primary parkinsonism or idiopathic. Idiopathic is a term describing a disorder for which a cause has not yet been found. In other forms of parkinsonism, either the cause is known or the disorder occurs as a secondary effect of another disorder that causes loss or interference with the action of dopamine in the basal ganglia (e.g., head trauma, postencephalitic parkinsonism, stroke, tumors, and toxin- and drug-induced parkinsonian syndrome). Older people are especially prone to the development of Parkinson's-like symptoms as a side effect of antipsychotic medications, and any older adult receiving these medications should be routinely screened for extrapyramidal symptoms (EPS). Box 21-9 lists symptoms of PD.

Pathophysiology. The pathogenesis of PD is unknown. Epidemiological data suggest genetic, viral, and toxic (pesticide exposure) causes. In more than one half of those with PD, atrophy and neuronal loss are found (Boss, 2006). The main feature is degeneration of the neurons of the substantia nigra. Lewy bodies and intracytoplasmic eosinophilic inclusions are found in those neurons remaining in the substantia nigra. New evidence suggests that PD is not limited to the nigrostriatal system and may actually originate from the dorsal motor nucleus of the glossopharyngeal and vagal nerves and anterior olfactory nucleus. The disease then spreads from the brain stem in an ascending course. This may explain the nonmotor complications of PD such as depression, memory loss, dysphagia, and sleep problems (Chan et al, 2008).

PD is progressive, and symptoms grow worse over time. Symptoms vary, and the intensity of symptoms also varies from person to person; some become severely disabled, and others experience only minor motor disturbances. The progression of symptoms may take 20 years or more. Older age at onset and the presence of rigidity or hypokinesia as an initial symptom may predict a more rapid rate of motor progression (American Academy of Neurology [AAN], 2006a). In late stages of the disease, complications such as pressure ulcers, pneumonia, aspiration, and falls can lead to death.

Box 21-9   Primary Symptoms of Parkinson's Disease (PD)

Resting Tremor

Occurs in approximately 50% to 75% of all PD patients and is often the initial symptom

Affects mainly hands and feet but may also involve the head, neck, face, lips, tongue, or jaw

Appears regular and rhythmic; approximately 4 to 6 beats per second

Rigidity

Sustained muscle contractions; often mistaken for common stiffness or achiness

Walking with arms held stiffly at the sides (rather than swinging naturally)

Most common types include:
- Cogwheeling: muscles move in a series of short jerks
- Lead-pipe: muscles move smoothly, yet stiffly

May affect breathing, eating, swallowing, and speech

Bradykinesia—*Brady "Slow" Kinesia "Movement"*

Slowing of ordinary movements, such as walking, sitting down, and getting dressed

Reduction in semiautomatic gestures, such as crossing the legs or scratching

Reduction of spontaneous facial movements, resulting in masklike stare

Handwriting begins large and becomes smaller as patient fatigues

Voice may become soft and trail off

Postural Instability

Difficulty maintaining balance when walking or standing

Leans forward in an effort to maintain center of gravity

May result in injuries from frequent falls

Data from The American Parkinson Disease Association, 60 Bay Street, Staten Island, NY 10301.

Clinical Signs. By the time a person becomes overtly symptomatic, 80% to 90% of the dopamine-producing cells are lost (Burke and Laramie, 2000). PD has such an insidious onset that it is very difficult to diagnose, particularly in the early stages. Diagnosis is one of exclusion, ruling out other possible causes of symptoms. Classic signs of PD are (1) tremor at rest, (2) rigidity (stiff muscles), (3) akinesia (poverty of movement), and (4) postural abnormalities. The American Academy of Neurology (AAN) recommends olfactory testing and administration of a levodopa or apomorphine and evaluating effect on symptoms (challenge test) as useful in confirming the diagnosis if there is doubt (AAN, 2006a). Early falls, poor response to levodopa, symmetry of motor symptoms, lack of tremor, and early autonomic dysfunction may be useful in distinguishing PD from other parkinsonian syndromes (AAN, 2006a).

The most conspicuous sign is the tremor—an asymmetrical, regular, rhythmic, low-amplitude tremor. It disappears briefly during voluntary movement. It can occur in the leg, but the arm is more commonly involved. Rarely is the head involved. All tremors are increased with stress and anxiety. Tremor is not present during sleep and when present is a pill-rolling movement. Tremor, however, is a minor part of the clinical picture. A greater cause of disability is the rigidity, slow movements, and postural instability. Other signs include soft-spoken voice, little facial animation (masked facies), infrequent blinking, restless legs, and greasy skin. The characteristic gait is called festination and consists of very short steps and minimal arm movements. Turning is difficult and may require many steps. If a person is off balance, correction is very slow, so falls are common. Other clinical signs include sleep difficulties, constipation, fatigue, excessive salivation, pain, loss of smell, depression, visual disturbances, psychosis, seborrhea, sweating, and hypotension, which is a considerable problem in PD and with the medications used to treat PD.

Rigidity impedes passive and active movement. It is a state of involuntary contraction of all skeletal muscles. Severe muscle cramps may occur in the toes or the hands. On examination, a limb may exhibit "lead pipe" resistance during passive movement. Akinesia (absence or poverty or movement) is an often overlooked symptom. All the striated muscles in the extremities, the trunk, the ocular area, and the face are affected, including the muscles of mastication (chewing), deglutition (swallowing), and articulation. Handwriting is small (micrographia). The person with PD has difficulty initiating movement. "Freezing" is a common problem and may be precipitated by trying to move, turning, or initiating tactile and visual contact. Postural reflexes are lost, and there is involuntary flexion of the head and neck, a stooped posture, and a tendency to fall backward.

Management. Management focuses on relieving symptoms with medication, increasing functional ability, preventing excess disability, and decreasing risk of injury. Many treatment options to manage the symptoms and the consequences of PD are available. The AAN has published comprehensive clinical practice guidelines related to PD, as well as excellent patient information tools (www.aan.com).

Drug therapy focuses on replacement, mimicking, or slowing dopamine breakdown. Choice of medication is based on patient preference, clinical history, and related comorbidities (Chan et al, 2008). Typically, individuals are maintained on a combination of carbidopa and levodopa (Sinemet), which are dopamine precursors. The AAN recommends either levodopa or a dopamine agonist (Parlodel) to treat initial symptoms. Selegiline (monoamine oxidase [MAO] inhibitor) also may be of mild benefit as an initial treatment (AAN, 2006b). Sinemet loses effectiveness since the amino acid l-dopa competes with other amino acids for absorption at both the intestinal wall and the blood-brain barrier. It also has a higher risk of dyskinesia side effects.

Other medications useful in management include the dopamine agonists; dopaminergics; catechol-O-methyltransferase (COMT) inhibitors; MAO inhibitors; antihistamines; and anticholinergics (for tremor relief). Medications may be used in combination and for specific effects. Most recently, rasagiline (Azilect) was approved as a single drug therapy and also to be used in combination with levodopa in advanced disease. The action of Azilect is to block the breakdown of dopamine. People taking this medication must avoid food or drinks that contain tyramine because of interactions causing sudden and severe rises in blood pressure causing stroke or death. Requip XL (ropinirole extended-release tablets), the first and only oral once-daily nonergot dopamine agonist agent indicated for PD, provides continuous delivery of ropinirole over 24 hours to provide smoother blood levels and seems effective in reducing "off" time associated with PD.

Medication therapy is complicated and should be closely supervised by a neurologist. The medications used to treat PD are not without serious side effects. Hypotension is a problem, as are dyskinesias, dystonia, end-of-dose deterioration, and the on-off phenomenon. Medications also cause hallucinations and sleep disorders, as does PD. Sinemet must be taken 1 hour before or 2 hours after a meal to minimize gastrointestinal (GI) side effects, and it must also be given routinely and on time to prevent fluctuations in symptoms. Anxiety and depression frequently occur in PD. Depression may be one of the earliest signs of PD and may occur 15 to 20 years before other symptoms. Medications of choice for depression are the selective serotonin reuptake inhibitors (SSRIs) such as venla-faxine. Bupropion, sertraline, paroxetine, trazodone, and mirtazapine also are used.

Approximately 14% of patients with PD will develop at least mild dementia (Galvin et al, 2007). The etiology of dementia in PD is not clearly understood. DLB (discussed earlier) and PDD have the same clinical symptoms. PDD is diagnosed if motor symptoms precede dementia by more than 12 months. DLB is diagnosed if dementia precedes or is concurrent with parkinsonism. Both DLB and PDD are classified as forms of LBD (Galvin et al, 2007).

Surgical procedures include ablation (pallidotomy, thalamotomy), deep brain stimulation (DBS), and cell transplantation. DBS is the most commonly performed surgery for PD and is used in patients who have not responded to drug therapy or have intractable motor fluctuations, dyskinesias, or tremor. Transplantation is in the experimental stage. Research is ongoing and has shown promising results for both DBS and transplantation. However, the AAN (2006c) states that evidence is insufficient to support or refute DBS at this time.

Nonpharmacological interventions such as exercise, relaxation, stress management, education, and self-care management may be beneficial in helping people cope with PD. Music therapy is being researched as a therapeutic intervention for people with PD, as is investigation of the use of different rhythms to assist in movement (www.pdtrials.org). At this time, the AAN (2006c) does not recommend any vitamin or food additive or other treatment such as acupuncture, biofeedback, or manual therapy as effective treatment of PD. Exercise therapy and speech therapy for patients with dysarthria should be considered.

Nursing Interventions. Persons with PD experience great functional problems in mobility, communication, and ADLs, and nursing interventions can contribute greatly to quality of life and functional ability. Comprehensive functional assessments with attention to self-care abilities in ADLs and nutritional assessment are important, as well as fall assessment and risk reduction interventions. The goal of treatment is to preserve self-care abilities and prevent complications. Exercise, range of motion (ROM), and balance work must begin early in the course of PD, and physical therapy evaluation and treatment are important. Rigidity of facial muscles and bradykinesia can affect eating ability, nutrition, swallowing, and communication. Occupational therapy can assist with adaptive equipment such as weighted utensils, non-slip dinnerware, and other self-care aids. Speech therapy is beneficial for dysarthria and

dysphagia, and patients can be taught facial exercises and swallowing techniques.

Regular pain assessments and appropriate pain management are also essential to address the often unnoticed problem of pain related to rigidity, contractures, dystonia, and central-pain syndromes of the disease itself. Other important interventions are assessment and treatment of postural hypotension, continence, GI distress, depression and anxiety, sleep disturbances, and constipation. Box 21-10 provides some suggestions for nursing interventions. Many resources are available for people with PD to provide practical information about living with the disease, as well as information related to new developments and treatment. The Resources section at the end of this chapter and resources at evolve.elsevier.com/Ebersole/gerontological provide further information that the nurse can use for referral.

Frontotemporal Dementia

Frontotemporal dementia (FTD) is described as a clinical syndrome associated with shrinking of the frontal and temporal anterior lobes of the brain. FTD was previously known as Pick's disease but now includes primary progressive aphasia and semantic dementia (National Institute of Neurological Disorders and Stroke, 2008a). FTD is linked to chromosomal abnormalities, and 30% to 40% of people with FTD have other family members with a neurodegenerative disease. Mean age at onset is between 52 and 56 years, but it has been reported in both younger and older individuals as well. The disease progresses rapidly, and the prognosis is poor. Similar to LBD, FTD is often not accurately diagnosed. Early symptoms are different from those seen in AD and are more often related to changes in personality and inappropriate or bizarre social behavior.

IMPLICATIONS FOR GERONTOLOGICAL NURSING AND HEALTHY AGING

Person-Centered Care

Irreversible dementias such as Alzheimer's disease have no cure, and although new medications offer hope for improved function, the most important treatment for the disease is competent and compassionate person-centered care. "Since Alzheimer's affects mind and personality, as well as physical function, there is a great danger that the person can become obscured by the disease, defined by symptoms rather than by her or his unique spirit and continuing sense of self" (Sifton, 2001, p. iv). Person-centered

Box 21-10	Nursing Interventions for Parkinson's Disease

Exercise
- Flexibility exercises, gentle stretching or yoga
- Range of motion twice a day
- Walking at least 4 times a day. Bring your toes up with every step you take. Use a wide base (legs 12 to 15 inches apart when walking); swing your arms freely when walking; if legs feel frozen or "glued" to the floor, a lift of the toes eliminates muscle spasm; if walking with a helper, have him or her walk by your side, never having the helper pull from the front; wear shoes with a firm sole (no rubber or crepe-soled shoes)
- Practice sitting down and getting up. Sit down slowly with your body bent sharply forward until you touch the seat; when getting up, try rising as quickly as possible; use a lift chair
- Balance exercises (tai chi)
- Proper use of assistive devices
- Try exercise in pool or in bed, or try crawling if balance is poor

Eating and Nutrition
- Small, frequent meals
- Drink ample water—drink by the clock to ensure intake of at least 6 to 8 cups/day
- Cut foods in smaller portions
- Exercise your face and jaw—blow kisses or read aloud; sing with forceful lip and tongue motion; practice making faces in the mirror; recite the alphabet (try these with your grandchildren)
- For upset stomachs linked to medication, try eating an oatmeal cookie or pretzel
- Chew food hard and move food around in the mouth; avoid just swallowing
- Eat sitting up, and remain upright for at least 30 minutes after eating
- Allow adequate time for meals; keep food at proper temperature (insulated cups, warming trays)
- Try non-slip china, swivel or weighted utensils, or wrist weights

Continence and Constipation
- Routine toileting
- Consider bedside commode
- Use raised toilet seat and grab bars
- Wear clothing that is easy to remove
- Drink 6 to 8 cups of water every day; seltzer water adds air and moisture to the bowel and can increase intestinal motility
- Increase fruits and vegetables in diet
- Weak hot tea or hot water with lemon first thing in the morning or prune juice with pulp can stimulate the bowel
- Use medications such a stool softener; avoid stimulant laxatives and bulk or fiber laxatives (unless you drink at least 48 ounces of water/day)

Sleep Difficulties
- Try relaxation exercises, meditation, music
- Use medication for pain or discomfort if present
- Avoid sleeping medications
- Use body pillows or bolsters for comfort in bed
- Try satin sheets to aid turning

Adapted from Parkinson Handbook, National Parkinson Foundation; Imke S: *Nutritional guidelines for people with Parkinson's disease and bowel hygiene: curing the GI blues,* presented at NCGNP Conference, 2005, Cleveland, Ohio; Parkinson disease: signs and symptoms. Available at www.helpguide.org. Accessed 7/8/08. Bonifazi W: A question of balance, *Nursing Spectrum,* June 19, 2006. Available at www.nursingspectrum.com. Accessed 7/8/08.

care looks beyond the disease and the tasks we must perform to the person within and our relationship with them. The focus is not on what we need to "do to the person" but rather on the person himself or herself and how to enhance well-being and quality of life.

Gerontological nurses know that the person, not the disease, is always the focus of care, and they practice from a belief that the person with dementia is still a whole person, someone who can think, feel, learn, grow, and be in a relationship (Touhy, 2004). "The person with dementia is not an object, not a vegetable, not an empty body, not a child, but an adult, who, given support, might exercise choices and respond to a respectful approach" (Woods, 1999, p. 35). Person-centered care fosters abilities, supports limitations, ensures safety, enhances quality of life, prevents excess disability, and offers hope. Care for persons with dementia is more than keeping their bodies alive, safe, and clean; performing tasks; and managing behavior—the care must also nourish their souls (Touhy, 2004). Person-centered care is care that establishes connections and a sense of security; respects and appreciates the person; and supports the person's need to love and be loved, to be known and accepted, to give and to share, and to be productive and successful (Bell and Troxel, 2001).

Despite a growing body of evidence on the importance of person-centered care and therapeutic work with people with dementia, the emphasis in the literature and in practice continues to be on the care of the body (bathing, feeding) and the management of aggressive and problematic behavior. Discussions of how to prevent catastrophic reactions and handle aggressive behavior are far more common than discussions of how to nurture personhood and quality of life. The emphasis on the decline associated with the disease, the catastrophic behaviors, and the loss of humanness promotes despair, hopelessness, and fear on the part of professional caregivers, patients, and families (Touhy, 2004). Special skills and attitudes are required to nurse the person with dementia, and caring is paramount. It is not an area of nursing that "just anyone can do" (Splete, 2008, p. 11). Williams et al (2005) provide a comprehensive set of nurse competencies to improve dementia care.

Nursing Models of Care for Persons with Dementia

Gerontological nurses often provide direct care for people with dementia in the community, hospitals, and long-term care facilities. They also work with families and staff, teaching best practice approaches to care and providing education and support. Much of the care of people with dementia takes place in the home and is provided by a spouse or other family member, or in a nursing home where it is provided by nursing assistants. Gerontological nurses will be most effective when they assist caregivers in all settings to understand the nature of dementia and the interventions likely to be most effective. Overall, interventions must match expectations with capacities, incorporate earlier life skills and interests, and provide a calm, caring, and structured environment. Several nursing models of care are useful in guiding practice and assisting families and staff in providing care to people with dementia.

PLST Model

The progressively lowered stress threshold (PLST) model (Hall and Buckwalter, 1987; Hall, 1994) was one of the first models used to plan and evaluate care for people with dementia in every setting. The PLST model categorizes symptoms of dementia into four groups: (1) cognitive or intellectual losses, (2) affective or personality changes, (3) conative or planning losses that cause a decline in functional abilities, and (4) loss of the stress threshold, causing behaviors such as agitation or catastrophic reactions. Symptoms such as agitation are a result of a progressive loss of the person's ability to cope with demands and stimuli when the person's stress threshold is exceeded. Five common stressors that may trigger these symptoms are fatigue; change of environment, routine, or caregiver; misleading stimuli or inappropriate stimulus levels; internal or external demands to perform beyond abilities; and physical stressors such as pain, discomfort, acute illness, and depression.

Using this model, care is structured to decrease the stressors and provide a safe and predictable environment. Outcomes reported when the model was used on an Alzheimer's special care unit included increased hours of sleep; decreased nighttime awakening; decreased sedative and tranquilizer use; increased food intake and weight; increased socialization; decreased episodes of anxious, agitated, combative behaviors; increased caregiver satisfaction with care; and increased functional level (Hall and Buckwalter, 1998).

Using principles of the PLST model, DeYoung et al (2003) designed a behavior management unit in a long-term care facility. Reported outcomes included a decrease in aggressive, agitated, and disruptive behaviors. Staff training was an important part of this program and included an emphasis on knowing the patient well and modifying the environment. McCloskey (2004) offers practical suggestions based on the PLST model in the acute care environment when caring for patients with dementia. Box 21-11 presents the principles of care derived from the PLST model.

Need-Driven, Dementia-Compromised Behavior Model

The need-driven, dementia-compromised behavior (NDB) model (Kolanowski, 1999; Richards et al, 2000; Algase et al, 2003) is a framework for the study and understanding of behavioral symptoms of dementia. All behaviors have meaning and are a form of communication, particularly as verbal communication becomes more limited (Ortigara, 2000). The NDB model proposes that the behavior of persons with dementia carries a message of need that can be addressed appropriately if the person's history and habits, physiological status, and physical and social

environment are carefully evaluated (Kolanowski, 1999). Rather than behavior being viewed as disruptive, it is viewed as having meaning and expressing needs. Behavior reflects the interaction of background factors (cognitive changes as a result of dementia, gender, ethnicity, culture, education, personality, responses to stress) and proximal factors (physiological needs such as hunger or pain, mood, physical environment [e.g., light, noise]) with social environment (e.g., staff stability and mix, presence of others) (Richards et al, 2000).

Optimal care is provided by manipulating the proximal factors that precipitate behavior and by maximizing strengths and minimizing the limitations of the background factors. For instance, sleep disruptions are common in people with dementia. If the person is not getting adequate sleep at night, agitated or aggressive behavior during the day may signal the need for more rest. Interventions to modify proximal factors interfering with sleep, such as noise, frequent awakenings during the night, and daytime boredom, can help meet the need for rest and sleep and decrease agitation or aggression.

Other authors have discussed the importance of viewing all behavior as meaningful rather than disruptive or problematic and encourage nurses to avoid labeling the behavior of persons with dementia as aggressive (Cohen-Mansfield, 2000; Smith and Buckwalter, 2005). Terms such as disruptive and aggressive focus on the caregiver's negative response (disturbed, disrupted) rather than on the perspective of the person with dementia (fearful, protective) (Talerico and Evans, 2000). Behavioral symptoms usually occur during personal care activities and are associated with higher levels of disability and communication deficits. Fear, pain, discomfort, unfamiliar surroundings and people, illness, fatigue, depression, need for autonomy and control, caregiver approaches, and environmental stressors are frequent precipitants of behavioral symptoms (Box 21-12).

Nurses must use appropriate assessment to understand the meaning of behavior and determine what interventions would be most helpful to meet the needs being expressed. Yet behaviors are frequently treated without appropriate assessment. Putting yourself in the place of the person with dementia and trying to see the world from his or her eyes will help you understand their behavior. Questions of *what, where, why, when, who,* and *what now* are important components of the assessment of behavior. Box 21-13 presents a framework for asking questions about the possible meanings and messages behind observed behavior. Federal documentation requirements in skilled nursing homes call

Box 21-11	Principles of Care Derived from PLST Model

1. Maximize functional abilities by supporting all losses in an assistive manner.
2. Establish caring relationship, and provide person with unconditional positive regard.
3. Use patient's behaviors indicating anxiety and avoidance to determine appropriate limits of activity and stimuli.
4. Teach caregivers to try to find out causes of behavior and to observe and evaluate verbal and nonverbal responses.
5. Identify triggers related to discomfort or stress reactions (factors in the environment, caregiver communication).
6. Modify the environment to support losses and promote safe function.
7. Evaluate care routines and responses on a 24-hour basis, and adjust plan of care accordingly.
8. Provide as much control as possible—encourage self-care, offer choices, explain all actions, do not push or force the person to do something.
9. Keep environment stable and predictable.
10. Provide ongoing education, support, care, and problem solving for caregivers.

PLST, Progressively lowered stress threshold.

Adapted from Hall GR, Buckwalter KC: Progressively lowered stress threshold: a conceptual model for care of adults with Alzheimer's disease, *Arch Psychiatr Nurs* 1(6):399-406, 1987.

Box 21-12	Conditions Precipitating Behavioral Symptoms in Persons with Dementia

- Communication deficits
- Pain or discomfort
- Acute medical problems
- Sleep disturbances
- Perceptual deficits
- Depression
- Need for social contact
- Hunger, thirst, need to toilet
- Loss of control
- Misinterpretation of the situation or environment
- Crowded conditions
- Changes in environment or people
- Noise, disruption
- Being forced to do something
- Fear
- Loneliness
- Psychotic symptoms
- Fatigue
- Environmental overstimulation or understimulation
- Depersonalized, rushed care
- Restraints
- Psychoactive drugs

Adapted from Talerico K, Evans L: Making sense of aggressive/protective behaviors in persons with dementia, *Alzheimers Care Q* 1(4):77-88, 2000.

Box 21-13	Framework for Asking Questions about the Meaning of Behavior

What?
What is being sought? What is happening? Does the behavior have a physical or emotional component or both? What are the person's responses? What would be done if the person was 20 years old instead of 80? What is the behavior saying? What is the emotion being expressed?

Where?
Where is the behavior occurring? Environmental triggers?

When?
When does the behavior most frequently occur? After what (e.g., activities of daily living [ADLs], family visits, mealtimes)?

Who?
Who is involved? Other residents, caregivers, family?

Why?
What happened before? Poor communication? Tasks too complicated? Physical or medical problem? Person being rushed or forced to do something? Has this happened before and why?

What Now?
  Approaches and interventions (physical, psychosocial)?
  Changes needed and by whom?
  Who else might know something about the person or the behavior or approaches?
  Communicate to all and include in plan of care.

Adapted from Hellen C: *Alzheimer's disease: activity focused care*, Boston, 1998, Butterworth-Heinemann; Ortigara A: Understanding the language of behaviors, *Alzheimer Care Q* 1(4):89-92, 2000.

for assessment of behavior and responses to any interventions. The Behave-AD, the Cohen-Mansfield Agitation Inventory, and the Neuropsychiatric Inventory for Nursing Homes are examples of monitoring instruments (Ault, 2007).

Pharmacological and Nonpharmacological Treatment of Behavior Expressions in Dementia

It is so very important that nurses who care for people with dementia use evidence-based practice guidelines to understand and respond to behavioral expressions. Many of the models discussed offer guidelines for appropriate practice. The overuse of the antipsychotic medications to treat behavioral responses is of serious concern in light of the side effects of such medications Approximately 70% of the 1.5 million long-term care residents have dementia, and of these, about 10% have

psychotic symptoms. Despite evidence that antipsychotic medications are effective less than 20% of the time, their continued use is common and often accepted. None of these medications are approved for use in treatment of behavioral responses in dementia. In a comprehensive study, Schneider and colleagues (2006) reported that the benefits of such medications are uncertain, and adverse effects offset any advantages. Yet nearly 21% of nursing facility residents are taking antipsychotic medications despite the absence of diagnosed psychosis. Medicaid has spent more on antipsychotic drugs than any other class of drugs (Pettey, 2008).

Medications should not be the first or even second line of response. When medications are considered appropriate, they must be reduced and discontinued as soon as possible. It is important to review all medications being taken by older people because the inappropriate or contraindicated use of medications is common and is associated with poor outcomes (Chapter 14). The increased sensitivity to drug effects on the central nervous system is a risk factor for adverse drug events in this population. A recent study reported that despite research evidence and recommendations to avoid CNS-active medications, these medications continue to be prescribed for older people with cognitive impairments. Commonly prescribed medications that are problematic include ben-

zodiazepines, oxybutynin, amitriptyline, fluoxetine, and diphenhydramine (Barton et al, 2008).

The focus must be on understanding that behavioral expressions communicate distress and the response is to investigate the possible sources of distress and intervene appropriately. This may include providing pain relief, treating depression, decreasing stimuli, attending to basic needs such as hunger or the need to eliminate, providing comfort measures, and ensuring safety. Positive outcomes of interventions using therapeutic and healing touch and massage to calm agitated behavior in persons with dementia have been reported (Kim and Buschmann, 2004; Kolcaba et al, 2006; Wang and Hermann, 2006). Further research on the use of these modalities is needed (Box 21-14). Touch is a powerful tool to promote comfort and well-being when working with older people.

Box 21-14 **Evidence-Based Practice: Pilot Study to Test the Effectiveness of Healing Touch on Agitation in People with Dementia**

Purpose
The purpose of this pilot study was to assess the effectiveness of Healing Touch (HT) in lowering agitation levels of residents with dementia.

Sample and Setting
A dementia special care unit, an 18-bed secured unit, at the Veterans Affairs Medical Center in Prescott, Arizona, was the site for the study. Fourteen male residents with similar average scores on the Cohen-Mansfield Agitation Inventory were placed in either a control group (8) (receiving usual care) or a treatment group (6) (receiving HT).

Method
A Healing Touch practitioner used 2 HT techniques (unruffling and modified mind clearance) for 10 minutes daily for 4 weeks with the treatment group. Mean agitation scores using the Cohen-Mansfield Agitation Inventory and t tests were used for data analysis. Qualitative results were obtained from a data sheet that the Healing Touch practitioner used to record her observations and comments from the participants. Data on use of psychotropic medication use were also obtained.

Results
HT significantly lowered the frequency of agitation behaviors in male dementia residents exhibiting higher agitation scores. Qualitative comments from the participants included feelings of relaxation, enjoyment. Five of six residents in the treatment group who were receiving psychotropic medications had dose reductions during the intervention, and two of the six had dose increases within the first 2 weeks after the HT interventions were stopped. The small sample size limits the inferences from the study, and the placebo effect is also to be considered, since the participants received extra attention as a result of the HT treatment. Another limiting variable is that all participants were men and the HT practitioner was a woman.

Implications
HT may be an effective intervention to reduce agitation levels in persons with dementia. Further study is indicated and should include larger and more gender-diverse samples, longer time periods, and comparison to other types of placebo treatments.

Data from Wang K, Hermann C: Pilot study to test the effectiveness of Healing Touch on agitation in people with dementia, *Geriatr Nurs* 27(1):34-40, 2006.

Teri and colleagues (2003) and Livingston and colleagues (2005) provide other resources on nonpharmacological approaches to deal with behavioral expressions including exercise training, behavioral management techniques, and psychological interventions. Nonpharmacological interventions and nursing responses derived from the use of the frameworks just described place the focus of care on understanding the person with the disease and what he or she is experiencing or trying to communicate to us. Gerontological nurses with this focus create environments and relationships that value and respect older adults with dementia rather than ones that punish or control.

All professionals working in any setting with people with dementia need the knowledge and skills to effectively treat these patients without the use of unapproved medications whose harm can outweigh their benefits. A team approach to care of persons with dementia is necessary. Results of a recent randomized clinical trial suggested that a collaborative care approach using care management led by a geriatric nurse practitioner decreased behavioral and psychological symptoms by 30% without increasing the use of antipsychotic medications. The intervention also resulted in significant decreases in caregiver distress and improvement of mood (Callahan et al, 2006). Chapter 15 discusses care models in more depth.

Therapeutic Activities

Meaningful and enjoyable activities for persons with dementia provide cognitive stimulation and opportunities for interaction with others. Participation in therapeutic activities enhances feelings of self-worth, promotes a sense of belonging and accomplishment, and encourages expression of feelings and thoughts. "Activities for persons with dementia should be considered rehabilitative if they can increase or prevent further decline in adaptation and functional levels" (Camp and Skrajner, 2004, p. 426). It is important for caregivers in the home, as well as those in assisted living and nursing homes, to provide meaningful and therapeutic activities for persons with dementia. Such activities are of benefit in enhancing communication and enjoyable interaction for both the caregiver and the person with dementia. Buettner and Kolanowski (2003) provide guidelines for recreation therapy in the care of persons with dementia.

Research has shown that activities for persons with dementia that involve "external memory aids and procedural learning assist in increasing engagement with the environment and more positive affect than standard activities programming" (Camp and Skrajner, 2004, p. 426). Camp and colleagues have created Montessori-based activities based on the work of Maria Montessori, an Italian educator who developed an educational method for children. The Montessori method uses task breakdown, guided repetition, progressions from simple to complex and concrete to abstract, extensive use of external cues, and reliance on procedural memory rather than explicit memory. These techniques are part of the principles that have been found useful in interventions for cognitive stimulation and therapeutic work with persons with dementia. Activities are structured to the person's functional and cognitive level and can be modified to accommodate a wide range of cognitive abilities. Camp has authored two training manuals to guide the implementation of Montessori-based activities (Camp, 2001).

Group work, such as reminiscence and storytelling, is another therapeutic approach to encouraging communication, providing opportunities for enjoying memories and conversation, and promoting interaction that enhances self-esteem. Chapter 3 discusses group work in more detail.

Exercise

The therapeutic benefit of exercise for older people was discussed in Chapter 10. Older people with dementia should have regular opportunities for exercise to maintain or improve function, prevent excess disability, and improve mood. Results of a recent study (Williams and Tappen, 2007a; 2007b) reported that nursing home residents with Alzheimer's disease who participated in a comprehensive 16-week exercise program exhibited higher positive and lower negative affect and mood. Results suggest that exercise programs with whole body movement (targeting balance, endurance and upper and lower extremity strength), rather than walking alone, may be more beneficial in improvement of mood. Yves et al (2007) reported a significantly slower decline in ADL score in patients with AD living in a nursing home who participated in a 1-hour twice weekly exercise program of walking, and strength, balance, and flexibility training conducted over a 12-month period. Further research is needed, but exercise has positive benefits for all older adults, regardless of condition or setting.

Interventions for MCI and Early-Stage Memory Loss

With increasing knowledge of Alzheimer's disease and other dementias, and recent advances in available medication, clinicians are diagnosing and working with people much earlier in the disease process. Earlier diagnosis provides opportunities to begin pharmacological and psychosocial interventions that may "lessen the devastation of the disease for both patients and families" (Teel and Carson, 2003, p. 39). However, there has been scant research to guide interventions in early-stage memory loss. Persons diagnosed with MCI and those with early-stage AD present different care needs, and further research is needed to determine what interventions are most helpful to them.

To date, the preponderance of research and intervention programs for caregivers has been directed toward persons and their families living with moderate to late-stage dementia and has focused on preparing caregivers to cope with later-stage concerns such as behavior problems, incontinence, ADL care, nursing home placement, depression, and burden (Whitlach et al, 2006). Many of the issues addressed are not relevant to those in the early stages, will not be of interest to them in the near future, and can be frightening and misleading as well (Adams, 2006; Zarit et al, 2004). Too much information, given too early, may over-burden families (Moniz-Cook et al, 2006). "The subtle onset and progression of caregiving responsibilities in early stage memory loss often necessitates that family members assume the role of caregiver without identifying themselves as such until the middle stages of the disease" (Garand et al, 2005, p. 512). Early-stage carers need help in "coming to terms with the impending decline and loss of the patient as opposed to requiring specific behavior management skills" (Kuhn and Fulton, 2004, p. 111).

Cummings (1998) described three primary emotional challenges of the early stage: 1) accepting the diagnosis; 2) accepting the prognosis; and 3) relinquishing the relationship as it was previously known (p. 31). Adams (2006) found that the stories of family carers of persons with early-stage memory loss focused on accommodating the impairments, taking on new instrumental and psychosocial tasks, and experiencing loss of support and reciprocity in their relationships. Different information and kinds of support are needed at different times, and matching interventions with the stage-specific needs of carers is essential (Kuhn and Fulton, 2004).

Common Care Concerns

Nutrition, ADLs, maintenance of health and function, safety, communication, and caregiver needs and support are the major care concerns for patients, families, and staff who care for people with dementia. Mary Opal Wolanin, a gerontological nursing pioneer, sug-

gested that nurses are not as interested in the neurofibrillary tangles in the brain as they are in trying to smooth out the environmental and relational tangles the person experiences. The overriding goals in caring for older adults with dementia are to maintain function and prevent excess disability, structure the environment and relationships to maintain stability, compensate for the losses associated with the disease, and create a therapeutic milieu that nurtures the personhood of the individual and maintains quality of life.

Two common care concerns for people with moderate to late-stage dementia are discussed in the remainder of this chapter—ADLs care and wandering. Nutrition is discussed in Chapter 8, communication in Chapter 3. Caregiving for persons with dementia is also discussed in more depth in Chapter 23. Interventions for early-stage dementia are discussed in the next section. The Hartford *Try This* Series provides many excellent resources for the care of persons with dementia. Examples of these and other useful resources are presented in Box 21-15.

Providing Care for Activities of Daily Living

The losses associated with dementia interfere with the person's communication patterns and ability to understand and express thoughts and feelings. Perceptual disturbances and misinterpretations of reality contribute to fear and misunderstanding. People with dementia often struggle to understand the world and to make their needs known. Often, bathing and the provision of other ADL care such as dressing, grooming, and toileting are the cause of much distress for both the person with dementia and the caregiver. Bathing and care for ADLs, particularly in nursing homes, can be perceived as an attack by persons with dementia who may respond by screaming or striking out. A rigid focus on tasks or institutional care routines, such as a shower three mornings each week, can contribute to the distress and precipitate distressing behaviors. Being touched or bathed against one's will violates the trust in caregiver relationships and can be considered a major affront (Rader and Barrick, 2000). The behaviors that may be exhibited by the person with dementia are not deliberate attacks on caregivers by a violent person. The message is, in the words of Rader and Barrick (2000, p. 49), "Please find another way to keep me clean, because the way you are doing it now is intolerable."

To care effectively for older adults with dementia, nurses and other caregivers need to try to put themselves

Box 21-15   Resources for Care of Persons with Dementia

Try This Series Resources (www.hartfordign.org)

Issue D1: Avoiding Restraints in Patients with Dementia

Issue D2: Assessing Pain in Persons with Dementia

Issue D4: Therapeutic Activity Kits

Issue D5: Recognition of Dementia in Hospitalized Older Adults (article and video)

Issue D6: Wandering in the Hospitalized Older Adult

Issue D7: Communication Difficulties: Assessment and Interventions

Issue D9: Decision Making in Older Adults with Dementia

Issue D10: Working with Families of Hospitalized Older Adults with Dementia

Issue D11.1: Eating and Feeding Issues in Older Adults with Dementia: Part 1: Assessment

Issue D11.2: Eating and Feeding Issues in Older Adults with Dementia: Part 2: Interventions

Other Resources:

Alzheimer's Association Campaign for Quality Residential Care: *Dementia care practice recommendations for assisted living residences and nursing homes*, 2005. Available at www.caassistedliving.org/information/dementia_care_practice_recommendations_051.pdf. Accessed 7/8/08.

Fletcher K: Nursing standard of practice protocol: recognition and management of dementia. In Capezuti E, Swicker D, Mezey M et al, editors: *Evidence-based geriatric nursing protocols for best practice,* ed 3, New York, 2008, Springer. Also available at www.consultgerirn.org.

Volicer L: *End-of-life care for people with dementia in residential care settings,* 2005, The Alzheimer's Association.

Williams C, Hyer K, Kelly A et al: Development of nurse competencies to improve dementia care, *Geriatr Nurs* 26(2):98-105, 2005.

Source: The Hartford Geriatric Nursing Institute (www. hartfordign. org/TryThis).

---

in the place of the person with dementia and try to see the world from his or her eyes. The following paragraph will illustrate:

> You are asleep in the chair at home when suddenly you are awakened by a person you have never seen before trying to undress you. Then he or she puts you naked into a hard, cold chair and wheels you down a hallway. Suddenly cold water hits you in the face and the person is touching your private areas. You don't understand why the person is trying to do this to you. You are embarrassed, frightened, cold, angry. You hit and scream at this person and try to get away.

It is very important to remember that behavior is an expression of needs, and as such, the focus must be on understanding what the person is trying to communicate through behavior. Family members and nurses caring for people with dementia must understand that they are the ones who must change their behavior, reactions, and approaches because the person with dementia cannot do this. In research in nursing homes, Rader and Barrick (2000) have provided comprehensive guidelines for bathing people with dementia in ways that are pleasurable and decrease distress. Asking the question "What is the easiest, most comfortable, least frightening way for me to clean the person right now?" guides the choice of interventions (Rader and Barrick, 2000, p. 42). Knowing the person's lifetime bathing routines and preferences; providing care only when the person is receptive; respecting refusals to participate in care; explaining all actions; realizing that a bath is not an essential intervention; encouraging self-care to the extent possible; making bathrooms and shower areas warm, comfortable, and safe; being attentive to pain and discomfort; and using alternative bathing methods such as a towel bath or sponge bath are some suggested responses.

Wandering

Wandering associated with dementia is one of the most difficult management problems encountered in home and institutional settings. Wandering is a complex behavior and not well understood. There is a need for more research on wandering as well as interventions for this behavior. Some research indicates that there may be a relationship between certain types of wandering and different presentations of dementia (Dewing, 2006). People with dementia who wander may have more visuospatial impairments, anxiety and depression, and a history of a prior active lifestyle.

Wandering does present safety concerns in all settings. Wandering can lead to falls, elopement (leaving the home or facility), disturbances in care routines such as eating, and interference with the privacy of others (Algase et al, 2003). The stimulus for wandering arises from many internal and external sources. Wandering can be considered a rhythm, intrinsically and extrinsically driven. The following excerpts about wandering from an article by Laurenhue (2001) provide a great deal of insight into this concern from the person's perspective:

> "Wandering and restlessness is one of the by-products of Alzheimer's disease…When the darkness and emptiness fills my mind, it is totally terrifying…Thoughts increasingly haunt me. The only way I can break the cycle is to move" (Davis, 1989, p. 96).
>
> "Very often, I wander around looking for something which I know is very pertinent, but then after awhile I forget all about what it was I was looking for. When I'm wandering around, I'm trying to touch base with—anything, actually. If anything appeared I'd probably enjoy it, or look at it or examine it and wonder how it got there. I feel very foolish when I'm wandering around not knowing what I'm doing and I'm not always quite sure how to do any better. It's not easy to figure out what the heck I'm looking for" (Henderson, 1998, p. 24).

Wandering behaviors can be predicted through careful observation and knowing the person's patterns. For example, if the person with dementia starts wandering or trying to leave the home around dinnertime everyday, meaningful activities such as music, exercise, and refreshments can be provided at this time. Research suggests that wandering may be less likely to occur when the person is involved in social interaction. Environmental interventions such as camouflaging doorways, providing enclosed outdoor gardens and paths for walking, and electronic bracelets that activate alarms at exits are some examples. There are also several instruments to assess risk for wandering as well as assessing wandering behavior (Algase, 2006).

Box 21-16 presents suggestions for additional interventions, but further research in needed to determine the nature of wandering and appropriate evidence-based interventions. A guideline for approaches to prevent and manage wandering in the hospitalized older adult can be found at www.hartfordign.org. An evidence-based protocol for wandering (Futrell and Mellilo, 2002) can be found at www.guidelines.gov.

Wandering behavior may also result in people with dementia going outside and getting lost, a phenomenon studied by Rowe (2003). The Alzheimer's Association estimates that 60% of people with dementia will wander and become lost in the community at some point (www.alz.org/living_with_alzheimers_wandering_behaviors.asp). Conclusions from Rowe's (2003) research, a retrospective review of the records of Safe Return (a nationwide federally funded identification program of the Alzheimer's Association), advised that all people with dementia should be considered capable of becoming lost. Caregivers must prevent people with dementia

from leaving homes or care facilities unaccompanied, register the person in the Safe Return program, and have a plan of action in case the person does become lost. Rowe also suggests that police must respond rapidly to requests for searches and the general public should be informed about how to recognize and assist people with dementia who may be lost (2003). Box 21-17 presents specific recommendations from this study.

Box 21-16   Interventions for Wandering or Exiting Behaviors

- Face the person, and make direct eye contact (unless this is interpreted as threatening).
- Gently touch the person's arm, shoulders, back, or waist if he or she does not move away.
- Call the person by his or her formal name (e.g., Mr. Jones).
- Listen to what the person is communicating verbally and nonverbally; listen to the feelings being expressed.
- Identify the agenda, the plan of action, and the emotional needs the agenda is expressing.
- Respond to the feelings expressed, staying calm.
- Repeat specific words or phrases, or state the need or emotion (e.g., "You need to go home, you're worried about your husband").
- If such repetition fails to distract the person, accompany him or her and continue talking calmly, repeating back phrases and the emotion you identify.
- Provide orienting information only if it calms the person. If it increases distress, stop talking about the present situations. Do not "correct" the person or belittle his or her agenda.
- At intervals, redirect the person toward the facility or the home by suggesting, "Let's walk this way now" or "I'm so tired, let's turn around."
- If orientation and redirection fail, continue to walk, allowing the person control but ensuring safety.
- Make sure you have a backup person, but he or she should stay out of eyesight of the person.
- Have someone call for help if you are unable to redirect. Usually the behavior is time-limited because of the person's attention span and the security and trust between you and the person.

Adapted from Rader J et al: How to decrease wandering, a form of agenda behavior, *Geriatr Nurs* 6(4):196-199, 1985.

Box 21-17	Recommendations to Prevent People with Dementia from Getting Lost

- Do not leave the person with dementia alone in the home.
- Secure the environment so that the person cannot leave by himself or herself while the caregiver is asleep or busy.
- If the person lives in a nursing facility, keep in supervised area; do frequent checks; use bed, chair, and door alarms and Wanderguard bracelets; identify potential wanderers by special arm bands; and disguise doorways.
- Place locks out of reach, hide keys, and lock windows.
- Consider motion detectors or home security systems that raise an alert when doors are opened.
- Register the person in the Safe Return program of the Alzheimer's Association, and ensure that the person wears the Safe Return jewelry or clothing tags at all times.
- Let neighbors know that a person with dementia lives in the neighborhood.
- Prepare a search and rescue plan in case the person becomes lost.
- Keep copies of up-to-date photos ready for distribution to searchers, police, hospital, and the media.
- Conduct a search immediately if the person becomes lost.
- Call the local law enforcement agency and the Safe Return program to report the missing person.
- If the person is not found within 6 to 12 hours (or sooner depending on weather conditions), search any wooded areas or fields near where the person was last seen. People with dementia may not seek help or respond to calls and may try to hide from searchers; search in an organized manner with as many searchers as possible.

Adapted from Rowe M: People with dementia who become lost, *Am J Nurs* 103(7):32-39, 2003.

Wandering is a complex behavior that calls for observation, investigation, and a variety of individualized approaches. The safety and comfort of the person are paramount so that wandering and getting lost do not result in injury or death. There must be an agenda of research looking at the meaning of wandering for persons with dementia, the benefits of wandering, and how safe wandering can be enabled through the use of assistive technology. Dewing (2006) suggests that there needs to be a "transformation from a culture of care and management where wandering is seen as a problem behaviour to be prevented or severely controlled to one that for most persons with dementia facilitates safe wandering" (p. 246). The following quote illustrates:

Can you seriously expect me to live—and I mean live, in one building or one part of a building for the remainder of my life, not being able to walk around as I wish, go out when I feel like it, feel the wind and rain on my skin and only be allowed out for special trips with a bunch of other people when someone else gives the OK? So what if I do wander and get lost? ... I will fight for my right to move about and fill up all the space I want to be me...–A.B. (Dewing, 2006, pp. 246-247.)

Environmental Alterations

Both home and institutional settings can be modified to be more supportive for people with dementia. The culture change movement has significantly changed the way care is delivered in long-term care facilities (Chapter 26). Many nursing homes resemble little hospitals and can be cold, impersonal, and confusing places for people with dementia. The culture change movement to humanize and make nursing home environments more person-centered and homelike is a welcome change to the more commonly found environments. Many facilities have established special care units, designed for the needs of people with dementia. In nursing homes, space can be designed to create a more homelike environment, with smaller areas more like rooms in a house. Family rooms, small-group dining rooms, kitchens on the unit where residents can participate in meal preparation and eat together, private spaces, natural light, elimination of noises such as overhead paging systems, spa-like bathrooms, and outdoor walking and sitting areas are some examples. There are many other ideas and descriptions of more appropriate designs for institutions (Eastman, 2001; Lindstrom, 2004).

CAREGIVING FOR PERSONS WITH DEMENTIA

In the United States, more than 5 million households are providing care for someone with dementia. 85% to 90% of people with dementia are cared for at home, and this care is particularly demanding (Robinson et al,

2005). These caregivers experience more adverse consequences than caregivers of those with other chronic illnesses and are more likely to experience depression and health problems than other caregivers (McCarty and Drebing, 2003; Robinson et al, 2005). Spousal caregivers comprise approximately 50% of all primary family caregivers. They are at most risk for adverse effects related to their own advanced age and the long duration of the illness (Dibartolo, 2002).

According to a recent Harris poll conducted by the Alzheimer's Foundation of America (2008), 68% of caregivers for persons with Alzheimer's disease agree that they are emotionally and physically exhausted from the experience. Factors that influence the stress of caregiving include grief over the multiple losses that occur, the physical demands and duration of caregiving (up to 20 years), and resource availability (Dibartolo, 2002). Behavioral symptoms, difficulties in providing ADLs care, and communication problems have been found to be the best predictors of caregiver distress and care-receiver institutionalization (Farran et al, 2004).

Peterson (2006) suggests that grief is a major dimension of caregiving for persons with dementia, beginning on the day of diagnosis and continuing long after the death of the person. "Losses come in smaller steps such as the day the doctor told her that her husband should not drive, the moment when he asked her his daughter's name, and the most excruciating, his placement in residential care" (Peterson, 2006, p. 15). Often, caregivers do not recognize grief and do not seek help. Marwit and Meuser (2002) reported on the development of an inventory to assess grief in caregivers of persons with Alzheimer's disease, and it may be useful in both practice and research.

Most research has focused on caregiving in the late stages of dementia and on the "burden" of caregiving. Many authors suggest that the "concept of burden alone does not adequately explain the complexities of caregiving for an older person with dementia" (Suwa, 2002, p. 5). Warmth, pleasure, comfort, spiritual growth, self-transcendence, and other positive dimensions of caregiving have also emerged in qualitative studies (Acton, 2002; Farran et al, 2004). In the study by the Alzheimer's Foundation of America (2008), 77% of survey participants reported that they have become stronger than they thought; 64% believed that they have become more compassionate as a result of caregiving; and 59% said they feel closer to the patient since they began caring for them. Further research is needed to help us understand how we can extend caring to both the caregiver and the person with dementia in ways that maintain personhood, enhance re-

lationships, promote quality of life, and balance the stresses with the joys (Haak, 2000). Additional information on caregiving is found in Chapter 23.

IMPLICATIONS FOR GERONTOLOGICAL NURSING AND HEALTHY AGING

Many of the interventions to prevent delirium and to care for people with cognitive impairment are achieved by applying the principles of good gerontological nursing care. An understanding of these principles and how to adapt responses and the environment to people with cognitive impairment will ensure the meeting of basic needs and enhance quality of care and quality of life. Some of these principles may seem like basic nursing, but they are often not practiced, leading to iatrogenesis, distress, and excess disability. Often these consequences are more problematic than the illnesses themselves. Our care, however well intentioned, must not increase disability. It must be based on knowledge and research to be considered best practice. We also have a responsibility to teach others about best practices.

The four roles of a successful caregiver for someone with dementia presented by Rader and Tornquist (1995) provide a framework for competent and compassionate care and promotion of healthy aging for older adults with cognitive impairment:

Magician role: To understand what the person is trying to communicate both verbally and nonverbally, we must be a magician who can use our magical abilities to see the world through the eyes, the ears, and the feelings of the person. We know how to use tricks to turn an individual's behavior around or prevent it from occurring and causing distress.

Detective role: The detective looks for clues and cues about what might be causing distress and how it might be changed. We have to investigate and know as much about the person as possible to be a good detective.

Carpenter role: By having a wide variety of tools and selecting the right tools for the job, we build individualized plans of care for each person.

Jester role: Many people with dementia retain their sense of humor and respond well to the appropriate use of humor. This does not mean making fun of but rather sharing laughter and fun. "Those who love their work and do it well employ good doses of humor as part of the care of others as well as for self-care" (Rader and Barrick, 2000, p. 42). The jester spreads joy, is creative, energizes, and lightens the burdens (Rader and Barrick, 2000; Laurenhue, 2001).

APPLICATION OF MASLOW'S HIERARCHY

Consistent with the philosophy of this book, the nursing care of older adults with dementia presented in this chapter is focused not only on meeting basic needs, but also on creating environments and relationships that promote growth, self-actualization, and quality of life. Despite their inability to express their thoughts and feelings in ways that we are accustomed to, people with cognitive impairment still have higher-order needs, such as those for belonging, self-esteem, and a meaningful life. The care relationships and the environment must support the meeting of all their needs. Surely we would want the same for ourselves. "The relationship between the caregiver and care recipient is the central determinant of quality of life and quality of care" (Rader and Barrick, 2000, p. 36).

Figure 21-1 presents a nursing situation that one nurse experienced in caring for a patient with dementia who was being admitted to a nursing home. Written from the perspective of the nurse and his knowing of the patient, the story provides insight into important nursing responses such as person-centered care, therapeutic communication, and establishing meaningful relationships. It is a lovely example of expert gerontological nursing for older adults with dementia and a fitting way to end this chapter.

KEY CONCEPTS

▶ Nurses must advocate for thorough assessment of any elder who appears to be experiencing cognitive decline and inability to function in important aspects of life.

▶ Delirium sometimes is the result of physiological imbalances and may be caused by a variety of biological disturbances. Delirium is characterized by fluctuating levels of consciousness, sometimes in a diurnal pattern, and frequent misperceptions and illusions. It often goes unrecognized and is attributed to age or dementia. People with dementia are more susceptible to delirium. Knowledge of risk factors, preventive measures, and treatment of underlying medical problems is essential to prevent serious consequences.

▶ Medications and pain are frequently the causes of delirious states in older people.

▶ Irreversible dementias follow a pattern of inevitable decline accompanied by decreased intellectual function, personality changes, and impaired judgment. The most common of these is Alzheimer's disease.

▶ Alzheimer's disease has been the subject of enormous research in attempts to understand the causes. Genes, latent viruses, enzyme and neurotransmitter deficiencies, environmental toxins, and psychosocial stressors have all been implicated to some degree. Research is continuing in attempts to discover ways to protect against or halt the progress of the disease. There is no known cure, although some medications seem to slow the progress of the dementia for a time.

▶ Vascular dementia refers to a group of heterogeneous disorders arising from cerebrovascular insufficiency or ischemic or hemorrhagic brain damage. VaD is the second most prevalent type of dementia in the United States and often coexists with AD. Hypertension, cardiac disease, diabetes, smoking, alcoholism, and hyperlipidemia are additional risk factors for VaD. Prevention and treatment of risk factors are important.

▶ Assessment of cognitive impairment is complex. Nurses may do a cursory assessment with any number of brief mental status examinations and must request more thorough assessment when there is an indication of dementia.

▶ Individuals with cognitive impairment respond best to calmness and patience, adaptations of communication techniques, and environments and relationships that enhance function, support limitations, ensure safety, and provide opportunities for a meaningful quality of life. Because cognitively impaired persons may be unable to express their feelings and needs in ways that are easily understood, the gerontological nurse must always try to understand the world from their perspective.

ACTIVITIES AND DISCUSSION QUESTIONS

1. What are the differences between delirium, dementia, and depression?
2. What are some of the risk factors for development of delirium?
3. Discuss communication strategies useful for the person experiencing delirium.
4. Why is it important to ensure that the person experiencing any change in mental status receives a thorough assessment and evaluation?
5. What would you say to a person who reports to you that he or she has had symptoms of a transient ischemic attack (TIA)?
6. How do the symptoms of Parkinson's disease affect functional abilities? What nursing interventions would be important when caring for a person with Parkinson's disease?

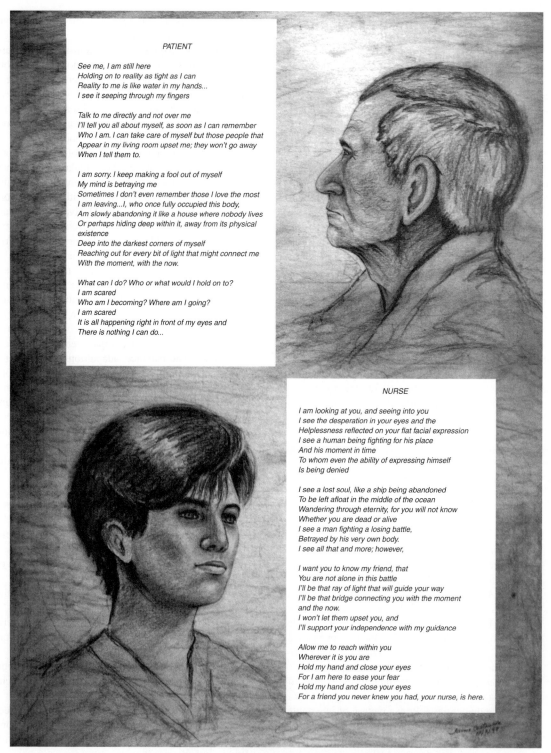

PATIENT

See me, I am still here
Holding on to reality as tight as I can
Reality to me is like water in my hands...
I see it seeping through my fingers

Talk to me directly and not over me
I'll tell you all about myself, as soon as I can remember
Who I am. I can take care of myself but those people that
Appear in my living room upset me; they won't go away
When I tell them to.

I am sorry. I keep making a fool out of myself
My mind is betraying me
Sometimes I don't even remember those I love the most
I am leaving...I, who once fully occupied this body,
Am slowly abandoning it like a house where nobody lives
Or perhaps hiding deep within it, away from its physical
existence
Deep into the darkest corners of myself
Reaching out for every bit of light that might connect me
With the moment, with the now.

What can I do? Who or what would I hold on to?
I am scared
Who am I becoming? Where am I going?
I am scared
It is all happening right in front of my eyes and
There is nothing I can do...

NURSE

I am looking at you, and seeing into you
I see the desperation in your eyes and the
Helplessness reflected on your flat facial expression
I see a human being fighting for his place
And his moment in time
To whom even the ability of expressing himself
Is being denied

I see a lost soul, like a ship being abandoned
To be left afloat in the middle of the ocean
Wandering through eternity, for you will not know
Whether you are dead or alive
I see a man fighting a losing battle,
Betrayed by his very own body.
I see all that and more; however,

I want you to know my friend, that
You are not alone in this battle
I'll be that ray of light that will guide your way
I'll be that bridge connecting you with the moment
and the now.
I won't let them upset you, and
I'll support your independence with my guidance

Allow me to reach within you
Wherever it is you are
Hold my hand and close your eyes
For I am here to ease your fear
Hold my hand and close your eyes
For a friend you never knew you had, your nurse, is here.

Fig. 21-1   Nurse and person. *(Copyright © 1998 by Jaime Castaneda, Lake Worth, Fla.)*

7. Brainstorm with fellow students how it would feel to be bathed by a total stranger.

8. The nursing assistants in a nursing home complain to you that Mr. G. hit them when they were trying to give him his required twice-weekly shower. How might you assist them in meeting Mr. G's need for bathing?

9. Describe how you would design a special care unit for individuals with dementia.

10. A family caregiver tells you that his or her loved one keeps trying to leave the house to find the children. What are some strategies you might share with the caregiver to deal with this situation?

RESOURCES

Websites

Accelerate Cure/Treatments for Alzheimer's Disease
www.act-ad.org

Alzheimer's Association
www.alz.org

Parkinson's Disease Foundation
www.pdf.org

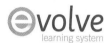

For additional resources, please visit evolve.elsevier.com/Ebersole/gerontological.

REFERENCES

Acton G: Self-transcendent views and behaviors: exploring growth in caregivers of adults with dementia, *J Gerontol Nurs* 28(12):22-30, 2002.

Adams KB: The transition to caregiving: the experience of family members embarking on the dementia caregiving career, *J Gerontol Soc Work* 47(3/4):3-27, 2006.

Algase D: What's new about wandering behavior? An assessment of recent studies, *Int J Older People Nurs* 1(4):226-234, 2006.

Algase D, Beel-Bates C, Beattie E: Wandering in long-term care, *Ann Long-Term Care* 11(1):33-29, 2003.

Alzheimer's Association: African-Americans and Alzheimer's disease, 2008. Available at www.alz.org/living_with_alzheimers_african_americans.asp. Accessed 11/7/08.

Alzheimer's Association: Alzheimer's disease, 2008. Available at www.alz.org. Accessed 7/7/08.

Alzheimer's Association: 2008 Alzheimer's disease facts and figures. Available at www.alz.org. Accessed 11/7/08.

Alzheimer's Foundation of America: I CAN3 Survey: life of a sandwich generation caregiver, January 29, 2008. Available at www.alzfdn.org. Accessed 11/6/08.

American Academy of Neurology (AAN), Practice Parameter: *Diagnosis and prognosis of new onset Parkinson's disease* (an evidence-based review), 2006a. Available at www.aan.com. Accessed 11/7/08.

American Academy of Neurology (AAN), Practice Parameter: *Treatment of Parkinson's disease with motor fluctuations and dyskinesia* (an evidence-based review), 2006b. Available at www.aan.com. Accessed 11/7/08.

American Academy of Neurology (AAN), Practice Parameter: Neuroprotective strategies and alternative therapies for Parkinson disease (an evidence-based review), 2006c. Available at www.aan.org. Accessed 11/7/08.

American Psychiatric Association (APA): *Diagnostic and statistical manual of mental disorders (DSM-IV),* ed 4, Washington, DC, 2000, The Association.

Atri A, Shaughnessy L, Locascio J, Growdon J: Long-term course and effectiveness of combination therapy in Alzheimer disease, *Alzheimer's Dis Assoc Disord* 22(3):209-221, 2008.

Balas B, Gale M, Kagan S: Delirium in older patients in surgical intensive care units, J *Nurs Scholarsh* 39(2):47-154, 2007.

Balas MC, Gale M, Kagan SH: Delirium doulas: an innovative approach to enhance care for critically ill older adults. *Crit Care Nurs* 24(4):36-46, 2004.

Barton C, Sklenicka J, Sayegh B, Yaffe K: Contraindicated medication use among patients in a memory disorders clinic, *Am J Geriatr Pharmacother* 6(3):147-152, 2008.

Beato CV: *Progress review: heart disease and stroke,* April 23, 2003, USDHHS. Available at www. healthypeople.gov/Data 2010/prog/focus12/. Accessed 7/22/06.

Bell V, Troxel D: Spirituality and the person with dementia: a view from the field, *Alzheimers Care Q* 2(2):31-45, 2001.

Bellelli G, Frisoni GB, Turco R et al; Delirium superimposed on dementia predicts 12-month survival in elderly patients discharged from a postacute rehabilitation facility, *J Gerontol A Biol Sci Med Sci* 63(10):1124-1125, 2008.

Bhidayasiri R: When it's not AD: atypical dementing illnesses. Part 1, *CNS Senior Care* 5(2):1, 17, 2006.

Boss B: Alterations in neurological function. In McCance KL, Huether SE, editors: *Pathophysiology: the biologic basis for disease in adults and children,* ed 5, St Louis, 2006, Mosby.

Bradley E, Webster T, Baker D et al: After adoption: sustaining the innovation: a case study of disseminating the Hospital Elder Life Program, *J Am Geriatr Soc* 53(9):1455-1461, 2005.

Braes T, Milisen K, Foreman M: Assessing cognitive function. In Capezuti E, Swicker D, Mezey M et al, editors: *Evidence-based geriatric nursing protocols for best practice,* ed 3, New York, 2008, Springer.

Buettner L, Kolanowski A: Practice guidelines for recreation therapy in the care of persons with dementia, *Geriatr Nurs* 24(1):18-25, 2003.

Burke MM, Laramie JA: *Primary care of the older adult: a multidisciplinary approach,* St Louis, 2000, Mosby.

Callahan C, Boustani M, Unverzagt F et al: Effectiveness of collaborative care for older adults with Alzheimer's disease in primary care: a randomized clinical trial, *JAMA* 295(18):2148-2157, 2006.

Camp C: *Montessori-based activities for persons with dementia*, Baltimore, 2001, Health Professions Press.

Camp C, Skrajner J: Resident-assisted Montessori programming (RAMP): training persons with dementia to serve as activity group leaders, *Gerontologist* 44(3)426-431, 2004.

Chan D, Cordato D, O'Rourke F: Management for motor and non-motor complications in late Parkinson's disease, *Geriatrics* 63(5):22-27, 2008.

Cohen-Mansfield K: Nonpharmacological management of behavioral problems in persons with dementia: the TREA model, *Alzheimers Care Q* 1(4):22-34, 2000.

Crowley SL: Aging brain's staying power, *AARP Bulletin* 37(4):1, 1996.

Dahlke S, Phinney A: Caring for hospitalized older adults at risk for delirium: the silent, unspoken piece of nursing practice, *J Gerontol Nurs* 34(6):41-47, 2008.

Davis R: *My journey into Alzheimer's disease,* Wheaton, Ill, 1989, Tyndale House.

deJonghe JF, Kalisvaart K, Timmers J et al: Delirium-O-Meter: a nurses' rating scale for monitoring delirium severity in geriatric patients, *Int J Geriatr Psychiatry* 20(12):1158-1166, 2005.

Dewing J: Wandering into the future: reconceptualizing wandering "A natural and good thing," *Int J Older People Nurs* 1(4):239-249, 2006.

DeYoung S, Just G, Harrison R: Decreasing aggressive, agitated, or disruptive behavior participation in a behavior management unit, *J Gerontol Nurs* 28(6):22-30, 2003.

Dibartolo M: Exploring self-efficacy and hardiness in spousal caregivers of individuals with dementia, *J Gerontol Nurs* 28(4):24-33, 2002.

Dosa D, Intrator O, McNicoll L et al: Preliminary derivation of a nursing home confusion assessment method based on data from the Minimum Data Set, *J Am Geriatr Soc* 55(7):1099-1105, 2007.

Eastman P: Environmental therapy aids Alzheimer's patients, *Caring for the Ages* 2(9):18, 2001.

Ely EW, Margolin R, Francis J et al: Evaluation of delirium in critically ill patients: validation of the Confusion Assessment Method for the intensive care unit (CAM-ICU), *Crit Care Med* 29(7):1370-1379, 2001.

Farran C, Loukissa D, Lindeman D et al: Caring for self while caring for others: the two-track life of coping with Alzheimer's disease, *J Gerontol Nurs* 30(5):38-46, 2004.

Fick D, Kolanowski A, Woller J, Inouye S: Delirium superimposed on dementia in a community-dwelling managed care population: a 3-year retrospective study of occurrence, costs, and utilization, *J Gerontol A Biol Sci Med Sci* 60A(6):748-753, 2005.

Fick D, Mion L (2005). Assessing delirium in persons with dementia, Geriatric Nursing Hartford Foundation *Try This Dementia Series*, 2005. Available at www.hartfordign.org/resources/education/tryThis.html. Accessed 7/25/08.

Figiel G, Sadowsky C: A systematic review of the effectiveness of rivastigmine for the treatment of behavioral disturbances in dementia and other neurological disorders, *Curr Med Res Opin* 24(1):157-166, 2008.

Fladd D: Subcortical vascular dementia, *Geriatr Nurs* 26(2):117-121, 2005.

Flaherty JH, Morley JE: A call to improve current standards of care, J *Am Geriatr Soc* 51(7):341-343, 2004.

Flaherty JH, Tariq S, Bakshi S et al: A model for managing delirious older inpatients, *J Am Geriatr Soc* 51(7): 1031-1035, 2003.

Fletcher K: Dementia. In Capezuti E, Swicker D, Mezey M et al, editors: *Evidence-based geriatric nursing protocols for best practice,* ed 3, New York, 2008, Springer.

Folstein MF, Folstein S, McHugh P: *Mini-mental state: a practical method for grading the cognitive status of patients for the clinician,* Oxford, 1975, Pergamon.

Foreman MD, Wakefield B, Culp K, Milisen K: Delirium in elderly patients: an overview of the state of the science. *J Gerontol Nurs* 27(4):12-20, 2001.

Futrell M, Mellilo KD: An evidence based protocol for wandering, 2002. Available at www.guidelines.gov. Accessed 7/25/08.

Galik E, Resnick B: Tips from CRNP perspective: *Caring for the Ages* 8(8):19, 2007.

Galvin J, Boeve B, Duda J et al: Current issues in Lewy body dementia: diagnosis, treatment and research, 2007. Accessed 7/7/08 from www.lbda.org/.

Garand L, Dew M, Eazor L et al: Caregiving burden and psychiatric morbidity in spouses of persons with mild cognitive impairment, *Int J Geriatr Psychiat* 20(6):512-522, 2005.

Haak N: One joy will scatter a hundred griefs, *Alzheimers Care Q* 1(4):1-3, 2000.

Hall GR, Buckwalter KC: Progressively lowered stress threshold: a conceptual model for care of adults with Alzheimer's disease, *Arch Psychiatr Nurs* 1(6):399-406, 1987.

Hall GR: Caring for people with Alzheimer's disease using the conceptual model of progressively lowered stress threshold in the clinical setting, *Nurs Clin North Am* 29(1):129-141, 1994.

Ham RJ: Dementias (and Delirium). In Ham RJ, Sloane P, Warshaw G, editors: *Primary care geriatrics*, St Louis, 2002, Mosby.

Hargrave R: Caregivers of African-American elderly with dementia: a review and analysis, *Ann Long-Term Care* 14(10):36-40, 2006.

Henderson C: Partial view: an Alzheimer's journal, Dallas, 1998, Southern Methodist Press.

Hustey FM, Meldon SW: The prevalence and documentation of impaired mental status in elderly emergency department patients, *Ann Emerg Med* 39(3):248-253, 2002.

Inouye SK, van Dyck CH, Alessi CA et al: Clarifying confusion: the confusion assessment method. A new method for detection of delirium, *Ann Intern Med* 113(12):941-948, 1990.

Inouye SK: Delirium in older persons, *N Engl J Med* 354(15):1157-1165, 2006.

Inouye SK, Bogardus ST Jr, Charpentier PA et al: A multi-component intervention to prevent delirium in hospitalized older patients, *N Engl J Med* 340(9):669-676, 1999.

Irving K, Foreman M: Delirium, nursing practice and the future, *Int J Older People Nurs* 1(2):121-127, 2006.

Kalisvaart K, deJohghe J, Bogaards M et al: Haloperidol prophylaxis for elderly hip-surgery patients at risk for delirium: a randomized placebo-controlled study, *J Am Geriatr Soc* 53(10):1658-1666, 2005.

Kim EJ, Buschmann MGT: Touch-stress model and Alzheimer's disease: using touch intervention to alleviate patients' stress, *J Gerontol Nurs* 30(12):33-39, 2004.

Knapp M, Thorgrimsen L, Patel A et al: Cognitive stimulation therapy for people with dementia: cost-effectiveness analysis, *Br J Psychiatry* 188:574-580, 2006.

Kuhn D, Fulton, B: Efficacy of an educational program for relatives of persons in the early stages of Alzheimer's disease, *J Gerontol Soc Work* 42(3/4):109-130, 2004.

Kolcaba K, Dowd T, Steiner R, Mitzel A: The effects of hand massage on comfort of nursing home residents, *Geriatr Nurs* 27(3):85-91, 2006.

Kolanowski AM: An overview of the Need-Driven Dementia–Compromised Behavior Model, *J Gerontol Nurs* 25(9):7-9, 1999.

Laurenhue K: Each person's journey is unique, *Alzheimers Care Q* 2(2):79-83, 2001.

Leira EC, Adams HP: Cerebrovascular disease. In Landefeld CS Palmer R, Johnson MA et al, editors: *Current geriatric diagnosis and treatment,* New York, 2004, McGraw Hill.

Lewy Body Dementia Association: *Lewy body update.* Accessed 7/7/08 from www.lbd.org.

Lindstrom A: Designer's challenge, *Caring for the Ages* 5(4):1, 16, 18, 27, 2004.

Livingston G, Johnston K, Katona C et al: Systematic review of psychological approaches to the management of neuropsychiatric symptoms of dementia, *Am J Psychiatry* 162(11):1996-2021, 2005.

Marcantonio ER, Simon SE, Bergmann MA et al: Delirium symptoms in post-acute care: prevalent, persistent, and associated with poor functional recovery, *J Am Geriatr Soc* 51(1):4-9, 2003.

Marwit S, Meuser T: Development and initial validation of an inventory to assess grief in caregivers of persons with Alzheimer's disease, *Gerontologist* 42(6):751-765, 2002.

McCarty E, Drebing C: Exploring professional caregivers' perceptions: balancing self-care with care for patients with Alzheimer's disease, *J Gerontol Nurs* 29(9):42-48, 2003.

McCloskey R: Caring for patients with dementia in an acute care environment, *Geriatr Nurs* 25(3):139-144, 2004.

McCusker J, Cole C, Dendukrui N et al: Delirium in older medical inpatients and subsequent cognitive and functional status: a prospective study, *Can Med Assoc J* 165(5):575-583, 2001.

McGowin DF: *Living in the labyrinth: a personal journey through the maze of Alzheimer's,* New York, 1993, Dell.

Moniz-Cook E, Manthorpe J, Carr I et al: Facing the future: a qualitative study of older people referred to a memory clinic prior to assessment and diagnosis, *Dementia* 5(3):375-395, 2006.

National Institute on Aging: Alzheimer's disease medications fact sheet, 2008. Accessed 7/7/08 from www.nia.nih.gov/Alzheimers/Publications/medicationsfs.htm.

National Institute of Neurological Disorders and Stroke: Frontotemporal dementia information page, 2008a. Accessed 7/7/08 from www.ninds.nih.gov/disorders/picks/picks.htm.

National Institute of Neurological Disorders and Stroke: NINDS Transient ischemic attack information page, 2008b. Accessed 7/7/08 from www.ninds.nih.gov/disorders/tia/tia/htm.

Neary S, Mahoney D: Dementia caregiving: the experiences of Hispanic/Latino caregivers, *J Transcult Nurs* 16(2):163-170, 2005.

Neelon VJ, Champagne M, Carlson J, Funk S: The NEECHAM confusion scale: construction, validation and clinical testing, *Nurs Res* 45(6):324-330, 1996.

Ortigara A: Understanding the language of behaviors, *Alzheimer Care Q* 1(4):89-92, 2000.

Ozbolt L, Paniagua M, Kaiser R: Atypical antipsychotics for the treatment of delirious elders, *J Am Med Dir Assoc* 9(1):19-28, 2008.

Pandharipande P, Shintani A, Peterson J et al: Lorazepam is an independent risk factor for transitioning to delirium in intensive care unit patients, *Anesthesiology* 104(1):21-26, 2006.

Peterson B: Grief and dementia, *Aging Today* 27(3):5,13, 2006.

Pettey S: Medical director puts use of antipsychotics in perspective, *Caring for the Ages* 9(1):1, 20, 2008.

Pisani M, Araujo K, Van Ness P et al: A research algorithm to improve detection of delirium in the intensive care unit, *Critical Care* 10(4): R121, 2006. Available at http://ccforum.com/content/10/4/R121/abstract. Accessed 11/7/08.

Rader J, Barrick A: Ways that work: bathing without a battle, *Alzheimer Care Q* 1(4):35-49, 2000.

Rader J, Tornquist E: *Individualized dementia care*, New York, 1995, Springer.

Rader J, Doan J, Schwab M: How to decrease wandering, a form of agenda behavior, *Geriatr Nurs* 6(4):196-199, 1985.

Richards K, Lambert C, Beck C: Deriving interventions for challenging behaviors from the need-driven, dementia-compromised behavior model, *Alzheimer Care Q* 1(4):62-76, 2000.

Rigney T: Delirium in the hospitalized elder and recommendations for practice, *Geriatr Nurs* 27(3):151-157, 2006.

Robinson K, Buckwalter K, Reed D: Response by Robinson, Buckwalter, and Reed, *West J Nurs Res* 27(20):145-147, 2005.

Rowe MA: People with dementia who become lost, *Am J Nurs* 103(7):32-39, 2003.

Rubin FH, Williams J, Lescisin D et al: Replicating the Hospital Elder Life Program in a community hospital and demonstrating effectiveness using quality improvement methodology, *J Am Geriatr Soc* 54(6):969-974, 2006.

Russo CA, Andrews AM: *Statistical brief #51: hospital stays for stroke and other cerebrovascular diseases, 2005,* 2008. Available at www.hcup-us.ahrq.gov/reports/statbriefs/sb51.jsp. Accessed 1/20/2009.

Sanders AB: Missed delirium in older emergency department patients: a quality-of-care problem, *Ann Emerg Med* 39(3):338-341, 2002.

Schneider LS, Tariot P, Dagerman K et al: Effectiveness of atypical antipsychotic drugs in patients with Alzheimer's disease, *N Engl J Med* 355(15):1525-1538, 2006.

Sifton C: Life is what happens while we are making plans, *Alzheimers Care Q* 2(2):iv-vii, 2001.

Smith M, Buckwalter K: Behaviors associated with dementia, *Am J Nurs* 105(7):40-52, 2005.

Solomon P, Murphy C: Should we screen for Alzheimer's disease? A review of the evidence for and against screeing for Alzheimer's disease in primary care practice, *Geriatrics* 60(11):26-29, 2006.

Splete H: Nurses have special strategies for dementia, *Caring for the Ages* 9(6):11, 2008.

Stefanacci R: Evidence-based treatment of behavioral problems in patients with dementia, *Ann Long-Term Care* 16(4):33-35, 2008.

Steis M, Fick D: Are nurses recognizing delirium? *J Gerontol Nurs* 34(9):40-48, 2008.

Sullivan M: Now is the time to prepare for the onslaught of Alzheimer's disease, *Caring for the Ages* 8(8):12, 2007.

Suwa S: Assessment scale for caregiver experience with dementia, *J Gerontol Nurs* 28(12):5-12, 2002.

Sweeny S, Bridges S, Wild L, Sayre C: Care of the patient with delirium, *AJN* 108(5):72CC-72FF, 2008.

Talerico K, Evans L: Making sense of aggressive/protective behaviors in persons with dementia, *Alzheimers Care Q* 1(4):77-88, 2000.

Teel CS, Carson P: Family experiences in the journey through dementia diagnosis and care, *J Fam Nurs* 9(1):38-58, 2003.

Teri L, Gibbons LE, McCurry SM et al: Exercise plus behavioral management in patients with Alzheimer disease: a randomized controlled trial, *JAMA* 290(15):2015-2022, 2003.

Touhy T: Dementia, personhood and nursing: learning from a nursing situation, *Nurs Sci Q* 17(1):43-49, 2004.

Truman B, Ely EW: Monitoring delirium in critically ill patients: using the Confusion Assessment Method for the intensive care unit, *Crit Care Nurs* 23(2):25-36, 2003.

Tullmann D, Mion LC, Fletcher K, Foreman MD: Delirium: prevention, early recognition, and treatment, In Capezuti E, Swicker D, Mezey M et al, editors *Evidence-based geriatric nursing protocols for best practice,* ed 3, New York, 2008, Springer.

Voelker R: Programs ease hospitalization experience for patients with dementia, *CNS Senior Care* 7(1):3, 17-18, 2008.

Wang K, Hermann C: Pilot study to test the effectiveness of healing touch on agitation in people with dementia, *Geriatr Nurs* 27(1):34-40, 2006.

Waszynski C, Petrovic K: Nurses' evaluation of the confusion assessment method: a pilot study, *J Gerontol Nurs* 34(4):49-56, 2008.

Whitlach C, Judge K, Zarit S, Femia E: Dyadic intervention for family caregivers and care receivers in early-stage dementia, *Gerontologist* 46(5):688-694, 2006.

Williams C, Byer K, Kelly A et al: Development of nurse competencies to improve dementia care, *Geriatr Nurs* 26(2):98-105, 2005.

Williams C, Tappen R: Exercise training for depressed older adults with Alzheimer's disease, *Aging Mental Health* 12(1):72-80, 2007a.

Williams C, Tappen R: Effect of exercise on mood in nursing home residents with Alzheimer's disease, *Am J Alz Dis Other Dementias* 22(5):389-397, 2007b.

Woods B: Dementia challenges assumptions about what it means to be a person, *Generations* 13(3):39, 1999.

Yves R, Pillard F, Klapouszczak A et al: Exercise program for nursing home residents with Alzheimer's disease: a 1-year randomized, controlled trial, *J Am Geriatr Soc* 55(2):158-165, 2007.

Zarit S, Femia E, Watson J et al: Memory club: a group intervention for people with early-stage dementia and their partners, *Gerontologist* 44(2): 262-269, 2004.

Economic and Legal Issues

22

LEARNING OBJECTIVES

Upon completion of this chapter, the reader will be able to:

- Describe the major methods of financing health care for older adults.
- Compare the costs to the consumer between Medicare and Medicaid.
- Explain the fundamentals of Medicare, Medicaid, and TRICARE sufficiently to assist elders in accessing the services needed.
- Discuss the potential impact of health care financing in long-term and home health care.
- Describe the roles of the nurse as case and care managers.

GLOSSARY

CMS The Centers for Medicare and Medicaid Services, the federal agency under the U.S. Department of Health and Human Services responsible for the administration of Medicare and Medicaid.

Custodial care The provision of personal assistance related to a person's inability to perform the activities needed in daily living. This care may be provided informally by family and friends or formally by nursing assistants.

Prospective payment system (PPS) A system in which the payment of a health service is calculated in advance and based on a number of factors, including diagnosis and age of the patient rather than the actual costs and length of the care needed.

Skilled care The provision of a level of care that requires professional expertise and training, such as that provided by licensed nurses, physical therapists, or occupational therapists.

The Social Security Act The legislation passed in 1935 that provides regular income for older persons.

Title XVIII of the Social Security Act The federal legislation providing for Medicare to all eligible persons over age 65 and to the disabled.

Title XIX of the Social Security Act The federal legislation providing for Medicaid to individuals over age 65 or the disabled with very low incomes.

Title XIV of the Social Security Act The federal legislation that established Supplementary Security to elders with extremely low incomes and few assets.

THE LIVED EXPERIENCE

When I was growing up life was hard. We were so poor we couldn't do much but to hold on tight. When I was lucky I could get work plowing a field and make $1.00 an acre. You work hard, and you make do. There were not such things as going to a doctor or a hospital, you just did the best you could do and pray you don't get sick. Then when I turned 65 I got a little check from the government and a red, white, and blue insurance [Medicare] card. The check isn't much, only about $564 a month, but you know I just consider myself blessed and better off than ever before. And now I don't worry about my health, I will be taken care of.

Aida, age 74

People growing up in the United States represent all levels of education, experience, and income. However, all have in common the potential need for health care. It is rare to meet an older adult who does not have experience in some way with both the past and the present health care systems in the United States. Today's is a system in a state of flux and stress as we find a way to care for the ever increasing number of older adults in the face of skyrocketing costs and increasing legal issues. For gerontological nurses to provide the best care to older adults, it is helpful to have a basic understanding of the heath care system and financing associated with the care they provide and a working knowledge of some of the legal issues older adults face.

SOCIAL SECURITY

The health care system of today and its financing began in 1935. There had been an exodus from the country and farms into the cities and the factories in the early 1900s, changing the social and financial basis of the family. In the country, an elder worked in some way until death, but this was not possible in cities given the exceedingly difficult work of the factories. For the first time people were retiring by reason of disability. The word *retiring,* which had meant "to withdraw from public" in the 1800s, now meant "no longer qualified," with dramatically different implications (Achenbaum, 1978).

The family, no longer able to provide all the care to their elders, looked to the federal government for help. In 1935 the Social Security Act was passed. The Social Security program, established at the time of the Great Depression, was considered by many to be one of the most successful federal programs. Its primary function was to provide monetary benefits to American citizens and legal residents over the age of 65 to prevent their dependency on their families

Social security (SS) was designed as a pay-as-you-go system. Payroll taxes collected from employees and employers are immediately distributed to beneficiaries (retirees, the disabled, or eligible spouses). In 2008 payroll taxes were withheld on the first $102,000 of income, collected from employees and employers, and immediately distributed to beneficiaries. Social Security funds, although individually deposited by employers and employees, are not reserved for any one individual. No one has an account set aside in his or her name. All funds that are not immediately paid out to beneficiaries are "borrowed" by the federal government for regular operating expenses.

As long as the amount of contributions from the workers exceeds those paid to the beneficiaries, the program as designed can continue. At the time of its inception the system was constructed to transfer funds from those believed to be relatively well off (workers) to those believed to be relatively poor (retirees). Social security and a number of programs that followed were set up as "age-entitlement" programs. This meant that an individual could receive the benefits simply because of age and regardless of need. In other words, the monetary support is available to those persons at a certain age regardless of other sources of personal income or assets. They were and are, however, limited to American citizens and legal residents older than a certain age or totally and permanently disabled who have paid into the system through payroll taxes for at least 10 years or are married to someone who is eligible.

The amount of benefit is calculated in part on the person's average salary during 35 of his or her working years. If 35 years were not worked, these nonworking years count as zero in the calculation, but the average is still reached by dividing by 35 (Hooyman and Kiyak, 2008). This has been most beneficial to older white men, who are more likely to have worked the most consistently and at higher salaries than all other groups of workers. It has been most disadvantageous for many women who took time off for child or parent care. The amount of benefit increases each year on January 1 as a cost-of-living adjustment (COLA). In 2008 the average Social Security benefit for the 39 million recipients was $1087.52/month (SSA, 2008a).

In an effort to save money the SS system has been increasing the age when one is eligible for full benefits. Those born in 1938 are eligible to begin receiving partial SS benefits at age 62; however, they must wait until age 65 if they want to receive their full benefit. The age at which one becomes eligible is increasing slowly and will transition to 67 years old for those born in 1960 or after (U.S. Social Security Administration [SSA], 1984).

Supplemental Security Income

Not all older persons living in the United States have Social Security benefits adequate to provide even the most basic necessities of life. This has been true especially for persons who have spent their lives employed in the agriculture industry or as domestic workers and were paid very low wages, often on a cash basis. Supplemental Security Income (SSI) was established in 1965 by Title XVI of the Social Security Act. SSI provides for a minimum level of economic support to older adults. Among the requirements is very low income; income includes monetary gifts, food, and shelter provided by others. SSI payments are calculated on total monthly income with supplementation to the maximum allowed by the state of residence. For example the 2008 California rates bring the person's monthly income to $870.00 if living in the community and to $658.67 if living in another's household (SSA, 2008b). If one's income or the contributions of others increases, the payment decreases accordingly.

MEDICARE AND MEDICAID

History

In 1934 President Franklin D. Roosevelt tried to organize a plan to provide universal health insurance in the United States. This was met with unbeatable opposition from groups such as the American Medical Association and, by poll, the majority of the American public (Cantril, 1951). Except for a few successful insurance plans for working people, health care was on a fee-for-service, out-of-pocket basis. This meant that each health care service could be purchased from one's own funds, or "pocket." When costs were reasonable, older adults could continue to pay for their care, especially since they had a guaranteed income of some kind through Social Security. However, as people began to live longer with more health problems, and as technology advanced and costs rose, paying for the costs of health care out-of-pocket grew harder and even impossible for many older adults who were entirely dependent on the limited incomes of Social Security.

In 1965, through the efforts of President Lyndon B. Johnson, legislation (Title XVIII of the Social Security Act) was passed creating an insurance plan (Medicare A) covering the costs of hospitalization for all persons eligible for Social Security, SSI, or railroad retirement benefits. A second policy (Medicare B) could be purchased, which was a subsidized medical policy to cover the costs of seeing health care providers. The costs of outpatient medications were not covered by Medicare until 2006, when Medicare D was created.

Medicare was meant to provide insurance coverage for medical care to the elderly and disabled regardless of their financial situation. Another amendment (Title XIX) to the Social Security Act created a second form of insurance for the elderly, the disabled, and children with low incomes, known as *Medicaid*. Medicaid was designed to defray expenses for those who did not

qualify or could not afford to purchase the supplemental policy (Medicare B) or to pay the copayments required. All persons eligible for SSI are automatically eligible for Medicaid.

Medicare

Medicare is administered by the Centers for Medicare and Medicaid Services (CMS) (www.cms.gov) and is a part of the Department of Health and Human Services, a special entity created to improve the administration of the programs. In 2007, over 44 million people were covered by Medicare. This included over 36 million people age 65 and over, and over 7 million who were disabled. This contrasts with the 19 million people who were covered in 1966 (when it was limited to persons 62 and older) (CMS, 2007).

To be eligible for Medicare, the adult must have legally worked 10 years (30 quarters) and be at least 65 years old or be younger than 65 with severe disabilities or end-stage renal disease (ESRD). If these criteria are not met, coverage may be purchased. Medicare consists of four parts (Box 22-1).

Medicare only covers select services and requires that these services be considered medically necessary. This means that the services are prescribed and are needed for the diagnosis or treatment of a medical condition, meet the standards of good medical practice, and are performed not for the convenience of the health care provider (CMS, 2009).

Medicare A

In the 3 months before one's sixty-fifth birthday, a person applies for Medicare. He or she is then automatically enrolled in Medicare A and receives a Medicare card (red, white, and blue) indicating coverage. If a person does not apply during that time, he or she has to wait for the next "open enrollment period," with the beginning of benefits July 1 of that year, and penalties may be charged (CMS, 2009). Medicare Part A is a hospital insurance plan covering acute care, acute and short-term rehabilitative care, some costs associated with hospice care, and home health care under certain circumstances.

In 2009, if a person has not worked the requisite time, he or she may be eligible to purchase Part A coverage for a monthly fee of up to $443 (CMS, 2009). The coverage and copayments under Medicare A vary by setting under the original fee-for-service plans. When acute care is needed, the patient responsibility can be quite high, including a deductible of $1068

Box 22-1   Medicare Basics

Medicare A

A hospital insurance plan that is automatically provided for all persons who qualify, with no premium attached. Covers part of the costs of acute care, acute and short-term rehabilitative care, some costs associated with hospice care, and home health care under certain circumstances. There are co-pays and deductibles for most services.

Medicare B

A purchased insurance plan to cover some of the costs of services provided by physicians; nurse practitioners; outpatient services (e.g., lab work); qualified physical, speech, and occupational therapy; and skilled home and hospice care. It also covers a growing number of health screens. One prevention and health screening–oriented visit within 6 months after one's sixty-fifth birthday is also covered. Persons can "opt out" of Medicare B and enroll in Medicare C.

Medicare C

Medicare C is also known as the Medicare Advantage Plan and includes covered services through either a PPO or MCPs, such as what are known as HMOs. The consumer "enrolls" to receive services from assigned specific locations and providers. In the MCP there are fewer out-of-pocket costs unless an individual decides to see a provider or seek a service without a referral or outside the system to which he or she has subscribed. Medical services are expected to emphasize preventive medicine, comprehensive care, periodic physical examinations, and immunizations.

Medicare D

Medicare D is not one plan but is a designation for dozens of private medication payment plans that meet certain criteria and are approved by the Centers for Medicare and Medicaid. The premiums vary by company and reflect the range of medications covered. All Medicare D plans have an annual deductible and a certain amount of coverage until a cap occurs, with no coverage until the next cap and then significant coverage for the rest of the year. The deductibles and caps change every year.

HMO, Health maintenance organization; *MCP,* managed care plan; *PPO,* preferred provider organization.
See www.cms.gov for the latest information about covered services and associated costs. These are all subject to change.

(as of 2009) for days 1 to 60 and a copay of $267/day for days 61 to 90. Each beneficiary has a 60-day lifetime reserve at the copay cost of $534 per day; there is no coverage after 90 days. These co-pays are repeated every time the person is readmitted to an acute care facility with the exception of the lifetime reserve (CMS, 2009).

Medicare A also pays 100% of the costs for the first 20 days in a skilled nursing facility for the purpose of rehabilitation. There is a co-pay of $133.50 for days 21-100, and no coverage after that (CMS, 2009).

When the assistance needed is limited to personal care or medication supervision, it is not covered by Medicare at all. Similarly, for home health care, for the costs to be paid by Medicare the care must be provided at the written direction of a physician. Ongoing supervision can be provided by either a physician or a nurse practitioner. It must be through a certified agency and for the purposes of active rehabilitation as seen in the nursing home setting. There are no co-payments for home health care and limited co-pays for hospice care.

Medicare B

A person who is eligible for Part A must apply for Part B through the local Social Security Administration office (www.socialsecurity.gov). At that time the person will be asked to choose one of the Medicare B plans that are available in his or her area. The possible plans include the Original Medicare Plan or one of the Medicare Advantage Plans (formerly called Medicare + Choice). Medicare B covers the costs associated with the services provided by physicians; nurse practitioners; outpatient services (e.g., lab work); qualified physical, speech, and occupational therapy; and some home health care. Medicare C replaces Medicare B and is a managed care plan similar to what we know as a health maintenance organization. Many older adults are being encouraged or directed to enroll in Medicare C plans rather than the Original Medicare.

The Original Medicare Plan is based on a traditional fee-for-service arrangement; the patient receives services from a provider for a medical problem, a bill for the costs of the care is sent to Medicare (through a carrier) or to the patient, who can submit the claims, and the provider or the patient is reimbursed. After a deductible of $135 a year, Medicare reimburses at a rate of 80% of what Medicare considers an "allowable charge" for medical services (mental health is limited to 50%). The patient is responsible for the remaining 20% (or 50%) of the charge. A provider who "accepts assignment" cannot charge a patient any more than the 20% of the "allowable charge." The number of physicians who accept assignment under the original Medicare system is decreasing rapidly (CMS, 2009).

A provider who does not accept assignment may charge the patient up to 15% above the allowable charge. With the Original Medicare Plan, the patient is responsible for an annual deductible, copays, coinsurance charges, and a monthly premium based on income and marital status. The premium is usually deducted directly from the monthly Social Security check. In 2009 the monthly premium for Part B is $96.40 a month. Beginning in 2009 individuals with incomes above $85,000 and couples with incomes above $170,000 pay slightly higher premiums (CMS, 2009).

The advantages of the Original Medicare Plan include choice and access. The person can seek the services of any provider of his or her choice, without a referral. Many people with the Original Medicare Plan purchase what are called Medigap policies to cover the deductibles and copays.

Medicare C

The *Medicare Advantage Plan (Medicare C)*, depends on location and may include a preferred provider organization (PPO) plan and/or any number of managed care plans (MCPs). Not all plans are offered at all locations. The plans provide extra benefits beyond those usually covered by the Original Medicare plan (e.g., limited drug coverage, which replaces Medicare D); they may require small copays, have special rules that must be followed, and may charge extra premiums for the added services. Referrals for services are always required.

The PPO plan works like the Original Medicare except that only specific providers can be used (those in the network) and the allowable charges are preset. Any additional services and fees or copays vary by plan. A patient may choose to be seen by a provider outside the PPO network for an additional charge.

In MCPs (also known as HMOs), the consumer "enrolls" to receive services from assigned specific locations and providers. There are fewer out-of-pocket costs unless an individual decides to see a provider or seek a service without a referral or outside the system to which he or she has subscribed. These are not usually covered at all. Medicare contracts with MCPs to provide comprehensive services for the elderly, financed by Medicare premiums. The best of these are complete health care systems with highly trained physicians, nurse practitioners, and nurses working out of single or regional completely equipped medical centers. Medical services are expected to emphasize preventive medicine, comprehensive care, periodic physical examinations, and immunizations.

Capitation is imposed on managed care plans by Medicare; this means that the plan is paid a certain fixed amount each day for each enrollee regardless of the amount of care given, and with this amount all needed care must be provided. While the intention of this design was to increase preventive care, in some cases, this has created abuses and horror stories in which elders were denied necessary treatments, presumably motivated by the plan's desire to lower its costs. Now patient protection laws are in place that allow consumers to lodge complaints and initiate legal action against the suspected abuse. The Center for Patient Advocacy supported a much-needed bill that became law in October 1999, which allows appeals when an MCP denies care, guarantees access to specialists when needed, ensures that health-related decisions are made by health care providers rather than bureaucrats, and holds MCPs legally accountable for medical decisions that cause harm.

HMOs that have been granted Medicare capitation cannot refuse applicants based on preexisting health conditions. The supplemental services offered may save the participant a considerable amount in the costs of medications, assistive devices, and professional consultation charges. The negative aspects of HMOs and managed care are the access barriers to specialists and high-tech procedures and treatments. Some HMOs provide extensive health education services, support groups, and telephone support services to the homebound.

Medicare D

Medicare D was created as part of the Medicare Modernization Act. This is an optional medication payment plan. People must enroll within 6 months of initial Medicare eligibility. Otherwise they have to wait until the next enrollment period, with a penalty based on the number of months they waited to enroll. Medicare D is not one plan but is a designation for dozens of private plans that meet certain criteria and are approved by the Centers for Medicare and Medicaid. The premiums vary by company and reflect the range of medications covered. The average premium is about $70 and can be deducted from one's Social Security check. In 2009 the annual deductible is $295. From $296 to $2700 in drug costs there is approximately 75% coverage. However there is no coverage between $2702 and $4350. This uncovered period is called the "donut hole" and is reached by many in the late fall of the year. After $4350 coverage is at about 95%. Individuals can purchase additional private insurance to supplement this. A challenging aspect of Medicare D has been in the limitations of approved medications in the standard plans, necessitating many persons to change their prescriptions. After considerable restrictions in the first year, there have been adjustments every year since (CMS, 2009; Resnick & Jett, 2005).

Medicaid

For elders with low incomes (including all persons receiving SSI), Medicaid may be available to offset the high Medicare copays and deductibles, as well as to provide additional health benefits.

In 2004 Medicaid provided health care insurance to 4.5 million persons 65 years of age or older (10% of all Medicaid beneficiaries) at a cost of over $11,345 per person, and for 7.5 million disabled persons at $10,040 per person. State Medicaid programs paid for 41% of all the nursing home and home health care in the United States. This included $37.2 billion ($21,898 per beneficiary) for 1.7 million of the people in nursing homes and $3.5 billion ($3475 per person) for 1 million at home (CMS, 2007).

Within the broad guidelines established by the federal government, each state establishes its own eligibility criteria, determines the types and extent of services to be covered, sets the payment rates to providers, and administers its own programs. In most cases, Medicaid covers more services than Medicare, including custodial care in nursing homes and preventive care with no copays or deductibles; however, this is highly variable by state and by the year and depends on the state's fiscal health and political priorities. States pay for half of the costs and determines who is eligible and which services are provided. This means that the Medicaid services available to the poorest of the elderly and the disabled are dependent on the affluence and the policy of a given state. Alabama, with one of the highest percentages of poor residents, also has one of the lowest state incomes and therefore one of the lowest levels of Medicaid services.

More states are turning to Medicaid MCPs, very similar to Medicare C, in an attempt to control costs. Sometimes the MCP is optional for the beneficiary, and sometimes enrollment is mandatory. Waiver programs are designed to allow the states to design and implement innovative delivery models to keep Medicaid-eligible elders out of nursing homes. Medicaid does not help the near-poor, who cannot qualify for aid but cannot afford basic health care, even with the partial aid of Medicare.

The premise of Medicare and Medicaid managed care is that better outcomes will result from systems of care that integrate professionals in responsive teams, maximize the use of subacute care, and provide incentives to reduce the reliance on institutional acute care. Managed care systems are most effective for individuals enrolled over a long period who use ongoing primary care and preventive strategies to maintain health and avoid high-cost emergency services and intensive treatment.

The American Association of Managed Care Nurses was established in 1994 to educate nurses regarding managed health care (www.aamcn.org).

CARE FOR VETERANS

The Veterans Health Administration (VA) system has long held a leadership position in gerontological research, medical care, and extended care. A great deal of the research that has guided gerontologists was generated through the VA system. In addition, the vast majority of geriatric fellowships have been provided through the Department of Veterans Affairs (VA) hospitals. The VA system has been a model for continuity of care in the various care provider systems in place. Early on, this system provided VA-run nursing homes, home care and community-based primary care programs, respite care, blindness rehabilitation, mental health, and numerous other services in addition to acute medical-surgical provisions. As a result of a combination of budget cuts and growth of the covered population, services have become more restricted.

Persons and their dependents that have been part of the uniformed services may be eligible for health care services through veterans' hospital networks or through TRICARE (see next section). At one time, veteran's hospitals and services were available on an as-needed basis for anyone who had served at any time. It was not necessary for individuals to use their Medicare benefits. However, this system has undergone significant change. One of the first changes was restrictions placed on the use of Veterans Hospitals and services. Instead of coverage for any health problems, priorities were set for those problems that were in some way deemed "service-connected"; in other words, the health care problem had to be linked to the time the person was on active duty.

TRICARE for Life

TRICARE is the health care insurance program provided by the Department of Defense for eligible beneficiaries. The TRICARE for Life (TFL) plan is for Medicare-eligible beneficiaries age 65 and older and their dependents or widows or widowers older than 65. This plan requires that the person enroll in both Medicare A and B and pay the premiums for Part B. As a Medigap policy, TFL covers those expenses not covered by Medicare, such as copays and prescription medicines. Dependent parents or parents-in-law may be eligible for pharmacy benefits if they turned age 65 on or after April 1, 2001 and are enrolled in Medicare B. For more information, see www.tricare.osd.mil.

LONG-TERM CARE INSURANCE

Some persons are electing to purchase additional insurance (long-term care insurance [LTCI]) for their potential long-term care needs. Ideally these policies cover both the expenses related to copays for nursing home and home care and for what is called custodial care, that is help with activities of daily living (ADLs). Traditionally these policies were limited to care in long-term care facilities and provided a flat-rate reimbursement to residents for their costs. However, these policies are becoming more creative and innovative and may cover home care costs instead, or in addition, under some circumstances. Since they do not receive any governmental funding support, the premium costs can be prohibitive.

Many plans are being marketed at present, although many do not reach the ideal. The purchaser must be cautioned to read the policy carefully and understand all the details, limitations, and exclusions. There are particular concerns related to Alzheimer's disease because many policies exclude these individuals from home benefits and include very limited institutional benefits. The best LTCI packages have been negotiated by a large employer or state organization or association (see www.ANA.org). It is also advisable to check consumer reports of the particular insurance company and its claims paid history before purchasing a policy.

IMPLICATIONS FOR GERONTOLOGICAL NURSING AND HEALTHY AGING

Nurses are increasingly at the frontlines of helping elders achieve the highest level of wellness possible. They also advocate for the best, most cost-effective care available.

Case and Care Management

Although the terms *case manager* and *care manager* have slightly different connotations, in real practice the roles are seldom that clear and there is much overlap. Both of these roles include that of an advocate, broker, leader, manager, counselor, negotiator, administrator, and communicator. Ideally the care manager follows the person through the entire continuum of care. Care managers must be experts regarding community resources and understand how these can best be used to meet the client's needs. They are expected to make appropriate referrals within the person's expectations and abilities and to monitor the quality of any arranged services. The care or case manager is a resource person whom the client can seek for advice and counsel and for brokering (negotiating, arranging) the flow of services. As a gatekeeper, the case or care manager controls the entrances and exits to services to make sure that the elder gets what is needed without wasting resources.

Care managers are usually paid privately. Those who cannot afford the out-of-pocket expenses of purchased case management services must rely on those available through Medicare-managed care plans and community agencies. As these are publically funded their availability varies by state and areas within the states. For further information see www.cmsa.org and www.rncasemanager.com.

Some frail and needy elders desire to remain in their homes even when few services and minimal assistance are available to them. This situation is often distressing to the nurse, but as competent adults, elders have a right to make their own life choices and may opt to stay home with less rather than going to a nursing home with more. However, nurses can continue to advocate for and support the elder in any way that is possible and acceptable to them.

Care that is well managed is believed to be a solution to both the spiraling cost and the fragmentation of care experienced by elders with multiple needs. The care manager works to optimize the resources and outcome for the client and the agency or community in which the person resides.

In response to the emergence of case management, the Case Management Society of America (CMSA), an international, nonprofit organization, was founded in 1990 (www.cmsa.org; www.aamcn.org). The CMSA developed the Standards of Practice for Case Management and the Standards of Practice and Ethics Statement. Education, research, and networking to create professionalism and accountability are top priorities of the organization (Box 22-2).

Multidisciplinary Care Team Planning

The nurse also influences health outcomes and promotes healthy aging through participating in and leading multidisciplinary care team meetings. This can be part of his or her responsibility as the care or case manager, as a representative of an insurer, or as a health care provider (e.g., nurse in a nursing home). The basic case management team for the care of an individual and family involves a physician and/or nurse practitioner, licensed nurse, rehabilitation specialist, and social worker. It also may include chaplains, dietitians, and certified nursing assistants.

As the health care system becomes more complex, the need for collaboration among these interested parties becomes more important. The special knowledge and skills of a dozen or more professionals may be required in working with a single elder and his or her family. A functioning multidisciplinary team will reduce care redundancy, fragmentation, and waste by making use of the resources available in a coordinated and cost-effective manner.

Ensuring Quality Of Care

Nurses are also influential in and responsible for ensuring continuous quality improvement and quality management in all health care settings regardless of the financial arrangements. Funders, licensing agencies, accrediting bodies, and patients all depend on the nurse to make sure that the care provided is the care that is actually needed, and that the care is of high quality. Funding sources, especially the federal government through Medicare, have taken steps to ensure that their standards are met and that their monies are not wasted; this is accomplished through audits, the required documentation of care, and performance incentives.

LEGAL ISSUES IN GERONTOLOGICAL NURSING

Basic knowledge of the most common legal issues that may arise when working with older adults is as important as the financial issues just discussed. Legal concerns are most often related to an individual's ability to make health care decisions and consent to treatment or research.

Box 22-2	Ten Commandments of Case Management During Hospitalization

1. Be visible in the acute care setting; the case manager must follow the client through any level of care.
2. Communicate routinely with the hospital discharge planner (HDP); when the client is hospitalized, immediately call the HDP to alert him or her to your involvement.
3. Provide support for the hospitalized client. Ideally, visit daily and keep the client informed of discharge plans.
4. Provide for necessary monitoring of the home while the client is absent, such as pet care.
5. Monitor the client's hospital progress and make staff aware of previous functional needs and abilities.
6. Recommend appropriate levels of discharge to the HDP.
7. Maximize benefits of hospitalization by initiating assessment and care of conditions that the client may have been neglecting before hospitalization.
8. Encourage early discharge.
9. Begin discharge planning on the day of hospital admission. Discuss with the HDP a package of potential services needed on discharge.
10. Make placement recommendations based on experience with the quality of care or special facilities in specific institutions; seek the least restrictive alternative. At times you must educate the physician or acute care staff regarding the differences in levels of long-term institutional care.

Modified from Peters B: The ten commandments of case management during hospitalization: a practice perspective. In Pelham AO, Clark WF, editors: *Managing home care for the elderly: lessons from community based agencies,* New York, 1986, Springer.

petepete
peterpeter

peterpeter

Competence (Capacity)

Competence and *capacity* are legal terms used to indicate the level of a person's ability to make decisions. This includes the ability to understand the consequences of one's actions and choices. This ability is presumed unless there is clear evidence indicating that the person cannot understand the information needed to make decisions.

Capacity is multifaceted. It includes the ability to handle finances and daily business, to take care of oneself, and, finally, to make medical and health-related decisions. Capacity includes the ability to agree to or to decline health care treatment and procedures. Giving consent to participate in research is more complex because it may or may not directly benefit the individual.

When the capacity of an individual to make informed decisions is believed to be impaired, only the courts can declare the person "incapacitated." He or she may be determined to have no or limited capacity in one area of his or her life but to have ability in another. For example, one may not be able to adequately take care of day to day personal business such as bill paying but may still be able to make personal health care decisions. For those who are unable to speak for themselves or not able to understand the consequences of their decisions for whatever reason, legal protection may be needed. However, every attempt should be made to match the level of protection to that which is needed. In other words, actions are taken that provide the needed protection at the lowest level of personal restriction.

Legal protection of the person with impaired capacity ranges from a general power of attorney, often limited to financial concerns, to guardianship, a mechanism in which the person becomes a "ward" under the complete protection of a guardian or conservator. Each is discussed below.

Power of Attorney

A power of attorney (POA) is a legal document and device in which one person designates another person (e.g., family member, friend, etc.) to act on his or her behalf. The two types are a general POA and a durable POA. The appointed person becomes known as the *attorney-in-fact*. The attorney-in-fact named in a general POA usually has the right to make financial decisions, pay bills, etc., in defined circumstances but not to make decisions related to health care.

The attorney-in-fact appointed in a durable POA usually has additional rights and responsibilities to make health-related decisions for persons when they are unable to do so themselves. This person is known as the *health care surrogate.* A health care surrogate is expected to use "substituted judgment" in making decisions; that is, the decision is expected to be that which the person would have made for herself or himself if able to do so and not what the surrogate would make for herself or himself in the same situation. Therefore it is always advisable that the choice of the surrogate is someone who knows and is willing to uphold the wishes and preferences of the person. Whether the health care surrogate is allowed to make end-of-life decisions is determined by state statutes (see Chapter 25).

Powers of attorney are in effect only at the specific request of the elder or, in the case of the durable POA, in the event that he or she is unable to act on his or her own behalf. As soon as the person regains abilities, the POA is no longer in force unless the individual requests it to continue. The elder retains all of the rights and responsibilities afforded by usual law. This is the least restrictive form of protection and assistance, providing decision making for persons with impaired capacity. An important aspect of the POA is that persons who are given decision-making rights are those who have been chosen by the elder rather than by a court. This type of advance planning is generally recommended because it is the least restrictive and the most likely to ensure that the wishes of the person are followed.

Guardians and Conservators

Guardians and conservators are individuals, agencies, or corporations that have been appointed by the court to have care, custody, and control of a disabled person and manage his or her personal or financial affairs (or both) when the person has been found (adjudicated) to lack capacity.

Whereas a *conservator* is appointed specifically to control the finances of the ward, the person appointed to be responsible for the person is usually called the *guardian,* although these terms are sometimes used interchangeably. The conservator or guardian continues in that role until the court rescinds the order. The appointment is made at a court hearing in which someone demonstrates the incapacity of the elder. Often the elder is not present. The elder is declared *incapacitated* (formerly called *incompetent*). How this is handled differs by state. In many states the ward, as a person without any legal standing is called, is unable to petition the courts to have his or her rights restored.

In some states, limits are set according to the degree of protection needed. Total dependency means the person cannot meet basic needs for survival and is unable to manage the environment in any self-sustaining way. Some dependency means the person may be able to manage certain challenges of life; health or judgment may interfere with management of other needs. In the latter situation, a limited guardian may be appointed to protect the person in very specific ways. There are considerable pros and cons in the use of conservatorships and guardianships, including high risk for exploitation.

IMPLICATIONS FOR GERONTOLOGICAL NURSING AND HEALTHY AGING

Although nursing has long recognized the need for gerontological specialization, the law and lawyers have only more recently done so. The National Elder Law Foundation (NELF) is one of the few specialty organizations that certify lawyers who have demonstrated knowledge pertinent to the legal needs of older adults (www.naela.org).

These categories of need relate to both legal and economic concerns of older adults and differ little from those with which nurses have been dealing for years as they care for their elderly clients. Gerontological nursing as a specialty has been evolving (see Chapter 2) and has become more important as the population of older adults has increased and their health care and other needs have been identified, and acknowledged. Nurses who are consulted by clients about legal issues should not attempt to provide legal advice, but instead should refer their clients to a NELF certified attorney. The state or local bar association is a resource for nurses and for elders and their advocates.

ELDER MISTREATMENT AND NEGLECT

Unfortunately, a person in need of the assistance of others is at risk for harm and injury at the hands of a frustrated, angry, fraudulent, careless, or disturbed caregiver. Mistreatment of older frail and vulnerable adults is found in all socioeconomic, racial, and ethnic groups in the United States. It can be seen in any configuration of family and in every setting. Mistreatment includes several types of abuse and neglect; however, the definitions of exactly what constitutes any of these vary somewhat by state. The most common types of abuse are physical, psychological, sexual, and financial (see Appendix 22-A). Medical abuse is also seen, wherein the person is subjected to unwanted treatments or procedures, or medical neglect is seen when desired treat-

ment is withheld. Neglect implies that the caregiver has not met his or her obligation. Self-neglect is recognized when a person is not caring for herself or himself in the manner in which most peers would do so. In all cases the vulnerable person is harmed.

In recognition of the escalating problem of elder mistreatment across the globe, countries are busy defining the problem and establishing plans for prevention. Federal definitions of elder abuse, neglect, and exploitation appeared for the first time in the 1987 Amendments to the Older Americans Act. These definitions were provided in the law only as guidelines for identifying the problems and not for enforcement purposes (Appendix 22-A). The specific definitions of elder abuse or mistreatment are now defined by state law and vary considerably from one jurisdiction to another. In 1992 the U.S. Congress passed the Family Violence Prevention and Services Act, mandating an analysis of the problem, and the Vulnerable Elder Rights Protection Act, which established the National Ombudsman Program (www.ltcombudsman.org). In December 2001, the first National Summit on Elder Abuse in the United States was held to identify future directions in the protection of abused elders. The National Center for Elder Abuse (NCEA) provides detailed information on the state of elder abuse and related laws (see www.elderabusecenter.org).

Just how much mistreatment is occurring is almost impossible to ascertain; estimates of abuse range from 4% to 6% of elders from several countries (Wang et al, 2006). In the United States, this number is estimated to be between 3% and 10% (Hall et al, 2005). In more contemporary times, defining mistreatment is becoming more difficult as our countries become more diverse. Cultural differences are numerous in the identification and definition of abuse. Given our diverse society, this must be considered (Simpson, 2005).

Most abuse occurs in the home setting, where the majority of caregiving occurs. Most abusers are spouses or adult children. The majority (84%) of the documented cases are among white elders (Meiner, 2006). The incidence of elder abuse is expected to increase with the increase in the numbers of persons in need of care, the increasingly conflicting demands on the caregiver's time, and the increased pressure to report suspicions of abuse (Gorbien and Eisenstein, 2005).

Elder abuse requires an abuser, an elder, and the context of caregiving (Lantz, 2006). The abuse tends to be episodic and recurrent rather than isolated. There are multiple risk factors for one to be or become an abuser or abused (Box 22-3). Persons who are abusing substances,

Box 22-3 Profiles of Abused and Abusers

Abused Elders
Woman age 80 years or older
Lives alone or with abuser
Has mental or physical disability
Is dependent on abuser

Abusers
Middle-aged male sibling or offspring
Has mental health and substance abuse problems
Is financially dependent on abused
Has history of abuse and being abused

Adapted from Utley R: Screening and intervention in elder abuse, *Home Care Provid* 4(5):198, 1999.

have emotional or mental illnesses, or have a history of abusing or being abused are more likely to be abusers, as are caregivers who are exhausted and frustrated. The abuser is usually the caregiver but may also be the care recipient. Caregivers, be they informal (e.g., spouses) or formal (e.g., nursing assistants), may be subjected to verbal and physical abuse by the person they are caring for. This may be a lifelong pattern that intensifies in the caregiving situation, or it may be the result of deep-seated prejudices (Gorbien and Eisenstein, 2005).

Older women are at particular risk for mistreatment (Box 22-4). In a recent cross-sectional study of abuse

Box 22-4 Women and Abuse

A study conducted by Bonnie Fisher and Saundra Regan examined the types of abuse, repeated abuse, and the experiences of multiple abuse by women over 60. A telephone survey was responded to by 842 women living in the community. Almost half the women have experienced some type of abuse since the age of 55; many of these reported repeated abuse. The abused women were more likely than the non-abused women to complain of health problems, including bone and joint problems, digestive problems, depression or anxiety, chronic pain, high blood pressure, or heart problems.

Data from Fisher BS, Regan SL: The extent and frequency of abuse in the lives of older women and their relationship with health outcomes, *Gerontologist* 46(2):200-209, 2006.

among community-dwelling women older than 55 years, nearly half reported having experienced some type of abuse, and many of them reported repeated abuse (Fisher and Regan, 2006). This risk is intensified if they have been abused in the past or if their behavior is aggressive, combative, or provocative; that is, they are viewed as overly demanding or unappreciative (Gorbien and Eisenstein, 2005). The level of dependency is also a factor; the more dependent the elder, the more vulnerable he or she is to being abused. Men or women who had abused the caregiver earlier in life are at risk for retaliation.

Since both the majority of caregiving and the majority of abuse occur within the family, this is the context. Caregiver–care recipient relationships that were conflicted earlier in life will continue to be so. However mistreatment and exploitation can also occur in any caregiving situation (Quinn and Zielke, 2005). When there are a number of providers, monitoring becomes especially difficult. Situations of potential formal caregiver abuse include those in which there is inadequate supervision of patient care, poor coordination of services, inadequate staff training, theft and fraud, drug and alcohol abuse by staff, tardiness and absenteeism, unprofessional and criminal conduct, and inadequate record keeping. Exploitation includes what is referred to as "undue influence" when it is suspected that a caregiver, companion, or home care provider has influenced an impaired elder to transfer assets to them without consultation with usually involved others (Hall et al, 2005). These situations are being examined more carefully in the courts, and some states are activating legal protections against undue influence (see Box 22-5). The nurse should pay particular attention to the caregiver, formal or informal, who is alone, with no support from others and no opportunities for respite.

Most often, older victims are unwilling or afraid to report the problem because of shame, embarrassment, intimidation, or fear of retaliation. The abuser may be the only caregiver available, and reporting or complaining could leave him or her without any care at all. The abuse may be part of a lifelong pattern in which the victim has always felt somewhat at fault and so he or she will remain in the situation.

IMPLICATIONS FOR GERONTOLOGICAL NURSING AND HEALTHY AGING

Nurses must be vigilant and sensitive to the potential for abuse, observing for signs and symptoms in all their interactions with vulnerable elders (Box 22-6). In

Box 22-5	Potential Indications of Undue Influence

- Elder takes actions inconsistent with his or her life history. Actions run counter to the person's previous long-time values and beliefs.
- Elder makes sudden changes with regard to financial management. Examples include cashing in insurance policies or changing titles on bank accounts or real property.
- Elder changes his or her will and previous disposition of assets.
- Elder is taken to practitioners different from those he or she has always trusted. Examples include bankers, stockbrokers, attorneys, physicians, and realtor.
- Elder is systematically isolated from or is continually monitored with others who care about him or her.
- Someone suddenly moves into the person's home, or the elder is moved into someone's home under the guise of providing better care.
- Someone attempts to get income checks directed differently from the usual arrangement.
- Documents are suddenly signed, frequently as the elder nears death.
- A history of mistrust exists in the elder's family, especially with financial affairs, and the elder places unusual trust in newfound acquaintances.
- Someone promises to provide lifelong care in exchange for receipt of property on the elder's death.
- Statements of the elder and the alleged abuser vary concerning the elder's affairs or disposition of assets.
- A power imbalance exists between the parties in matters of finances or health.
- Someone shows unfairness to the weaker party in a transaction. The stronger person unduly benefits by the transaction.
- The elder is never left alone with anyone. No one is allowed to speak to the elder without the alleged abuser having a way of finding out about it.
- Unusual patterns arise in the elder's finances. For instance, numerous checks are written out to "cash," always in round numbers, and often in large amounts.
- The elder reports meeting a "wonderful new friend who makes me feel young again." The elder then becomes suspicious of family and begins to avoid family gatherings.
- The elder is pressed into a transaction without being given time to reflect or contact trusted advisors.

From Quinn M: Undue influence and elder abuse: recognition and intervention strategies, *Geriatr Nurs* 23(1):11-16, 2002.

addition to the physical signs (see Appendix 22-A), the nurse looks for more subtle signals. Is there an unusual delay between the beginning of a health problem and when help is sought? Are appointments often missed without reasonable explanations? Are there inconsistencies between the history given by the elder and that by the caregiver?

There also may be behavioral indications suggestive of an abusive situation. Does the caregiver do all of the talking in a situation, even though the elder is capable? Does the caregiver appear angry, frustrated, or indifferent while the elder appears hesitant or frightened? Is the caregiver or the care recipient aggressive toward the other or the nurse?

If abuse is suspected, a full assessment should be done, including a determination of the safety of the victim and the desires of the victim if competent. Assessment of mistreatment involves several components. Terry Fulmer at the Hartford Institute for Geriatric Nursing (www.hartfordign.org) presents a detailed assessment that is considered one of the

best practice protocols. Her tool can be found in Appendix 22-B.

Intervention

The goals of intervention are to stop mistreatment and neglect of elders, to protect the victim and society from inappropriate and illegal acts, to hold abusers accountable, to rehabilitate the offender, and to order restitution of property and payment for expenses incurred as a result of exploitation. However, most of these are beyond the nurse's usual scope of practice. The most important information for nurses to know is how to participate in the prevention and early recognition of potential abuse as well as the requirements for mandatory reporting in their states (Box 22-7).

Mandatory Reporting

In most states and U.S. jurisdictions, licensed nurses are required to report suspicions of abuse to the state, usually to a group called "adult protective services." Most often

Box 22-6	Signs of and Responses to Elder Mistreatment

Signs and Signals

Obvious physical signs of violence

Feeling of the victim that he or she has done something wrong

Isolation from others outside the relationship

Restriction of elder's contact with others

Perpetrator easily irritated or agitated and demonstrates poor control of anger

Verbalized threats toward elder or caregiver

Actions to be Taken

Assess the presence of physical danger

Identify appropriate options:

- Seek legal advice
- Get a protective order
- Have the abuser arrested
- Support victim's decision to leave or stay
- Develop a workable safety plan

Reestablish contact with family and friends

Identify emergency actions that will assist the victim:

- Give specific information on places of sanctuary

Modified from Davey P, Davey D: Domestic violence: a clinical view, *Home Health Focus* 2(10):78-79, 1996.

Box 22-7	Tips for the Prevention of Elder Mistreatment

Make professionals aware of potentially abusive situations.

Educate the public about normal aging processes.

Help families develop and nurture informal support systems.

Link families with support groups.

Teach families stress management techniques.

Arrange comprehensive care resources.

Provide counseling for troubled families.

Encourage the use of respite care and day care.

Obtain necessary home health care services.

Inform families of resources for meals and transportation.

Encourage caregivers to pursue their individual interests.

these reports are anonymous. Allegations of abuse should not be made on the basis of casual suspicion but on that of solid evidence. If the nurse believes the elder to be in immediate danger, the police must be notified and the person protected from harm. How the nurse accomplishes this varies with the work setting. In hospitals and nursing homes this is often first reported internally to the facility social worker or supervisor. In the home care setting, the report is made to the nursing supervisor. It would be very unusual for the nurse not to go through his or her employer. However, the nurse who is a neighbor, friend, or privately paid caregiver may be under obligation to make the report. In the nursing home or licensed assisted living facility, the nurse has the additional resource of calling the state long-term care ombudsman for help. In each state, ombudsmen are either volunteers or paid state employees who are responsible for acting as advocates for vulnerable elders in institutions. All reports, either to the state ombudsman or to adult protective services, will be investigated. A unique aspect of elder abuse compared with child abuse is that the physically frail but mentally competent adult can refuse assessment and intervention and often does. Abused but competent elders cannot be removed from harmful situations without their permission, much to the frustration of the nurse and other health care providers. As discussed earlier, an older adult continues to have the right to make all personal decisions unless declared otherwise in a court of law.

Prevention of Mistreatment

In the ideal situation, gerontological nurses are alert to situations of risk for mistreatment of vulnerable elders and take steps to prevent the occurrence of abuse or neglect (Box 22-7). In some situations the abuse may be preventable, and in others, it is not preventable. If the abuse is the result of psychopathological conditions, especially if the situation is long-standing, the nurse is unlikely to be able to prevent the abuse. However, nurses can make sure that the potential victims know how to get help if it is needed and know what resources are available to them, and nurses can provide support and encouragement that it is possible to leave the situation, if this is the case. Unfortunately there are very few shelters that will accept a frail older adult. The nurse can also work with the elder, the caregiver, and community supports to increase the exposure of the elders to others. If the abusive behavior is learned or a response to stress, the situation may allow for change. Learned abuse, theoretically, can be unlearned and may respond to a close working relationship with a mentoring professional who can model positive problem solving and new ways of managing difficult situations.

If the abuse is based on the stress of caregiving, nurses can be very proactive and help all involved do things to lessen the stress. This may include finding respite services, changing the situation entirely (giving permission to the caregiver to give up the role), referring to support groups for ventilation of frustrations and peer support, teaching people how to use crisis hotlines, professional consultation, victim support groups, victim volunteer companions, and, above all, thoughtful and compassionate care for both.

It has become clear as we face the burgeoning population of very old survivors and the entry of the baby boomers into the ranks of older persons that many aspects of the health care system must be modified. Because nurses are pivotal players within the system and occupy diverse roles, there are abundant opportunities for professional growth and gratification in working with the aged in our ever-shifting health care system. Nurses are case managers and primary care coordinators in the home. We expect that nurses will continue to occupy a pivotal role in home care as advocates and to carefully evaluate care plans, quality outcomes, and costs.

APPLICATION OF MASLOW'S HIERARCHY

At the most basic levels of Maslow's Hierarchy, nurses are expected to provide safety and security to the persons under their care to the extent possible regardless of the capacity of the person; this responsibility increases as the limitations of the elder decreases. The nurse is often the one who provides much of the information that elders and their significant others need to make informed decisions. When doing so it is essential that this exchange is documented in the health care record (see Chapter 5). The nurse often deals with the difficult and problematic legal and ethical issues in the provision of culturally appropriate care. Providing culturally appropriate care within the context of a patient's changing cognitive capacity and judgment is at the core of many ethical and legal dilemmas in gerontological nursing.

KEY CONCEPTS

▶ Health care and its systems are undergoing profound changes, including the increase in the number of managed care organizations and changes in the roles of health care providers. All of these changes affect the care of the older adult.

▶ A combination of Social Security and Supplementary Security Income payments provide eligible persons with a regular income after the age of 65 or earlier if disabled. The total amount varies greatly and is dependent on qualified earned income during the working years.

▶ Medicare, Medicaid, and TRICARE are insurance plans for specific groups of people.

▶ Medicaid pays for a large portion of the cost associated with long-term home and nursing home care.

▶ There may be substantial out-of-pocket costs associated with the receipt of health care today.

▶ In order for Medicare to pay for the expenses related to long-term care or home health care, strict criteria of medical necessity must be met.

▶ Good care management is a mode of care management that considers cost, quality, and coordination of services for the benefit of the client.

▶ Nurses have key roles in the assurance of quality care to older adults.

▶ Protective measures are available for persons with limited or absent capacity through power-of-attorney, guardians, and conservators.

▶ The nurse has a responsibility to ensure the safety and security of those persons to whom care is provided. This responsibility does not change with the change in the persons' legal status or capacity.

▶ Elder abuse requires a situation of caregiving; however either the care recipient or the caregiver may be the perpetrator.

▶ In most jurisdictions the nurse is required to report suspicions of abuse of the elderly and any person who is vulnerable.

ACTIVITIES AND DISCUSSION QUESTIONS

1. Interview a nurse case manager, and ask about the components of the position that are gratifying and those that are the most difficult.
2. Discuss your thoughts about specific activities that are different for case managers and care managers.
3. Describe the role of the nurse-advocate in relation to health and consumer protections.
4. Explain the fundamentals of Medicare and Medicaid sufficiently to assist elders in obtaining more specific information.
5. Interview an elder in a rehabilitation center, and ask about his or her experiences with acute hospitalization, long-term care, and Medicare.
6. Discuss with this elder his or her thoughts about Medicare and how it does or does not meet his or her needs. Write a brief summary, and present it to the class.

RESOURCES

Books and Publications

Consumers' Guide to Health Plans. Publication that has rated health care maintenance organizations (HMOs) across the nation as excellent, very good, good, fair, or poor. This guide also gives information on keeping costs down and getting the best care when enrolled in a plan. Contact Health Plan Guide, 733 15th Street NW, Suite 821, Washington, DC 20005.

Medicaid at a Glance, 2005. Available at http://www.cms.hhs.gov/medicaidgeninfo/Downloads/MedicaideAtAGlance2005.pdf.

Organizations

American Association of Managed Care Nurses
4435 Waterfront Drive, Suite 101
PO Box 4975
Glen Allen, VA 23058

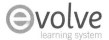

For additional resources, please visit evolve.elsevier.com/Ebersole/gerontological

REFERENCES

Achenbaum WA: *Old age in a new land,* Baltimore, 1978, Johns Hopkins Press.

Cantril H: *Public opinion 1935-1946,* Princeton, NJ, 1951, Princeton University Press.

Center for Medicare and Medicaid Services (CMS): Medicare Enrollment: National Trends, 2007. Available at www.cms.hhs.gov/MedicareEnRpts/Downloads/HISMI07.pdf. Accessed 7/25/08.

Center for Medicare and Medicaid Services (CMS): Medicare and you, 2009. Available at www.medicare.gov/publications/pubs/pdf/10050.pdf. Accessed 1/9/09.

Fisher BS, Regan SL: The extent and frequency of abuse in the lives of older women and their relationship with health outcomes, *Gerontologist* 46(2):200-209, 2006.

Gorbien MJ, Eisenstein AR: Elder abuse and neglect: an overview. *Clin Geriatr Med,* 21(2):279-292, 2005.

Hall RC, Hall RCW, Chapman MJ: Exploitation of the elderly: undue influence as a form of elder abuse, *Clin Geriatr* 13(2):28-36, 2005.

Hooyman N, Kiyak H: *Social gerontology: a multidisciplinary approach,* New York, 2008, Pearson.

Lantz MS: Elder abuse and neglect: help starts with recognizing the problem, *Clin Geriatrics* 14(9):10-13, 2006.

Meiner S: Legal and ethical issues. In Meiner S, Lueckenotte A, editors: *Gerontologic nursing,* ed 3, St Louis, 2006, Mosby.

Quinn K, Zielke H: Elder abuse, neglect, and exploitation: policy issues. *Clin Geriatr Med,* 21(2):440-457, 2005.

Resnick B, Jett K: *The Medicare Modernization and Improvement Act: the Medicare Part D drug benefit tips for nurses,* 2005. Available at www.consultgerirn.org/advocacy/medicare_part_d_drug_benfit_tips_for_nurses. Accessed 12/25/08.

Simpson AR: Cultural issues and elder mistreatment. *Clin Geriatr Med,* 21(2):355-364, 2005.

U.S. Social Security Administration (SSA): *Summary of P.L. 98-21,* (HR 1900). 1984. Available at www.socialsecurity.gov/history/1983amend.html. Accessed 7/25/08.

U.S. Social Security Administration (SSA): *How are my retirement benefits calculated?* 2008a. Available at www.ssa.gov. Accessed 7/25/08.

U.S. Social Security Administration (SSA): *Supplementary security income (SSI) in California.* 2008. Available at http://www.ssa.gov/pubs/11125.html. Accessed 7/25/08.

Wang JJ, Lin J-N, Lee F-P: Psychologically abusive behavior by those caring for the elderly in domestic context, *Geriatr Nurs* 27(5):284-291, 2006.

The National Elder Abuse Incidence Study

DEFINITIONS OF ELDER ABUSE, EXPLOITATION, AND NEGLECT

The following definitions of abuse, exploitation, and neglect pertain to elders. The perpetrator of this abuse may or may not be the caregiver of an elderly person or a member of the elderly person's family. Furthermore, some signs and symptoms are characteristic of several kinds of maltreatment and should be regarded as indicators of possible maltreatment. These are most important:

▶ An elder's frequent unexplained crying
▶ An elder's unexplained fear of or suspicion of a particular person(s)

Physical abuse is defined as the use of physical force that may result in bodily injury, physical pain, or impairment. Physical abuse may include but is not limited to such acts of violence as striking (with or without an object), hitting, beating, pushing, shoving, shaking, slapping, kicking, pinching, and burning. In addition, the inappropriate use of drugs and physical restraints, force-feeding, and physical punishment of any kind also are examples of physical abuse.

Signs and symptoms of physical abuse include but are not limited to the following:

▶ Bruises, black eyes, welts, lacerations, and rope marks
▶ Bone fractures, broken bones, and skull fractures
▶ Open wounds, cuts, punctures, untreated injuries, and injuries in various stages of healing
▶ Sprains, dislocations, and internal injuries or bleeding
▶ Broken eyeglasses or frames, physical signs of being subjected to punishment, and signs of being restrained
▶ Laboratory findings of medication overdose or underutilization of prescribed drugs
▶ An elder's report of being hit, slapped, kicked, or mistreated
▶ An elder's sudden change in behavior
▶ The caregiver's refusal to allow visitors to see an elder alone

Sexual abuse is defined as nonconsensual sexual contact of any kind. Sexual contact with any person incapable of giving consent also is considered sexual abuse. It includes but is not limited to unwanted touching, all types of sexual assault or battery such as rape or sodomy, coerced nudity, and sexually explicit photographing.

Signs and symptoms of sexual abuse include but are not limited to the following:

▶ Bruises around the breasts or genital area
▶ Unexplained venereal disease or genital infections
▶ Unexplained vaginal or anal bleeding
▶ Torn, stained, or bloody underclothing
▶ An elder's report of being sexually assaulted or raped

Emotional or psychological abuse is defined as the infliction of anguish, pain, or distress through verbal or nonverbal acts. Emotional and/or psychological abuse includes but is not limited to verbal assaults, insults, threats, intimidation, humiliation, and harassment. In addition, treating an older person like an infant; isolating an elderly person from his or her family, friends, or regular activities; giving an older person a "silent treatment"; and enforced social isolation also are examples of emotional or psychological abuse.

Signs and symptoms of emotional and/or psychological abuse may manifest themselves in such behaviors of an elderly person as the following:

▶ Being emotionally upset or agitated
▶ Being extremely withdrawn and uncommunicative or unresponsive
▶ Unusual behavior usually attributed to dementia (e.g., sucking, biting, rocking)
▶ An elder's report of being verbally or emotionally mistreated

Neglect is defined as the refusal or failure to fulfill any part of a person's obligations or duties to an elder. Neglect may also pertain to a person who has fiduciary responsibilities to provide care for an elder (e.g., pay for necessary home care services), or to the failure on the part of an in-home service provider to provide necessary care. Neglect typically means the refusal or failure to provide an elderly person with such life necessities as food, water, clothing, shelter, personal hygiene, medicine, comfort, personal safety, and other essentials included in the responsibility or agreement to an elder.

Signs and symptoms of neglect include but are not limited to the following:

- Dehydration, malnutrition, untreated bedsores, and poor personal hygiene
- Unattended or untreated health problems
- Hazardous or unsafe living conditions or arrangements (e.g., improper wiring, no heat, or no running water)
- Unsanitary and unclean living conditions (e.g., dirt, fleas, lice on person, soiled bedding, fecal and/or urine smell, inadequate clothing)

Abandonment is defined as the desertion of an elderly person by an individual who has assumed responsibility for providing care for an elder, or by a person with physical custody of an elder.

Signs and symptoms of abandonment include but are not limited to the following:

- The desertion of an elder at a hospital, a nursing facility, or other similar institution
- The desertion of an elder at a shopping center or other public location
- An elder's own report of being abandoned

Financial or material exploitation is defined as the illegal or improper use of an elder's funds, property, or assets. Examples would include but are not limited to cashing an elderly person's checks without authorization or permission; forging an older person's signature; misusing or stealing an older person's money or possessions; coercing or deceiving an older person into signing any document (e.g., contracts, a will); and the improper use of conservatorship, guardianship, or power of attorney.

Signs and symptoms of financial or material exploitation include but are not limited to the following:

- Sudden changes in bank account or banking practice, including an unexplained withdrawal of large sums of money by a person accompanying the elder
- The inclusion of additional names on an elder's bank signature card
- Unauthorized withdrawal of the elder's funds using the elder's ATM card

- Abrupt changes in a will or other financial documents
- Unexplained disappearance of funds or valuable possessions
- Substandard care being provided or bills going unpaid despite the availability of adequate financial resources
- Discovery of an elder's signature being forged for financial transactions and for the titles of his or her possessions
- Sudden appearance of previously uninvolved relatives claiming their rights to an elder's affairs and possessions
- Unexplained sudden transfer of assets to a family member or someone outside the family
- The provision of services that are not necessary
- An elder's report of financial exploitation

Self-neglect is characterized as the behaviors of the person that threaten his or her own health or safety. Self-neglect generally manifests itself in an older person's refusal or failure to provide himself or herself with adequate food, water, clothing, shelter, personal hygiene, medication (when indicated), and safety precautions. The definition of self-neglect excludes a situation in which a cognitively or mentally competent older person (who understands the consequences of his or her decisions) makes a conscious and voluntary decision to engage in acts that threaten his or her health or safety as a matter of personal preference.

Signs and symptoms of self-neglect include but are not limited to the following:

- Dehydration, malnutrition, untreated or improperly attended medical conditions, and poor personal hygiene
- Hazardous or unsafe living conditions or arrangements (e.g., improper wiring, no indoor plumbing, no heat or running water)
- Unsanitary or unclean living quarters (e.g., animal or insect infestation, no functioning toilet, fecal and/or urine smell)
- Inappropriate and/or inadequate clothing, lack of the necessary medical aids (e.g., eyeglasses, hearing aid, dentures)
- Grossly inadequate housing or homelessness

From National Center on Elder Abuse: *Major types of elder abuse,* 2007. Available at www.ncea.aoa.org/NCEAroot/main_site/FAQ/basics/Types_of_Abuse.aspx.

Abuse and Neglect Assessment

1. General Assessment	Very Good	Good	Poor	Very Poor	Unable to Assess
a. Clothing					
b. Hygiene					
c. Nutrition					
d. Skin integrity					
Additional Comments:					

2. Possible Abuse Indicators	No Evidence	Possible Evidence	Probable Evidence	Definite Evidence	Unable to Assess
a. Bruising					
b. Lacerations					
c. Fractures					
d. Various stages of healing of any bruises or fractures					
e. Evidence of sexual abuse					
f. Statement by elder re: abuse					
Additional Comments:					

3. Possible Neglect Indicators	No Evidence	Possible Evidence	Probable Evidence	Definite Evidence	Unable to Assess
a. Contractures					
b. Decubiti					
c. Dehydration					
d. Diarrhea					
e. Depression					
f. Impaction					
g. Malnutrition					
h. Urine burns					
i. Poor hygiene					
j. Failure to respond to warning of obvious disease					
k. Inappropriate medications (under/over)					
l. Repetitive hospital admissions due to probable failure of health care surveillance					
m. Statement by elder re: neglect					
Additional Comments:					

From Fulmer T: Elder abuse and neglect assessment. *Try this: best practices in nursing care to older adults,* Hartford Institute for Geriatric Nursing, no. 15, May 2002.

Relationships, Roles, and Transitions

LEARNING OBJECTIVES

Upon completion of this chapter, the reader will be able to:

- Identify the variations of relationships that people identify as constituting "family."
- Examine family relationships in late life.
- Describe the various roles of grandparents.
- Explain the issues involved in adapting to a major transition such as retirement or widowhood.
- Identify the range of caregiving situations and the potential challenges and opportunities of each.
- Discuss nursing responses with older adults and their families who are assuming caregiver roles or experiencing other transitions.
- Discuss intimacy and sexuality in late life and appropriate nursing responses.

GLOSSARY

Caregiving The act of providing assistance to those who are unable to care entirely for themselves. Caregivers may be informal (family, friends, and others who volunteer this service) or formal (those persons hired to provide the care).

Competent The status of being able to make some decisions alone. There is a wide range of levels of competence from minimal to complex.

Respite A relief in caregiving, providing benefit to both the caregiver and the care recipient.

THE LIVED EXPERIENCE

It is so irritating when Madge tries to help me do things. After all, I have lived 85 years and have done very well. I think she wants to put me away somewhere. I wish she would just leave me alone. I'm sure I could manage if she just wouldn't interfere.

John, the father

I just can't stand watching as my father becomes weaker and is unable to do the things he always did so naturally and well. Yesterday he got lost on his way to the market. He was always my guide and protector. I knew I could count on him no matter what. It makes me feel sort of alone in the world.

Madge, the daughter

RELATIONSHIPS, ROLES, AND TRANSITIONS

This chapter focuses on the various relationships, roles, and transitions that characteristically play a part in late life. Concepts of family structure and function and of intimacy and sexuality, and the transitions of retirement, widowhood, widowerhood, and caregiving are examined. Nursing responses to support older adults in maintaining fulfilling roles and relationships are discussed.

FAMILIES

The idea of family evokes strong subjective impressions according to what an individual believes the typical family should be. Because everyone comes from a family, these impressions have powerful symbolic meaning. However, in today's world, the definition of a family is in a state of flux. As recently as 100 or so years ago, the norm was the extended family made up of parents, their grown children, and the children's children, often living together and sharing resources, strengths, and challenges. As cities grew and adult children moved to them in pursuit of work, parents did not always come along, and the primacy of the nuclear family evolved. The norm in the United States became two parents and their two children, or at least this was the norm in what has been considered mainstream America. This pattern was not as common, nor is it yet, in many families of color, especially living in what are called "ethnic neighborhoods," where the extended family is still the norm.

Other variations on the idea of family have developed. Approximately 42% of today's families are married couples without children. The high divorce and remarriage rate results in households of blended families with children from both previous marriages and the new marriage. Single-parent families, blended families, childless families, and fewer families altogether are common. Four- and five-generation families are also becoming common. Still other families are composed of same-gender couples, which may or may not include children. Others without biological families, either by choice or circumstance, have created their own "families" through communal living with siblings, friends, or others. Indeed, it is not unusual for childless persons residing in long-term care facilities to refer to the staff as their "family."

Family members, however they are defined, form the nucleus of relationships for the majority of older adults and their support system if they become dependent.

A long-standing myth in society is that families are alienated from their older family members and abandon their care to institutions. However, nearly 94% of elders have living family members; the majority (97%) live within an hour of the elder, and nearly 65% of them visit at least once a week (Hooyman and Kiyak, 2008). Most older adults possess a large intergenerational web of significant people, including sons, daughters, step-children, in-laws, ex–in-laws, nieces, nephews, grandchildren, and great-grandchildren, as well as partners and former partners of their offspring. All these people may play an important part in maintaining satisfaction in late life.

In coming to know the older adult, the gerontological nurse comes to know the family as well, learning of their special gifts and their life challenges. The nurse works with the elder within the unique culture of his or her family of origin, present family, and support networks, including friends.

Roles and Relationships

As families change, the roles of the members or their expectations of one another may change as well. Grandparents may assume parental roles for their grandchildren if their children are unable to care for them; or grandparents and older aunts and uncles may assume temporary caregiving roles while the children, nieces, and nephews work. Adult children of any age may provide limited or extensive caregiving to their own parents or aging relatives who become ill or impaired. A spouse or sometimes a sibling may become a caregiver as well when needed. This caregiving may be temporary or long term.

Close-knit families are more aware of the needs of their members and work to resolve problems and find ways to meet the needs of members, even if they are not always successful. Emotionally distant families are less available in times of need and have greater potential for conflict. If the family has never been close and supportive, it will not magically become so when members have unmet needs. Resentments long buried may crop up and produce friction or psychological pain. Long-submerged conflicts and feelings may return if the needs of any one family member exceed those of the others.

Traditional Couples

The traditional couple in the United States is husband and wife or, for the purposes of discussion, the long-standing unmarried heterosexual couple (formerly called "common-law"). Although this relationship is often the most solid if it extends into late life, the chance of a couple going through old age together is exceedingly slim. In 2006, older men were much more likely to be married than older women (72% of men versus 42% of women). Almost half of all older women are widows and there are over 4 times as many widows as widowers (U.S. Administration on Aging, 2008). Men who survive their spouse into old age ordinarily have multiple opportunities to remarry if they wish. A woman is less likely to have an opportunity for remarriage in late life.

Couple relationships are becoming more diverse, involving varying degrees of habit, culture, intimacy, shared backgrounds, and instrumental and emotional support. In late marriages or remarriage, it is an enormous challenge to develop an intimate, sharing relationship between individuals who have had 75 or 80 years of separate experiences and who often bring conflicting ideologies into the new relationship. Older people who remarry usually choose someone they have previously known and with whom they share similar backgrounds and interests. Often, older couples live together but do not marry because of economic and inheritance reasons (Hooyman and Kiyak, 2008).

Couples in late life have needs, tasks, and expectations that differ from those in their earlier years. Some couples have been married more than 60 or 70 years. These years together may have been filled with love and companionship, or abuse and resentment or anything in between. However, in general, marital status (or the presence of a long-time partner) is positively related to health, life satisfaction, and well-being. For all couples, the normal physical and sociological circumstances in late life present challenges. Some of the issues that strain many of these relationships include (1) the deteriorating health of one or both partners, (2) limitations in income, (3) conflicts with children or other relatives, (4) incompatible sexual needs, and (5) mismatched needs for activity and social activities.

Nontraditional Couples

As the variations in families grow, so do the types of coupled relationships. Among the types of couples we see today are lesbian, gay, bisexual, and transgender (LGBT) couples. Although the number of LGBT people of any age has remained elusive, there are an estimated 3 million LGBT people in the United States. The number is projected to increase to as many as 4 million by 2030 (DeVries, 2005-2006). These couples are less

often seen in the aging population, but even though they but may not allow themselves to be obvious because of long-standing discrimination and fear, they are nonetheless still there. Many older LGBT individuals have been part of a live-in couple at some time during their life (Hooyman and Kiyak, 2008).

Some research has suggested that older lesbian women and gay men may adapt more successfully to old age as a result of coping over a lifetime with discrimination and prejudice (Wojciechowski, 1998; Jones and Nystrom, 2002; DeVries, 2005-2006). However, the experience of discrimination and prejudice may also deter older lesbian women and gay men from accessing health care services. As society becomes more willing to accept persons in these relationships, they may be more willing to share with us who they are. The majority of research has involved lesbian and gay couples, and much less is known about bisexual and transgender relationships.

Although the issue of same-gender couples marrying is before the courts, it is not legal in most states to do so. In some cases the couples enter into a marriage type of commitment and, where possible, legally register as "domestic partners." Lesbian women and gay men in long-term committed relationships often share homes, resources, and professional interests. Their families may include children (biological and adoptive), parents, siblings, and friends. In some cases the couples may be estranged from families of origin and come to late life with a network of close friends who make up their "family." These nonrelatives become surrogate family and take on the instrumental and affective attributes of family. Because these family members are not relatives in the traditional sense, they may not be recognized by the health care system, leading to considerable stress to all involved.

Other issues such as Social Security and pension benefits, health insurance, and access to appropriate housing and services for future care needs have been identified as concerns by both older lesbian women and gay men (DeVries, 2005-2006). Interest in and availability of retirement and long-term care communities designed to meet the needs of lesbian and gay older men and women have increased (DeVries, 2005-2006) (see Chapter 26). Much more knowledge of cohort, cultural, and generational differences among age-groups is needed to understand the recent, dramatic changes in the lives of lesbians and gays in family lifestyles. Issues of concern to society and the LGBT community that need further investigation are the impact of homophobia on late-life health, retirement, and leisure issues, and the hidden incidence of abuse and neglect (Claes and Moore, 2000). The sexual health needs of older LGBT individuals are discussed later in this chapter.

Elders and Their Adult Children

In adulthood, relationships between the generations become increasingly important for most people. Older parents enjoy being told about the various activities and successes of their offspring, and these adult children begin to see aspects of themselves that have developed from their parents. At times, the relationships may become strained because the younger adults are more concerned with their own spouses, partners, and children. The parents are no longer central to their lives, though offspring may be central to the lives of their parents (Fingerman, 2001a). The most difficult situations occur when the elder parents are openly critical or judgmental about the lives of their offspring. In the best of situations, adult children shift to the role of friend, companion, and confidant to the elder, a concept known as filial maturity.

Contrary to popular opinion, older people are not neglected by families, and most older people see their children on a regular basis. Even children who do not live close to their older parents maintain their close connections, and "intimacy at a distance" can occur (Hooyman and Kiyak, 2008). By and large, elders and their children have relationships that are reciprocal in nature and characterized by affection and mutual support. These relationships are both the most important and potentially the most conflicted. Family resources are shared from birth and usually in some way until and after death. These resources may be tangible, such as money, belongings, and housing. Intangible resources may include advice, support, guidance, and day-to-day assistance with life. Elders provide a family history perspective, models for growing old, assistance with grandchildren, a sense of continuity, and a philosophy of aging.

Grandparenting

The role of grandparenthood, and increasingly, great-grandparenthood, is experienced by most older adults. Nearly 90% of parents age 90 years and older are grandparents, and nearly 50% are great-grandparents. Approximately 80% of grandparents see their grandchild weekly. Fifty percent of grandparents are under the age of 60, and some women experience grandparenthood for more than 40 years. There is wide diversity among grandparents, who range in age from their late 30s to over 100 years old. Grandchildren can range in age from newborns to retirees (Hooyman and Kiyak, 2008).

As the term implies, the "grands" are a step beyond parents in their concerns, exposure, and responsibility. The age, vitality, and proximity of both grandchild and grandparent produce a kaleidoscope of possible activities and interactions as both progress through their aging processes. Younger grandparents typically live closer to their grandchildren and are more involved in child care and recreational activities. Older grandparents with higher incomes may provide more financial assistance and other types of instrumental assistance (Hooyman and Kiyak, 2008). Among racially and culturally diverse families, there may be greater interactions and more grandparent responsibility for childrearing. More and more grandparents are assuming the role of primary caregivers to their grandchildren. This phenomenon is discussed later in the chapter.

Historically, the emphasis has been on the progressive aging of the grandparent as it affects the affinity, but little is said about the effects of the growth and maturation of the grandchild as these affect the relationship. Chan and Elder (2000) note a great matrilineal advantage in grandparenting relationships, but the role of grandfathers is also significant in the lives of many children. This area needs further study. "Overall, the grandparent role and identity tends to be associated with embeddedness in the family, along with life satisfaction, and psychological well-being" (Hooyman and Kiyak, 2008, p. 354). Box 23-1 provides a set of guidelines for grandparents. The views of a grandmother as seen by an 8-year-old child are presented in Box 23-2.

Siblings

Late-life sibling relationships are poorly understood and have been neglected by researchers. As individuals age, they often have more contact with siblings than they did in the years when family and work demands were more pressing. About 80% of older people have at least one sibling. For many elders, these relationships became increasingly important because they have a long history of memories and have in common the same generation, similar backgrounds, and the often ambivalent early relationship (Bedford and Avioli, 2001). Sibling relationships become particularly important when they are part of the support system, especially among single or widowed elders living alone.

Box 23-1	Guidelines for Grandparenting

- Grandchildren need your attention and interest in their activities.
- Celebrating special times creates memories and continues traditions.
- Grandchildren need help exploring their world while they are young.
- Offering assistance without interference is recommended.
- Rule-making is not a grandparent's task.
- Do not give advice about child rearing.
- Give the child undivided attention during projects, games, and reading.
- Be a link with the past; tell grandchildren about their parents and about you when you were a child.
- Support the parents in their decisions; never undermine.
- Offer the gift of your time: nature walks, baking cookies, and so on.

Long-Distance Grandparenting
- Brief and frequent cards and letters are useful; send clippings, cartoons, and riddles; use colorful stickers and stamps.
- Audiotapes and videotapes that you produce are appreciated, as are storytelling, reading, or singing.
- Celebrate special days and "firsts" (first lost tooth, first day of school, mastery of a new situation).
- Telephone frequently.
- Visit as often as you can.

From Good grandparenting, *Mayo Clin Health Lett* 11(1):6, 1993.

Box 23-2	Grandmother as Seen by an 8-Year-Old Child

"A grandmother is a woman who has no children of her own. That is why she loves other people's children."

"Grandmothers have nothing to do. They are just there: when they take us for a walk they go slowly, like caterpillars along beautiful leaves. They never say, 'Come on, faster, hurry up!'"

"Everyone should try to have a grandmother, especially those who don't have a TV."

From *Ageing in Focus*, March 2006.

The loss of siblings has a profound effect in terms of awareness of one's own mortality, particularly when those of the same gender die. When an elder reaches the age of the sibling who died, the reaction can be quite disruptive. Not only is grieving activated, but also rehearsal for one's own death may occur. In some cases in which an elder sibling survives younger ones, there may be not only a deep grief but also pangs of guilt: "Why them and not me?" (see Chapter 25).

Other Kin

Interaction with collateral kin (cousins, aunts, uncles, nieces, nephews) generally depends on proximity, preference, and the general availability of primary kin. The quality of relationships varies but is still a potential source of joy, support, assistance, or conflict. Maternal kin (related through female bloodlines) may be emotionally closer than those in one's paternal line (Jett, 2002). These relatives may provide a reservoir of kin from which to find replacements for missing or lost intimate relationships for singles or childless people as they grow older.

LATE LIFE TRANSITIONS

Role transitions that occur in late life include retirement, grandparenthood, divorce, widowhood, and becoming a caregiver or recipient of care. These transitions may occur predictably or may be imposed by unanticipated events. Retirement is an example of a predictable event that can and should be planned long in advance, although for some, it can occur unexpectedly as a result of illness, disability, or being terminated from a job. Divorce or becoming a widow or widower may occur unexpectedly and create emotional chaos in the transitional phase for some older people. To the degree that an event is perceived as expected and occurring at the right time, a role transition may be comfortable and even welcomed. Those persons who must retire "too early" or are widowed "too soon" will have more difficulty adapting than those who are at an age when these events are expected.

The speed and intensity of a major change may make the difference between a transitional crisis and a gradual and comfortable adaptation. Most difficult are the transitions that incorporate losses rather than gains in status, influence, and opportunity. The move from independence to dependence and becoming a care recipient is particularly difficult. Conditions that influence the outcome of transitions include personal meanings, expectations, level of knowledge, preplanning, and emotional and physical reserves. Cohort, cultural, and gender differences are inherent in all of life's major transitions. Those transitions that make use of past skills and adaptations may be less stressful. The ideal outcome is when gains in satisfaction and new roles offset losses. This section of the chapter discusses retirement, widowhood and widowerhood, divorce, grandparenting, and caregiving.

Retirement

Retirement is no longer just a few years of rest from the rigors of work before death. It is a developmental stage that may occupy 30 or more years of one's life and involve many stages. The transitions are blurring because numerous pursuits and opportunities may occur after one has "retired." Tafford (2002) addressed this relatively new segment of adult life. She examines the unprecedented aging in the life cycle and contends that people know as little about it as they did about adolescence at the turn of the century. The numerous patterns and styles of retiring have produced more varied experiences in retirement. The most significant factors in adaptation to retirement are health, income, and social involvement. More older people are working longer or changing careers after formal retirement. Some do so because of economic need, whereas others have a desire to remain involved and productive. With recent events that have seriously threatened pension security and portability, as well as a declining economy, more workers are remaining in the workforce. "The long-term trend toward ever-earlier retirement has halted" (Ekerdt and Dennis, 2002, p. 1).

Older people who did not expect retirement at the time when they left the workforce may suffer detrimental effects and be in need of counseling or assistance. They may experience job separation as a crisis and a traumatic role transition triggered by an unplanned job termination; this could be the result of illness or company downsizing, a euphemism for cutting out jobs. Others, given the opportunity to work past retirement age, must weigh the benefits. Part-time work during retirement is viewed by the working public of all ages as a desirable option. Employers value older workers because they are dependable. Seniors older than 65 years can now earn any amount without endangering Social Security benefits. Obviously, health and financial status affect decisions and abilities to work or engage in new work opportunities.

Retirement Planning

Decisions to retire are often based on financial resources, attitude toward work, chronological age, health, and self-perceptions of ability to adjust to retirement (Box 23-3). Retirement planning is advisable during early adulthood and essential in middle age. However, people differ in their focus on the past, present, and future and their realistic ability to "put away something" for future needs. Retirement preparation programs are usually aimed at employees with high levels of education and occupational status, those with private pension coverage, and government employees. Thus the people most in need of planning assistance may be those least likely to have any available, let alone the resources for an adequate retirement. Individuals who are retiring in poor health, culturally and racially diverse persons, and those in lower socioeconomic levels may experience greater concerns in retirement and may need specialized counseling. These groups are often neglected in retirement planning programs.

Working couples must plan together for retirement. Decisions will depend on their career goals, shared future interests, and the quality of their interpersonal relationship. The following are some questions one must weigh when deciding to retire or continue working:

▶ What do I want to do?
▶ Who needs me, and what are my best opportunities?
▶ What am I best able to do?
▶ What is the meaning of my life?
▶ What should my life accomplish or contribute?
▶ Am I financially secure for the rest of my life if I live 30 or more years?
▶ Can I afford to completely retire from paid work?

Retirement education plans are supplied through group lectures, individual counseling, booklets, DVDs, and computerized modules. However, at this juncture and in light of the many hazards experienced by preretirees, planning is often insufficient. Dennis (2002) notes that many individuals have very high expectations for the final third of their lives. Although federal laws encourage increased participation in company-sponsored 401(k) plans, many of these plans are unreliable. The proposals for the privatization of Social Security also contribute to uncertainty about retirement benefits. When considering retirement, Dennis notes that areas for consideration include the adequacy of (1) company-provided retirement benefits; (2) Social Security and Medicare benefits; (3) company-provided postretirement health care; and (4) financial planning.

Box 23-3	Potential Issues in Retirement

1. Financial need versus resources available
2. Employability
3. Rewards derived from employment:
   • Wages sufficient for needs and morale
   • Satisfaction level, possibility for resolution of job frustrations
   • Meaning of job, contact with friends, source of prestige
4. Psychosocial characteristics—attitudes toward retirement:
   • Attitudes of significant others (advising? directing?)
   • Strength of work ethic
   • Effect of retirement on prestige
5. Personality factors:
   • Time orientation (past, present, future)
   • Active versus passive stance in planning
   • Rationalism versus fatalism as life stance
   • Type A versus type B personality (hard-driving, easy-going)
   • Inner-directed versus other-directed (enjoyment of self or need for high level of external motivation)
6. Level of information about retirement:
   • Planning programs on the job, adult education, or community programs
   • Awareness of friends and family who have retired and how influenced by them
7. Pressures to retire:
   • Compulsory, age-discriminatory
   • Unemployment (how long?)
   • Job retrogression (being moved down the ladder)
   • Skill obsolescence (opportunities for developing other skills?)
   • Peer pressure (organized or informal)
   • Employer pressure (reduced incentives to continue work, increased incentives to retire)
   • Family pressure (spouse's working status)
   • Health, discomfort, or disability interfering with job performance and dependability

The adequacy of retirement income depends not only on work history but also on marital history. The poverty rates of older women are excessively high. Couples who had previous marriages and divorces may have significantly lower economic resources available than those in first marriages. Child support, divorce settlements, and pension apportionment to ex-spouses may have diminished retirement income. This problem is an ever-increasing impediment to retirement because, among couples presently approaching retirement age, fewer than half are in a first marriage (U.S. Divorce Statistics, 2002). Policies have been based on the traditional lifelong marriage, and this is no longer appropriate.

Dennis (2002) notes that retirement planning is really life planning and that the process is best accomplished when, early on, individuals determine their goals, values, and motivations in life. This assessment calls for personal reflection and thought about the choices in everyday life that provide satisfaction and that the individual will wish to continue in late life

(Shagrin, 2002). Retirement planning has become a highly specialized professional field. For people who can afford it, engaging a retirement planner in early adulthood is wise. Nurses must be familiar with these sources of information and discuss the need for retirement planning with their clients.

Special Considerations In Retirement

Retirement security depends on the "three-legged stool" of Social Security pensions, savings, and investments (Stanford and Usita, 2002). Older people with disabilities, those who have lacked access to education or held low-paying jobs with no benefits, and those not eligible for Social Security are at economic risk during retirement years. Culturally and racially diverse older persons, women—especially widows and those divorced or never married—immigrants, and gay and lesbian men and women often face greater challenges related to adequate income and benefits in retirement (Price and Joo, 2005; Angel et al, 2007). The traditional idea of retirement as a time of increased leisure, new interests, and relaxation and enjoyment may not be possible for many older people. "Future retirement policies will need to consider the rapidly changing demographics of the aging population and the special barriers faced by older people of color, women, immigrants, and gays and lesbians" (Stanford and Usita, 2002, p. 47).

Inadequate coverage for women in retirement is common because their work histories have been sporadic and diverse. Women are often called on to retire earlier than anticipated because of family needs. Whereas most men have always worked outside the home, it has been only within the past 30 years that this has been the expectation of women. Therefore large cohort differences exist. Traditionally, the variability of women's work histories, interrupted careers, the residuals of sexist pension policies, Social Security inequities, and low-paying jobs created hazards for adequacy of income in retirement. The scene is gradually changing in many respects, but the gender bias remains.

Basing retirement calculations on gender and projected survival statistics is now illegal, though until the early 1980s, women were allotted less pension income based purely on their expected longevity compared with men. Although this is no longer in force, women who retired 20 or 25 years ago remain penalized because of gender (Kingson et al, 2007). Older women are likely to have several years of no earnings calculated into the averages that determine the amount of their Social Security benefits. Some women find that they will receive more if their Social Security benefits are calculated on their husband's earnings; this may be true even though widowed or divorced. The Social Security Administration must be contacted regarding these matters because many variables must be considered.

Barriers to equal treatment for LGBT couples include job discrimination, unequal treatment under Social Security, pension plans, and 401(k) plans (Cahill and South, 2002). LGBT couples are not eligible for Social Security survivor benefits, and unmarried partners cannot claim pension plan rights after the death of the pension plan participant. These policies definitely place LGBT elders at a disadvantage in retirement planning.

IMPLICATIONS FOR GERONTOLOGICAL NURSING AND HEALTHY AGING

Successful retirement adjustment depends on socialization needs, energy levels, health, adequate income, variety of interests, amount of self-esteem derived from work, presence of intimate relationships, social support, and general adaptability. Nurses may have the opportunity to work with people in different phases of retirement or participate in retirement education and counseling programs (Box 23-4). Talking with clients older than 50 years about retirement plans, providing anticipatory guidance about the transition to retirement, identifying those who may be at risk for lowered income and health concerns, and referring to appropriate resources for retirement planning and support are important nursing interventions.

It is important to build on the strengths of older adults' life experiences and coping skills and to provide appropriate counseling and support to assist older people to continue to grow and develop in meaningful ways during the transition from the work role. In ideal situations, retirement offers the opportunity to pursue interests that may have been neglected while fulfilling other obligations. However, for too many older people, retirement presents challenges that affect both health and well-being, and nurses must be advocates for policies and conditions that allow all older people to maintain quality of life in retirement.

Widows and Widowers

Losing a partner after a long, close, and satisfying relationship is the most difficult adjustment one can face, aside from the loss of a child. The loss of a spouse is a stage in the life course that can be anticipated but seldom is. Nearly 50% of all women and 12% of all men ages 65 years and older are widowed (DeVries, 2001). The death of a life partner is essentially a loss of self. The mourning is as much for oneself as for the individual

Box 23-4	Phases of Retirement

Remote: Future anticipation with little real planning
Near: Preparation and fantasizing regarding retirement
Honeymoon: Euphoria and testing of the fantasies
Disenchantment: Letdown, boredom, sometimes depression
Reorientation: Developing a realistic and satisfactory lifestyle
Stability: Personal investment in meaningful activities
Termination: Loss of role resulting from illness or return to work

who has died. A core part of oneself has died with the partner, and even with satisfactory grief resolution, that aspect of self will never return. Even those widows and widowers who reorganize their lives and invest in family, friends, and activities often find that many years later they still miss their "other half" profoundly.

With the loss of the intimate partner, several changes occur simultaneously that involve social status, economics, and self-image. Individuals who have been self-confident and competent seem to fare best. The transitional phase of grief, if handled appropriately, leads to the confirmation of a new identity, the end of one stage of life and the beginning of another. Seldom in life is there such an abrupt and distinct breach that creates intense pain but offers the opportunity for the emergence of a new identity. Patterns of adjustment can be seen in Box 23-5. Knowing the stages of the transition to a new role as a widow or widower may be useful, although each individual is unique in this respect. Individuals respond to losses in ways that reflect the nature and meaning of the relationships as well as the unique characteristics of the bereaved.

Gender differences are found in the literature on widowhood. Bereaved husbands may be more socially and emotionally vulnerable. Many studies have found that widowers adapt more slowly than widows to the loss of a spouse and often remarry quickly. Loneliness and the need to be cared for is a factor influencing widowers to seek out new partners. Association with family and friends, being members of a church community, and continuing to work or engage in activities can all be helpful in the adjustment period following the death of a wife (Rushton, 2007). Common bereavement reactions of widowers are listed in Box 23-6 and should be discussed with male clients.

Box 23-5   Patterns of Adjustment to Widowhood

Stage One: Reactionary
(First Few Weeks)
Early responses of disbelief, anger, indecision, detachment, and inability to communicate in a logical, sustained manner are common. Searching for the mate, visions, hallucinations, and depersonalization may be experienced.
Intervention: Support, validate, be available, listen to talk about mate, reduce expectations.

Stage Two: Withdrawal
(First Few Months)
Depression, apathy, physiological vulnerability occur; movement and cognition are slowed; insomnia, unpredictable waves of grief, and anorexia occur.
Intervention: Protect against suicide, and involve in support groups.

Stage Three: Recuperation
(Second 6 Months)
Periods of depression are interspersed with characteristic capability. Feelings of personal control begin to return.
Intervention: Support accustomed lifestyle patterns that sustain person and assist him or her to explore new possibilities.

Stage Four: Exploration
(Second Year)
Individual begins new ventures, testing suitability of new roles; anniversaries or holidays, birthdays, and date of death may be especially difficult.
Intervention: Prepare individual for unexpected reactions during anniversaries. Encourage and support trials of new roles.

Stage Five: Integration
(Fifth Year)
Individual will feel fully integrated into new and satisfying roles if grief has been resolved in a healthy manner.
Intervention: Assist individual to recognize and share own pattern of growth through the trauma of loss.

Box 23-6	Common Widower Bereavement Reactions

- The search for the lost mate
- The neglect of self
- The inability to share grief
- The loss of social contacts
- The struggle to view women as other than wife
- The erosion of self-confidence and sexuality
- The protracted grief period

IMPLICATIONS FOR GERONTOLOGICAL NURSING AND HEALTHY AGING

Nurses working with the bereaved will need to review Lindemann's classic grief studies to understand the initial somatic responses of the bereaved (Lindemann, 1944). Feelings of the bereaved one are not orderly or progressive; they are conflicted, ambivalent, suicidal, full of rage, and often suspicious. Widows and widowers may exhibit personality disorganization that would be considered mentally aberrant or frankly psychotic under other circumstances. Some people handle grief with less apparent decompensation. Grief reactions must be accepted as personally valid and useful evidences of healing. DeVries (2001) discusses the signs of ongoing bonds and connections (dreaming of the deceased, ongoing daily communication, "checking in") with the deceased that persist long after death and counsels professionals to reexamine the idea that there is a timetable for "resolution" of grief.

With adequate support, reintegration can be expected in 2 to 4 years. People with few familial or social supports may need professional help to get through the early months of grief in a way that will facilitate recovery. To support the grieving person it is necessary to extend one's own self to reconnect the severed person with a world of warmth and caring. No one nurse or family member can accomplish this task alone. Hundreds of small, caring gestures build strength and confidence in the grieving person's ability and willingness to survive. Additional information about dying, death, and grief can be found in Chapter 25.

Divorce and the Elderly

In the past, divorce was considered a stigmatizing event; however, today it is so common that a person is inclined to forget the ostracizing effects of divorce from 60 years ago. Divorced and separated (including married with spouse absent) older persons represented only 11.8% of all older persons in 2006 (U.S. Administration on Aging, 2008). However, this percentage has increased since 1980, when approximately 5.3% of the older population were divorced or separated with spouse absent. There are large generational and individual differences in expectations from marriage, but older couples are becoming less likely to stay in an unsatisfactory marriage. Health care professionals must avoid making assumptions and be alert to the possibility of marital dissatisfaction in old age. Nurses should ask, "How would you describe your marriage?"

Long-term relationships are varied and complex, with many factors forming the glue that holds them together. Marital breakdown may be more devastating in old age because it is often unanticipated and may occur concurrently with other significant losses. Health care workers must be concerned with supporting a client's decision to seek a divorce and with assisting him or her in seeking counseling in the transition. A nurse should alert the client that a divorce will bring on a grieving process similar to the death of a spouse and that a severe disruption in coping capacity may occur until the client adjusts to a new life. The grief may be more difficult to cope with because no socially sanctioned patterns have been established, as is the case with widowhood. In addition, tax and fiscal policies favor married couples, and many divorced elderly women are at a serious economic disadvantage in retirement.

CAREGIVING

Mary Lund (2005, p. 152), quoting Rosalyn Carter, offers the following reflection on caregiving:

There are four kinds of people in the world: those who have been caregivers, those who are currently caregivers, those who will be caregivers, and those who will need caregivers.

Lund (2005) suggests the following of assuming a caregiving role:

[It] is a time of transition that requires a restructuring of one's goals, behaviors, and responsibilities. It requires taking on something new but it is also about loss—of what was and what could have been. Caregiving responsibilities often create conflicts with obligations to work or family. There is the emotional pain of seeing a parent or spouse become physically or cognitively incapacitated. Caregivers experience the whole range of human emotions: guilt, anger, frustration,

exhaustion, anxiety, fear, grief, sadness, love, and the not-to-be underestimated satisfaction of having done a good job (p. 152).

Gerontological nurses are most likely to encounter elders and their family and friends who are in situations involving caregiving of some kind. Family members provide 80% of care for older adults in the United States (Curry et al, 2006). The face of informal caregiving has changed and may include family, friends, and paid and unpaid workers, as well as volunteers in the home. "Researchers estimate that family caregiving for older adults in 2000 had an economic value of $257 billion. Without the involvement of informal caregivers caring for older relatives, the cost of providing care would stagger the health care system" (Schumacher et al, 2006, p. 42). In 2007, nearly 10 million Americans provided 8.4 billion hours of unpaid care to people with Alzheimer's disease (AD), 4 times what Medicare pays for nursing home care for people with AD and other dementias (www.alz.org/national/documents/report_alzfactsfigures2008.pdf).

Even though generally considered a women's issue, in more and more cases, male caregivers, including those other than spouses (e.g., brothers, nephews, sons), are assuming a full range of caregiving roles (Houde, 2001; Hooyman and Kiyak, 2008). Family caregiving has become a normative experience (similar to marriage, working, or retirement) for many of America's families and cuts across racial, ethnic, and social class distinctions (Lund, 2005). In 17% percent of white households and 15% of African-American households, at least one person is providing care to an adult 50 years of age or older (Schumacher et al, 2006).

Although caregiving is a means to "give back" to a loved one and can be an instance of finding joy in the giving, it is also stressful and can be physically and emotionally demanding, leading to increased medical illnesses and a greater risk of mortality (Zarit, 2006). Caregivers are considered to be "the hidden patient" (Schulz and Beach, 1999, p. 2216). Caregivers frequently experience depression and physical and emotional exhaustion (Box 23-7). Not all caregivers experience stress as a consequence of their role, it is true; however, the circumstances that are more likely to cause problems with caregiving include competing role responsibilities (e.g., work, home), advanced age of the caregiver, high-intensity caregiving needs, insufficient resources, dementia of the care recipient, and prior relational conflicts between the caregiver and care recipient (Navaie-Waliser et al, 2002). Box 23-8 presents caregiver needs.

Box 23-7   Suggestions to Reduce Caregiver Stress

To reduce caregiver stress, nurses are advised to use all means and resources at their disposal to do the following:
- Restore a sense of control and effectiveness in the situation.
- Reinforce any social supports that are available to the caregiver.
- Find opportunities for group participation with other caregivers.
- Advise routine times of respite, and assist caregiver in finding respite sources.

Schmall and Stiehl* suggest the following:
- Tailor programs and services to the unique situation of caregiver and care recipient.
- Urge the caregiver to take care of self.
- Encourage caregiver to maintain activities important to his or her well-being.
- Allow the caregiver to express negative and angry feelings he or she may have about the care recipient and the caregiving experience.
- Encourage the caregiver's efforts to use all available resources and assistance.
- Include all directly involved parties in decisions about care.
- Praise whatever is being done well, and encourage letting go of things that have not gone well.

*Schmall VL, Stiehl R: Coping with caregiving: how to manage stress when caring for older relatives, Corvallis, OR, 2003, Pacific Northwest Extension. Available at http://extension.oregonstate.edu/catalog/PDF/PNW/PNW315.pdf. Accessed 7/6/08.

Earlier studies have suggested that caregiver burden may be less in African Americans and that ethnic minority caregivers rely less on formal support than do whites. Results of a metaanalysis of ethnic differences in stressors, resources, and psychological outcomes of family caregiving (Pinquart and Sorensen, 2005) raise questions about assumptions that ethnic minority caregivers rely less on formal support or that they experience less caregiver burden or depression. Study results suggested that minority caregivers do not rely less on formal support services than do white caregivers as a result of differences in value systems. A lack of culturally competent caregiver support services and a lack of education about available resources may influence caregiving trends more than ethnicity or culture. This study points out the need for further

Box 23-8	Caregiver Needs

- Finding time for myself
- Keeping the person I care for safe
- Balancing work and family responsibilities
- Managing emotional and physical stress
- Finding easy and satisfying activities to do with the care recipient
- Learning how to talk to physicians
- Making end-of-life decisions
- Moving or lifting the care recipient; bathing and dressing
- Managing the challenging behaviors of the care recipient
- Negotiating health care and home- and community-based services
- Managing complex medication schedules or high-tech medical equipment
- Choosing a home health agency or assisted living or skilled nursing facility
- Managing incontinence or toileting problems
- Finding non-English educational material

From Curry L, Walker C, Hogstel MO: Educational needs of employed family caregivers of older adults: evaluation of a workplace project, *Geriatr Nurs* 27(3):166-173, 2006; Family Caregiver Alliance: Caregiver assessment: principles, guidelines and strategies for change, Report from a National Consensus Development Conference (vol 1), San Francisco, 2006, The Alliance.

research into ethnic differences in caregiving, an area of particular need in light of the increasing number of ethnically and racially diverse elders.

The positive benefits of caregiving have been given more attention in recent years, but further research is needed to help understand what factors influence how caregivers perceive the experience. Positive benefits of caregiving may include enhanced self-esteem and well-being, personal growth and satisfaction, and finding or making meaning through caregiving (Chappell and Reid, 2002; Hunt, 2003; Pinquart and Sorensen, 2005). "Giving and receiving care among family members involves complex interactions that can be stressful, with potentially positive and negative consequences for each member of the dyad" (Sebern, 2005, p. 170). Most attention in caregiving research has been given to the caregiver with less to the care recipient or the relationship between caregiver and care recipient.

Patricia Archbold and her colleagues have studied caregiving as a role, examining how the relationships between the caregiver and care recipient (mutuality) and the preparation of the caregiver (preparedness) influence reactions to caregiving (Archbold et al, 1990). Mutuality is defined as "an enduring quality of a relationship with four components: shared values, love, shared activities, and reciprocity (Sebern, 2005, p. 175). Caregivers who have a positive relationship with the care recipient experience less stress and find caregiving more meaningful. Ethnically and racially diverse caregivers, particularly African-American caregivers, seem to use more cognitive and emotion-focused coping and report better psychological health (Pinquart and Sorensen, 2005). However, it is nonetheless important to attend to the physical and psychological health and resources available to these caregivers.

Nursing interventions to assist in preparing the caregiver for the caregiving role, particularly at the time of discharge from the hospital, also seem to prevent or reduce role strain. Nurses working with older people and their caregivers must assess both the quality of the caregiver–care recipient relationship and how prepared the caregiver is for assuming the role (Archbold et al, 1990). Sebern (2005) suggests the construct of shared care as a framework for understanding both the caregiving and receiving aspects of the relationship and individualizing interventions to assist in enhancing the relationship to promote positive outcomes. Further research is needed to understand the complexities of the caregiving and the care receiving roles and provide a theory base for nursing interventions. Box 23-9 presents some suggestions for caregivers.

Box 23-9	Suggestions for Caregivers

- Educate yourself about the disease or medical condition
- Find a health care professional who understands the disease
- Consult with other experts to help plan for the future (legal, financial aspects)
- Tap your social resources for assistance
- Find a confidante
- Take time for relaxation and exercise
- Use community resources
- Maintain your sense of humor
- Explore religious beliefs and spiritual values
- Set realistic goals

From U.S. Department of Health and Human Services Administration on Aging, National Family Caregiver Support Program Resources: Taking care of yourself. Available at www.aoa.gov. Accessed 6/28/07.

With the increase in the older adult population, declining household size, and a shortage of direct–health care workers, projections are that there will be fewer caregivers for older people in the future. A new American Association of Retired Persons (AARP) Public Policy Institute report (2006), *Who's Caring for the Caregivers?* found that "the use of paid, formal care by older persons with disabilities in the community has been decreasing, while their sole reliance on family caregivers has been increasing."

Caregiving is considered in some depth here because it is one of the most crucial phenomena today. Caregiving for older people with Alzheimer's disease and other dementias presents some unique challenges and is discussed in Chapter 21.

Caring for Parents

The role of elders with adult children is usually studied as a caregiving issue. Adult children are sometimes said to reverse roles with parents when the parents become older and dependent. This scenario has a demeaning connotation, as if the elder becomes a child again. In illness and deterioration of the elder, the adult child may at times feel parental, but the inner child always remains in need of the protective and guiding parent. No matter how mature a person becomes, the parent symbolizes security and acceptance, regardless of the reality or facts. These dynamics often make the caregiving role very complex and difficult.

Caregivers are generally adult children (41%) followed by partners or spouses (23%). The "typical" caregiver is a 46-year-old woman (61%), married, and working outside the home earning an income of $35,000 (Hooyman and Kiyak, 2008). The number of male caregivers is increasing, but caregiving still remains a primarily female issue. Fifty percent of all women will provide care for elders at some point in their lives (Hooyman and Kiyak, 2008). In most cases, adult daughters are providing care for their older mothers, although caregiving for elders occurs across the life span, as discussed in this chapter. The "sandwich generation" (middle-aged caregivers) often struggle to balance the demands of work and parenting with caregiving for an older relative. Fingerman (2001b) provides research-based findings of the positive and negative emotions that occur between older mothers and their adult daughters, one of the most frequently encountered caregiving relationships.

Filial obligation is associated with a sense of duty toward one's parents that is inherent in the relationship. In some cultures and in many ethnic groups, this sense of duty is strong. As a result, it is expected that children will set aside their own needs to meet those of the parent. If the children have active lives and demanding careers or face multiple needs of their own children, conflicts with the needs of the parents are fairly certain. Many children find ways to overcome the conflicts and provide a substantial amount of elder care as just noted. The major concerns arise when the child caregiver is not available or willing to assume these responsibilities if he or she is needed.

Spousal Caregiving

Spouses provide a great deal of caregiving; about 22% of those caring for older adults are themselves 65 years of age or older. Elderly spouses caring for disabled partners have special needs and may face many role changes. "An older woman may need to learn to drive, manage money, or make decisions by herself. Male caregivers may need to take on unfamiliar household chores such as cooking or laundry, or helping their partner with personal hygiene" (Lund, 2005, p. 152). At present, more wives than husbands over the age of 65 care for a partner with a chronic illness, but husbands comprise nearly 40% of spousal caregivers. This trend is expected to grow as life expectancy for men increases (Hooyman and Kiyak, 2008).

Older spouses are at greater risk for negative consequences, and the nurse should be alert to situations in which health care personnel may be able to provide supports and resources that make it possible for an individual to assume new responsibilities without being totally overwhelmed. When a spouse is ill and the mate needs to take over functions for both, someone must be available to give reinforcement, encouragement, and relief. An adult day program, respite care services, routine visits from a community health nurse, or periodic assistance from a home health aide or a housekeeper may make it possible for the couple to continue to live together. It is important to pay attention to the physical and mental health needs of the caregiver as well as the care recipient.

Aging Parents Caring for Developmentally Disabled Children

Although we tend to think of caregivers as middle-aged adults caring for elders, an unknown number of elders are caring for their middle-aged children who are physically and mentally disabled. Earlier in the past century these developmentally disabled children usually died before reaching adulthood; now, with improved care, they are surviving. An estimated 4.3 million people in the United States with developmental disabilities live at home, and a quarter of them are being cared for by a family member who is at least 60 years old (Ansberry, 2004). Often this has been a burden carried by parents for their entire adult life and will end only with the death of the parent or the adult child. The phenomenon of an aging parent caring for an aging child is beginning to receive attention by both organizations for aging and organizations for developmentally disabled individuals. The Planned Lifetime Assistance Network (PLAN), available in some states through the National Alliance for the Mentally Ill (NAMI), provides lifetime assistance to individuals with disabilities whose parents or other family members are deceased or can no longer provide for their care (Hooyman and Kiyak, 2008; www.nami.org).

Grandparents Raising Grandchildren

In recent years, more grandparents have become, by default, the primary caregivers of grandchildren because the parents are unable to provide the care needed as a result of child abuse, teen pregnancy, imprisonment, joblessness, military deployment, drug and alcohol addictions, illness, death, and other social problems (AARP, 2005; Butler and Zakari, 2005; Hooyman and Kiyak, 2008). In the United States, the number of grandparents raising grandchildren has increased by more than 30% since 1990 and continues to grow. Over 670,000 grandparents have primary responsibility for grandchildren (U.S. Administration on Aging, 2008). National studies indicate that the majority of sole grandparent caregivers are white (62%), but Latinos (10%) and African Americans (30%) are disproportionately represented in light of their percentage of the total population (Hooyman and Kiyak, 2008). Unmarried older women and African-American grandparents are more likely to assume a primary caregiver role with their grandchildren. AARP (2003) reports on research related to African-American, Hispanic, and Native American caregiving grandparents (www.aarp.org/research/family/grandparenting/aresearch-import-483.html).

Grandparents raising grandchildren is a global phenomenon as well. The AARP report, *Intergenerational Relationships: Grandparents Raising Grandchildren,* states that although the number of children being raised by grandparents in the United States is significantly high, it is much less than the millions of children in Africa and other developing countries who are being raised by grandparents or other relatives. Grandparents in these developing countries face great challenges in providing basic subsistence for their grandchildren, and often for themselves. The Grandmother Project (www.aarp.org/research/family/grandparenting/may_06_gubser_grandmother.html) is a U.S. nonprofit organization working to strengthen the leadership role of grandmothers in improving health for women and children in Laos, Senegal, Mali, Uzbekistan, and Albania. Outcomes of the project include greater confidence among grandmothers, increased community respect for elder women, and improvements in advice to young women on pregnancy, infant feeding, and neonatal health.

Research is lacking related to the physical and mental health consequences of grandparents raising grandchildren, and no clear data are available on the effect of grandparent caregiving on health status (Grinstead et al, 2003; Butler and Zakari, 2005). As with other types of caregiving, there are both blessings and burdens (Davidhizar et al, 2000). For many grandparents, however, economic, health, and social challenges associated with caregiving may include limited income and financial support through the welfare system, lack of informal support systems, loss of leisure and social activities in retirement, and shame or guilt related to their children's inability to parent (Grinstead et al, 2003; Butler and Zakari, 2005; Hooyman and Kiyak, 2008).

The economic costs of grandparents caring for grandchildren are significant. Compared to noncustodial grandmothers, custodial grandmothers are more likely to live in poverty (Hooyman and Kiyak, 2008). Too often, both the children and their grandparents are in need of help. As expected, many of these children have multiple loss and grief issues and need mental health services (Brown-Standridge and Floyd, 2000). Interventions must be adapted to the wide variety of grandparenting issues in terms of "race, culture, socioeconomic status, age, and social class" (Hooyman and Kiyak, 2008, p. 357). Box 23-10 provides research-based suggestions for nursing interventions with older adults who are providing primary care to their grandchildren.

The U.S. government has recognized that increasing numbers of older adults are raising grandchildren, great-grandchildren, and other younger relatives. However, there is a continued need to develop services that support grandparents as sole caregivers. Some of the funds distributed through the Older Americans Act have been earmarked to support this group. Nurses can refer the grandparents to their local area agency on aging to inquire about available resources. The AARP

Box 23-10	Suggested Nursing Interventions with Grandparent Caregivers

- Early identification of at-risk grandparents
- Comprehensive assessment of physical, psychosocial, and environmental factors affecting those in the caregiving role for grandchildren
- Anticipatory guidance and counseling about child growth and development and other child-raising issues
- Referral to resources for support and counseling
- Advocacy for policies supportive of grandparents who have assumed a caregiving role for grandchildren

Data from Butler F, Zakari N: Grandparents parenting grandchildren: assessing health status, *J Gerontol Nurs* 31(3):43-54, 2005.

also provides resources for grandparents (see the Resources section at the end of this chapter and at evolve.elsevier.com/Ebersole/gerontological).

Long-Distance Caregiving

Because of the increasing mobility of today's society, more children move away from home for education or employment and do not return home. When the parent needs help, it must be provided "long distance." In 2004 the National Alliance for Caregiving (NAC) estimated that more than 7 million caregivers lived more than 1 hour away from the care recipient. Of these caregivers, 70% were employed full time and most lost work hours regularly because of their added responsibilities. This is perhaps one of the most difficult situations, and it presents unique challenges. Chapter 26 discusses residential care options for older people, including moving in with an adult child.

A profession and industry have emerged to assist the geographically distant family member to ensure that an elderly relative will be cared for; this profession is made up of geriatric care managers, some of whom are nurses or social workers. A care manager can be hired to do everything a family member would do if able, from being available in an emergency, to helping with estate planning, to making arrangements for a move to a nursing home. Often care managers know of resources that can assist the elder to remain independent and yet assure the family that safety and other needs are

being met. These services are available primarily to those who are able to pay for them, since they are not covered by private insurance, Medicare, or any public agencies. Although these services are expensive, they are far less expensive than alternative living arrangements or institutional placement. Similar services may be obtainable for persons with very low incomes by asking the local area agency on aging about the local "Community Care for the Elderly" programs. When incomes are too high to qualify for Medicaid, and too low to pay for private care managers, the persons and their families must do the best they can. Long-distance care then depends on the goodness of neighbors, local friends, and apartment managers and frequent trips by the long-distance caregiver to the elder.

Role of Nonfamily Caregivers

Close relationships often develop between older adults and their nonfamily caregivers. Over 50% of family caregivers use nurses, homemakers, and other personal care providers to assist in the care of their elder dependents (Piercy, 2001). These providers may include friends and hired or volunteer caregivers from a church or agency. The caregivers not only provide substantial physical care but also are involved with the elder, when possible, in social activities such as dining, concerts, and church events. Conditions that foster closeness include continuity of caregiver, social isolation of the elder, homogeneity of the client and caregiver, and the caregiver performing extra tasks and small personal attentions. The client will sometimes describe a paid caregiver as "my family." Elders and their caregivers in nursing homes often describe their relationship "like family" as well (Touhy et al, 2005). A caveat should be added (further explained in Chapter 22): dependent and lonely elders with assets may be victimized by apparently doting caregivers who may exert undue influence.

IMPLICATIONS FOR GERONTOLOGICAL NURSING AND HEALTHY AGING

Nurses are often the primary care providers and case managers for elders and their families, both in the home and in the institutional setting. The nurse monitors progress and manages chronic disorders of the elder within the context of the family. Support for families in the caregiving role is an important nursing intervention and one that needs continued attention by policymakers.

Assessment

Family Assessment

A comprehensive assessment of the elder includes assessing the family for the following: who are the members; what is the family history; what are their usual roles and their strengths and contributions; and what are the deterrents to the function of the family unit. Assessing the family's needs and strengths and the meaning it assigns to caregiving, as well as its sources of stress, particular methods of coping, cultural values, support system, and family dynamics, will help the nurse know the family and design responses that may strengthen the family unit.

Often, nurses see families in the times of crisis when an older family member needs care. It is important to encourage the expression of feelings from all involved family members, as well as the older person, and maintain a nonjudgmental attitude. It is important for the nurse to be aware of his or her vision of what a family "should" be and do. Our values should not enter into assessment and intervention with clients. Meiner and Lueckenotte (2006, p. 137) remind us that we should not "label families as 'dysfunctional' but rather build upon the strengths within each family and provide support and resources for limitations." Thus the nurse's role is to teach, monitor, and strengthen the family system so as to maintain health and wellness of the entire family structure.

A mutually constructed, written assessment of a family's needs and coping capacities can be both comprehensive and specific and becomes a document of the family's strengths to be consulted in times of stress. Including the family in the discussion of the outcome of the assessment is recommended for all settings, especially in long-term care facilities and home care.

Caregiver Assessment

Family members who assume the caregiving role, as just discussed, experience both stressors and benefits. The stresses, expectations of future needs and problems, and the positive aspects of the caregiving situation should be explored. Caregiver assessment includes how the family member can help the care recipient and how the health care team can help the person providing care. In light of the physical and emotional stressors often associated with the caregiving role, nurses must monitor the physical and emotional health of both the caregiver and the care recipient and provide support as necessary. A partnership model, combining the "nurse's professional expertise with the caregiver's knowledge

of the family member, is recommended" (Schumacher et al, 2006, p. 47). Box 23-11 presents a research-based model to guide nursing interventions with caregivers.

The Family Caregiver Alliance (2006) principles to guide caregiver assessment include the following: (1) caregiver assessment should include the needs and preferences of both the care recipient and the family caregiver; (2) caregiver assessment should reflect culturally competent practice; (3) caregiver assessment should be multidimensional and conducted with a multidisciplinary approach; and (4) caregiver assessment should result in a plan of care developed collaboratively with the caregiver that specifies the provision of services and intended measurable outcomes. Several validated caregiver assessment instruments are available, including the Preparedness for Caregiving Scale and the Mutuality Scale (Archbold et al, 1992) (website: www.consultgerirn.org) and the Caregiver Strain Index developed by Robinson (1983) (Figure 13-2).

Interventions

The New York University (NYU) Spouse Caregiver Intervention Study reported by Mittleman (2002) found the most useful of the interventions studied included a

---

Box 23-11   Nursing Actions to Create and Sustain a Partnership with Caregivers

- Surveillance and ongoing monitoring
- Coaching: helping caregivers apply knowledge and develop skills
- Teaching: providing information and instruction
- Fostering partnerships: fostering communication and collaboration between the caregiver and the care recipient and between them and the nurse
- Providing psychosocial support: attending to psychosocial well-being
- Rescuing: providing a safety net by stepping in to provide direct care and making clinical decisions
- Coordinating: orchestrating the work of other health care team members and the activities of the caregiver

Data from Eilers J, Heermann JA, Wilson ME: Independent nursing actions in cooperative care, *Oncol Nurs Forum* 32(4):849-855, 2005; Schumacher K, Beck C, Marren J: Family caregivers: caring for older adults working with their families, *Am J Nurs* 106(8): 40-49, 2006.

Box 23-12	Goals of Family Support Groups

- Learn to accept the elder as he or she is now; let go of the past.
- Learn the balance between protectiveness and smothering.
- Recognize one's own needs as fundamental to caring for others.
- Learn to share and cope with disappointment.
- Discuss resurgence of feelings of loss during holidays and anniversaries.
- Share knowledge of how to deal with family and community.
- Develop a caring and sharing network within the group.
- Deal with feelings of guilt, helplessness, and hopelessness.
- Identify realistic ways to assist in the care of the elder.

Modified from Richards M: Family support groups, *Generations* 10(4):68, 1986.

Box 23-13	Topics for Workplace Caregiver Assistance Programs

- Normal and healthy aging
- Communicating effectively with older adults
- Medication use
- Caring for the caregiver
- Specific health information
- Community resources
- Supplemental services
- Housing and long-term care options
- Medicare, Medigap, and other insurance (e.g., long-term care)
- Support groups
- End-of-life and legal information (e.g., advance directives)

From Curry L, Walker C, Hogstel MO: Educational needs of employed family caregivers of older adults: evaluation of a workplace project, *Geriatr Nurs* 27(3):166-173, 2006.

few sessions of counseling with the caregiver and other involved family members and a support group for primary caregivers, as well as ongoing telephone support. These interventions, when available, can alleviate much of the stress of caregiving (Box 23-12). Since many caregivers are trying to balance caregiving responsibilities while still working, educational programs offered in the workplace can be beneficial for both the caregiver and the employer (Curry et al, 2006). Box 23-13 presents suggested topics for programs. Several caregiver education and support programs are also available online (see the Resources section at the end of this chapter and at evolve.elsevier.com/Ebersole/gerontological).

Respite care is the provision of temporary relief to the caregiver and is perhaps the most significant intervention to assist family caregivers. Respite may be in many forms, including the temporary stay of the elder in a care facility, participation in an adult day program, or in-home relief by an informal or formal relief caregiver. Adult day services are a valuable resource for community-dwelling elders and can also provide needed respite for caregivers (see Chapter 26). Local area agencies on aging can provide information on adult day services and other forms of respite care. Respite care is also offered by many long-term care

facilities. Nurses should encourage caregivers to use this resource to provide needed relief from caregiving and to restore their energy and well-being.

An innovative intervention that may help caregivers obtain some relief from care is video respite. The care recipient in the home or institution can view videotapes of music, memories, and pictures that were developed by researchers at the Gerontology Center at the University of Utah for persons with dementia (Lund et al, 1995; Meiner and Lueckenotte, 2006). The researchers report that persons with AD watch and participate with the tapes, and nursing home staff report that the tapes have a calming effect on the residents (see the Resources section at the end of this chapter and at evolve.elsevier.com/Ebersole/gerontological). Families can also make their own videos or DVDs with family memories or messages from loved ones that can be played for care recipients.

Interventions with caregivers must always be made with consideration of the great variability in family structures, resources, traditions, and history. The range of adaptations is enormous, and the goal is always to restore the balance of the system to the greatest extent possible and support caregivers in their caring. The family can be visualized as a mobile with many parts: when one is touched, each part shifts to regain the balance. The intrusion of professionals into a family system will temporarily unbalance the system and may provide an opportunity to restore the balance in a healthier manner, sometimes by adding an element or increasing the weight of one or decreasing the weight of another. When the nurse works with a family from a different culture and that may have rituals and routines unfamiliar to him or her, the nurse must be particularly careful to respect these differences. The nurse can work with the family to make the best use of their strengths, whatever they may be. Each family member can be valued for what he or she brings to the situation. "Family members must not be allowed to 'fail' while providing care; a nurse should be available to step in when demands of the situation exceed family members' capabilities. And the nurse should be prepared to step back when the family's support is what's needed" (Schumacher et al, 2006, p. 48).

IMPLICATIONS FOR GERONTOLOGICAL NURSING AND HEALTHY AGING

Role transitions and losses often characterize the aging experience. For some older adults, these can be devastating and will necessitate support from nurses and other health professionals. Nurses can provide anticipatory guidance to assist older people in preparing for these transitions. It is important to build upon the strengths of older adults' life experiences and coping skills and to provide appropriate counseling and support to assist older people to continue to grow and develop in meaningful ways. During the transition from familiar roles to new ones, an individual needs the freedom to try various possibilities in an accepting atmosphere that encourages success, tolerates failure, and recognizes that progress is not accomplished by slow, even steps. In reality, progress follows a more wayward, uneven course. One is easily distracted and often falls back to the familiar. The nurse is most helpful in providing an accepting milieu that encourages independence and exploration, as well as the awareness that transitions all create some anxiety. Useful nursing interventions will assist the older adult in maintaining self-esteem and developing new and satisfying roles. Future generations of older adults will redefine what we now consider "norms" for aging and roles for older people. Research is needed to provide the foundation for nursing interventions with family caregivers, particularly among racially and ethnically diverse families and nontraditional families.

INTIMACY AND SEXUALITY

Intimacy

Although intimacy is often thought of in the context of sexual performance, it encompasses more than sexuality and includes five major relational components: commitment, affective intimacy, cognitive intimacy, physical intimacy, and interdependence (Blieszner and DeVries, 2001; Troll, 2001; Youngkin, 2004). "Intimacy is from a Greek work meaning 'closest to; inner lining of blood vessels'" (Steinke, 2005, p. 40). It is a warm, meaningful feeling of joy. Intimacy includes the need for close friendships; relationships with family, friends, and formal caregivers; spiritual connections, knowing that one matters in someone else's life, and the ability to form satisfying social relationships with others (Blieszner and DeVries, 2001; Piercy, 2001; Ramsey, 2001; Steinke, 2005).

Youngkin (2004) points out that older people may be concerned about changes in sexual intimacy, but "social relationships with people important in their lives, the ability to interact intellectually with people who share similar interests, the supportive love that grows between human beings (whether romantic or platonic), and physical nonsexual intimacy are equally—and in many instances more—important than the physical intimacy of direct sexual relations. All of these facets of intimate life are integrally woven into the fabric of aging, along with other influences that can make life rewarding" (p. 46). Intimacy needs with others change over time, but the need for intimacy and satisfying social relationships is an important component of successful aging (Steinke, 2005).

Sexuality

Sexuality is defined as a central aspect of being human throughout life and encompasses sex, gender identities and roles, sexual orientation, eroticism, pleasure, intimacy, and reproduction (World Health Organization, 2004). As a major aspect of intimacy, sexuality includes the physical act of intercourse, as well as many other types of intimate activity. Sexuality provides the opportunity to express passion, affection, admiration, and loyalty. It can also enhance personal growth and communication. Sexuality also allows a general affirmation of life (especially joy) and a continuing opportunity to search for new growth and experience (Butler and Lewis, 2002).

Sexuality, similar to food and water, is a basic human need, yet it goes beyond the biological realm to include psychological, social, and moral dimensions. The constant interaction among these spheres of sexuality work to produce harmony. The linkage of the four dimensions composes the holistic quality of an individual's sexuality. The social sphere of sexuality is the sum of cultural factors that influence the individual's thoughts and actions related to interpersonal relationships, as well as sexuality related to ideas and learned behavior. Television, radio, literature, and the more traditional sources of family, school, and religious teachings combine to influence social sexuality. The belief of what constitutes masculine and feminine is deeply rooted in the individual's exposure to cultural factors.

The psychological domain of sexuality reflects a person's attitudes, feelings toward self and others, and learning from experiences. Beginning with birth, the individual is bombarded with cues and signals of how a person should act and think about the use of "dirty words" or body parts. Conversation is self-censored in the presence of or in discussion with certain people. The moral aspect of sexuality, the "I should" or "I shouldn't," makes a difference that is based in religious beliefs or in a pragmatic or humanistic outlook.

The final dimension, biological sexuality, is reflected in physiological responses to sexual stimulation, reproduction, puberty, and growth and development.

Because of the interrelatedness, these dimensions affect each other directly or indirectly whenever an aspect of sexuality is out of harmony. Figure 23-1 illustrates the interrelationship of the sexuality dimensions.

Sexuality is a vital aspect to consider in the care of the older person regardless of the setting. Sexuality exists throughout life in one form or another in everyone. All older people have a need to express sexual feelings, whether the individuals are healthy and active or frail. Sexuality can be envisioned as part of Maslow's Hierarchy of Needs, with physical reproduction the lowest level and a progression to the higher levels with increased communication, trust, sharing, and pleasure with or without a physical action. Sexuality in the older person shifts its focus from procreation to an emphasis on companionship, physical nearness, intimate communication, and a pleasure-seeking physical relationship. Some researchers have coined the phrase "from procreation to recreation," which refers to this change in sexual emphasis. Figure 23-2 focuses on the hierarchy of sexuality.

Sexual Health

The World Health Organization defines sexual health as a state of physical, emotional, mental, and social well-being related to sexuality (World Health Organization,

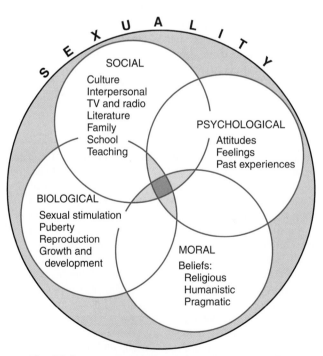

Fig. 23-1 Interrelationship of dimensions of sexuality.

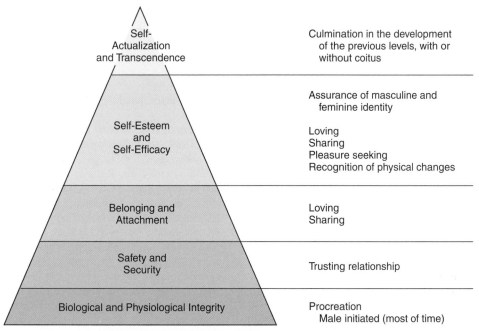

Fig. 23-2   Progression of sexual emphasis through life.

2004). This definition illustrates the multifaceted nature of the biological, psychosocial, cultural, and spiritual components of sexuality and implies that sexual behavior has the capacity to enhance self and others. Sexual health is individually defined and wholesome if it leads to intimacy (not necessarily coitus) and enriches the involved parties.

Expectations. Factors affecting a person's attitudes on intimacy and sexuality include family dynamics and upbringing and cultural and religious beliefs (Youngkin, 2004). Older people often internalize the broad cultural proscriptions of sexual behavior in late life that hinder the continuance of sexual expression. Much sexual behavior stems from incorporating other people's reactions. Older adults may not feel asexual until they are continually treated as such. American society continues to struggle with open acceptance of sexual expression for the young but continues to remain hostile to the attempts of older people to do the same. Sexual interest and activity in the elderly are sometimes regarded as deviant behavior and described in such terms as "dirty old man," "lecher," and "old biddy." The same activity attempted by a younger person would be viewed as appropriate. An often quoted statement by Alex Comfort (1974) sums it up nicely: "In our experiences, old folks stop having sex for the same reasons they stop riding a bicycle—general infirmity, thinking it looks ridiculous, no bicycle." Box 23-14 presents some of the myths about sexuality in older people that may be held by older people themselves and by society in general.

Box 23-14	Sexuality and Aging: Common Myths

- Masturbation is an immature activity of youngsters and adolescents, not older women.
- Sexual prowess and desire wane during the climacteric, and menopause is the death of a woman's sexuality.
- Hysterectomy creates a physical disability that results in the inability to function sexually.
- Sex has no role in the lives of the elderly, except as perversion or remembrance of times past.
- Sexual expression in old age is taboo.
- The elderly are too old and frail to engage in sex.
- The young are considered lusty and virile; the elderly are considered lecherous.
- Sex is unimportant or over when a person is older.
- Elderly women do not wish to discuss their sexuality with professionals.

Activity Levels. For both heterosexual and homosexual individuals, research supports that "liberal and positive attitudes toward sexuality, greater sexual knowledge, satisfaction with a long-term relationship or a current intimate relationship, good social networks, psychological well-being, and a sense of self-worth are associated with greater sexual interest, activity, and satisfaction" (Zeiss and Kasl-Godfrey, 2001, p. 20). Both early studies of sexual behavior in older adults and more recent ones indicate that men and women remain sexually active and find their sexual lives satisfying.

Results of the first comprehensive national survey of sexual attitudes, behaviors, and problems among 3005 community-living older adults in the United States revealed that about three quarters of individuals 57 to 85 years of age are married or living with a partner and three quarters of those are sexually active. The prevalence of sexual activity declined with age: 73% of people between 57 and 64 years of age reported being sexually active; 53% of those between 65 and 74; and 26% of those between 75 and 85. Sexual activity was closely tied to overall health, and people whose health was rated as excellent or very good were nearly twice as likely to be sexually active as those who rated their health as poorer. The most common reason for sexual inactivity among those with a partner was the male partner's health. Men are more sexually active than women, most likely because women live longer and may not have a partner. Women, especially those not in a relationship, were more likely than men to report lack of interest in sex (Lindau et al, 2007).

Cohort and Cultural Influences. The era in which a person was born influences his or her attitudes about sexuality (Youngkin, 2004). Women in their eighties today may have been strongly influenced by the prudish, Victorian atmosphere of their youth and may have experienced difficult marital adjustments and serious sexual problems early in their marriages. Sexuality was not openly expressed or discussed. The next generation of older people ("baby boomers") has experienced other influences, including more liberal attitudes toward sexuality, the women's movement, a higher number of divorced adults, the human immunodeficiency virus (HIV) epidemic, and increased numbers of gay and lesbian couples, all of which will affect their views and attitudes as they age. The boomers and generations beyond, as they find themselves experiencing sexuality beyond the age they had assigned to their elders, may alter current perceptions.

Most of what is known about sexuality in aging has been gained through research with well-educated, healthy, white older adults. Further research is needed among culturally, socially, and ethnically diverse older people, those with chronic illness, and gay, lesbian, and bisexual older people (Zeiss and Kasl-Godley, 2001). It is important to come to know and understand the older person within his or her social and cultural background and not make judgments based on one's own belief system.

Alternative Sexual Lifestyles: Lesbian, Gay, Bisexual, and Transgender. Knowledge is lacking about aging lesbian, gay, bisexual, and transgender (LGBT) individuals. Reasons for this include difficulties in studying the LGBT population because of problems with definition, differences in self-identification, societal attitudes, and a lack of support for research with this population. Research has been conducted primarily with middle-class white gay men and lesbians in urban areas (Blando, 2001). As a result of invisibility and discrimination, the needs of gay and lesbian elders and their families receive limited recognition in health and social services (Brotman et al, 2003). Even less is known about bisexual and transgender older people.

Older gay men and lesbians are as diverse as the remainder of the heterosexual elder population. Many gay men and lesbians age successfully, are healthy, and are active, with satisfied lives. Some gay and lesbian people are coupled, have children, and are open about their sexual orientation, and some are not. Some of these individuals have only recently "come out"; others have been "out" most of their lives; and some find themselves isolated in the larger society. Older gays and lesbians are more likely to have kept their relationships hidden than those who grew up in the modern-day gay liberation movement (Brotman et al, 2003).

Older lesbians have been labeled the "invisible minority" (Hooyman and Kiyak, 2008, p. 268). These women tend to keep a very low profile, although conservative estimates are that over 2 million now reside in the United States, preferring rural settings, whereas gay men prefer urban areas. An interesting note is that approximately one third of the lesbians "come out" after the age of 50 years. Most lesbians married, raised children, divorced, and lead double lives (Butler and Lewis, 2002).

Younger gay men have been found to have had multiple liaisons, but the number of gay men with partners does increase with age, peaking among those 46 to 55 years old. However, with the impact of acquired immunodeficiency syndrome (AIDS) on this population, a decrease in multiple liaisons has become evident. Older gay men are less likely to engage in short-term relationships and are more likely to be in a long-term relationship (average 10 years or more) or no relationship at all (Hooyman and Kiyak, 2008). After age 60, the percent of gay men in relationships decreases. The situation has been attributed to several factors, for example, the death of a loved one and rejection of the idea of a single lifelong partner.

Health care providers lack sufficient information and sensitivity when caring for older LGBTs. This sensitivity is of utmost importance when attempting to obtain a health history. Using open-ended questions such as "Who is most important to you?" or "Do you have a significant other?" is much better than asking "Are you married?" This form of the question allows the nurse to look beyond the rigid category of family. Euphemisms are frequently used for a life partner (roommate, close friend). Asking individuals if they consider themselves as primarily heterosexual, homosexual, or bisexual is also better. This question conveys recognition of sexual variety. An older lesbian woman in a health care situation may refer to herself indirectly by saying "people like us." Nurses must become more aware of these nuances and try to understand the fear of discovery that is apparent in the older gay man and lesbian woman. These elders are of a generation in which they were and may still be closeted because of the homophobic experiences they had through their younger years.

Better support and care services for gays and lesbians by care providers should include working through homophobic attitudes and discomfort discussing sexuality, learning about special issues facing older gay men and lesbians, and becoming aware of the gay and lesbian resources in the community. Programs to increase awareness of the needs of LGBT elders and reduce discrimination are necessary (Brotman et al, 2003). LGBT elders living in metropolitan areas may find organizations particularly designed for them, such as Senior Action in a Gay Environment (SAGE), (SAGE-Net is now in nine states and Ontario, Canada); New Leaf Outreach to Elders (formerly GLOE, San Francisco); Rainbow Project (Los Angeles); Gay and Lesbians Older and Wiser (GLOW, Ann Arbor, Mich.); and the Lesbian and Gay Aging Issues Network (LGAIN). Several of the major gerontological organizations have established special interest groups focusing on LGBT issues (see Resources section at the end of the chapter and at evolve.elsevier.com/Ebersole/gerontological).

Biological Changes with Age. Acknowledgement and understanding of the age-related changes that influence coitus may partially explain alteration in sexual behavior to accommodate these changes and facilitate the continuation of pleasurable sex (see Chapter 6). Characteristic physiological changes during the sexual response cycle do occur with aging, but these vary from individual to individual depending on general health factors. The "use it or lose it" phenomenon also applies here: the more sexually active the person is, the fewer changes he or she is likely to experience in the pattern of sexual response. Illnesses and medications also affect sexual response. Changes in the appearance of the body (wrinkles, sagging skin) may also affect the older person's security about their sexual attractiveness (Arena and Wallace, 2008). Physical alteration is one variable in the total picture of sexuality and is therefore included as one of the main factors that influence the act of intercourse. Many texts explain biological changes in depth.

Older people who do not understand the physical changes that affect sexual activity become concerned that their sex life is approaching its natural conclusion with the onset of menopause or, for men, when they discover a change in the firmness of their erection or the decreased need for ejaculation with each orgasm or when the refractory period is extended between episodes of intercourse. Although biological changes do affect sexual functioning, attitudes may be a more significant influence on sexual desire (DeLamater and Sill, 2005). A major nursing role is to provide information about these changes, as well as appropriate assessment and counseling within the context of the individual's needs. Assessment and interventions are discussed later in the chapter.

Sexual Dysfunction

Sexual dysfunction is defined as an impairment in normal sexual functioning and can have many causes, both physical and psychological. Sexual disorders have not been well studied among older people, but generally the following four categories are described: hypoactive sexual desire disorder; sexual arousal disorder; orgasmic disorder; and sexual pain disorders (Arena and Wallace, 2008). Aging changes, sexual disorders, and a number of medical conditions are associated with sexual dysfunction. Since sexuality is an important human need that does not change with age, it is important for nurses to be knowledgeable about factors affecting sexual health in aging and interventions to improve sexual health.

Male Dysfunction. Impotence (erectile dysfunction [ED]) is defined as the inability to achieve and sustain an erection sufficient for satisfactory sexual intercourse in at least 50% or more attempts. ED has become recognized as a common problem among men older than 50 years. Until recently, ED had been a neglected area of health that is fraught with myths and superstition. ED transiently occurs to men of all ages at some point in their life; however, the prevalence of ED increases with age, with estimates that 50% of men ages 40 to 70 and nearly 70% of those ages 70 and older experience ED (Agronin, 2004). Thirty-seven percent of the men who participated in the national survey (Lindau et al, 2007) reported erectile dysfunction, and 14% reported taking medication to improve their sexual function.

For most older men, ED is caused by an underlying medical diagnosis. Nearly one third of ED is a complication of diabetes. Alcoholism, medications, depression, and prostate disease and treatment are also causes of ED in older men. An erection is governed by the interaction among the hormonal, vascular, and nervous systems. A problem in any of these systems can cause ED. Various medications that affect the sympathetic and parasympathetic nervous system interfere with the man's capacity to have an erection or to ejaculate. Two of the major groups of medications are antidepressants and antihypertensives.

Because of professionals' discomfort discussing sexuality, or lack of knowledge about sexuality in older people, medications are often prescribed to both older men and women without attention to the sexual side effects. If medications that affect sexual function are necessary, adjustment of doses, use of alternative agents, and prescription of antidotes to reverse the sexual side effects are important (Agronin, 2004; Arena and Wallace, 2008). For a list of medications that affect sexual health, see http:www.netdoctor.co.uk/menshealth/feature/medicinessex.htm.

Most men who undergo surgical procedures such as transurethral resection and other types of prostatectomies, Y-V–plasty of the bladder neck, resection of the colon for cancer, or a sympathectomy may experience ED or have retrograde ejaculations caused by interference with autonomic innervation in the pelvis. Particularly after a prostatectomy, a space remains where the enlarged prostate had been. The principle that fluid travels the path of least resistance applies here. At the point of ejaculation, the semen moves backward into the bladder rather than forward through increased resistance, which produces a retrograde, or dry, ejaculation. A lack of knowledge regarding this physiological change further convinces men that their sexual activity is over when, in fact, it is not. Erection can be attained and orgasmic pleasure achieved. Any surgery that involves the male perineum has a high

risk of causing ED resulting from potential nerve damage in that area. Newer surgical procedures that spare the nerves may result in less effect on sexual functioning.

The use of phosphodiesterase inhibitors such as sildenafil (Viagra), vardenafil (Levitra), and tadalafil (Cialis) has revolutionized treatment for ED regardless of cause (Agronin, 2004). Use of these medications to treat female arousal disorders has been inconclusive to date, but they may be helpful for select women. Further research is needed and may lead to the development of better drug therapies for women (Mayer et al, 2005). Contraindications to the use of these medications include nitrate therapy, heart failure with low blood pressure, certain antihypertensive regimens, and other medications and cardiovascular conditions. See Chapter 14 for further discussion of contraindications and side effects. Before the availability of these medications, intracavernosal injections with the drugs papaverine and phentolamine, and vasoactive agents that reduce resistance of arteriolar and cavernosal smooth muscle tissue of the penis were used. Penile implants of the semirigid, adjustable-malleable, or hinged and inflatable types are available when impotence does not respond to other treatments or is irreversible. The hinged and inflatable types, which are inserted in the testicular area, are the most popular.

Female Dysfunction. Female dysfunction is considered a "persistent impediment to a person's normal pattern of sexual interest, response, or both" (Kaiser, 2000, p. 1174). Female sexual function can be influenced by factors such as culture, ethnicity, emotional state, age, and previous sexual experiences, as well as changes in sexual response with normal aging. For heterosexual women, frequency of intercourse depends more on the age, health, and sexual function of the partner, or the availability of a partner, rather than on their own sexual capacity. Lack of desire was reported by 43% of the women in the recent national survey, and 39% of the female participants reported vaginal dryness as a problem (Lindau et al, 2007). Pain resulting from anatomical changes and vaginal dryness can result in painful intercourse (dyspareunia) and avoidance of sexual activity. The use of water-soluble lubricants such as K-Y, Astroglide, Slip, and H-R lubricating jelly can help with vaginal dryness.

Women can experience arousal disorders resulting from drugs such as anticholinergics, antidepressants, and chemotherapeutic agents and from lack of lubrication caused by radiation, surgery, or stress. Orgasmic disorders also may result from drugs used to treat depression. Prolapse of the uterus, rectoceles, and cystoceles can be surgically repaired to facilitate continued sexual activity. Urinary incontinence (UI) is another condition that may affect sexual activity for both men and women. Appropriate assessment and treatment are important because many causes of UI are treatable (Chapter 9).

Intimacy and Chronic Illness

Chronic illnesses and their related treatments may bring many challenges to intimacy and sexual activity. Steinke (2005), in an excellent article discussing intimacy needs and chronic illness, suggests that although some research has been done on the effects of myocardial infarction on sexual function, less information is available for patients with heart failure, implantable cardioverter-defibrillators (ICDs), hypertension, arthritis, chronic pain, or chronic obstructive pulmonary disease (COPD). Often, patients and their partners are given little or no information about the effect of illnesses on sexual activity or strategies to continue sexual activity within functional limitations. Timing of intercourse (mornings or when energy level is highest), oral or anal sex, masturbation, appropriate pain relief, and different sexual positions are all strategies that may assist in continued sexual activity (Table 23-1). Tabloski (2006) provides age-appropriate illustrations of coital positions for older people with cardiovascular disease that can be used in teaching. Steinke (2005) also provides specific suggestions and teaching plans that will be very useful for nurses working with older people for sexual counseling after myocardial infarction and for older people with congestive heart failure (CHF), COPD, ICDs, and hypertension.

For individuals with cardiac conditions, manual stimulation (masturbation) may be an alternative that can be used early in the recovery period to maintain

Table 23-1   Chronic Illness and Sexual Function: Effects and Interventions

CONDITION	EFFECTS AND PROBLEMS	INTERVENTIONS
Arthritis	Pain, fatigue, limited motion Steroid therapy may decrease sexual interest or desire	Advise patient to perform sexual activity at time of day when less fatigued and most relaxed Suggest use of analgesics and other pain-relief methods before sexual activity Encourage use of relaxation techniques before sexual activity such as a warm bath or shower, application of hot packs to affected joints Advise patient to maintain optimum health through a balance of good nutrition, proper rest, and activity Suggest that he or she experiment with different positions, use pillows for comfort and support Recommend use of a vibrator if massage ability is limited Suggest use of water-soluble jelly for vaginal lubrication
Cardiovascular disease	Most men have no change in physical effects on sexual function; one fourth may not return to pre–heart attack function; one fourth may not resume sexual activity Women do not experience sexual dysfunction after heart attack Fear of another heart attack or death during sex Shortness of breath	Encourage counseling on realistic restrictions that may be necessary Instruct patient and spouse on alternative positions to avoid strain Suggest that patient avoid large meals for several hours before sex Advise patient to relax; plan medications for effectiveness during sex

(Continued)

CONDITION	EFFECTS AND PROBLEMS	INTERVENTIONS
Cerebrovascular accident (stroke)	Depression May or may not have sexual activity changes Often erectile disorders occur; decrease in frequency of intercourse and sexual relations Change in role and function of partners Decreased physical endurance, fatigue Mobility and sensory deficits Perceptual and visual deficits Communication deficit Cognitive and behavioral deficits Fear of relapse or sudden death	Encourage counseling Instruct patient to use alternative positions Suggest use of a vibrator if massage ability is limited Suggest use of pillows for positioning and support Suggest use of water-soluble jelly for lubrication Instruct patient to use alternative forms of sexual expression
Chronic obstructive pulmonary disease (COPD)	No direct impairment of sexual activity although coughing, exertional dyspnea, positions, and activity intolerance can have impact Medications may lead to erectile difficulties	Encourage patient to plan sexual activity when energy is highest Instruct patient to use alternative positions Advise patient to plan sexual activity at time medications are most effective Suggest use of oxygen before, during, or after sex, depending on when it provides the most benefit
Diabetes	Sexual desire and interest unaffected Neuropathy and/or vascular damage may interfere with erectile ability. About 50% to 75% of men have erectile disorders; a small portion have retrograde ejaculation Some men regain function if diagnosis of diabetes is well accepted, if diabetes is well controlled, or both Women have less sexual desire and vaginal lubrication Decrease in orgasms and/or absence of orgasm can occur; less frequent sexual activity; local genital infections	Recommend possible candidates for penile prosthesis Instruct patient to use alternative forms of sexual expression Recommend immediate treatment of genital infections
Cancers		
Breast cancer	No direct physical affect. There is a strong psychological effect: • Loss of sexual desire • Body-image change • Depression • Reaction of partner	Encourage individual or group counseling
Most other cancers	Men and women may lose sexual desire temporarily Men may have erectile dysfunction; dry ejaculation; retrograde ejaculation Women may have vaginal dryness, dyspareunia Both men and women may experience anxiety, depression, pain, nausea from chemotherapy, radiation, pelvic surgery, hormone therapy, nerve damage from pelvic surgery	

sexual function if the practice is not objectionable to the patient. Studies show that masturbation is less taxing on the heart and creates less oxygen demand. Although self-stimulation is steeped in myth and fear, masturbation is a common and healthy practice in late life. Individuals without partners or those whose spouses are ill or incapacitated find that masturbation is helpful. As children, today's older population was discouraged from practicing this pleasurable activity with stories of the evils of fondling one's own genitals. Masturbation provides an avenue for resolution of sexual tensions, keeps sexual desire alive, maintains lubrication and muscle tone of the vagina, provides mild physical exercise, and preserves sexual function in individuals who have no other outlet for sexual activity and gratification of their sexual need. In the study by Lindau and colleagues (2007), more than 50% of male participants and 25% of female participants acknowledged masturbating, regardless of whether or not they had a sexual partner.

Intimacy and Sexuality in Long-Term Care Facilities

Research is needed on sexuality in assisted living facilities and nursing homes, but surveys suggest that a significant number of older people residing in those settings might choose to be sexually active if they had privacy and an available partner (Messinger-Rapport et al, 2003). Intimacy and sexuality among nursing home residents include the opportunity to have not only coitus but also other forms of intimate expressions such as hugging, kissing, hand holding, and masturbation. Wallace (2003a) commented that the sexual needs of older adults in long-term care facilities should be addressed with the same priority as nutrition, hydration, and other well-accepted needs. The institutionalized older person has the same rights as noninstitutionalized elders have to engage in or abstain from sexual activity.

Nursing homes are required by federal regulation to allow married spouses to share a room if they desire, but no other requirements related to sexual activity in nursing homes exist (Messinger-Rapport et al, 2003). However, what about unmarried individuals in intimate relationships or gay and lesbian partners? In research with older gays and lesbians and their families (Brotman et al, 2003), participants reported being terrified of going into care facilities and having to hide their relationships or losing their partners and friends. One lesbian couple who had been living together for several decades were separated by health care professionals and family members who were not aware of the nature of their partnership. Another partner in a lesbian relationship changed her last name to her partner's so that they would be taken for sisters and put in the same room.

Privacy is a major issue in nursing homes that can prevent fulfillment of intimacy and sexual needs. Suggestions for providing privacy and an atmosphere accepting of sexual activity include the availability of a private room, not interrupting when doors are closed and sexual activity is taking place, allowing residents to have sexually explicit materials in their room, and providing adaptive equipment such as siderails or trapezes and double beds (Zeiss and Kasl-Godley, 2001; Wallace, 2003a). For safety, Wallace (2003a) suggests that a trusted staff member should be informed about the sexual activity and the call light should be within reach.

Attitudes about intimacy and sexuality among nursing home staff and, often, family members may reflect general societal attitudes that older people do not have sexual needs or that sexual activity is inappropriate. Wallace (2003a) suggests that families may have difficulty understanding that their older relative may want to have a new relationship. Caregivers often view residents' sexual acts as problems rather than expressions of the need for love and intimacy. Reactions may include disapproval, discomfort, and embarrassment, and caregivers may explicitly or implicitly discourage or deny intimacy needs. A lack of knowledge about intimacy and sexuality in late life and a lack of knowledge in handling related issues are major reasons for staff reactions (Zeiss and Kasl-Godley, 2001; Low et al, 2005; Bauer et al, 2007).

Staff, family, and resident education programs to promote awareness, provide education on sexuality and intimacy in late life, involve residents in discussions of sexuality, and discuss interventions to respond to residents' needs are important in long-term care settings (Ward et al, 2005). Staff education should include the opportunity to discuss personal feelings about sexuality, normal changes of aging, and the impact of diseases and medications on sexual function, as well as role playing and skill training in sexual assessment and intervention (Zeiss and Kasl-Godley, 2001; Wallace, 2003a; Low et al, 2005; Steinke, 2005; Arena and Wallace, 2008).

Intimacy, Sexuality, and Dementia

Intimacy and sexuality remain important in the lives of persons with dementia and their partners throughout the illness. Intimacy and sexuality may "serve as a nonverbal form of communication and intimacy when other cognitive skills and functions have declined" (Agronin, 2004, p. 13). As dementia progresses, particularly in persons living in long-term care facilities, intimacy and sexuality issues may present challenges, especially regarding the impaired person's ability to consent to sexual activity (Messinger-Rapport et al, 2003; Wallace, 2003a; Agronin, 2004; Ward et al, 2005), which necessitates accurate assessment and documentation.

Determination of a cognitively impaired person's ability to consent to participation in a sexual activity involves concepts of voluntary participation, mental competence, and the understanding of the risks and benefits (Messinger-Rapport et al, 2003). It is important for the person to understand the potential physical risks but also the "psychological risks including risk of loss through transfer, death, or discharge of his or her partner" (Messinger-Rapport et al, 2003, p. 52). "If it is determined that an individual is incapable of decision making, health care staff must prevent the cognitively impaired resident from unsolicited sexual advances by a spouse, partner, or other residents" (Arena and Wallace, 2008, p. 634). Resources and guidelines for determination of competent decision making for sexual activity in persons with cognitive impairment can be found in Gordon and Sokolowski (2004) and Gwyther and Willer (2004). Guidelines for practice guidelines and policy for intimacy, sexuality, and sexual behavior in dementia in long-term care facilities can be found at www.fhs.mcmaster.ca/mcah/cgec/toolkit.pdf.

Inappropriate sexual behavior such as exposing oneself, masturbating in public, or making inappropriate sexual advances or sexual comments may also occur in the nursing home setting and is most distressing to staff. Messinger-Rapport et al (2003) suggest that these behaviors may be triggered by unmet intimacy needs. Encouraging family and friends to touch, hug, kiss, and hold hands when visiting may help to meet touch and intimacy needs and decrease inappropriate sexual behavior. Also, allowing the person to stroke a pet or hold a stuffed animal may be helpful. Providing an environment for expression of sexuality in private may also be a solution (Arena and Wallace, 2008). When sexually inappropriate behavior does occur, it should be assessed like any other behavior as to cause, precipitating factors, and response to interventions. Aggressive or violent behavior may require limit setting, working with the resident and family, providing for sexual expression in a nonharmful manner, and pharmacological treatment if indicated (Messinger-Rapport et al, 2003). Staff will need opportunities for discussion and assistance with interventions.

AIDS AND THE ELDERLY

Individuals ages 50 years and older account for 12% to 15% of AIDS cases in the United States. The number of AIDS cases in this age-group has increased 22% since 1991 (Older Americans and HIV, 2001). After leveling off in the late 1990s after the introduction of the highly active antiretroviral treatment (HAART), the number of individuals older than 50 years diagnosed with HIV-AIDS is rising again, particularly among the African-American and Latino populations. In the context of reporting HIV statistics, the Centers for Disease Control and Prevention (CDC) considers an older adult to be older than 50 years rather than the commonly used 65 years (Uphold et al, 2004). AIDS is rising faster among the older population than it is in those ages 24 years and younger. Women older than 60 years make up one of the fastest growing risk groups (Goodroad, 2003). The incidence of HIV in older people is expected to continue to increase "as more individuals become infected later in life and as those who were infected in early adulthood live longer" (Uphold et al, 2004, p. 16).

The compromised immune system of an older individual makes him or her even more susceptible to HIV or AIDS than a younger person. AIDS is not exclusively a young person's disease, but it is frequently underreported in the elderly because the symptoms of fatigue, weakness, weight loss, and anorexia are common to other elder disease conditions or may be attributed to "normal aging." In addition, the idea that elders are not sexually active limits physicians' and other care providers' objectivity and thus their ability to recognize HIV-AIDS as a possible diagnosis.

Contrary to popular belief, HIV-AIDS in the elderly population is not the result of blood transfusions alone, nor is it confined to the homosexual population. Research shows that elders are sexually active and thus at risk for HIV-AIDS. People older than 50 years were one sixth as likely to use condoms during sex and one fifth as likely to have been tested for HIV. Because procreation is not an issue with elders, they are the least likely to use condoms. Responsible sexual behavior is a leading health indicator in *Healthy People 2010* (U.S. Department of Health and Human Services, 2001) and applies to young as well as older individuals. Lack of awareness about HIV in older people often results in late diagnosis and treatment. This is especially problematic for older people since HIV tends to progress faster in older persons (Older Americans and HIV, 2001).

Older women who are sexually active are at high risk for HIV-AIDS (and other sexually transmitted infections) from an infected partner, resulting in part from normal age changes of the vaginal tissue—a thinner, drier, more friable vaginal lining. Older men may frequent prostitutes (a potentially high-risk group for HIV-AIDS). Gay men may increase their risk of HIV exposure after the death of a long-term mate by turning to a more available younger partner, who may have HIV. In general, elders lack adequate knowledge about HIV-AIDS and believe that HIV-AIDS "just does not happen in my generation." This view places elders at high risk for HIV and AIDS. Further, older people may have limited access to HIV tests and age-appropriate information.

The U.S. Preventive Services Task Force (USPSTF) advises that all adults at high risk for HIV be screened. A study at the University of California, San Francisco, of 3200 predominantly heterosexual Americans older than 50 years, found that approximately 10% had at least one risk factor for HIV infection. Assessment and screening for other sexually transmitted infections (gonorrhea, chlamydia, syphilis, trichomonas, human papillomavirus [HPV]) should also be a part of primary care for sexually active elders. If symptoms of another disease such as herpes arise, testing should occur as well.

AIDS in older adults has been called the "Great Imitator." In addition to the vague signs mentioned earlier, symptoms include dementia with increased neurological abnormalities and unexplained diffuse encephalopathy that is demonstrated in progressive and chronic dementia. Elders may be misdiagnosed as having Alzheimer's disease (AD) instead of AIDS—the actual problem. AIDS dementia is rapid in onset, as opposed to the slow, progressive decline associated with AD. Educational materials and programs must be developed that include information about what HIV-AIDS is and how it is and is not transmitted, the need to use condoms for protection when engaging in sexual activity, symptoms of which to be aware, and the treatments that are available. Physicians, nurse practitioners, and other health professionals must become comfortable taking a complete sexual history and talking about sex with the elderly. In addition, the myth that elders do not engage in sexual activity must be put to rest. Websites with specific information about HIV and older people that can be used in prevention and education can be found in the Resources section at the end of this chapter and at evolve.elsevier.com/Ebersole/gerontological.

IMPLICATIONS FOR GERONTOLOGICAL NURSING AND HEALTHY AGING

Nurses have multiple roles in the area of sexuality and older people. The nurse is a facilitator of a milieu that is conducive to the older person asking questions and expressing his or her sexuality. The nurse has the responsibility to help maintain the sexuality of older people by offering opportunity for discussion. Nusbaum et al (2005) reported that older women had a similar number of sexual concerns as younger women but were less likely to be asked about sexual health during health care visits. Older women wanted health care providers to ask about their sexual functioning, although participants reported some discomfort discussing the topic with younger physicians. Some older people remain or want to remain sexually active, whereas others do not see this as an important part of their life. Nurses should open the door to discussions of sexual concerns in a nonjudgmental manner, helping those who want to continue to be sexually active and making it clear that stopping sex is an acceptable option for others (Lindau et al, 2007).

Assessment

To assist and support older people in their sexual needs, nurses should be aware of their own feelings about sexuality and their attitudes towards intimacy and sexuality in older people (single, married, and homosexual). Only after confronting one's own attitudes, values, and beliefs can the nurse provide support without being judgmental (Bauer et al, 2007). Rarely are sex histories elicited from the older person. Physical examinations often do not include the reproductive system unless it is directly involved in the present illness. However, when questions about sexual issues are asked or when older people are examined, the nurse needs to be particularly cognizant of the era and culture in which the individual has lived to understand the factors affecting conduct.

The nurse should be an educator and provide information and guidance to older people who need it. Older persons should be asked about their sexual satisfaction, because they may not mention it voluntarily. Anticipation of problems in older individuals' sexual experiences can ward off anxiety, misconceptions, and an arbitrary cessation of pleasurable sexual activity. Validation of the normalcy of sexual activity or a discussion of the physiological changes that occur with age or the effect of illness and treatment that may interfere with sexual activity by altering the routine or interfering with physical performance may be needed. Counseling may also be needed for the older person to adapt to natural physiological changes and image-altering surgical procedures. Assessment of any medical conditions or medications that are associated with poor sexual health and functioning, screening for HIV-AIDS and other sexually transmitted disease, and education about safe sexual practices is also important.

Discussion of sexuality and sexuality problems may be uncomfortable for both nurse and elder. Nonetheless, learning the significance that sexual function has for the elder and the perception of sexual function the elder has, without bringing the nurse's own biases into the interaction, is important. Lindau et al (2007) noted that older people were very willing to discuss their intimate lives with the researchers and often more likely to refuse questions about income than about sex.

The PLISSIT model (Annon, 1976) (www.hartfordign. org) is a helpful guide for discussion of sexuality (Box 23-15 and a Nursing Standard of Practice Protocol: Sexuality in Older Adults [Arena and Wallace, 2008] is available at www.consultgerim.org/).

Youngkin (2004) provides suggestions for use of the PLISSIT model with older people:

▶ **Permission**: Obtain permission from the client to initiate sexual discussion (Wallace, 2003b). Allow the person to discuss concerns related to sexual issues, and gather information about what might have changed in the person's life to affect

sexual needs and response. Questions such as "What concerns or questions do you have about fulfilling your sexual needs?" (Wallace, 2003b) or "In this era of HIV and other sexually transmitted infections, I ask all my patients about sexual practices and concerns. Are there any questions I can answer for you?" (Nusbaum et al, 2005).

▶ **Limited Information**: Limit the information provided to that needed for sexual function (Wallace, 2003b). Offer teaching about the normal age-associated changes that affect sexual performance or how illness may affect sexuality. Encourage the person to learn more about the concern from books and other sources.

▶ **Specific Suggestions**: Offer suggestions for dealing with problems such as lubricants for atrophic vaginitis; use of condoms to prevent sexually transmitted infections; proper use of ED medications; how to communicate sexual and other needs; ways to increase comfort with coitus or ways to be intimate without coital relations.

▶ **Intensive Therapy**: Refer as appropriate for complex problems that call for specialist intervention.

Interventions

Interventions will vary depending on the needs identified from the assessment data. A variety of suggested interventions for maintaining sexual function for older people with chronic conditions was presented in Table 23-1, and ED was discussed with available options of treatment. Perhaps one of the most important interventions is education regarding normal changes of aging related to sexual function and the dimensions of sexuality that provide pleasure. Following a comprehensive assessment, interventions may center on the following categories: (1) education regarding age-associated change in sexual function; (2) compensating for normal aging changes; (3) effective management of acute and chronic illness affecting sexual function; (4) removal of barriers associated with difficulty in fulfilling sexual needs; and (5) special interventions to promote sexual health in cognitively impaired older adults (Arena and Wallace, 2008).

Although older people do seek counseling on sexuality and sexual concerns, we do not always hear them, and many of us are not well enough prepared to help them. Successful and continuing sexual activity is but one sign of healthy aging. Some nurses have extensive education in sexuality and can provide intensive therapy

Box 23-15	PLISSIT Model

P	Permission from the client to initiate sexual discussion
LI	Providing the Limited Information needed to function sexually
SS	Giving Specific Suggestions for the individual to proceed with sexual relations
IT	Providing Intensive Therapy surrounding the issues of sexuality for the clients (may mean referral to specialist)

Compiled from Annon J: The PLISSIT model: a proposed conceptual theme for behavioral treatment of sexual problems, *J Sex Educ Ther* 2(2):1-15, 1976; Wallace M: Best practices in nursing care to older adults: sexuality, *Dermatol Nurs* 15(6):570-571, 2003; Youngkin E: The myths and truths of mature intimacy: mature guidance for nurse practitioners, *Adv Nurse Pract* 12(9):45-48, 2004.

for people with sexual problems. Although the nurse in the acute or long-term care facility may not be well prepared to engage in sex therapy, being knowledgeable about sexual changes that occur in aging or with illness, providing information about sexual issues in anticipation of questions or in response to questions asked, treating expressions of sexuality as normal, and referring individuals with complex problems to specialists are important nursing responses. Elders whose sexuality needs are fulfilled will consider their sexual life with satisfaction. This attitude will be apparent through verbal and nonverbal expression, the individual's self-image, and involvement and concern about others.

KEY CONCEPTS

▶ Elders and their family members carry a long history. Current family dynamics must be understood within the context of family history.
▶ Sibling relationships may increase in importance during old age as individuals cope with various losses.
▶ Grandparenting is a significant role among elders. In an increasing number of families, grandparents are the primary providers for young children and function as parents.
▶ Caregiving of impaired elders is one of the major social issues of our times. Most spouses will spend some time caring for one another, and most adult children will spend some time caring for aged parents. Many of the children travel long distances to provide care.
▶ Sexuality is love, sharing, trust, and warmth, as well as physical acts. Sexuality provides an individual with self-identity and affirmation of life.
▶ Sexuality continues in late life, though adaptations are needed for the age-related changes and the effects of chronic illness.
▶ Further research is needed to promote knowledge and understanding of the sexual health of older adults with alternative lifestyles, such as gay men, lesbians, and bisexual and transgender individuals.
▶ AIDS awareness and the practice of safe sex among older adults is still lacking. Older adults and health professionals may not consider older adults at risk for AIDS even though the incidence of AIDS in the older population is rapidly increasing.
▶ The major role of the nurse in older adult sexuality in the community or long-term care setting is education and counseling about sexual function, adaptations for age-related changes and chronic conditions, and the maintenance of sexuality for the older adult who desires this.

ACTIVITIES AND DISCUSSION QUESTIONS

1. Discuss your position in the family and how that has affected your relationship with siblings and parents.
2. What do you suppose your role will be when your parent or parents need help?
3. Write a brief essay discussing the ways in which your grandparents have affected your life.
4. What would you find most difficult in regard to assisting your older parent?
5. With a classmate, role play how you would conduct a review of systems in the area of sexual health with an older adult. What would be the most important factors to consider when providing education about sexuality and sexual health?
6. What resources are available for older LGBT individuals in your community?

RESOURCES

Sexuality
Organizations

National Council on Aging: Love and life: a healthy approach to sex for older adults (brochures, training materials, video)
www.ncoa.org

Family and Transitions
Organizations

National Center on Grandparents Raising Grandchildren
http://chhs.gsu.edu/nationalcenter/

U.S. Department of Health and Human Services (USDHHS) Administration on Aging
National family caregiver support program
www.aoa.gov

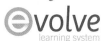

For additional resources, please visit evolve.elsevier.com/Ebersole/gerontological.

REFERENCES

Agronin M: Sexuality and aging: an introduction, *CNS Long-Term Care,* Summer:12-13, 2004.
AIDS Action: *Older Americans and HIV,* 2001. Available at www.aidsaction.org/. Accessed 11/8/08.
American Association of Retired Persons (AARP) Public Policy Institute: *Lean on me: support and minority outreach for grandparents raising grandchildren,* Washington, DC, 2003, The Association. Available at www.aarp.org. Accessed 7/8/08.

American Association of Retired Persons (AARP) Public Policy Institute: *Intergenerational relationships: grandparents raising grandchildren*, Washington, DC, 2005, The Association. Available at www.aarp.org. Accessed 7/8/08.

American Association of Retired Persons (AARP) Public Policy Institute: *Who's caring for the caregivers?* Washington, DC, 2006, The Association. www.aarp.org/research/press-center/presscurrentnews/caring_for_caregivers.html. Accessed 8/13/06.

Angel J, Jimenez M, Angel R: The economic consequences of widowhood for older minority women, *Gerontologist* 47(2):224-234, 2007.

Annon J: The PLISSIT model: a proposed conceptual scheme for behavioral treatment of sexual problems, *J Sex Educ Ther* 2(2):1-15, 1976.

Ansberry C: Parents devoted to a disabled child confront old age, *Wall Street Journal Online,* January 7, 2004. Available at www.onlinewsj.com. Accessed 1/20/09.

Archbold PG, Stewart BJ, Greenlick MR, Harvath TA: Mutuality and preparedness as predictors of caregiver role strain, *Res Nurs Health* 13(6):375-384, 1990.

Archbold PG, Stewart BJ, Greenlick MR. Harvath TA: Clinical assessment of mutuality and preparedness in family caregivers to frail older people. In Funk SG, Tornquist EM, Champagne MT, Capp LA, editors: *Key aspects of elder care: managing falls, incontinence, and cognitive impairment*, New York, 1992, Springer.

Arena J, Wallace M: Issues regarding sexuality. In Capezuti E, Swicker D, Mezey M et al, editors: *Evidence-based geriatric nursing protocols for best practice*, New York, 2008, Springer.

Bauer M, McAuliffe L, Nay R: Sexuality, health care and the older person: an overview of the literature, *Int J Older People Nurs* 2(1):63-68, 2007.

Bedford VH, Avioli PS: Variations in sibling intimacy in old age, *Generations* 25(2):34, 2001.

Blando J: Twice hidden: older gay and lesbian couples, friends and intimacy, *Generations* 25(2):87-89, 2001.

Blieszner R, DeVries B: Perspectives on intimacy, *Generations* 25(2):7-8, 2001.

Brotman S, Ryan B, Cormier R: The health and social service needs of gay and lesbian elders and their families in Canada, *Gerontologist* 43(2):172-202, 2003.

Brown-Standridge MD, Floyd CW: Healing bittersweet legacies: revisiting contextual family therapy for grandparents raising grandchildren in crisis, *J Marital Fam Ther* 26(2):185-197, 2000.

Butler R, Lewis M: *The new love and sex after 60,* New York, 2002, Ballantine Books.

Butler FR, Zakari N: Grandparents parenting grandchildren: assessing health status, *J Gerontol Nurs* 31(3):43-54, 2005.

Cahill S, South K: Policy issues affecting lesbian, gay, bisexual, and transgender people in retirement, *Generations* 26(11):49, 2002.

Chan CG, Elder GH: Matrilinear advantage in grandchild-grandparent relations, *Gerontologist* 40(2):189, 2000.

Chappell N, Reid R: Burden and well-being among caregivers: examining the distinction, *Gerontologist* 42(6):772-780, 2002.

Claes JA, Moore W: Issues confronting lesbian and gay elders: the challenge for health and human services providers, *J Health Hum Serv Adm* 23(2):181-202, 2000.

Comfort A: Sexuality in old age, *J Am Geriatr Soc* 22(10):440-442, 1974.

Curry L, Walker C, Hogstel MO: Educational needs of employed family caregivers of older adults: evaluation of a workplace project, *Geriatr Nurs* 27(3):166-173, 2006.

Davidhizar R, Bechtel GA, Woodring BC: The changing role of grandparenthood, *J Gerontol Nurs* 25(1):24-29, 2000.

DeLamater JD, Sill M: Sexual desire in later life, *J Sex Res* 42(2):138-149, 2005.

Delaney S, Delaney E: *Having our say: the Delaney sisters' first 100 years*, New York, 1993, Kodansha International.

Dennis H: The current state of retirement planning, *Generations* 13(2):38, 2002.

DeVries B: Grief: intimacy's reflection, *Generations* 25(2):75-79, 2001.

DeVries B: Home at the end of the rainbow, *Generations* 29(4):64-68, 2005-2006.

Ekerdt D, Dennis H: Introduction to retirement: new chapters in American life, *Generations* 26(11):entire issue, 2002.

Family Caregiver Alliance: *Caregiver assessment: principles, guidelines and strategies for change,* Report from a National Consensus Development Conference (vol 1), San Francisco, 2006, The Alliance.

Fingerman KL: A distant closeness: intimacy between parents and their children in later life, *Generations* 25(2):26, 2001a.

Fingerman KL: *Aging mothers and their adult daughters: a study in mixed emotions*, New York, 2001b, Springer.

Goodroad BK: HIV and AIDS in people older than 50, *J Gerontol Nurs* 29(4):18, 2003.

Gordon M, Sokolowski M: Sexuality in long-term care: ethics and action, *Ann Long-Term Care* 12(9):45-48, 2004.

Grinstead L, Leder S, Jensen S, Bond L: Review of research on the health of caregiving grandparents, *J Adv Nurs* 44(3):318-326, 2003.

Gwyther L, Willer L: Ask the expert: how do we assess and determine the mental capacity of our patients with Alzheimer's disease and dementia for consent to conjugal visits with their spouse? *Ann Long-Term Care* 12(4):27-28, 2004.

Hooyman N, Kiyak HA: *Social gerontology: a multidisciplinary perspective*, ed 8, Boston, 2008, Pearson.

Houde SC: Men providing care to older adults in the home, *J Gerontol Nurs* 27(8):13, 2001.

Hunt C: Concepts in caregiver research, *J Nurs Scholarsh* 35(1):27-32, 2003.

Jett KF: Making the connection: seeking and receiving help by elderly African Americans, *J Qualitative Health Res* 12(3):373-387, 2002.

Jones T, Nystrom M: Looking back … looking forward: addressing the lives of lesbians 55 and older, *J Women Aging* 14(3/4):59-76, 2002.

Kaiser F: Sexual function and the older woman, *Clinics in Geriatric Medicine* 19(3):463-472, 2000.

Kingson ER, Calhoun G, Morse M, Brown M: Options to liberalize Social Security disabled widows(er)s benefits, *J Aging Soc Pol* 19(1):39-60, 2007.

Lindemann E: Symptomatology and management of acute grief, *Am J Psychiatry* 101(2):141-148, 1944.

Lindau ST, Schumm LP, Laumann EO et al: A study of sexuality and health among older adults in the United States, *N Engl J Med* 357(8):762-744, 2007.

Low L, Lui M, Lee D, Thompson DR: Promoting awareness of sexuality of older people in residential care, *Elec J Hum Sex* 8(Aug 24): 2005. Available at www.ejhs.org/volume8/sexuality_of_older_people.htm. Accessed 11/7/08.

Lund DA, Hill RD, Caserta MS, Wright SD: Video respite: an innovative resource for family, professional caregivers, and persons with dementia, *Gerontologist* 35(5):683-687, 1995.

Lund M: Caregiver, take care, *Geriatr Nurs* 26(3):152-153, 2005.

Mayer M, Stief C, Truss M et al: Phosphodiesterase inhibitors in female sexual dysfunction, *World J Urol* 23(6):393-397, 2005.

Meiner S, Lueckenotte A: *Gerontological nursing*, St Louis, 2006, Mosby.

Messinger-Rapport B, Sandhu SK, Hujer ME: Sex and sexuality: is it over after 60? *Clin Geriatr* 11(10):45-53, 2003.

Mittleman MS: Family caregiving for people with Alzheimer's disease: results of the NYU spouse caregiver intervention study, *Generations* 26(1):104, 2002.

National Alliance for Caregiving (NAC) and AARP: *Caregiving in the U.S.*, 2004. Available at www.caregiving.org. Accessed 11/7/08.

Navaie-Waliser M, Feldman P, Gould D et al: When the caregiver needs care: the plight of vulnerable caregivers, *Am J Public Health* 92(3):409, 2002.

Nay R: Sexuality and the aged women in nursing homes, *Geriatr Nurs* 13(6):312, 1992.

Piercy KW: We couldn't do without them: the value of close relationships between older adults and their nonfamily caregivers, *Generations* 25(2):41-47, 2001.

Pinquart M, Sorensen S: Ethnic differences in stressors, resources, and psychological outcomes of family caregiving: a meta-analysis, *Gerontologist* 45(1):90-106, 2005.

Price C, Joo E: Exploring the relationship between marital status and women's retirement satisfaction, *Int J Aging Hum Dev* 61(1):37-55, 2005.

Ramsey J: Spiritual intimacy in later life: implications for clinical practice, *Generations* 25(2):59-63, 2001.

Robinson B: Validation of a caregiver strain index, *J Gerontol* 38(3):344, 1983.

Rushton P: Widower responses to the death of a wife: the impact of family members, *Topics Adv Pract Nurse eJournal* 7(2), 2007. Available at www.medscape.com/viewarticle/560196_print. Accessed 7/14/08.

Schulz R, Beach SR: Caregiving as a risk factor for mortality: the Caregiver Health Effects Study, *JAMA* 282(23):2215-2219, 1999.

Schumacher K, Beck C, Marren J et al: Family caregivers: caring for older adults, working with their families, *Am J Nurs* 106(8):40-49, 2006.

Sebern M: Shared care, elder and family member skills used to manage burden, *J Adv Nurs* 52(2):170-179, 2005.

Shagrin S: Retirement saving and financial planning: different from a decade ago, *Generations* 26(2):40-44, 2002.

Stanford P, Usita P: Retirement: who is at risk? *Generations* 26(11):45-48, 2002.

Steinke E: Intimacy needs and chronic illness, *J Gerontol Nurs* 31(5):40-50, 2005.

Tabloski P: *Gerontological nursing*, Boston, 2006, Pearson Prentice Hall.

Tafford A: *The bonus decades*, New York, 2002, Basic Books.

Touhy T, Brown C, Strews W: Expressions of caring as lived by nursing home staff, families and residents, *Int J Human Caring* 9(3):31-37, 2005.

Troll L: When the world narrows: intimacy with the dead? *Generations* 25(2):55-58, 2001.

Uphold CR, Maruenda J, Yarandi HN, Sleasman JW: HIV and older adults, *J Gerontol Nurs* 30(7):16-24, 2004.

U.S. Administration on Aging: *A statistical profile of older Americans aged 65 and over*, 2008. Available at www.aoa.gov. Accessed 11/11/08.

U.S. Divorce Statistics: *DivorceMagazine.com,* December 2002. Available at www.divorcemag.com/statistics/statsUS.shtml. Accessed 1/20/09.

U.S. Department of Health and Human Services: *Healthy People 2010. understanding and improving health*, Washington, DC, 2001, Author.

Wallace M: Sexuality and aging in long-term care, *Ann Long-Term Care* 11(2):53-59, 2003a. Available at www.annalsoflongtermcare.com/article/315. Accessed 8/8/06.

Wallace M: Best practices in nursing care to older adults: sexuality, *Dermatol Nurs* 15(6):570-571, 2003b.

Ward R, Vass A, Aggarwal N: A kiss is still a kiss? The construction of sexuality in dementia care, *Dementia* 4(1):49-72, 2005.

Wojciechowski C: Issues in caring for older lesbians, *J Gerontol Nurs* 24(7):28-33, 1998.

World Health Organization: *Sexual health: A new focus for WHO*, 2004, Progress in Reproductive Health Research. Available at www.who.int/en/. Accessed 7/18/08.

Youngkin E: The myths and truths of mature intimacy, *Adv Nurse Prac* 12(9):45-48, 2004.

Zarit SH: Assessment of family caregivers: a research perspective. In Family Caregiver Alliance: *Caregiver assessment: voices and views from the field,* Report from a National Consensus Development Conference (vol II), San Francisco, 2006, The Alliance.

Zeiss A, Kasl-Godley J: Sexuality in older adults' relationships, *Generations* 25(2):18-25, 2001.

Mental Health and Wellness in Late Life

24

GLOSSARY

Dysthymia At least 2 years of depressed mood for more days than not, accompanied by additional depressive symptoms, but symptoms do not meet the criteria for a major depressive episode.

Hallucination A false sensory perception in the absence of a real stimulus (e.g., hearing voices that no one else can hear).

Idiosyncratic A peculiarity of constitution or temperament: an individualizing characteristic or quality; individual hypersensitivity (as to a drug or food)

Illusion Misinterpretation of a real experience (e.g., thinking a curled rope is a snake).

THE LIVED EXPERIENCE

An elderly man wrote his philosophy succinctly:

"I have no ideas about what would constitute happiness for anyone else, considering the differences in taste and preferences, and no spate of ideas about improving the lot of the aged. But I am sure that among other things, a calm acceptance of the facts of life is a great help. I consider serenity and peace of mind two of the greatest gifts I have, although I cannot tell you where they come from or how to get them."

From Burnside IM: Listen to the aged, Am J Nurs 75(10):1800-1803, 1975.

Mental health is not different in late life, but the level of challenge may be greater. Developmental transitions, life events, physical illness, cognitive impairment, and situations calling for psychic energy may interfere with mental health in older adults. These factors, though not unique to older adults, often influence adaptation. However, anyone who has survived 80 or so years has been exposed to many stressors and crises and has developed tremendous resistance. Most older people face life's challenges with equanimity, good humor, and courage. It is our task to discover the strengths and adaptive mechanisms that will assist them to cope with the challenges.

What it means to be mentally healthy is subject to many interpretations and familial and cultural influences. Mental health, as with physical health, can be thought of as being on a fluctuating continuum from wellness to illness. Mental health in late life is difficult to define because a lifetime of living results in many variations of personality, coping, and life patterns. One can say what 5-year-olds or 15-year-olds in general are like, but the same is not true for older people. Each individual becomes, the older he or she gets, more uniquely himself or herself. Well-being in late life can be predicted by cognitive and affective functioning earlier in life. Thus, it is very important to know the older person's past patterns and life history (see Chapter 3).

Qualls (2002) offered the following comprehensive definition of mental health in aging: A mentally healthy person is "one who accepts the aging self as an active being, engaging available strengths to compensate for weaknesses in order to create personal meaning, maintain maximum autonomy by mastering the environment, and sustain positive relationships with others" (p. 12).

Erikson et al (1986) proposed that autonomy, intimacy, integrity, and generativity were all aspects of mentally healthy adult adaptation (see Chapter 7). Using Maslow's (1970) hierarchial need model (see Chapter 1), the higher one rises in terms of needs met, the more likely one is to be emotionally healthy (self-actualization). Older adults with physical and cognitive illnesses causing functional impairments may have difficulty meeting basic-level needs. This may affect their ability to move up the hierarchy toward finding meaning and fulfillment in life. It is important for nurses caring for older adults to create relationships and environments that not only meet basic needs, but also contribute to health, happiness, and meaning throughout life, even at the end of life.

Healthy People 2010 (U.S. Department of Health and Human Service [USDHHS], 2000) has set goals and objectives for mental health and substance abuse. Box 24-1 presents some of these objectives as they relate to adults.

The focus of this chapter is on the differing presentation of mental health problems that may occur in older adults and appropriate assessment and treatment interventions. Readers should refer to a comprehensive psychiatric-mental health text for more in-depth discussion of mental health disorders. A discussion of cognitive impairment and the behavioral symptoms that may accompany this disorder is found in Chapter 21.

MENTAL HEALTH AND WELLNESS IN LATE LIFE

Stress and Stressors

To understand mental health and mental health disorders in aging, it is important to be aware of stressors and their effect on the functioning of older people. The experience of stress is an internal state accompanying

---

Box 24-1	*Healthy People 2010:* **Mental Health and Substance Abuse Goals and Objectives**

- Increase the proportion of adults with recognized depression who receive treatments.
- Reduce deaths and injury caused by alcohol- or drug-related motor vehicle crashes.
- Reduce number of cirrhosis deaths.
- Reduce alcohol-related hospital emergency department visits.
- Reduce intentional injuries resulting from alcohol-related violence.
- Reduce the proportion of adults using any illicit drug during the past 30 days.
- Reduce the proportion of adults who engaged in binge drinking of alcohol beverages during the past month.
- Reduce average annual alcohol consumption.
- Reduce the treatment gap for alcohol problems.
- Increase the number of people referred for follow-up care for alcohol problems.

From U.S. Department of Health and Human Services: *Healthy People 2010, ed 2,* Washington, DC: 2000, U.S. Government Printing Office.

threats to self. Healthy stress levels motivate one to-wards growth, whereas stress overload diminishes one's ability to cope effectively. As a person ages, many situations and conditions occur that may create disruptions in daily life and drain one's inner resources or create the need for new and unfamiliar coping strategies. The narrowing range of biopsychosocial homeostatic resilience and changing environmental needs as one ages may produce a stress overload. Some stressors that may be experienced by older people are listed in Box 24-2.

Older people often experience multiple, simultaneous stressors. Some older people are in a chronic state of grief because new losses occur before prior ones are fully resolved; stress then becomes a constant state of being (see Chapter 25). Stress tolerance is variable and based on current and ongoing stressors as well as coping ability. For example, if an elder has lost a significant person in the previous year, the grief may be manageable. If he or she has lost a significant person and developed painful, chronic health problems, the consequences may be quite different and can cause stress overload.

In the older adult, stress may appear as a cognitive impairment or behavior change that will be alleviated as the stress is reduced to the parameters of the individual's adaptability. Older people may also be reluctant to seek help because of pride of independence, stoic acceptance of difficulty, unawareness of resources, and fear of being "put away."

Assessment of mental health in older people is often complex and calls for an understanding of past and present history, the person's coping abilities, and the effect of life events. Most importantly, it calls for a nurse who believes that wellness is possible in old age and implements interventions to promote the highest quality of life, no matter the circumstances.

Mental Health Care

Nearly 20% of people older than 55 years experience mental health disorders that are not part of normal aging, and these figures are expected to rise significantly in the next 25 years with the aging of the population. The figures may be even higher because mental health disorders are both underreported and not well researched. The most prevalent mental health problems in late life are anxiety, severe cognitive impairment, and mood disorders. Alcohol abuse and dependence is also a growing concern among older adults.

Stigma about having a mental health disorder ("being crazy"), particularly for older people, discourages many from seeking treatment. Estimates are that 63% of older adults with a mental health disorder do not receive the services they need, and only about 3% report seeing mental and behavioral health professionals for treatment (American Psychological Association, 2003). The rate of utilization of mental health services for elders, even when available, is less than that of any other age-group. Lack of knowledge on the part of health care professionals about mental health in late life presents another barrier to appropriate diagnosis and treatment.

In July 2008, the U.S. Senate passed a bill to phase out Medicare's discriminatory practice of imposing a 50% coinsurance requirement for outpatient mental health services instead of the 20% required for other medical services. The reduction of this coinsurance to 20% over a period of 6 years will bring payments for mental health care in line with those required for all

---

Box 24-2	Stressors in Late Life

- Incompetency proceedings
- Inheritance conflicts
- Abandonment: fear of dying alone and/or not being found and/or painful death
- Hospitalization
- Institutionalization
- Separation from personal physician
- Sensory changes (vision and hearing)
- Housing and home maintenance
- Lack of protection when frail and vulnerable
- Limited mobility and lack of transportation
- Unnamed concerns about the future
- Functional impairment, inability to be independent in activities of daily living (ADLs)
- Fear of dementia
- Social losses, loss of driver's license
- Acute and chronic pain
- Medications
- Abuse and neglect
- Loss of pet
- Rent increases or increases in other living expenses
- Caregiving of a partner with dementia
- Illness
- Relocation
- Loss of children
- Loss of cohorts
- Loss of siblings
- Loss of friends
- Dispersal of significant belongings

other Medicare Part B services. The passage of this legislation will significantly improve the lives of older adults by providing them with improved access to mental health care (American Association for Geriatric Psychiatry, 2008).

Nursing homes and, increasingly, assisted living facilities (ALFs), although not licensed as psychiatric facilities, are providing the majority of care given to older adults with psychiatric conditions. Eighty-nine percent of older people with serious mental illness who are institutionalized reside in nursing homes (Madhusoodanan and Brenner, 2007).

An insufficient number of trained personnel affects the quality of mental health care in nursing homes and often causes great stress for staff. Some of the obstacles to mental health care in this setting include: (1) shortage of trained personnel; (2) limited availability and access for psychiatric services; (3) lack of staff training related to mental health and mental illness; and (4) inadequate Medicaid and Medicare reimbursement for mental health services. The implementation of the Minimum Data Set (MDS) (see Chapter 13) and the reduction of chemical and physical restraints have resulted in more resident-oriented care, but more attention must be paid to the mental health of older people in these settings.

Geropsychiatric nursing is a master's-level subspecialty within the adult-psychiatric mental health nursing field. Few educational programs focus on this specialty and, unfortunately, few professional curricula include adequate content on mental health and aging. The American Psychiatric Nurses Association (APNA) is the recipient of a geropsychiatric grant as part of the Nursing Competence in Aging Initiative (see Chapter 2) and is developing a web-based geropschiatric education program to assist better preparation in the field of geropsychiatric nursing (Mellilo et al, 2005).

Advanced practice nurses are lobbying for parity in reimbursement for providing mental health services and there are efforts underway to increase the Medicare coinsurance rate for mental health services for all providers. These efforts, as well as increased attention to preparation of mental health professionals, are important initiatives to improve mental health care delivery for the growing numbers of older adults.

Cultural and Ethnic Disparities

Lack of knowledge and awareness of cultural differences about the meaning of mental health, differences in the way concerns may become apparent, the lack of culturally competent mental health treatment, and limited research is this area must be addressed in light of the rapidly increasing numbers of culturally and ethnically diverse older adults. These populations have less access to mental health services and receive poorer quality mental health care. Some identified barriers to the use of services include a lack of bilingual staff and a lack of awareness of the existence of services.

It is important to include a cultural assessment and a discussion of what culturally and ethically diverse older adults believe about their mental health problems in all assessment situations. Culturally appropriate education about mental health concerns is also important. Research on all aspects of culture and mental health is critically needed. Chapter 4 discusses culture and aging in depth.

Anxiety Disorders

A general definition of anxiety is unpleasant and unwarranted feelings of apprehension, which may be accompanied by physical symptoms. Anxiety itself is a normal human reaction and part of a fear response; it is rational, within reason. Anxiety becomes problematic when it is prolonged, is exaggerated, and interferes with function.

Anxiety disorders are not considered part of the normal aging process, but the changes and challenges that older adults often face (e.g., chronic illness, cognitive impairment, emotional losses) may contribute to the development of anxiety symptoms and disorders. Many anxious older people have had anxiety disorders earlier in their lives, but late-onset anxiety is not a rare phenomenon (Wetherell et al, 2005).

Epidemiological studies indicate that anxiety disorders are common in older adults; however, relatively few patients are diagnosed with these disorders in clinical practice. The occurrence of anxiety meeting the criteria for a diagnosable disorder ranges from 3.5% to 10% of older people—a higher prevalence than late-life depression has. Anxiety symptoms that may not meet the *Diagnostic and Statistical Manual of Mental Disorders* (DSM-IV) (American Psychiatric Association [APA], 2000) criteria (subthreshold symptoms) are even more prevalent, with estimated rates from 15% to 20% in community samples, with even higher rates in medically ill populations (Ayers et al, 2006).

Anxiety symptoms and disorders are significant yet understudied conditions in older adults. Anxiety in older people is not often thought of as a serious problem, and there is little research or empirical data on anxiety in older people. Similar to other mental health problems, the diagnostic criteria and treatment methods for anxiety disorders are largely based on data from young and middle-aged adults and may not reflect the unique problems of older adults (Smith, 2005; Wetherell et al, 2005).

Older people are less likely to report psychiatric symptoms or acknowledge anxiety, and often attribute their symptoms to physical health problems. Separating a medical condition from the physical symptoms of an anxiety disorder may be difficult. The presence of cognitive impairment also makes diagnosis complicated. It is estimated that 40% to 80% of older people with Alzheimer's disease or related dementias experience anxiety-related symptoms that may be expressed with behavior, such as agitation, irritability, pacing, crying, and repetitive verbalizations (Smith, 2005) (see Chapter 21). Anxiety symptoms are frequently associated with depression, but anxiety disorders without comorbid depression are also common (Wetherell et al, 2005). Risk factors for anxiety disorders in older people include the following: female; urban living; history of worrying or rumination; poor physical health; low socioeconomic status; high-stress life events; and depression and alcoholism.

Older people frequently have coexistent medical conditions that mimic symptoms of generalized anxiety. Some of the medical disorders that cause anxiety responses include cardiac dysrhythmias, delirium, depression, dementia (probably the most common cause of anxiety), congestive heart failure, hyperthyroidism, hypoglycemia, postural hypotension, pulmonary edema, and pulmonary emboli. Many medications also cause anxiety reactions: anticholinergics, caffeine, digitalis, theophylline, antihypertensives (clonidine), beta blockers, beta-adrenergic stimulators (albuterol), corticosteroids, and over-the-counter (OTC) drugs such as appetite suppressants, nicotine, and cough and cold preparations containing ephedrine. Withdrawal from alcohol, sedatives, and hypnotics will cause also symptoms of anxiety.

Geriatric anxiety is associated with more visits to primary care providers and increased average length of visit. Anxiety symptoms and disorders are associated with many negative consequences including decreased physical activity and functional status, decreased life satisfaction, and increased mortality rates (Wetherell et al, 2005; Ayers et al, 2006). Unidentified or untreated anxiety disorders in older people adversely affect well-being and quality of life.

Generalized anxiety disorder (GAD) is the most common anxiety disorder in older people (APA, 2000). Most older people with GAD have a history from childhood or adolescence, but 30% to 40% report an onset later in life (Wetherell et al, 2005). Other anxiety disorders that occur in older people include phobic disorder, obsessive-compulsive disorder, panic disorder, and posttraumatic stress disorder (PTSD) (discussed later in this chapter). PTSD associated with trauma earlier in life and phobias, particularly agoraphobia, which may be associated with a specific event such as falling, are increasingly recognized as important conditions that may emerge for the first time in late life (Smith, 2005).

IMPLICATIONS FOR GERONTOLOGICAL NURSING AND HEALTHY AGING

Assessment

Mental health problems in older adults are frequently unrecognized and untreated. Accurate and appropriate assessment is critical. Chapter 13 discusses assessment tools for gerontological nursing, and more specific information on instruments appropriate for assessment of depression, suicide, and substance abuse are presented in this chapter.

General issues in the psychological and mental health assessment of older adults involve distinguishing among normal, idiosyncratic, and diverse characteristics of aging and pathological conditions. Baseline data are often lacking from an individual's earlier years. Using standardized tools and functional assessment is valuable, but the data will be meaningless if not placed in the context of the patient's early life and hopes and expectations for the future. Distinguishing normal from pathological aging in a particular individual depends on these factors. Although some age-appropriate assessment instruments are available, many of the available tools were developed for younger people. Further research is needed in developing appropriate tools, especially for culturally and ethnically diverse elders and those with dementia.

Assessment of mental health includes examination of cognitive function, functional abilities, and the specific conditions of anxiety and adjustment reactions, depression, substance abuse, and suicidal risk. Assessment of mental health must also focus on social intactness and affective responses appropriate to the situation. Obtaining assessment data from older people is best done during short sessions after some rapport has been established. Performing repeated assessments at various times of the day and in different situations will give a more complete psychological profile. It is important to be sensitive to a patient's anxiety, special needs, and disabilities and be vigilant in protecting privacy. The interview should be focused so that attention is given to strengths and skills, as well as deficiencies.

Data suggest that approximately 70% of all primary care visits are driven by psychological factors (e.g., panic, generalized anxiety, somatization) (American Psychological Association, 2003). This means that nurses often encounter anxious older people and can identify "anxiety-related symptoms and initiate assessments that will lead to appropriate treatment and management... Whether symptoms represent a diagnosable anxiety disorder is perhaps less important than the fact that the individual will suffer needlessly if assessment and treatment are not addressed" (Smith, 2005, p. 169).

Assessment of anxiety in older people focuses on physical, social, and environmental factors, as well as past life history and recent events. Older people more often report somatic complaints rather than cognitive symptoms such as excessive worrying. It is important to remember that expressed fears and worries may be realistic or unrealistic, so the nurse must investigate and obtain collateral information from family or caregivers. For example, fear of leaving the home may be related to frequent falling or crime in the neighborhood. Worries about financial stability may be related to the current economic situation or financial abuse by other people.

It is important to investigate other possible causes of anxiety, such as medical conditions and depression. Diagnostic and laboratory tests may be ordered as indicated to rule out medical problems. Cognitive assessment, brain imaging, and neuropsychological evaluation are included if cognitive impairment is suspected (see Chapter 21). When comorbid conditions are present, they must be treated. A review of medications, including OTC and herbal or home remedies, is essential, with elimination of those that cause anxiety.

Few assessment instruments are designed and evaluated for older adults and if such instruments used, they should be weighed carefully with other data—complaints, physical exam, history, and collateral interview data (Smith, 2005). Box 24-3 presents suggested questions to identify anxiety disorders in older people.

When assessing anxiety reactions, look for daily disturbances, such as with staff or caregiver changes, room changes, or events over which the individual feels a lack of control or influence. By themselves, these circumstances seldom provoke an anxiety reaction, but they may be "the straw that breaks the camel's back,"

Box 24-3   Suggested Questions to Identify Anxiety in Older People

1. Have you been concerned about or fretted over a number of things?
2. Is there anything going on in your life that is causing you concern?
3. Do you find that you have a hard time putting things out of your mind?

Other questions useful in identifying how and when physical symptoms began:

1. What were you doing when you noticed the chest pain?
2. What were you thinking about when you felt your heart start to race?
3. When you can't sleep, what is usually going through your head?

From: The Anxiety Disorder Association of America (www.adaa.org/GettingHelp/FocusOn/Elderly.asp; accessed 7/8/08).

---

particularly in frail elders. Anxiety embodies an overwhelming sense of being out of control of one's life and destiny. Restoring the individual's sense of control as quickly as possible is critical. Providing a structured environment may alleviate anxiety in older people experiencing dementia. Nurses must be alert to the signs of anxiety in frail older people or those with dementia, since they may be unable to tell us how they are feeling. Carefully observing behavior and searching for possible reasons for changes in behavior or patterns is important (see Chapter 21).

Interventions

Although further research is needed to provide evidence to guide treatment, existing studies suggest that anxiety disorders in older people can be treated effectively. Treatment choices depend on the symptoms, the specific anxiety diagnosis, comorbid medical conditions, and any current medication regimen. Nonpharmacological interventions are preferred and are often used in conjunction with medication (Smith, 2005).

Pharmacological

Research on the effectiveness of medication in treating anxiety in older people is limited. Age-related changes in pharmacodynamics and issues of polypharmacy (see

Chapter 14) make prescribing and monitoring in older people a complex undertaking. Antidepressants in the form of selective serotonin reuptake inhibitors (SSRIs) are usually the first-line treatment. Within this class of drugs, those with sedating rather than stimulating properties are preferred (e.g., citalopram, paroxetine, sertraline, venlafaxine).

Second-line treatment may include short-acting benzodiazepines (alprazolam, lorazepam) or mirtazapine. Treatment with benzodiazepines should be used for short-term therapy only (less than 6 months) and relief of immediate symptoms, but must be used carefully in older adults. Use of older drugs such as diazepam or chlordiazepoxide should be avoided because of their long-half lives and the increased risk of accumulation and toxicity in older people. All these medications can have problematic side effects, such as sedation, falls, cognitive impairment, and dependence (see Chapter 14). Nonbenzodiazepine anxiolytic agents (buspirone) may also be used. Buspirone has fewer side effects but requires a longer period of administration (up to 4 weeks) for effectiveness (Smith, 2005).

Nonpharmacological

Cognitive behavioral therapy (CBT), either in individual or group formats, is being used increasingly in treating anxiety in older adults. CBT is designed to modify thought patterns, improve skills, and alter the environmental states that contribute to anxiety. CBT may involve relaxation training and cognitive restructuring (replacing anxiety-producing thoughts with more realistic, less catastrophic ones), and education about signs and symptoms of anxiety (Anxiety Disorders Association of America, www.ada.org/GettingHelp/FocusOn/Elderly.asp).

Significant decreases in anxiety and depression over time have been reported when older women participated in a course using psychoeducation and skills training (Smith, 2005). Attention to the principles of geragogy and additional adaptations for older adults may be necessary depending on the unique characteristics of the group. These include increased structure during sessions, a slower rate of progression, use of memory aids and prompts, frequent reinforcement of learning, use of age-relevant coping statements, and attention to vision and hearing impairments (Smith, 2005) (see Chapter 7).

The therapeutic relationship between the patient and the health care provider is the foundation for any intervention. Family support, referral to community resources, support groups, and sources of educational materials are other important interventions.

Other Anxiety Disorders

Obsessive-Compulsive Disorder.

Obsessive-compulsive disorder (OCD) is characterized by recurrent and persistent thoughts, impulses, or images (obsessions) that are repetitive and purposeful, and intentional urges of ritualistic behaviors (compulsions) that improve comfort level but are recognized as excessive and unreasonable. OCD is an anxiety disorder that significantly impairs function and consumes more than 1 hour each day (APA, 2000). Among older adults, symptoms are often not sufficient to seriously disrupt function and thus may not be considered a true disorder but rather a coping strategy. If symptoms progress to a point at which they disrupt function, the elder will need clinical attention. Recommended treatments include exercise and CBT in combination with pharmacological treatment (SSRIs) if indicated.

Posttraumatic Stress Disorder (PTSD).

According to DSM-IV, PTSD was recognized over 20 years ago as a syndrome characterized by the development of symptoms after an extremely traumatic event that involves witnessing, or unexpectedly hearing about, an actual or threatened death or serious injury to oneself or another closely affiliated person. Individuals often reexperience the traumatic event in episodes of fear and experience symptoms such as helplessness, flashbacks, intrusive thoughts, memories, images, emotional numbing, loss of interest, avoidance of any place that reminds of the traumatic event, poor concentration, irritability, startle reactions, jumpiness, and hypervigilance.

Individuals with PTSD may have ongoing sleep problems, somatic disturbances, anxiety, depression, and restlessness. Over the long term, individuals with PTSD may be impaired in work, may have maladaptive lifestyles, and do not develop close relationships. Avoidance or numbing, dissociation, intrusive symptoms, and survivor guilt seem to occur less frequently in older people as symptoms of PTSD, whereas estrangement from others may occur more often. (Wetherell et al, 2005). An instrument to assess PTSD can be found at www.hartfordign.org.

PTSD is fairly common with a lifetime prevalence of 7% to 12% of adults. It occurs increasingly in women. Rape is the most likely specific trauma that will result in long-lived PTSD in women, followed by child abuse, being threatened with a weapon, being molested, being neglected as a child, and physical violence. For men, the greatest trauma is also rape, followed by abuse as a child, combat, and being molested.

PTSD has become a part of our national vocabulary and reminds us of the deep and lasting toll that war and natural disasters take. PTSD was first recognized as an outcome of overwhelmingly stressful experiences of individuals in the war in Vietnam and is now a growing concern among Gulf War and Iraq War veterans. Only recently realized is the fact that many World War II veterans have lived most of their lives under the shadow of PTSD without its being recognized.

Seniors in our care now have also experienced the Great Depression, the Holocaust, racism, and the Korean conflict, events that also may precipitate PTSD. Although they may have managed to keep symptoms under control, a person who becomes cognitively impaired may no longer be able to control thoughts, flashbacks, or images. This can be the cause of great distress that may be exhibited by aggressive or hostile behavior.

Older individuals who are Holocaust survivors may experience PTSD symptoms when they are placed in group settings in institutions. Bludau (2002) described this as the concept of second institutionalization. Older women with a history of rape or abuse as a child may also experience symptoms of PTSD when institutionalized, particularly during the provision of intimate bodily care activities such as bathing. Box 24-4 provides some clinical examples of PTSD.

PTSD prevention and treatment are only now getting the research attention that other illnesses have received over the years. The care of the individual with PTSD involves awareness that certain events may trigger inappropriate reactions, and the pattern of these reactions should be identified when possible. Knowing the person's past history and life experiences is essential in understanding behavior and implementing appropriate interventions.

Effective coping with traumatic events seems to be associated with secure and supportive relationships; the ability to freely express or fully suppress the experience; favorable circumstances immediately following the trauma; productive and active lifestyles; strong faith, religion, and hope; a sense of humor; and biological integrity. CBT with pharmacological therapy will be useful for supporting the person with PTSD. Sertraline and paroxetine have U.S. Food and Drug Administration (FDA) approval to treat PTSD.

Psychosis and Psychiatric Symptoms in Late Life

Psychosis is characterized as a syndrome or constellation of psychiatric symptoms that occur in a number of physical and mental health disorders. Predominating

---

Box 24-4   Clinical Examples of PTSD in Older Adults

Ernie's Story
Ernie may have had PTSD, though it was only speculative after his suicide. On his eighteenth birthday, Ernie joined the U.S. Army Air Corps (precedent to our present U.S. Air Force) in 1941. He was quickly trained and sent to Burma, China, and India. During his 3-year stint, Ernie survived two airplane crashes, saw several of his companions mutilated in crashes, watched the torture of captured Japanese, and witnessed the capture of some of his friends. When Ernie returned to the United States, his hair had turned from deep auburn to pure white. He retired from the service after 20 years but was never really able to work after his retirement.

Ernie's life was filled with episodes of alcoholic binges, outbursts of anger, and episodes of abusing others, all seemingly quite out of his control. One friend remained from his service days and visited him periodically until his death in 1996. Other relationships seemed to have been superficial and to have had little meaning for Ernie. On his seventy-eighth birthday, which he spent alone, Ernie shot himself. One must wonder how many of the elderly veterans of World War II, the most highly suicidal group in the United States, are suffering from PTSD.

Jack's Story
An 80-year-old WWII veteran resident with dementia was admitted to a large Veterans Administration (VA) nursing home. He became very agitated and attempted to hit other residents around him when placed in the large day room. The staff recognized this as a PTSD reaction from his years as a prisoner of war. They always placed him in a smaller dayroom near the nursing station away from other residents, where he remained calm and pleasant. The aggression stopped without the need for medication.

PTSD, Posttraumatic stress disorder.

symptoms include hallucinations and delusions. Two types of psychosis occur in older adults:

- ▶ Chronic psychosis in people who have had life-long schizophrenia, major depression, or bipolar disorder with psychosis
- ▶ Older people who develop psychotic symptoms for the first time in late life (Mentes and Bail, 2005) (Box 24-5).

The onset of true psychotic disorders is low among older people, but psychotic manifestations may occur as a secondary syndrome in a variety of disorders, the most common being Alzheimer's disease and other dementias, as well as Parkinson's disease. Often, behaviors of persons with dementia such as wandering, disruptive vocalizations, hallucinations, illusions, and delusions are misidentified and treated as psychotic behavior. Antipsychotic medications may be given that do little to improve the behaviors and cause serious side effects. Psychotic symptoms in dementia necessitate different assessment and treatment than do long-standing psychotic disorders (see Chapter 21). Temporal lobe epilepsy, untreated endocrine disorders, and systemic lupus erythematosus also may have psychotic symptomatology (Mentes and Bail, 2005).

Paranoia

Paranoid behavior can be induced by medications, alcoholism, and hearing impairment. Fear and a lack of trust originating from a basis in reality may become magnified, especially when one is isolated from others and does not receive reality feedback. It is important to assess for causes of paranoid behavior, especially hearing impairment. Paranoia is an early symptom of Alzheimer's disease, appearing approximately 20 months before diagnosis.

In his description of a woman with a peculiar disease of the cerebral cortex, Dr. Alois Alzheimer described the first noticeable symptoms of the illness as suspiciousness of her husband and the belief that people were out to murder her. Memory loss and forgetfulness may result in the elder being convinced that items are being stolen or that medications are not the correct ones. The dynamics seem to be loss of control, inability to evaluate the social milieu appropriately, and the feeling of external forces controlling one's life, which in many instances may be true. It is sometimes difficult to determine the reality of an apparent paranoid or delusional reaction. Many cases have been encountered in which plots against an older person or beliefs of wrong-doing or threats were real.

Delusions

Delusions are beliefs that guide one's interpretation of events and help make sense out of disorder, even though they are inconsistent with reality. The delusions may be comforting or threatening, but they always form a structure for understanding situations that otherwise might seem unmanageable. A delusional disorder is one in which conceivable ideas, without foundation in fact, persist for more than 1 month.

Common delusions of older adults are of being poisoned, of children taking their assets, of being held prisoner, or of being deceived by a spouse or lover. In older adults, delusions often incorporate significant persons rather than the global grandiose or persecutory delusions of younger persons. Many delusions related to family members and their actions or intentions occur among institutionalized older people. Some may aid in coping, whereas others may be troubling to the person. One study found that 21% of 125 new nursing home residents had delusions (Grossberg, 2000) (Box 24-6).

Hallucinations

Hallucinations are best described as sensory perceptions of a nonexistent object and may be spurred by the internal stimulation of any of the five senses. Although not attributable to environmental stimuli, hallucinations may occur as a combined result of environmental factors. Hallucinations arising from psychotic disorders are less common among older adults, and those that are

---

Box 24-5	Possible Causes of Psychosis and/or Psychotic Symptoms in Older Adults

- Schizophrenia
- Delusional disorder
- Mood disorders with psychotic features (bipolar disorder, major depression)
- Delirium
- Psychotic symptoms associated with Alzheimer's disease, vascular dementia, Lewy body disease, frontal lobe dementias
- Parkinson's disease
- Substance abuse
- Polypharmacy; medication reactions and toxicity

Data from: Mentes J, Bail J: Psychosis in older adults. In Mellilo K, Houde S, editors: *Geropsychiatric and mental health nursing,* Sudbury, MA, 2005, Jones and Bartlett, pp. 174-175.

Box 24-6	Clinical Examples of Delusions in Older Adults

Maggie's Story

Maggie persistently held onto the delusion that her son was a very important attorney and was coming to force the administration to discharge her from the nursing home. Her son, a factory worker, had been dead for 10 years. The events of her day, her hopes, and her status were all organized around this belief. It is clear that without her delusion she would have felt forlorn, lost, and abandoned.

Herman's Story

Herman was an 88-year-old man in a nursing home who insisted that he must go and visit his mother. His thoughts seemed clear in other respects (often the case with people who are delusional), and one of the authors (P.E.) suspected that he had some unresolved conflicts about his dead mother or felt the need of comforting and caring. I did not argue with him about his dead mother, since arguing is never a useful approach to persons with delusions. Rather, I used the best techniques I could think of to assure him that I was interested in him as a person and recognized that he must feel very lonely sometimes. He continued to say that he must go and visit his mother. When I could delay his leaving no longer, I walked with him to the nurses' station and found that his 104-year-old mother did indeed live in another wing of the institution and that he visited her every day.

generated are thought to begin in situations in which one is feeling alone, abandoned, isolated, or alienated. To compensate for insecurity, a hallucinatory experience is stimulated, often an imaginary companion. Imagined companions may fill the immense void and provide some security, but they may also become accusing and disturbing.

The character and stages of hallucinatory experiences in late life have not been adequately defined. Many hallucinations are in response to physical disorders, such as dementia, Parkinson's disease, physiological and sensory disorders, and medications. Hallucinations of older adults most often seem mixed with disorientation, illusions, intense grief, and immersion in retrospection, the origins being difficult to separate. Older people with hearing and vision deficits may also hear voices or see people and objects that are not actually present (illusions). Some have explained this as the brain's attempt to create stimulation in the absence of adequate sensory input. If illusions or hallucinations are not disturbing to the person, they do not necessitate treatment.

One older woman in a nursing home who had Alzheimer's disease and was experiencing agnosia would look in the mirror and talk to "the nice lady I see in there." "Do you want to eat or go out for a walk with me?" she would ask. It was comforting to her, and therefore she did not need medication for her "hallucination," as some would have labeled her behavior. As is the case with many disease symptoms, frail elders do not typically manifest the cardinal signs we have been taught to associate with certain physical and mental

disorders. Diagnostic criteria, and often evidence-based practice guidelines, have been developed out of observation and research with younger people and may not always fit the older person. Until knowledge and research on the unique aspects of aging increase, nurses and other health care professionals are urged to individualize their assessment and treatment of older people using guidelines specific to older people.

The assessment dilemma is often one of determining if paranoia, delusions, and hallucinations are the result of medical illnesses, medications, dementia, psychoses, deprivation, or overload—because the treatment will vary accordingly. Treatment must be based on a comprehensive assessment and a determination of the nature of the psychotic behavior (primary or secondary psychosis) and the time of onset of first symptoms (early or late). Treating the underlying cause of a secondary psychosis caused by medical illnesses, dementia, substance abuse, or delirium, is a priority (Mentes and Bail, 2005). It is never safe to conclude that someone is delusional or paranoid or experiencing hallucinations unless you have thoroughly investigated his or her claims, evaluated physical and cognitive status, and assessed the environment for contributing factors to the behaviors.

Frightening hallucinations or delusions, such as feeling that one is being poisoned, usually arise in response to anxiety-provoking situations and are best managed by reducing situational stress, being available to the person, providing a safe, nonjudgmental environment, and attending to the fears more than the content of the delusion or hallucination. Direct confrontation is likely to increase anxiety and agitation and the sense of vulnerability; it also may disrupt the relationship. A more useful approach is to establish a trusting relationship that is nondemanding and not too intense.

It is important to identify the client's strengths and build on them. Demonstrating respect and a willingness to listen to complaints and fears is important. It is important that the nurse be trustworthy, give clear information, and present clear choices. Do not pretend to agree with paranoid beliefs or delusions, but rather ask what is troubling to the person and provide reassurance of safety. It is important to try to understand the person's level of distress as well as how he or she is experiencing what is troubling. Other suggestions are to avoid television, which can be confusing, especially if the person awakens and finds it on or has a hearing or vision impairment. In addition, reduce clutter in the person's room, eliminate large mirrors, and eliminate shadows that can appear threatening. Provide glasses and hearing aids to maximize sensory input and decrease misinterpretations.

If symptoms are interfering with function and interpersonal and environmental strategies are not effective, antipsychotic drugs may be used. The newer atypical antipsychotics (risperidone, olanzapine) are preferred but must be used judiciously, with careful attention to side effects and monitoring of response. None of the antipsychotic medications are approved for use in treatment of behavioral responses in dementia. The benefits are uncertain, and adverse effects offset any advantages (Schneider et al, 2006) (see Chapter 21).

Schizophrenia

Schizophrenia is a severe mental disorder characterized by two or more of the following symptoms: delusions, hallucinations, disorganized thinking, disorganized or catatonic behavior (called positive symptoms) and affective flattening, poverty of speech, or apathy (called negative symptoms) that cause significant social or occupational dysfunction, are not accompanied by prominent mood symptoms or substance abuse, or attributed to medical causes (APA, 2000; U.S. Department of Health and Human Services [USDHHS], 1999). The diagnostic criteria for schizophrenia are the same across the life span.

The onset of schizophrenia usually occurs between adolescence and the mid-thirties, but it can extend into and first appear in late life. Prevalence of schizophrenia in older people is estimated to be approximately 0.6%, about half of the prevalence in younger adults. Distinction

is made between early onset schizophrenia (EOS), occurring before the age of 40; midlife onset (MOS), between 40 and 60 years of age; and late onset (LOS), after 60 years of age. There is some suggestion that there may be neurobiologic differences between LOS and EOS, and further investigation is needed.

Patients with LOS are more likely to be women, with paranoia as a dominant feature of the illness; they tend to have a greater prevalence of visual hallucinations, less prevalence of a formal thought disorder, fewer negative symptoms, and less family history of schizophrenia. Women with LOS are also at greater risk for tardive dyskinesia; have less impairment in the areas of learning and abstraction; and require lower doses of neuroleptic medications for symptom management (USDHSS, 1999; Smith, 2005). Individuals with EOS who have grown older may experience fewer hallucinations, delusions, and bizarre behavior as well as inappropriate affect. Positive symptoms may wane whereas negative symptoms tend to persist into late life (Mentes and Bail, 2005).

Treatment for schizophrenia includes both medications and environmental interventions. Conventional neuroleptic medications (e.g., haloperidol) have been effective in managing the positive symptoms but are problematic in older people and carry a high risk of disabling and persistent side effects such as tardive dyskinesia (TD). The abnormal involuntary movement scale (AIMS) is useful for evaluating early symptoms of TD (see Chapter 14). The newer atypical antipsychotic medications (risperidone, olanzapine, quetiapine), given in low doses, are associated with a lower risk of extrapyramidal symptoms (EPS) and TD. Federal guidelines for the use of antipsychotic medications in nursing homes provide the indications for use of these medications in schizophrenia.

Other important interventions include a combination of support, education, physical activity, and CBT. Families of older people with schizophrenia experience the burden of caring for a family member with a chronic disability as well as dealing with their own personal aging. Community-based support services are needed that include assistance with housing, medical care, recreation services, and services that help the family plan for the future of their relative. There are relatively few services in the community for older persons with schizophrenia. The National Alliance for the Mentally Ill (NAMI) (www.nami.org) is an important resource for clients and their families (Mentes and Bail, 2005).

Individuals with severe persistent mental illnesses such as schizophrenia form a disenfranchised group whose access to medical care has been limited, leading to greater functional declines and mortality, as demonstrated by statistics that individuals with schizophrenia have a life expectancy 20% lower than the general population (Davis, 2004). An estimated 41% of older people with schizophrenia now reside in nursing homes. "Schizophrenia is one of the most expensive disorders across the adult life span and interventions to improve independent functioning irrespective of age and in conjunction with community services would decrease expenditure of institutionalization" (Madhusoodanan and Brenner, 2007, p. 30).

Bipolar Disorder

Bipolar disorder is not common in late life, but with the growing numbers of older people, more cases will be seen. Bipolar disorders, characterized by periods of mania and depression, often level out in late life, and individuals tend to have longer periods of depression. Mania is a more frequent cause of hospitalization than depression, but depression may account for more disability (Kennedy, 2008). Lithium, the most commonly used substance for individuals with bipolar disorders, has neurological effects that make it difficult for older people to tolerate; it also has a long half-life (more than 36 hours). Careful monitoring of blood levels and patient response is important. Recommended treatment consists of a combination of one or more mood stabilizers and aggressive psychosocial intervention. Antidepressants (SSRIs) may be used for individuals with little or no history of mania.

Patients and family education and support is essential, and the family must understand that the individual is not able to control mania and irritating behaviors because of a chemical imbalance in the brain. It is hoped that results of a large scale study of bipolar disorder (Systematic Treatment Enhancement Program for Bipolar Disorder-STEP BD) that included an older adult segment will provide additional evidence upon which to base treatment decisions (Kennedy, 2008). Other resources for bipolar disorder can be found at the end of the chapter and at evolve.elsevier.com/Ebersole/gerontological.

Depression

Depression is not a normal part of aging, and studies show that most older people are satisfied with their lives, despite physical problems (National Institute of Mental Health [NIMH], 2008). To understand depression, the nurse must understand the influence of late-life stressors and changes, culture, and the beliefs older people, society, and health professionals may have about depression and its treatment. The stigma associated with depression may be more prevalent in older people, and they may not acknowledge depressive symptoms or seek treatment. Many elders, particularly those who have survived the depression, world wars, the Holocaust, and other tragedies, may see depression as shameful, evidence of flawed character, self-centered, a spiritual weakness, and sin or retribution.

Health professionals often expect older people to be depressed and may not take appropriate action to assess for and treat depression. The differing presentation of depression in older people, as well as the increased prevalence of medical problems that may cause depressive symptoms, also contributes to inadequate recognition and treatment. Up to one in four primary care patients suffer from depression, but primary care physicians identify only one-third of these patients (Chizobam et al, 2008).

Ethnically and culturally diverse elders receive substantially less follow-up for mental health problems following hospitalization (Kurlowicz and Harvath, 2008a). Ethnicity and cultural background affect both recognition and treatment of depression in ways not yet completely understood. Depression may be seen as a sign of weakness or deficiency of character, and fear of being ostracized may make individuals less likely to seek help, particularly among South Asian and black Caribbean elders (Lawrence et al, 2006).

African American and black Caribbeans who experience a major depressive episode are more likely to be untreated, and they experience more disabling effects than non-Hispanic whites. The availability of culturally competent mental health services, mentioned earlier in the chapter, is a growing concern in light of the increasing numbers of ethnically and culturally diverse elders and evidence of disparities in health outcomes (Kurlowicz and Harvath, 2008a).

Prevalence and Consequences

Depression is the most common mental health problem of late life and remains underdiagnosed and undertreated. Major depressive disorder (MDD) is undiagnosed in approximately half of older persons with this disorder (Das et al, 2007). The prevalence of major depressive disorders in late life is estimated to be 1% to 5%; however, the prevalence of depression in general is much higher. Estimates of prevalence vary radically depending on the qualitative variables being considered and the definition being used. The prevalence of depressive symptoms in community-dwelling older adults is 3% to 26%, with homebound older adults having much higher rates of depressive symptoms (Box 24-7).

For elders in nursing homes, the prevalence of depressive symptoms may be as high as 54%, with even higher rates in older adults with Alzheimer's disease and other dementias (Kurlowicz and Harvath, 2008a). Nursing home residents who are female, black, or cognitively impaired are less likely to receive treatment for depression (Byrd, 2005). More than 15% of older adults with chronic physical conditions are

depressed, and depression has been called "the unwanted cotraveler" accompanying many medical illnesses (Byrd, 2005, p. 132). Many medications that older people may take also can also cause depression. The rate of depression is twice as high in older women than older men.

Depression and depressive symptomatology are associated with negative consequences such as increased disability, delayed recovery from illness and surgery, excess use of health services, cognitive impairment, malnutrition, decreased quality of life, and increased suicide and non–suicide-related death (Kurlowicz and Harvath, 2008b). Failure to treat depression increases

---

Box 24-7   Evidence-Based Practice: Depression and Social Support
Effective Treatment for Homebound Older Adults

Purpose
The purposes of this pilot study were to identify the prevalence of depression in homebound elderly adults receiving home care services and to examine the relationship between depression and social support systems.

Sample and Setting
A convenience sample was used of 25 older people (75-98 years of age) receiving home health services in the Chicago area. Of the participants, 80% were white and 20% were African American; 19 were female, and 6 were male.

Method
Participants were screened for depression using the long form of the GDS. Social support was defined as the quantity and quality of social interaction. Participants indicated the number of formal social support services they received and completed the short form of the social support questionnaire, which measures perceived social support. The reliability of both instruments has been demonstrated with older adult populations. Chi square was used to determine statistical associations between depression severity and perceived quality and quantity of social support using the SPSS program.

Results
In the study, 55% of the white and 40% of the African-American participants reported depressive symptoms, with more men than women reporting mild depression. Formal measures of social support and living alone were not found to be related to depression. Using Pearson's correlation, depression was positively associated with being a man, being unmarried, and needing formal social supports in the home.

Implications
The nonrandom sample and small sample size limit the interpretation and generalizability of the findings. The prevalence of depression found in this study is similar to other studies of homebound older adults and indicates a need to address depression in this population. Findings that functional decline contributed more to depression than lack of social support have also been reported in other studies in this population. Further research is needed to examine the relationship between social support and depression in older adults. Identifying and treating depression in homebound elders are important roles for home health nurses and nurse practitioners working in home settings. A team approach involving nurses, social workers, families, primary care providers, and the patient is recommended. Education in self-management skills to cope with chronic illness is suggested as an effective nursing intervention to prevent depression.

GDS, Geriatric depression scale; *SPSS,* Statistical Package for the Social Sciences.
Data from Loughlin A: Depression and social support: effective treatment for homebound older adults, *J Gerontol Nurs* 30(5):11-15, 2004.

morbidity and mortality. Depression is often reversible with prompt and appropriate treatment, and 60% to 80% of older people will improve with appropriate medication, psychotherapy and psychosocial interventions, or a combination (Kurlowicz and Harvath, 2008a). It is highly likely that nurses will encounter a large number of older people with depressive symptoms in all settings. Recognizing depression and enhancing access to appropriate mental health care are important nursing roles to improve outcomes for older people.

Etiology

The causes of depression in older adults are complex and must be examined in a biopsychosocial framework. Factors of health, gender, developmental needs, socioeconomics, environment, personality, losses, and functional decline are all significant to the development of depression in later life. Biologic causes such as neurotransmitter imbalances or dysregulation of endocrine function have also been proposed as factors influencing the development of depression in late life (Kurlowicz and Harvath, 2008a).

Some of the medical disorders that cause depression are cancers; cardiovascular disorders; endocrine disorders, such as thyroid problems; neurological disorders, such as Alzheimer's disease, stroke, and Parkinson's disease; metabolic and nutritional disorders, such as Vitamin B_{12} deficiency and malnutrition; viral infections such as herpes zoster and hepatitis; and advanced macular degeneration. Among patients who have suffered a cerebral vascular accident, the incidence of MDD is approximately 25%, with rates being close to 40% in patients with Parkinson's disease (Das et al, 2007). Vascular depression is a term being used to describe a late-life depression associated with vascular changes in the brain and characterized by executive dysfunction (Thakur and Blazer, 2008).

Medications may also result in depressive symptoms including hypertensives, angiotensin-converting enzyme (ACE) inhibitors, methyldopa, reserpine, guanethidine, antidysrhythmics, anticholesteremics, antibiotics, analgesics, corticosteroids, digoxin, and L-dopa (Kurlowicz and Harvath, 2008b).

Other important factors influencing the development of depression are alcohol abuse, loss of a spouse or partner, loss of social supports, lower income level, caregiving stress (particularly caring for a person with dementia), and gender. Some psychological traits such as neuroticism, pessimistic thinking, and those with less open attitudes to new experiences have been found to be associated with higher rates of depression and

suicide (Das et al, 2007). Some common risk factors for depression are presented in Box 24-8).

Differing Presentation of Depression in Elders

The DSM-IV (APA, 2000) provides criteria for the diagnosis of major depression, dysthymia, and minor (subsyndromal) depression. Depression can be considered a syndrome consisting of an array of affective, cognitive, and somatic or physiological symptoms. Depression may range in severity from mild symptoms to more severe forms, both of which can persist over long periods. Suicidal ideation and psychotic features (delusional thinking) accompany more severe depression (Kurlowicz and Harvath, 2008a).

The DSM-IV criteria "do not capture symptoms distinctive of geriatric depression" (Byrd, 2005, p. 136). The criteria stipulate that for a diagnosis of major depression, dysthymia, or minor depression, the symptoms must not be the result of a medical condition or a substance (medication, alcohol). Comorbid medical conditions are, however, the "hallmark of depression in older people and

---

Box 24-8   Common Risk Factors for Depression in Older Adults

- Chronic medical illnesses, disability, functional decline
- Alzheimer's disease and other dementias
- Bereavement
- Caregiving
- Female (2:1 risk)
- Lower SES
- Family history of depression
- Previous episode of depression
- Admission to long-term care or other change in environment
- Medications
- Alcohol or substance abuse
- Living alone
- Widowhood
- New stressful losses, including loss of autonomy; loss of privacy; loss of functional status; loss of independence; loss of body part; loss of family member, roommate, or pet

SES, Socioeconomic status.

Adapted from Tanner E: Recognizing late-life depression: why is this important for nurses in the home setting? *J Gerontol Nurs* 26(3):145-148, 2005.

a major difference from depression in younger people" (Kurlowicz and Harvath, 2008a, p. 63).

Symptoms of depression are different in older people. Older people who are depressed report more somatic complaints, such as physical symptoms, insomnia, loss of appetite and weight loss, memory problems, or chronic pain. They are less likely to have the feelings of guilt and worthlessness seen in younger depressed individuals. The somatic complaints "are often difficult to distinguish from the physical symptoms associated with chronic physical illness" (Kurlowicz and Harvath, 2008a, p. 59). Patients with late-life depression are also less likely to have a family history of depression than younger individuals (Das et al, 2007).

Hypochondriasis is also common, as are constant complaining and criticism, which may actually be expressions of depression. Decreased energy and motivation, lack of ability to experience pleasure, hopelessness, increased dependency, poor grooming and difficulty completing activities of daily living (ADLs), withdrawal from people or activities enjoyed in the past, decreased sexual interest, and a preoccupation with death or "giving up" are also signs of depression in older people (Meiner and Lueckenotte, 2005). Table 24-1 presents some symptoms of depression and related behavior in older adults.

Depression may be an early-presenting symptom of dementia, but it is unclear if it is a prodrome for the onset of dementia, a risk factor for dementia, or an independent event (Das et al, 2007). Results of a recent study suggest that a history of depression, particularly an early onset (before 60 years of age), but not presence of depressive symptoms, increases the risk for Alzheimer's (Geerlings et al, 2008). Symptoms such as agitated behavior and repetitive verbalizations in persons with dementia may be a symptom of depression. It is important that older people with memory impairment be evaluated for depression. (See Chapters 7 and 21).

Table 24-1 Symptoms of Depression and Related Behaviors in Older Adults	
SYMPTOMS OF DEPRESSION	BEHAVIOR
Decrease of energy, motivation, interest, social engagement	Decreased self-care ability: (1) refuses to do tasks requiring physical exertion; (2) asks staff to do total care when not medically indicated; (3) change in socialization patterns and attendance at activities
Frequent somatic complaints, worry	Frequently uses signal light; numerous physical complaints that do not resolve with usual nursing-measures
Decreased or increased appetite	Takes inadequate nutrition, refuses food and fluids, overeats
Perceived cognitive deficits	Complains of being forgetful; loses familiar objects but performs well on mental status examination; poor on concentration; gives "I don't know" answers
Critical and envious of others	Complains about poor care, criticizes family and staff; may tell you others are getting better treatment
Decreased concentration and indecisiveness	Cannot keep his or her mind on what you are saying, especially patient teaching; has difficulty with decisions (e.g., "When would you like your bath?"—"I don't know, I don't care, leave me alone.")
Loss of self-esteem, decreased sense of lifelong accomplishments	Ignores appearance; has no positive feelings about his or her life, hobbies, marriage, family, accomplishments; shares pessimism about future, little about self
Combative or resistive behavior	May strike out at staff or be verbally abusive when being cared for or may lash out verbally or physically at another patient. Aggressive and agitated behavior and repetitive vocalizations are frequently signs of depression in elders with cognitive impairment.
"Model patient" who never uses signal light	"Don't bother with me"; rarely complains or asks for anything, passive and apathetic

Adapted from Dreyfus JK: Depression assessment and intervention in medically frail elderly, *J Gerontol Nurs* 14(9):27-36, 1988; Tanner E: Recognizing late-life depression: why is this important for nurses in the home setting? *J Gerontol Nurs* 26(3):145-149, 2005.

Recognition and treatment of minor (subsyndromal) depression in older adults is emerging as a significant concern. Minor depression is 2 to 4 times as common as major depression in older adults. Minor depression is associated with clinically significant distress and impairment and imposes an increased risk of developing major depression. Twenty-five percent of persons with minor depression will go on to experience a major depressive episode (Byrd, 2005).

IMPLICATIONS FOR GERONTOLOGICAL NURSING AND HEALTHY AGING

Assessment

Both health care providers and patients have difficulty identifying signs of depression (NIMH, 2007). Assessment involves a systematic and thorough evaluation using a depression screening instrument, interview, history and physical, functional assessment, cognitive assessment, laboratory tests, medication review, determination of iatrogenic or medical causes, and family interview as indicated. Assessment for depressogenic medications and for related comorbid physical conditions that may contribute to or complicate treatment of depression must also be included. A comprehensive guide to assessment and treatment of depression in older adults, *Nursing Standard of Practice Protocol* (Kurlowicz and Horvath, 2008b) is available at www. consultgerirn.org.

Screening of all older adults for depression should be incorporated into routine health assessments across the continuum of care—in hospitals, primary care, long-term care, home care, and community-based settings (Kurlowicz and Harvath, 2008a). The Short Form of the Geriatric Depression Scale (GDS-SF) (see Appendix 24-A) has been validated and used extensively with older adults (Sheikh and Yesavage, 1986). It takes approximately 5 minutes to administer, and although it is not a substitute for individualized assessment, it is an effective screening tool for older adults, including those with mild to moderate cognitive impairment or those who are institutionalized (Kurlowicz and Harvath, 2008a). The GDS is also available in Spanish (Ortiz and Romero, 2008).

Byrd (2005) notes that one drawback of the GDS-SF is that it does not include a question on suicidal intent or thoughts. A GDS-SF score of 11 or greater is almost always indicative of depression, and a score of 6 to 9 indicates possible depression. An article on the use of the GDS-SF can be found at www.nursingcenter.com/ prodev/ce_article.asp?tid=743421, and a video illustrating its use can be found at www.nursingcenter.com/ prodev/ce_article.asp?tid=743421.

The Center for Epidemiological Studies Depression Scale (CES-D) (see Appendix 24-A) was developed for use in studies of depression in community samples and is frequently used in the research. The CES-D contains 20 items. Respondents are asked to report the amount of time they have experienced symptoms during the past week. Typically, a threshold of 17 and above is taken as indicating depression although a higher cutoff point (24 and above) has been suggested.

The Cornell Scale for Depression in Dementia (Alexopoulos et al, 1988), a caregiver report tool, is also used to screen for depression in elders with late-stage dementia. Compared to the GDS, it has better validity in patients with dementia, but it has not been specifically validated in patients with dementia in nursing homes (Thakur and Blazer, 2008). The Dementia Mood Picture Test (Tappen and Barry, 1995), a series of faces depicting moods, is another instrument being evaluated for assessment of depression in dementia. In most cases, older people with dementia should be assessed using the self-report instruments because many are able to provide accurate information (Pautex et al, 2007).

Interventions

If depression is diagnosed, treatment should begin as soon as possible, and appropriate follow-up should be provided. Depressed people are usually unable to follow through on their own and without appropriate treatment and monitoring may be candidates for deeper depression or suicide. For severe depression (GDS-SF score of 11 or above), five to nine depressive symptoms, and other positive responses on individualized assessment (suicidal thoughts, psychosis, substance abuse), the individual should be referred for psychiatric evaluation. For less severe depression (GDS-SF score of 6 or greater), fewer than five depressive symptoms and other positive responses on individualized assessment, refer to mental health services for psychotherapy or counseling, and evaluation of the need for medication (Kurlowicz and Harvath, 2008b).

The major treatments options for depression are pharmacotherapy, psychotherapy, psychosocial interventions, and electroconvulsive (ECT) therapy. ECT is being used more frequently for older people with psychotic depression or those who do not respond to antidepressant medications. People who received no treatment, treatment of short duration, or treatment with inadequate doses of medication may respond quite well to ECT. It is hypothesized that people who suffer depression for a long time may experience neuronal degeneration that impairs their ability to recover.

ECT is much improved, but older people will need a careful explanation of the treatment since they may have many misconceptions. The relapse rate using ECT with antidepressant medication therapy is 10% to 20%. ECT is contraindicated in patients with increased intracranial pressure, severe heart disease, recent myocardial infarction, and aortic aneurysm (Tabloski, 2006).

In one of the largest studies examining treatment preferences of older, depressed primary care patients, most of the participants desired active treatment, particularly counseling, although it was rarely available. The most effective treatment is a combination of pharmacological therapy and psychotherapy or counseling. Interventions are individualized and are based on history, severity of symptoms, concomitant illnesses, and level of disability. Family and social support, education, grief management, exercise, humor, spirituality, CBT, brief psychodynamic therapy, interpersonal therapy, reminiscence, life review therapy (see Chapter 3), and problem-solving therapy have all been noted to be helpful in depression. Box 24-9 presents suggestions for families and professionals caring for older adults with depression.

An interdisciplinary approach with team members prepared in geropsychiatry, collaborative models of care, and care management, often involving advanced practice nurses, has been successful in improving outcomes of depression as well as lowering costs of care (Unutzer et al, 2008). Chapter 15 discusses care models in more depth. Outcomes of treatment are as follows:

1. Patient safety will be maintained.
2. Patients with severe depression will be evaluated by psychiatric services.
3. Patients will report a reduction of symptoms that are indicative of depression. A reduction in the GDS score will be evident, and suicidal thoughts or psychosis will resolve.
4. The patient's daily functioning will improve (Kurlowicz and Harvath, 2008b).

Medications

Drug therapies are very effective in managing depression. The most commonly prescribed are the SSRIs, serotonin-norepinephrine reuptake inhibitors (SNRIs), and drugs related to the tricyclic antidepressants (TCAs). These agents work selectively on neurotrans-

| Box 24-9 | Interpersonal Support by Family and Professionals |

- Provide relief from discomfort of physical illness
- Enhance physical function (i.e., regular exercise and/or activity; physical, occupational, recreational therapies)
- Develop a daily activity schedule that includes pleasant activities
- Increase opportunities for socialization and enhance social support
- Provide opportunities for decisions and to exercise control
- Focus on spiritual renewal and rediscovery of meanings
- Reactivate latent interests, or develop new ones
- Validate depressed feelings as aiding recovery; do not try to bolster the person's mood or deny his or her despair
- Help the person become aware of the presence of depression, the nature of the symptoms, and the time limitation of depression
- Provide an accepting atmosphere and an empathic response
- Share yourself
- Demonstrate faith in the person's strengths
- Praise any and all efforts at recovery, no matter how small
- Assist in expressing and dealing with anger
- Do not stifle the grief process; grief cannot be hurried
- Create a hopeful environment where self-esteem is fostered and life is meaningful
- Assist in dealing with guilt, real or neurotic
- Foster development of connections with others

mitters in the brain to alleviate depression. The SSRIs are generally well tolerated in older people. Common side effects include nausea, vomiting, dizziness, drowsiness, and hyponatremia (see Chapter 14).

Medications must be closely monitored for side effects and therapeutic response. As with other medications for older people, doses should be lower at first and titrated as indicated while adequate treatment effect is ensured (Kurlowicz and Harvath, 2008b). Most medications take about 6 weeks to completely resolve symptoms, and inadequate dosing or duration of treatment is common. Current recommendation for people age 70 years and over is for long-term treatment (for at least 2 years) after the person is symptom-free to prevent future depressive episodes (Reynolds et al, 2006). More severe depression complicated by psychosis or suicidal intent may necessitate lifelong medication therapy.

Choice of medication depends on comorbidities, drug side effects, and the type of effect desired. People with agitated depression and sleep disturbances may benefit from medications with a more sedating effect, whereas those who are not eating may do better taking medications that have an appetite-stimulating effect. If depression is immobilizing, psychostimulants may be used.

SUICIDE

Elders comprise only 12% of the U.S. population but account for 16% of the suicide deaths. The rate of suicide among older adults is higher than that for any other age group—and the suicide rate for persons 85 years and older is the highest of all, twice the overall national rate (www.consultgerirn.org). Non-Hispanic white men with MDD are 5 times more likely to commit suicide than the general population (Das et al, 2007). Older African Americans have a much lower suicide rate; however, suicide rates of elderly black males is increasing, so attention must be paid to assessment in this group (Joe et al, 2006).

In most cases, depression and other mental health problems contribute significantly to suicide risk. Eighty percent of suicides are related to depression (Das et al, 2007). Suicide may have some familial tendencies, with estimates that a suicide of one parent in the family is associated with a sixfold increase of suicide in the children (Kennedy, 2008). One of the major differences in suicidal behavior in the old and the young is lethality of method. Of men older than 65, 8 of 10 suicides were with firearms. Older people rarely threaten to commit suicide; they just do it.

Up to 75% of older adults who die by suicide visited a physician within 1 month before death; 20% visited the physician on the day of the suicide; and 40% visited within 1 week of the suicide (National Institute of Mental Health, 2007). These statistics suggest that opportunities for assessment of suicidal risk are present but the need for intervention is not seen as urgent or not even recognized. Consequently, it is very important to implement depression screening for all older people, assess for suicidal thoughts and ideas based on depression assessment, and recognize warning signs and risk factors for suicide.

Common precipitants of suicide include physical or mental illness, death of a spouse or partner, substance abuse, and pathological relationships. Contrary to popular opinion, the majority of older people who committed suicide were not physically ill. Most of these individuals were depressed (65%) or had other mental health problems (Mitty and Flores, 2008). Other behavioral clues and risk and recovery factors are presented in Box 24-10.

IMPLICATIONS FOR GERONTOLOGICAL NURSING AND HEALTHY AGING

Assessment

Older people with suicidal intent are encountered in many settings. It is our professional obligation to prevent, whenever possible, an impulsive destruction of life that may be a response to a crisis or a disintegrative reaction. The lethality potential of an elder must always be assessed when elements of depression, disease, and spousal loss are evident. Any direct, indirect, or enigmatic references to the ending of life must be taken seriously and discussed with the elder.

The most important consideration for the nurse is to establish a trusting and respectful relationship with the person. Since many older people have grown up in an era when suicide bore stigma and even criminal implications, they may not discuss their feelings in this area. It is also important to remember that in older people, typical behavioral clues such as putting personal affairs in order, giving away possessions, and making wills and funeral plans are indications of maturity and good judgment in late life and cannot be construed as indicative of suicidal intent. Even statements such as "I won't be around long" or "I'm ready to die" may be only a realistic appraisal of the situation in old age.

If there is suspicion that the elder is suicidal, use direct and straightforward questions such as the following:
▶ Have you ever thought about killing yourself?
▶ How often have you had these thoughts?
▶ How would you kill yourself if you decided to do it?

The following must also be considered in assessing lethality potential:
▶ Internal resources (personality factors, coping strategies)
▶ External resources (money, family, friends, services)
▶ Communication skills (ability to ask for help and express feelings)

Interventions

It is important to have a suicide protocol in place that clearly defines how the nurse will intervene if a positive response is obtained from any of the questions (Byrd,

Box 24-10	Suicide Risk and Recovery Factors

Risk Factors and Warning Signs
Being male
Physical illness
Functional impairment
Depression
Alcohol and substance misuse and abuse
Major loss, such as the death of a spouse or partner
History of major losses
Recent suicide attempt
History of suicide attempts
Major crises or transitions such as retirement or relocation to an assisted living or nursing facility
Major crises in the lives of family members
Social isolation
Preoccupation with death
Poorly controlled pain
Expression of the belief that one is in the way, a burden
Giving away favorite possessions, money

Recovery Factors
A capacity for the following:
    Understanding
    Relating
    Benefiting from experience
    Benefiting from knowledge
    Accepting help
    Being loving
    Expressing wisdom
    Displaying a sense of humor
    Having a social interest
    Accepting a caring and available family
    Accepting a caring and available social network
    Accepting a caring, available, and knowledgeable professional and health network

2005). Patients at high risk should be hospitalized, especially if they have current psychological stressors and/or access to lethal means. Patients at moderate risk may be treated as outpatients provided they have adequate social support and no access to lethal means. Patients at low risk should have a full psychiatric evaluation and be followed up carefully (Das et al, 2007). Box 24-11 presents interventions if suicidal intent has been established.

Suicide is a taboo topic for most of us, and there is a lingering fear that the introduction of the topic will be suggestive to the patient and may incite suicidal action. Precisely the opposite is true. By introducing the topic, we demonstrate interest in the individual and open the door to honest human interaction and connection on the deep levels of psychological need. Superficial interest

and mechanical questioning will not, of course, be meaningful. It is the nature of our concern and our ability to connect with the alienation and desperation of the individual that will make a difference. Working with isolated, depressed, and suicidal elders challenges the depths of nurses' ingenuity, patience, and self-knowledge.

SUBSTANCE MISUSE AND ALCOHOL USE DISORDERS

Alcohol

Substance abuse often arises in old age as a coping mechanism to deal with loss, anxiety, depression, or boredom. Misuse of alcohol and prescription medications appears to be a more common problem among

Box 24-11	Interventions for the Older Adult with Suicidal Intent

If suicidal intent has been established, the following interventions, arranged in order of immediacy, are necessary:

1. Reduce immediate danger by removing hazardous articles.
2. Do not leave the person alone; evaluate the need for constant attendance; and arrange for family, friend, or professional to be present during the period of immediate danger.
3. Provide an honest expression of concern, such as "I do not want you to take your life. I will help you with this troubling situation."
4. Evaluate the need for consultation with a mental health professional and possible hospitalization.
5. Sometimes a no-suicide contract can be initiated. If the person demonstrates a high risk of suicide, a no-suicide contract cannot be relied on as a preventive measure.
6. Evaluate the need for medication.
7. Focus on the current hazard or crisis that gives the client the most present distress.
8. Mobilize internal and external resources by getting the person reinvolved with external supports and reconnected with internal capabilities. The health professional or the family or caregiver may have to take the initiative to find activities, support systems, transportation, and other resources for the individual.
9. Implement a specific plan of action with an ongoing structured program. Develop a lifeline of individuals who can be called on at any hour of distress, and plan regular calls and follow-up for the individual.

older adults than abuse of illicit drugs. The most common type of substance-use disorder is heavy drinking (Naegle, 2008). Alcohol-related problems in the elderly often go unrecognized, although the residual effects of alcohol abuse complicate the presentation and treatment of many chronic disorders of older people. The current DSM-IV (APA, 2000) criteria for abuse (failure to fulfill major role obligations at work, school, or home; substance use in physically hazardous situations; substance-related legal problems; or recurrent social or interpersonal problems) was developed and validated on young and middle-aged adults and may not adequately describe consequences of alcohol use in older adults (USDHHS, 1999; Finfgeld-Connett, 2004). In the general population, alcohol abuse is readily recognized because of social or work problems; however, elders may live alone and not come under scrutiny at work. They may easily hide their drinking.

The misuse and abuse of alcohol is prevalent among older adults and constitute significant public health concerns. The exact extent of alcohol abuse is not known, but prevalence estimates of unhealthy drinking among older adults range from 1% to 15% and higher. Men age 65 and over have a higher prevalence of unhealthy drinking than women, ranging from 10% to 15% compared to 2% to 5%. Prevalence is likely to increase with the aging of the "baby boomers," who had more access to drugs, alcohol, and other substances (Epstein et al, 2007; Merrick et al, 2008).

An estimated 35% of older primary care patients consume alcohol at levels that place them at risk for harm, and up to 50% of nursing home patients have a history of alcohol abuse. Hospital admissions for alcohol-related problems may be equal to admission rates for myocardial infarction (Masters, 2003). The actual prevalence of alcohol-related hospitalizations is most likely greater than reported, and many studies have shown that older adults are less likely to receive a primary diagnosis of alcoholism than are younger adults (Culberson, 2006a).

Most severe alcohol abuse is seen in people ages 60 to 80 years, not in those older than 80 years. Two thirds of elderly alcoholics are early-onset drinkers (alcohol use began at 30 or 40 years of age), and one third are late-onset drinkers (use began after age 60 years). Late-onset drinking may be related to situational events such as illness, retirement, or death of a spouse and includes a higher number of women (Finfgeld-Connett, 2005).

Gender Issues

Men (particularly older widowers) are 4 times more likely to abuse alcohol than women, but prevalence in women may be underestimated. The number and impact of older female drinkers is expected to increase over the next 20 years as the disparity between men's and women's drinking decreases (Epstein et al, 2007). Women of all ages are significantly more vulnerable to the effects of alcohol misuse including drug interactions, physical injury from alcohol-related falls and accidents, cognitive impairment, and liver and heart disease. Older women also experience unique barriers to detection of and treatment for alcohol problems.

Health care providers often assume that older women do not drink problematically and do not screen for this. Often, alcohol abuse in women is undetected until the consequences are severe (Epstein et al, 2007).

Drug Effects

Many drugs that elders use for chronic illnesses cause adverse effects when combined with alcohol. Alcohol interacts with at least 50% of prescription drugs (Naegle, 2008). Medications that interact with alcohol include analgesics, antibiotics, antidepressants, benzodiazepines, H_2 receptor antagonists, nonsteroidal anti-inflammatory drugs (NSAIDs), and herbal medications (echinacea, valerian) (Masters, 2003). Also, some mouthwash and cough and cold preparations have up to 40% alcohol content (Letizia and Reinboltz, 2005). Acetaminophen taken on a regular basis, when combined with alcohol, may lead to liver failure. Alcohol diminishes the effects of oral hypoglycemics, anticoagulants, and anticonvulsants. All older people should be given precise instructions regarding the interaction of alcohol with their medications.

Other effects of alcohol in older people include urinary incontinence, which results from rapid bladder filling and diminished neuromuscular control of the bladder; gait disturbances from alcohol-induced cerebellar degeneration and peripheral neuropathy; depression and suicide; sleep disturbances and insomnia; and dementia or delirium. Elders who drink to excess are susceptible to cognitive decline, physical decline, functional decline, and increased risk for injury.

Physiology

Older people develop higher blood alcohol levels because of age-related changes (increased body fat, decreased lean body mass and total body water content) that alter absorption and distribution of alcohol (Culberson, 2006a). Reduced liver and kidney function slow alcohol metabolism and elimination. A decrease in the gastric enzyme alcohol dehydrogenase results in slower metabolism of alcohol and higher blood levels for a longer time. Risks of gastrointestinal ulceration and bleeding may be higher in older people because of the decrease in gastric pH that occurs in aging (Letizia and Reinboltz, 2005). Older women are more susceptible to the effects of alcohol since they have less body water than men, less mean muscle mass, and lower levels of the enzyme that breaks down alcohol. Even low-risk drinking levels (no more than one standard drink/day) can be hazardous for older women (Epstein et al, 2007).

IMPLICATIONS FOR GERONTOLOGICAL NURSING AND HEALTHY AGING

Assessment

A comprehensive medical history, physical exam, cognitive assessment, functional assessment, review of medications, and screening for alcohol use and depression is important. Diagnostic tests should include a complete blood count (CBC), liver function tests, chemistries, and an electrocardiogram.

Screening for alcohol abuse is not routinely conducted in primary or long-term care settings. Reasons for the low rates of alcohol detection among older adults by health care professionals include poor symptom recognition, inadequate knowledge about screening instruments, lack of age-appropriate diagnostic criteria for abuse in older people, and ageism. Alcohol-related problems may be overlooked in older people because they do not disrupt their lives or are not clearly linked to physical disorders. Health care providers may also be pessimistic about the ability of older people to change long-standing problems (Naegle, 2008). Finfgeld-Connett (2004) reported that 37% of primary care physicians overlooked alcohol abuse among older women because "it is one of the few pleasures they have left" (p. 32).

Alcoholism is a disease of denial and not easy to diagnose, particularly in older people with psychosocial and functional decline from other conditions that may mask decline caused by alcohol. Health care providers tend to overlook substance abuse disorders and misuse among older people, mistaking the symptoms for those of dementia, depression, or other problems common to older adults. Early signs such as weight loss, irritability, insomnia, and falls may not be recognized as indicators of possible alcohol problems and may be attributed to "just getting older." Box 24-12 presents signs and symptoms that may indicate the presence of alcohol problems in older adults.

The possible health benefits of alcohol in moderation have been reported in the literature (reduced risk of coronary artery disease, ischemic stroke, Alzheimer's disease, and vascular dementia). As a result, older people may not perceive alcohol use as potentially harmful, but clinically significant adverse effects can occur in some individuals consuming as little as two to three drinks per day over an extended period.

Alcohol screening with older adults suggests that 15% of men regularly drink more than 14 drinks per week and that 12% of women regularly drink more than

Box 24-12	Signs and Symptoms of Potential Alcohol Problems in Older Adults

Anxiety
Irritability (feeling worried or "crabby")
Blackouts
Dizziness
Indigestion
Heartburn
Sadness or depression
Chronic pain
Excessive mood swings
New problems making decisions
Lack of interest in usual activities
Falls
Bruises, burns, or other injuries
Family conflict, abuse
Headaches
Incontinence
Memory loss
Poor hygiene
Poor nutrition
Insomnia
Sleep apnea
Social isolation
Out of touch with family or friends
Unusual response to medications
Frequent physical complaints and physician visits
Financial problems

Adapted from National Institute on Alcohol Abuse and Alcoholism: Older adults and alcohol problems, Participant Handout, 2005. Available at www.niaaa.nih.gov. Accessed 7/9/08; and Geriatric Mental Health Foundation: Substance abuse and misuse among older adults: prevention, recognition and help, 2006. Available at www.gmhfonline.org. Accessed 7/8/08.

Alcohol users often reject or deny the diagnosis, or they may take offense at the suggestion of it. Feelings of shame or disgrace may make elders reluctant to disclose a drinking problem. This may be especially true among ethnically or culturally diverse older women from a background in which alcohol use is highly discouraged (Finfgeld-Connett, 2004). Families of older people with substance abuse disorders, particularly their adult children, may be ashamed of the problem and choose not to address it. Health care providers may feel helpless over alcoholism or uncomfortable with direct questioning or may approach the person in a judgmental manner.

Many of the traditional ways of dealing with alcoholism emphasize a confrontational or punitive approach that may have "little impact on a person who views him or herself at the final stage of life" (Naegle, 2008, p. 207). A caring and supportive approach that provides a safe and open atmosphere is the foundation for the therapeutic relationship. It may also be helpful to discuss the issue factually. For example, "Many elders find that the stresses, loneliness, and losses of aging are very hard to bear. Some retreat into alcohol use as a way of coping. There are treatments and groups that assist individuals in these difficult adjustments. If this is a problem for you or if it becomes a problem, please let us know so we may provide resources or referrals for you." It is always important to search for the pain beneath the behavior. Box 24-13 presents some suggested questions to be used in assessment.

Box 24-13	Questions Regarding Abuse of Alcohol

- How many times a week do you drink alcoholic beverages? (If answer is none, ask how many times a month.)
- Are you upset when people criticize your drinking? How do you handle that?
- Do you believe that you sometimes drink too much? Are there particular occasions when that occurs?
- Do you feel disturbed about your alcohol consumption?
- Do you drink when you are feeling lonely?
- Have you identified a pattern regarding your drinking?
- Would you like to stop drinking?

7 drinks per week (National Institute on Alcohol Abuse and Alcoholism, 2005). Because of the increased risk of adverse effects from alcohol use, the National Institute on Alcohol Abuse and Alcoholism (NIAAA) has recommended that individuals over the age of 65 limit alcohol consumption to no more than one standard drink per day. The Substance Abuse and Mental Health Services Administration (SAMSHA) recommends a maximum of two drinks on any drinking occasion (holidays or other celebrations) and somewhat lower limits for women. Health professionals must share information with older people about safe drinking limits and the deleterious effects of alcohol intake.

Culberson (2006b) suggests that a simple question—"Have you had a drink containing alcohol within the past 3 months?"—be included in an assessment to identify clients in whom further screening is indicated. This may be followed by administration of a screening instrument such as the Michigan Alcoholism Screening Test—Geriatric Version (MAST-G) (available at www.hartfordign.org) or the Alcohol Use Disorders Identification Test (AUDIT) to identify problem drinking or dependence. The AUDIT has good validity in ethnically mixed groups and in older adults (Naegle, 2008).

Assessment of depression is also important, as discussed on p. 17. Alcohol and depression screenings should be offered routinely at health fairs and other sites where older people may seek health information and should be included as part of the annual assessment of all older adults. Screening should also be done before prescribing any new medications that may interact with alcohol and as needed after life-changing events (Epstein et al, 2007).

Interventions

Alcohol problems affect physical, mental, spiritual, and emotional health. Interventions must address quality of life in all of these spheres and be adapted to meet the unique needs of the older adult (Box 25-14). Abstinence from alcohol is seen as the desired goal, but a focus on education, alcohol reduction, and reducing harm is also appropriate. Increasing the awareness of older adults about the risks and benefits of alcohol consumption in the context of their own situation is an important goal (Merrick et al, 2008). Treatment and intervention strategies include cognitive-behavioral approaches, individual and group counseling, medical and psychiatric approaches, referral to Alcoholics Anonymous, family therapy, case management and community and home care services, and formalized substance abuse treatment. Treatment outcomes for older people have been shown to be equal to or better than for younger people (Naegle, 2008).

Unless the person is in immediate danger, a stepped-care intervention approach beginning with brief interventions followed by more intensive therapies if necessary should be used. Brief interventions may range from one meeting to four or five short sessions. Brief intervention is a time-limited, patient-centered strategy focused on changing behavior and assessing patient readiness to change. Sessions can range from one meeting of 10 to 30 minutes to 4 or 5 short sessions. The goals of brief intervention are to (1) reduce or stop

---

Box 24-14	Adapting Alcohol Treatment Interventions for Older Adults

- Accommodate for vision, hearing, and other functional impairments
- Provide easy access and transportation if needed
- Address issues older adults tend to face such as loss, grief, health problems
- Including relevant topics to older adults such as worries about the future of independent living, grandparenting, retirement, fixed income
- Consider using life review and reminiscence techniques
- Use a respectful rather than confrontational approach
- Slow the pace of treatment
- Use case management and interdisciplinary approaches
- Address spiritual needs
- Tailor treatment to level of cognitive function
- Provide opportunities for interesting activities and socialization opportunities that don't involve drinking
- Focus on strengths and past coping skills used during hard times
- Demonstrate faith in the person's ability to change, and avoid ageist attitudes
- Consider groups designed for women only, since their needs are different

Adapted from: Epstein E, Fischer-Elber K, Al-Otaiba Z: Women, aging, and alcohol use disorders, co-published simultaneously in *J Women Aging* 19(1/2):31-48, 2007 and Malatesta V, editor: *Mental Health Issues of Older Women: A Comprehensive Review for Health Care Professionals*, Florence, Ken, 2007, Routledge.

---

alcohol consumption, and (2) facilitate entry into formalized treatment if needed. Research results indicate that this type of intervention has positive outcomes when used by primary care providers. Older people may be more likely to accept treatment given by their primary care provider (Culberson, 2006b).

Long-term self-help treatment programs for elders show high rates of success, especially when social outlets are emphasized and cohort supports are available. A significant concern is the lack of programs designed specifically for older people, particularly older women, whose concerns are very different from those of a younger population who abuse drugs or alcohol. The cost of care is another issue, since Medicare covers only hospital-based detoxification and limits coverage of outpatient counseling services to 50%. Health status, availability of transportation, and mobility impairments further may limit access to treatment. Epstein and colleagues (2007) suggest the development of treatment sites in senior centers, and assisted living facilities. Additional information on late-life addictions can be found in the Substance Abuse Among Older Adults Treatment Improvement Protocol (TIP), available from www.samhsa.gov.

Acute Alcohol Withdrawal

When there is significant physical dependence, withdrawal from alcohol can become a life-threatening emergency. Detoxification should be done in an inpatient setting because of the potential medical complications and because withdrawal symptoms in older adults can be prolonged (USDHHS, 1999).

Older people who drink are at risk of experiencing acute alcohol withdrawal if admitted to the hospital for treatment of acute illnesses or emergencies. All patients admitted to acute care settings should be screened for alcohol use and assessed for signs and symptoms of alcohol-related problems. Older people with a long history of consuming excess alcohol, previous episodes of acute withdrawal, and/or a history of prior detoxification are at increased risk of acute alcohol withdrawal (Letizia and Reinboltz, 2005). Symptoms of acute alcohol withdrawal vary but may be more severe and last longer in older people. Minor withdrawal (withdrawal tremulousness) begins 6 to 12 hours after a patient has consumed the last drink. Symptoms include tremor, anxiety, nausea, insomnia, tachycardia, and increased blood pressure and frequently may be mistaken for common problems in older adults. Major withdrawal is seen 10 to 72 hours after cessation of alcohol intake, and symptoms include vomiting, diaphoresis, hallucinations, tremors, and seizures (Letizia and Reinboltz, 2005).

Delirium tremens (DTs) is the term used to describe alcohol withdrawal delirium; it usually occurs 24 to 72 hours after the last drink but may occur up to 10 days later. DTs occur in 5% of patients with acute alcohol withdrawal and is considered a medical emergency with a mortality rate from respiratory failure and cardiac arrhythmia as high as 15%. Other signs and symptoms include confusion, disorientation, hallucinations, hyperthermia, and hypertension. The Clinical Institute Withdrawal Assessment (CIWA) scale is recommended as a valid and reliable screening instrument (www.pubs.niaa.nih.gov) (Letizia and Reinboltz, 2005).

Recommended treatment is the use of short-acting benzodiazepines at one half to one third the normal dose around the clock or as needed during withdrawal. Disulfiram use in older adults to promote abstinence is not recommended because of the potential for serious cardiovascular complications (USDHHS, 1999). The use of oral or intravenous alcohol to prevent or treat withdrawal is not established.

The CIWA aids in medication adjustments. Other interventions include assessing mental status, monitoring vital signs, and maintaining fluid balance without overhydrating. Calm and quiet surroundings, no unnecessary stimuli, consistent caregivers, frequent reorientation, prevention of injury, and support and caring are additional suggested interventions. Nutritional assessment is indicated, as well as addition of a multivitamin containing folic acid, pyridoxine, niacin, vitamin A, and thiamine (Letizia and Reinboltz, 2005).

Other Substance Abuse Concerns

Misuse of alcohol and prescription medications appears to be a more common problem among older adults than abuse of illicit drugs. Older adults infrequently use illicit drugs (USDHHS, 1999). However, few studies have been conducted, and projections are that the use of illicit drugs will increase significantly in the coming years, largely as a result of the aging of the baby boomers. This has implications for education and proactive treatment planning (Naegle, 2008).

A more common concern seen among older people is the misuse of prescription and OTC medications. Drug misuse is defined as use of a drug for reasons other than those for which it was prescribed. Older people are prescribed more than 33% of all prescription drugs, and the nonmedical use of prescription drugs is increasing in people over 60 years of age. The negative effects of polypharmacy are often increased by an older person's use of alcohol (Naegle, 2008). The inappropriate use of benzodiazepines and barbiturates is especially problematic for older women, who are more likely than men to receive prescriptions for these drugs (Epstein et al, 2007). Benzodiazepines represent 17% to 23% of drugs prescribed to older adults (Morgan et al, 2005). Opiates are ranked second only to benzodiazepines among abused prescription drugs in the older adult population (Naegle, 2008). Increases in illness and mortality are associated with misusing prescription and nonprescription medications, although this is not considered a disorder by DSM-IV (Blow et al, 2002).

Some of the reasons for the abuse of psychoactive prescription medications may be inappropriate prescribing and ineffective monitoring of response and follow-up. In many instances, older people are given prescriptions for benzodiazepines or sedatives because of complaints of insomnia or nervousness, without adequate assessment for depression, anxiety, or other conditions that may be causing the symptoms. Older people may not be informed of the side effects of these medications including interactions with alcohol, dependence, and withdrawal symptoms. More important, conditions such as anxiety and depression may not be recognized and treated appropriately.

Risk, prevention, assessment, and treatment of alcohol and substance abuse have not been sufficiently studied among older people. Diagnostic criteria to identify alcohol and prescription drug misuse among older adults, particularly older women and culturally and ethnically diverse elders, also need further investigation (Finfgeld-Connett, 2004). This is a particularly salient issue for gerontological nursing research in light of the growing numbers of older people, many of whom have a history of alcohol and drug use. Nurses in contact with older adults in institutionalized and community settings must be competent in assessment for mental health disorders as well as in screening, assessment, and counseling about the use of alcohol, prescription, illicit, and OTC drug use. Providing education to older people and their families and referring to specialists and community resources are also important nursing roles and essential to "best practices" (Naegle, 2008, p. 661).

IMPLICATIONS FOR GERONTOLOGICAL NURSING AND HEALTHY AGING

The development of holistic and humanistic models of care for elders experiencing mental health disturbances is critically important in gerontological nursing. Much of the distress associated with mental health disorders in late life can be relieved through competent, caring, and compassionate gerontological nursing care. Awareness of appropriate assessment and treatment of the distressing reactions that can occur in late life, as presented in this chapter, is a very important component of best practice care. However, knowing and appreciating each elder's uniqueness, his or her past and present experiences, and how they color the present may contribute far more to mental health and wellness than medications or therapy.

Believing in and supporting the strength and wisdom of older people restores self-confidence and feelings of worth, an important component of mental health and wellness. Appreciating the nature of loss and grief in old age means that gerontological nurses listen,

really listen, and offer support to weather the storm. Our work must focus on the development of environments of care that enhance both physical and mental health and wellness, create conditions of hope, and support elders in the often difficult journey in late life.

APPLICATION OF MASLOW'S HIERARCHY

Using Maslow's hierarchy of needs model, satisfaction of basic needs is a significant component of mental health. Attention to basic needs of biological integrity, safety and security, belonging and attachment, self-esteem, and self-efficacy in the daily lives of elders is essential to mental health and wellness. The higher one rises in terms of needs met, the more likely one is to be mentally healthy.

KEY CONCEPTS

▶ Mental health in late life is difficult to determine because the accrual of life experiences makes for great variation. Mental health in late life must be determined by the gratification and satisfaction that individuals feel in their particular situations.
▶ Mental health is a fluctuating situation for most individuals, with peaks and valleys of happiness and pain.
▶ Elders are not well served within the mental health system as it exists today.
▶ The incidence of psychotic disorders with late-life onset is low among older people, but psychotic manifestations can occur as secondary symptoms in a variety of disorders, the most common being Alzheimer's disease. Psychotic symptoms in Alzheimer's disease necessitate different assessment and treatment than long-standing psychotic disorders.
▶ Anxiety disorders are common in late life and reestablishing feelings of adequacy and control is the heart of crisis resolution and stress management.
▶ PTSD is finally being recognized in older adults who have been subjected to extremely traumatic events.
▶ Depression is the most common emotional disorder of aging and likewise the most treatable. Unfortunately, it is often neglected or assumed to be a condition of aging that one must "learn to live with." An important nursing intervention is assessment of depression.
▶ Suicide is a significant problem among older men. Assessment of suicidal intent is important especially

in light of loss. Many come to be seen by the health care professional with physical complaints shortly before they commit suicide.

▶ Substance abuse, particularly alcohol, and misuse of prescription drugs are often under-recognized and undertreated problems of older adults, particularly older women. Screening and appropriate assessment and intervention are important in all settings.

▶ Further research is needed to fully understand the cultural and ethnic differences in mental health concerns, as well as appropriate assessment and treatment in culturally and ethnically diverse older people.

ACTIVITIES AND DISCUSSION QUESTIONS

1. List the various stressors you have encountered with the older people you have cared for and then discuss what was done about them.
2. Discuss the three most common mental health disturbances that elders are likely to experience and describe appropriate assessment and treatment.
3. What is likely to be different in the appearance of depression in a person who is 70 years old compared to its appearance in a person who is 20 years old?
4. What behaviors are indicative of suicidal intent in an older adult? Discuss the methods of assessment and your reactions to these.
5. Discuss the various situations that may result in elder substance abuse and ways to effectively intervene.
6. What type of teaching would you provide to an older adult related to the use of alcohol and medications?
7. Formulate strategies that may be used to promote mental health and wellness in late life.

RESOURCES

Organizations
American Association for Geriatric Psychiatry
   www.aagponline.org
National Coalition on Mental Health and Aging
   www.ncmha.org

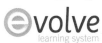

For additional resources, please visit evolve.elsevier.com/Ebersole/gerontological.

REFERENCES

Alexopoulos G, Young J, Shamoian C: Cornell Scale for Depression in Dementia, *Biol Psychiatry* 23:271-284, 1988.

American Association for Geriatric Psychiatry: Action alert: Medicare parity, 2008. Available at http://capwiz.com/aagp/issues/alert/?alertid=11593391. Accessed 7/30/08.

American Psychiatric Association (APA): *Diagnostic and statistical manual of mental disorders (DSM-IV)*, ed 4, Washington, DC, 2000, The Association.

American Psychological Association (APA): *Mental health care and older adults: facts and policy recommendations,* July 2003. Available at www.apa.org. Accessed 4/22/08.

Antai-Otong D: Schizophrenia in the elderly, *Adv NP* 8(3):39, 2000.

Anxiety Disorders Association of America: *Anxiety disorders in older adults.* Accessed 6/22/08 from www.adaa.org

Ayers C, Loebach J, Wetherell E et al: Treating late-life anxiety, *Psychiatr Times* 23(3 March 1):1-2, 2006. Available at www.psychiatrictimes.com/display/article/10168/46976?pageNumber=1. Accessed 6/27/08

Blow F, Oslin D, Barry K: Misuse and abuse of alcohol, illicit drugs, and psychoactive medications among older people, *Generations* 26(1):50-54, 2002.

Bludau J: Second institutionalization: impact of personal history on patients with dementia, *Caring Ages* 3(5):3-4, 2002.

Burnside IM: Listen to the aged, *Am J Nurs* 75(10):1800-1803, 1975.

Byrd E: Nursing assessment and treatment of depressive disorders of late life. In Mellilo K, Houde S, editors: *Geropsychiatric and mental health nursing*, Sudbury MA, 2005, Jones and Bartlett.

Chizobam A, Bazargan M, Hindman D et al: Depression symptomatology and diagnosis: Discordance between patients and physicians in primary care settings, *BMC Family Practice* 9(1), 2008. Available at http://www.biomedcentral.com/1471-2296/9/1/abstract. Accessed 7/17/08.

Culberson J: Alcohol use in the elderly: beyond the CAGE. Part 1 of 2: prevalence and patterns of problem drinking, *Geriatrics* 61(10):23-27, 2006a.

Culberson J: Alcohol use in the elderly: beyond the CAGE. Part 2 of 2: screening instruments and treatment strategies, *Geriatrics* 61(11):20-26, 2006b.

Das B, Greenspan M, Muralee S et al: Late-life depression: a review, *Clin Geriatr* 15(10):35-44, 2007.

Davis B: Assessing adults with mental disorders in primary care, the nurse practitioner, *Am J Primary Health Care* 29(5):19-27, 2004.

Epstein E, Fischer-Elber K, Al-Otaiba Z: Women, aging, and alcohol use disorders, *J Women Aging* 19(1-2):31-48, 2007.

Erikson EH, Erikson JM, Kivnick HQ: *Vital involvement in old age: the experience of old age in our time,* New York, 1986, WW Norton.

Finfgeld-Connett DL: Treatment of substance misuse in older women: using a brief intervention model, *J Gerontol Nurs* 30(8):31-37, 2004.

Finfgeld-Connett DL: Self-management of alcohol problems among older adults, *J Gerontol Nurs* 31(5):51-58, 2005.

Fitzwater E: *Gero gems: older adults and mental health,* Part 2, Anxiety disorder, Center for Aging with Dignity, Cincinnati OH, University of Cincinnati College of Nursing, February 2008. Available at www.CareAdvocate.org. Accessed 7/8/08.

Frampton K: The state of geriatric mental health services in LTC, *Caring Ages* 5(4):47-51, 2004.

Geerlings MI, denHeijer T, Koudstaat P et al: History of depression, depressive symptoms, and medical temporal lobe atrophy and risk of Alzheimer's disease, *Neurology* 70:1258-1264, 2008.

Grossberg GT: Diagnosis and treatment of late-life psychosis in the elderly, *Long-Term Care Forum* 1(3):7, 2000.

Joe S, Baser R, Breeden G et al: Prevalence of and risk factors for lifetime suicide risks among blacks in the United States, *JAMA* 296(17):2112-2123, 2006.

Kennedy GJ: Prevention of suicide in older persons: lessons and limitations of evidence-based interventions, *Ann Long-Term Care* 12(8):43-48, 2004.

Kennedy GJ: Bipolar disorder in late life: depression, *Prim Psychiatry* 15(3):30-34, 2008.

Kurlowicz L, Harvath T: Depression. In Capezuti E, Swicker D, Mezey M et al, editors: *Evidence-based geriatric nursing protocols for best practice,* ed 3, New York, 2008a, Springer.

Kurlowicz L, Harvath T: *Depression: nursing standard of practice protocol,* New York, 2008b, Hartford Institute for Geriatric Nursing. Available at www.consultgerirn.org. Accessed 7/8/08.

Lawrence V, Murray J, Banerjee S et al: Concepts and causation of depression: a cross-cultural study of the beliefs of older adults, *Gerontologist* 46(1):25-32, 2006.

Letizia M, Reinboltz M: Identifying and managing acute alcohol withdrawal in the elderly, *Geriatr Nurs* 26(3):176-183, 2005.

Madhusoodanan S, Brenner R: Caring for the chronically mentally ill in nursing homes, *Ann Long-Term Care* 15(9):29-32, 2007.

Maslow A: *Motivation and personality,* ed 2, New York, 1970, Harper & Row.

Masters J: Moderate alcohol consumption and unappreciated risk for alcohol-related harm among ethnically diverse urban-dwelling elders, *Geriatr Nurs* 24(3):155-161, 2003.

Meiner S, Lueckenotte A: *Gerontological Nursing,* St. Louis, Mosby, 2005.

Mellilo K, Hoff L, Huff M: Geropsychiatric nursing as a subspecialty. In Mellilo K, Houde S, editors: *Geropsychiatric and mental health nursing,* New York, 2005, Springer.

Mentes J, Bail J: Psychosis in older adults. In Mellilo K, Houde S, editors: *Geropsychiatric and mental health nursing,* Sudbury MA, 2005, Jones and Bartlett.

Merrick E, Hodgkins D, Garnick D et al: Unhealthy drinking patterns in older adults: prevalence and associated characteristics, *J Am Geriatr Soc* 56(2):214-223, 2008.

Mitty E, Flores S: Suicide in late life, *Geriatr Nurs* 29(3):160-165, 2008.

Moorhead SA, Brighton VA: Anxiety and fear. In Maas ML, Buckwalter K, Hardy M et al, editors: *Nursing care of older adults: diagnoses, outcomes, and interventions,* St. Louis, 2001, Mosby.

Morgan B, White D, Wallace A: Substance abuse in older adults. In Mellilo K, Houde S, editors: *Geropsychiatric and mental health nursing,* Sudbury, MA, 2005, Jones and Bartlett.

Naegle M: Substance misuse and alcohol use disorders. In Capezuti E, Swicker D, Mezey M et al, editors: *Evidence-based geriatric nursing protocols for best practice,* ed 3, New York, 2008, Springer.

National Institute on Alcohol Abuse and Alcoholism: Older adults and alcohol problems, Participant Handout, 2005. Available at www.niaaa.nih.gov. Accessed 7/8/08.

National Institute of Mental Health (NIMH): *Older adults: depression and suicide facts,* 2007. Available at www.nimh.gov/publicat/bipolstory08.cfm. Accessed 7/8/08.

National Institute of Mental Health (NIMH): *How do older adults experience depression?* 2008. Available at www.nimh.nih.gov. Accessed 10/2/08.

Ortiz I, Romero L: Cultural implications for assessment and treatment of depression in Hispanic elderly individuals, *Ann Long-Term Care* 16(8):45-48, 2008.

Pautex S, Michon A, Emond H et al: Pain in severe dementia: self-assessment of observational scales? *Ann Long-Term Care* 15(9):46, 2007.

Qualls S: Defining mental health in later life, *Generations* 26(7):9-13, 2002.

Reynolds C, Dew A, Pollock B et al: Maintenance treatment of major depression in old age, *N Engl J Med* 354(11):1130-1138, 2006.

Schneider LS, Tariot P, Dagerman K et al: Effectiveness of atypical antipsychotic drugs in patients with Alzheimer's disease, *N Engl J Med* 355(15):1525-1538, 2006.

Sheikh JI, Yesavage JA: Geriatric depression scale (GDS): recent evidence and development of a shorter version, *Clin Gerontol* 5:165-173, 1986.

Smith M: Nursing assessment and treatment of anxiety in late life. In Mellilo K, Houde S, editors: *Geropsychiatric and mental health nursing,* Sudbury, MA, 2005, Jones and Bartlett.

Tabloski P: *Gerontological nursing,* Upper Saddle River NJ, 2006, Pearson Prentice Hall.

Tappen R, Barry C: Assessment of affect in advanced Alzheimer's disease: the dementia mood picture test, *J Gerontol Nurs* 21(3):44-46, 1995.

Thakur M, Blazer D: Depression in long-term care, *JAMDA* 9(2):82-87, 2008.

Unutzer J, Katon W, Callahan C et al: Long-term cost effects of collaborative care for late-life depression, *Am J Managed Care* 14(2):95-100, 2008.

U.S. Department of Health and Human Services (USDHHS): *Mental health: a report of the surgeon general—executive summary,* Rockville, MD, 1999, The Department.

U.S. Department of Health and Human Services (USDHHS): *Healthy people 2010,* ed 2, Washington, DC: 2000, US Government Printing Office.

Wetherell J, Maser J, Balkom A: Anxiety disorders in the elderly: outdated beliefs and a research agenda, *Acta Psychiatr Scand* 111(6):401-402, 2005 (editorial).

Appendix 24-A — *Depression Rating Scales*

THE SHORT FORM OF THE GERIATRIC DEPRESSION SCALE

1. Are you basically satisfied with your life?
2. Have you dropped many of your activities and interests?
3. Do you feel that your life is empty?
4. Do you often get bored?
5. Are you in good spirits most of the time?
6. Are you afraid that something bad is going to happen to you?
7. Do you feel happy most of the time?
8. Do you often feel helpless?
9. Do you prefer to stay at home, rather than going out and doing new things?
10. Do you feel you have more problems with memory than most?
11. Do you think it is wonderful to be alive?
12. Do you feel pretty worthless the way you are now?
13. Do you feel full of energy?
14. Do you feel that your situation is hopeless?
15. Do you think that most people are better off than you?

From Yesavage J, Brink TL, Rose TL et al: Development and validation of a geriatric depression screening scale: a preliminary report, *J Psychiatr Res* 17(1):37, 1982-1983.

CENTER FOR EPIDEMIOLOGIC STUDIES DEPRESSION SCALE

INSTRUCTIONS FOR QUESTIONS: Below is a list of the ways you might have felt or behaved. Please tell me how often you have felt this way during the past week.

Rarely or none of the time (less than 1 day)
Some or a little of the time (1-2 days)
Occasionally or a moderate amount of time (3-4 days)
Most or all of the time (5-7 days)

During the past week:

1. I was bothered by things that usually don't bother me.
2. I did not feel like eating; my appetite was poor.
3. I felt that I could not shake off the blues even with help from my family or friends.
4. I felt that I was just as good as other people.
5. I had trouble keeping my mind on what I was doing.
6. I felt depressed.
7. I felt that everything I did was an effort.
8. I felt hopeful about the future.
9. I thought my life had been a failure.
10. I felt fearful.
11. My sleep was restless.
12. I was happy.
13. I talked less than usual.
14. I felt lonely.
15. People were unfriendly.
16. I enjoyed life.
17. I had crying spells.
18. I felt sad.
19. I felt that people dislike me.
20. I could not get "going."

From Center for Epidemiologic Studies, National Institutes of Mental Health.

Loss, Grief, Dying, and Death in Late Life

LEARNING OBJECTIVES

Upon completion of this chapter, the reader will be able to:

- Differentiate between loss and grief.
- Explain the different types of grief and the dynamics of the grieving process.
- Explain the characteristics required of the nurse to be able to effectively intervene in grief and bereavement.
- Identify and discuss the needs of the dying and appropriate interventions.
- Explain the role and responsibility of the nurse in advance directives.
- Explain the difference between passive and active euthanasia.

GLOSSARY

Bereavement overload A number of grief situations in a short period of time (weeks, months, 1 year).
Euthanasia Death that is unrelated to the natural life processes or random accident.

Grief An emotional response to loss.
Mourning The process by which grief is experienced.

THE LIVED EXPERIENCE

When we were in our sixties my friends and I met over cards, went on trips, and experienced all of the joys of retirement. We didn't have much time to worry about aches and pains. In our seventies we had less time to play because we were busy visiting one another in the hospital or in nursing homes. In our eighties we met frequently again, but it was usually at our friends' funerals, leaving little time for cards or travel. Now that I am in my nineties hardly any of my friends are still alive; you know it gets kind of lonely, so you just have to make new younger friends!

Theresa, age 93

Life is like a pinwheel, a thing of beauty and change. Loss, like the wind, sets it in motion, beginning the life-changing process of grieving. Throughout one's life the winds of loss will gently stir recurrent episodes of grief through sights, sounds, smells, anniversary dates, and other triggers. The arms of the pinwheel suggest movement by the bereaved, reaching out of the experience of grief by surrendering through resting, or lowering one's defenses toward life and being open to reality, or the acceptance of the life event and reaching out to others and rejoining life through change. Each gust of wind may generate a resurgence of grief, but the pinwheel will never lose its beauty.

Loss, dying, and death are universal, incontestable events of the human experience. Some loss is associated with the normal changes with aging, such as the loss of flexibility in the joints. Some is related to the normal changes in everyday life and life transitions, such as moving and retirement. Other losses are those of loved ones through death. Some deaths are considered normative and expected, such as older parents and friends. Other deaths are considered nonnormative and unexpected, such as the death of adult children or grandchildren.

Regardless of the type of loss, each one has the potential to trigger grief and a process we call bereavement or mourning. Grief and mourning are usually used synonymously. However, grief is an individual's response to a loss and mourning is an active and evolving process that includes those behaviors used to incorporate the loss experience into one's life after the loss. Mourning behaviors are strongly influenced by social and cultural norms that prescribe the appropriate ways of both reacting to the loss and coping with it (Chow et al, 2007; Gerdner et al, 2007). There is no single way to grieve or respond to loss; each person grieves in his or her own way.

Although there are cultural expectations related to grief behaviors for loss through death, there are no guidelines for behavior when the loss is of another type. For example, an individual who is seriously ill, who moves to a nursing home (loses one's home), or who retires (willingly or unwillingly) may be very sad, irritable, and forgetful. The person may be suspected of developing dementia when he or she is actually grieving. When the losses accumulate in quick succession, a state of bereavement overload may result. The griever may become incapacitated and require careful and skilled support and guidance.

Gerontological nurses need to have basic knowledge of the grieving process and how to comfort and care for grievers, including one another. Additional knowledge about the dying process is needed as are skills related to care of the dying person and his or her survivors. In this chapter we hope to provide the basic information necessary to promote effective grieving, peaceful dying, and good and appropriate deaths.

The Grieving Process

Researchers have tried for years to understand the grieving process, and their efforts have resulted in a number of proposed models to explain and predict the experience. The majority of the models developed between the early 1970s and early 1980s, influence what caregivers and society in general have been taught about grief. Although intended to describe death-related grief, these same models can be applied to any of the losses in the lives of older adults that are considered significant or meaningful.

All models recognize similar physical and psychological manifestations of acute grief (when it is first felt), a middle period in which the manifestations of grief (e.g., despair, depression) affect the person's day-to-day functioning, and an ending phase where the person learns to adjust to life in a new way without which has been lost. At the same time it is also recognized that the grieving process is not rigidly structured and that a predictable pattern of responses does not always occur.

Worden

Worden's (2003) model has been frequently cited and adapted. He represents the grieving process as a series of evolving tasks, repeated for all losses or parts of losses. For example, the person diagnosed with Alzheimer's (and a loss of his or her former self, plans for the future, etc.) may, at some point, (1) accept the reality of the loss (diagnosis); (2) work through the physical and emotional pain associated with the diagnosis and all of its implications, such as loss of driving ability; (3) adjust to a change in environment (e.g., may no longer be able to go to work); and (4) emotionally relocate the loss and move on with life (continuing to live with the new diagnosis).

If this model is applied to someone who has lost a loved one, such as a life partner, the nurse may look for signs of the person accepting the reality of the death when the deceased person is referred to in the past tense rather than the present. For example, Helen may speak of Chris as someone who "just loved to garden" rather than "just loves to garden."

Although working through the pain is an individual process, Helen has a support network of family, friends and church members. They encourage her to "tell her story" of not only Chris's life but also their life together, and gently move her to thinking of her life without Chris. In working through acute grief, the grief-pain will not lessen if avoided with the regular use of medications such as tranquilizers. Although these may be necessary to enable the griever to accomplish some needed tasks, they are not recommended for everyday use since they actually interfere with what we call resolution.

Adjusting to loss may take a considerable period of time, especially if the relationship with the deceased was a long and close one. Changes in the environment may be physical, emotional, or spiritual, such as re-arrangement of furniture or a different seating pattern at the dinner table.

As Helen proceeds through the grieving process, her memories of life with Chris will be those of the past, and she will be able to develop new memories of her life without Chris. Although there may be a lot of pain associated with the first birthday, anniversary, holiday, and so on, it will lessen with subsequent years as the loss is relocated from the present to the past.

A Loss Response Model

Jett's Loss Response Model is a modification of that proposed by Barabara Giacquinta for families facing cancer (Giacquinta, 1977). It incorporates a systems approach that leads to a framework for the design of nursing interventions.

When loss occurs within a system, such as a family, the impact is experienced as acute grief. The system's equilibrium is in chaos and is seen as a functional dis-ruption; that is, the system cannot perform its usual activities. Either the person or the members are in a state of disequilibrium. The loss seems unreal. The grieving family searches for meaning: why did this happen? How will they survive the loss? If an elder is reacting to the loss of a child or a grandchild, thoughts of "why wasn't it me?" are common. The family then may become active in informing others. Each time the story is repeated, the loss becomes more real and the system moves toward a new steady state. The story is also different each time it is told, as it is told from a new perspective. Informing others involves engaging emotions that may have been previously withheld or subdued because of the shock of the impact. The ex-pression of emotions can release energy that can be used to reorganize the family structure. As roles change, adaptation and accommodation are necessary. Someone else steps in to perform the roles of the per-son who is now absent or to complete the tasks no longer possible in the presence of the loss. For exam-ple, when the elder patriarch dies, the eldest son may step up and assume some of his father's roles and re-sponsibilities. Finally, if the system is to survive, it will need to redefine itself. One of the ways that it does this is by reframing its memories; that is, families accept that portraits and reunions are still possible, just differ-ent than they were before the loss; or they accept that a person can still be vital, active, and important even

after the loss of the ability to drive a car, to walk unas-sisted, or to live alone (Figure 25-1).

Types of Grief

Grieving takes enormous amounts of physical and emo-tional energy. It is the hardest thing anyone can do and may be especially hard for older adults. Emotions can be intense, and this intensity may manifest as confusion, depression, or preoccupation with thoughts of the de-ceased or the loss. This reaction may be mistaken for other conditions, such as dementia, when it probably is a type of delirium, something that requires care. The ge-rontological nurse is most likely to work with elders who are experiencing anticipatory grief, acute grief, or chronic grief. A fourth type, disenfranchised grief, may be hid-den, but when it occurs it is nonetheless significant.

Anticipatory Grief

Anticipatory grief is the response to a real or perceived loss before it actually occurs, a dress rehearsal, so to speak. One observes this grief in preparation for potential loss, such as loss of belongings (e.g., selling of a home), moving (e.g., into a nursing home), or knowing that a body part or function is going to change (e.g., a mastec-tomy), or in anticipation of the loss of a spouse or oneself either through dementia or through death. Behaviors that may signal anticipatory grief include preoccupation with the loss, unusually detailed planning, or a sudden change in attitude toward the thing or person to be lost (Lewis and McBride, 2004). End-of-life communication has been found to be associated with anticipatory grief and im-proved bereavement-related outcomes (Metzger and Gray, 2008).

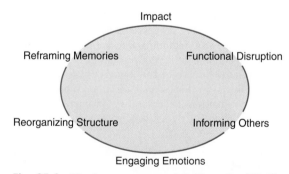

Fig. 25-1 The loss response model. *(From Jett KF: The loss response model, unpublished manuscript, 2004. Adapted from Giacquinta B: Helping families face the crisis of cancer, Am J Nurs 77(10):1585-1588, 1977.)*

The grieving process described by the models may occur in the context of anticipatory grief with one significant difference: the loss has not yet occurred. If the loss is certain but no one can say when it will occur, or if it does not occur when or as expected, those awaiting the actual loss or death may become irritable, hostile, or impatient, not because they want the loss to occur but in response to the emotional ups and downs of the waiting. Researchers Glaser and Strauss (1968) described what they call an interruption in the sentimental order of a nursing unit when this occurs—no one quite knows how to behave. Professionals who are grieving, such as nurses, as well as family and friends, usually deal much more easily with anticipated losses when they occur at an expected time or in a set manner.

Anticipatory grief can result in the phenomenon of premature detachment from an individual who is dying or detachment of the dying person from the environment. Pattison (1977) called the premature withdrawal of others sociological death, and the premature withdrawal of the person, psychological death. In either case, the person who is dying is no longer involved in day-to-day activities of living and essentially suffers a premature death.

Acute Grief

Acute grief is a crisis. It has a definite syndrome of somatic and psychological symptoms of distress that occur in waves lasting varying periods of time. These symptoms may occur every time the loss is acknowledged, others are informed, or another person offers condolences. Preoccupation with the loss is a phenomenon similar to daydreaming and is accompanied by a sense of unreality. Depending on the situation, feelings of self-blame or guilt may be present and manifest themselves as hostility or anger toward friends, depression, or withdrawal.

It is often difficult for persons who are acutely grieving to accomplish their usual activities of daily living or meet other responsibilities (functional disruption). Even if the tasks are accomplished, the person may complain of feeling distracted, restless, and "at loose ends." Common, simple activities such as deciding what to wear may seem too complex a task. Fortunately the signs and symptoms of acute grief do not last forever, or else none of us could survive. Acute grief is most intense in the months immediately following the loss, especially the first 3 months, with the intensity of feelings lessening over time (Taylor et al, 2008). To follow the example of Helen: in the first months she may cry any time her partner is mentioned. Later, she will still be grieving, but the tears are replaced with a surging sense of loss and sadness, and still later by more fleeting reactions.

Chronic Grief

Grief may temporarily inhibit some activity but is considered a normal response. The intermittent pain of grief is often exacerbated on anniversary dates (birthdays, holidays, and wedding anniversaries). For the survivors of tragedies, such as war, the Oklahoma City bombing, the 9/11 or some other terrorist attack, the grief may never completely go away. This type of lingering grief has been described as "shadow grief," or that which resurfaces from time to time but does not persist; it produces temporary grief, usually triggered by a sight, smell, or sound (see Box 25-1) (Coryell, 2007).

Some chronic grief is more than that of shadow grief and crosses the boundary to what we call impaired, pathological, abnormal, dysfunctional, or maladaptive grief. It has been thought that pathological chronic grief begins with normal grief responses, whose normal evolution toward adjustment, toward the reestablishment of equilibrium, is blocked by some obstacle. The memories resist being reframed. Reactions are exaggerated, and memories are experienced as recurrent acute grief—over and over again, months and years later. Signs of possible pathological grief include excessive and irrational anger, outbursts in social settings, and insomnia that lingers for an extended time or surfaces months or years later, or a grief episode that triggers a major depressive episode. The families who have had a loved one who has committed suicide have been found to be among those who have a greater risk for complicated grief (Starks et al, 2007). This type of grief necessitates the professional intervention of a grief counselor, a psychiatric nurse

---

Box 25-1   The Carved Birds

One day as I was browsing at an art show, I came across a booth of carved birds, a favorite design of my beloved mother. I turned to remark to her. Except she was not there: she had died 15 years earlier in my home. Sadness passed over me like a cloud, and I wished she were there—I would buy her one as a special gift. Instead, I turned to my husband and shared reminiscences as I had done before, and he listened patiently. As the wind blows, so did the cloud pass, and I moved on, enjoying the day.

Kathleen Jett at 40

practitioner, or a psychologist who has skills at helping grieving elders and their loved ones.

Disenfranchised Grief

Disenfranchised grief is an experience of the person whose loss cannot be openly acknowledged or publicly mourned. The grief is socially disallowed or unsupported (Doka, 2002). The person does not have a socially recognized right to be perceived or function as a bereaved person. In other words, a relationship is not recognized; the loss is not sanctioned, or the griever is not recognized or cannot be made public. Disenfranchised grief has frequently been associated with domestic partnerships in which the family of the deceased does not acknowledge the partner or in secret relationships in which the involved party cannot tell others of the meaning or depth of the attachment. Disenfranchised grief can also occur in situations of family discord in which a member of the family is considered the "black sheep." Older adults can experience this disenfranchisement when persons close to them do not understand the full meaning of a retiree's retirement or the impact of a pet's death, or when gradual losses occur that are caused by chronic conditions that have great impact on the elder but are not seen as important to others. Families coping with a member who has Alzheimer's disease may also experience disenfranchised grief, particularly when others perceive the death of the elder as a blessing and fail to support the griever or caregiver who has struggled for years with anticipatory grief and now must cope with the acute grief of the actual death (Doka, 2002).

Factors Affecting Coping with Loss

Coping as it relates to loss and grief is the ability of the individual or family to find ways to deal with the stress. In the language of the Loss Response Model (Jett, 2008), it is the ability to move from a state of chaos and disequilibrium to one of renewed order, equilibrium, and peace (see www.youtube.com, *Grief and Sorrow*). Many factors affect the ability to cope with loss and grief (Box 25-2).

Those at special risk for significantly adverse effects of grief are older spouses and life partners of any kind. Intense grief may cause a temporary decrease in cognitive function that can be misinterpreted as dementia, isolating the griever (Ward et al, 2007).

Another classic authority on death and dying was psychiatrist Avery Weisman (1979). He described those who are more likely to effectively deal as "good

---

> **Box 25-2   Factors Influencing the Grieving Process**
>
> - If the illness causes a number of losses
> - If each loss can be identified
> - How important the loss is to the person
> - If psychotropic drugs are used appropriately
> - Level of health and fitness before the loss, e.g., nutritional status, sleep, and exercise
> - Coping skills and types of coping responses available to the person
> - Past experience with loss or death
> - Immediate circumstances surrounding loss
> - Timing of the loss
> - Number, type, and quality of secondary losses occurring at the same time
>
> ### Additional Factors Specific to Dying and Death
>
> - Role that deceased occupied in family or social system
> - Amount of unfinished business
> - Perception of deceased's fulfillment in life
> - Immediate circumstances surrounding death
> - Length of illness before death
> - Anticipatory grief and involvement with dying patient
>
> Modified from Hess PA: Loss, grief, and dying. In Beare PG, Myers JL, editors: *Principles and practice of adult health nursing*, ed 2, St Louis, 1994, Mosby.

---

copers" (p. 42). These are individuals or families who have experience with the successful management of crisis. They are resourceful and are able to draw on coping strategies that have worked in the past. Weisman (1979, pp. 42-43; 1984) found persons who cope effectively with cancer do the following:

- ▶ Avoid avoidance
- ▶ Confront realities, and take appropriate action
- ▶ Focus on solutions
- ▶ Redefine problems
- ▶ Consider alternatives
- ▶ Have good communication with loved ones
- ▶ Seek and use constructive help
- ▶ Accept support when offered
- ▶ Can keep up their morale

In other words, the effective copers are those who can acknowledge the loss and try to make sense of it. They are able to maintain composure, use generally good judgment, and are able to remain optimistic without denying the loss. These good copers seek good guidance when they need it.

In contrast, those who cope less effectively have few if any of these abilities. They tend to be more rigid and pessimistic, are demanding, and are given to emotional extremes. They may be dogmatic and expect perfection from themselves and others. Ineffective copers are also more likely to be individuals who live alone, socialize little, and have few close friends or an ineffective support network. They may have a history of mental illness, or they may have guilt, anger, and ambivalence toward the individual who has died or that which has been lost. Those at risk for pathological grief will more likely have unresolved past conflicts or be facing the loss and other, secondary stressors simultaneously. They will have fewer opportunities as a result of the loss. They are the elders who are most in need of the expert interventions of grief counselors and skilled gerontological nurses.

IMPLICATIONS FOR GERONTOLOGICAL NURSING AND HEALTHY AGING

The goal of the nurse is not to prevent grief but to support those who are grieving. Although the loss will never change, the potential long-term detrimental effects can be lessened. Working with grieving elders is part of the normal workday of gerontological nurses, who are professional grievers in our own way. It is one of the few areas in nursing where small actions can make a large difference in the quality of life for the person to whom we provide care and with whom we work.

Assessment

The goal of the grief assessment is to differentiate those who are likely to cope effectively from those who are at risk for ineffective coping, so that appropriate interventions can be planned. A grief assessment is based on knowledge of the grieving process and the subsequent mourning. Data are obtained through observation of behavior of the individual and are assessed within the framework of the cultural context (National Cancer Institute [NCI], 2006).

A thorough grief assessment includes questions about recent significant life events, life or religious values, and relationship to that which has been lost. How many other stressful or demanding events or circumstances are going on in the griever's life? Information about these concurrent life stresses will help determine

who is at risk for impaired grieving. The more concurrent stressors in the person's life, the more he or she will need the nurse or other grief specialists. The nurse determines what stress management techniques have been used in the past, and whether they were helpful (e.g., talking) or potentially harmful (e.g., substance use or abuse). Was the griever's identity closely tied to that which is lost, such as a lifelong athlete who is faced with never walking again? If the loss is of a partner, how was the relationship? The loss of an abusive or controlling partner may liberate the survivor, who may feel guilty for not feeling the amount of grief that is expected. For many older women who have been dependent financially on their spouses, death may leave them impoverished, significantly complicating their grief. Knowing more about the loss and the effect of the loss on the elder's life will enable the nurse to construct and implement appropriate and caring responses.

Interventions

One goal of intervention is to assist the individual (or family) in attaining a healthy adjustment to the loss experience and reestablishing equilibrium. Actions that can meet this goal are basic and simple; however, the emotional overlay makes the simple difficult. For the new nurse who is confronted with a person's grief for the first time, there may be discomfort, fear, and insecurity. The tendency is to be sympathetic rather than empathetic. Questions arise in one's mind: What do I say? Should I be cheerful or serious? Should I talk about or even mention the dead person's name?

Nursing interventions, especially when elders are in crisis, begin with the gentle establishment of rapport. Nurses introduce themselves, explain the nature of their roles (e.g., charge nurse, staff nurse, medication nurse) and the time available. If it is the time of *impact* (e.g., just after a new serious diagnosis, at the death of a family member, or upon becoming a new but resistant resident of a long-term care facility), the most we can do is to provide support and a safe environment and ensure that basic needs, such as meals, are met. The nurse can soften the despair by fostering reasonable hope, such as, "You will make it through this time, one moment at a time, and I will be here to help."

Nurses observe for *functional disruption* and offer support and direction. They may have to help the family figure out what has to be done immediately and find ways to do it—either the nurse offers to complete the task or finds a friend or family member who can step in so the disruption does not have any deleterious effects.

As grievers *search for meaning*, they may need help finding what they are looking for. Sometimes it is information about a disease, a situation, or a person. Sometimes it is a spiritual search and help in finding a resource or a place of peace, such as the chapel. Often what is needed most is someone to listen to the "whys" and "hows"—questions that cannot be answered.

Sometimes nurses offer to contact others for those who are grieving, thinking that this is something that will help. However it is far more therapeutic for grievers to be the ones who *inform others* because it helps the reality of the loss become real. The nurse can offer to find a phone number or hold the griever's hand during the conversation or just "be there" when the news is being shared. In this way the nurse can be available to provide support when the griever's emotions engage.

As the elder moves forward in adjusting to the loss, such as a move from home to a nursing home, the nurse can help the person *reorganize the structure* of life. The nurse talks with the elder about what was most valued about living at home and what habits were comforting, and finds ways to incorporate these in a new way into the new environment. If the elder does not have access to a kitchen and always had a cup of tea before bed, this can become part of the individualized plan of care.

According to the Loss Response Model, *memories are reframed* in order for the cycle of grieving to be completed. The grandmother who had always hosted her eldest daughter's birthday party can still do that even if she is now a resident in a long-term care facility. When the nurse has the information about this important ritual, she or he can help the person reserve a private space, send out invitations, and have the birthday party as always, just reframed in that it is catered by the facility in the elder's new "home."

Countercoping

Avery Weisman (1979) also described the work of health care professionals related to grief as "countercoping." Although he was speaking of working with people with cancer, it is equally applicable to working with people who are grieving for any loss. "Countercoping is like counterpoint in music, which blends melodies together into a basic harmony. The patient copes; the therapist [nurse] countercopes; together they work out a better fit" (Weisman, 1979, p. 109). Weisman suggests four very specific types of interventions or countercoping strategies: (1) clarification and control, (2) collaboration, (3) directed relief, and (4) cooling off.

Clarification and Control. The nurse helps the person cope with loss by helping him or her confront the loss by getting or receiving information, considering alternatives, and finding a way to make the grief manageable. The nurse helps the person resume control by encouraging him or her to avoid acting on impulse.

Collaboration. The nurse collaborates by encouraging the griever to share stories with others and repeat the stories as often as is necessary as he or she "talks it out." The nurse as a collaborator is more directive than usual; it may be acceptable to say, "No, this is not a good time to make any major decisions."

Directed Relief. Some temporary directed relief may be necessary, especially during acute grief. Catharsis may be helpful. In many instances it is the nurse who encourages the griever to cry or otherwise express feelings such as hurt or anger. The nurse may have to say something like, "Expressing your feelings might help." Activity may also be recommended as a natural extension of feelings. Intense physical activity gives one emotional relief. In some cultures, people may tear their clothes or cut their hair. Today, there are numerous ways of acting out feelings—from throwing things, to taking a walk, to busying oneself with tasks, to expressing feelings through creative works.

Cooling Off. From time to time the griever might be encouraged to temporarily avoid active mourning through diversions that worked in the past during times of stress, especially when things have to be done or decisions have to be made. The nurse may need to suggest new tactics that may prove helpful. Although there is considerable cultural variation, cooling off also means encouraging the person to modulate emotional extremes and to think about ways to make sense of the loss, to build a new sense of self-esteem after the loss, and help reestablish life patterns.

In all interventions related to grief, the nurse must have skills in therapeutic communication. Active listening is greatly preferable to giving advice. When listening, the nurse soon discovers that it is not the actual loss that is of utmost concern, but rather the fear associated with the loss. If the nurse listens carefully to both the stated and the implied, what will be heard may be expressions such as the following: "How will I go on?" "What will I do now?" "What will become of me?" "I don't know what to do." "How could he (she) do this to me?" Because the nurse knows there will be resolution of some kind, such comments may seem exaggerated or melodramatic, but to the one who is grieving there seems to be no resolution. The person who is actively grieving cannot yet look ahead and know that the despair and other feelings will resolve. Like good copers, good gerontological nurses must be flexible, practical, resourceful, and abundantly optimistic.

DEATH AND DYING

Many people have said that death is not the problem, it is the dying that takes the work. This is true for all involved: the person who is dying, the loved ones, and the professional caregivers, such as the nurses and, in long-term care facilities, the nursing assistants.

Dying is both a challenging life experience and a private one. How one deals with dying is a reflection of one's culture and the way the person has handled earlier losses and stressors. Most people probably do die as they have lived. Although not all older adults have had fulfilling lives or have a sense of completion, transcendence, or self-actualization, their deaths at the age or after that of their parents are considered normative. If the dying process is particularly long or the death occurs after a painful illness, we may rationalize it or view it as a relief, at least in part. Death at a younger age or as the result of trauma or catastrophe is viewed as tragic and sometimes incomprehensible. After 9/11 no one rationalized the deaths of the older victims as a relief; all deaths were considered an unacceptable loss of human potential.

Conceptual Models

As models have been proposed to explain the grieving process, so have they been proposed for the process of dying. One of the most well known has been that of Dr. Elizabeth Kübler-Ross. In her book *On Death and Dying* (1969) she reported on her observations of inpatients on the psychiatric ward where she did her psychiatry residency. She proposed the stages of dying as denial, anger, bargaining, depression, and acceptance. Nurses and many others have tried to help the dying work through denial to achieve acceptance before their deaths. However, we have come to realize that the "stages" are actually types of emotional reactions to dying that people experience, and not a model at all. An alternative model that has been very useful to nursing practice is presented below.

The Living-Dying Interval

Whereas physically we may begin dying early in life, as proposed by the theories of aging (see Chapter 6), in personal terms dying begins at a moment called the "crisis knowledge of death" (Pattison, 1977, p. 44) and ends at the moment of physiological death. Pattison (1977) calls the time between these two points the living-dying interval, made up of the acute, chronic, and terminal phases. The chronological time of the living-dying interval is accordion-like because of remissions and exacerbations in the terminal diagnosis; it may last days, weeks, months, or years. The manner in which one faces dying is an expression of personality, circumstances, illness, and culture.

The "crisis knowledge of death" occurs when someone receives the information that he or she will not live as long as previously anticipated. Certainly it would appear that the greater the discrepancy between the previously assumed length of life and the newly projected length of life, the greater the adjustment and perhaps the intensity of the grief experienced.

The point of crisis is a moment in time that is followed by an acute phase. It is usually the peak time of stress and anxiety since the life and future of the individual and the family is thrown into disequilibrium. Crisis intervention is most effective here because the individual, the family, and the caregivers are struggling to come to terms with the knowledge. A significant amount of anticipatory grieving may be observed.

Since no one can withstand a crisis indefinitely, most of the dying time is spent in the chronic phase. During this time the dying and those about them are forced to resume some sense of normalcy. Bills still need to be paid, dishes still need to be done, and life can still be lived. The challenge for persons with terminal diagnoses and their families is to work toward living while dying and not dying while still living. Entertainment, work, and relationships can be maintained as normally as the individual's condition permits. Life goes on despite the anticipation of its end.

The terminal phase is reached when the speed of the physical dying is accelerated and the person no longer has the energy to maintain the activities of everyday life. The person may withdraw or turn away from the outside world; or the person may engage in coded communication, such as saying "good-bye" instead of the usual "good night," giving away cherished possessions as gifts, or urgently contacting friends and relatives with whom he or she has not communicated for a long time. The focus then turns to preserving energy and completing life's journey. In some cultures this period of time is called the "death watch" and is associated with prescribed rituals.

The living-dying interval can reflect an integrated or disintegrated trajectory (Figure 25-2) (Pattison, 1977). The interval is integrated when each new crisis occurs, is dealt with effectively, and the quality of life while dying is preserved. The interval is disintegrated

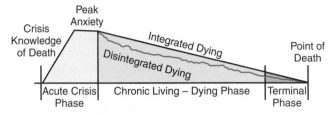

Fig. 25-2 The living-dying interval. *(From Pattison EM: The experience of dying, Englewood Cliffs, NJ, 1977, Prentice-Hall.)*

if one crisis tumbles on to the next one without any effective resolution and the quality of life while dying is compromised.

THE NEEDS OF THE DYING AND THEIR FAMILIES AND IMPLICATIONS FOR GERONTOLOGICAL NURSING

The needs of the dying are like threads in a piece of cloth. Each thread is individual but necessary to the integrity and completeness of the fabric. If one thread is pulled, it affects the other threads, and the material's appearance, the thread placement, and the stability of the cloth. When one need is unmet it will affect all others because they are interdependent and interwoven.

The responsibility of the nurse is to provide safe conduct as the dying and their families navigate through unknown waters to a good and appropriate death. A good and appropriate death is one that a person would choose if choosing were possible. A good and appropriate death is one in which one's needs are met to the extent possible. There are several ways to approach an understanding of the needs of persons who are dying and the responsibilities of the nurse. The approaches discussed here can be called the 6 C's approach.

The 6 C's Approach

Weisman (1984) identified six needs of the dying: *c*are, *c*ontrol, *c*omposure, *c*ommunication, *c*ontinuity, and *c*losure.

Care

Persons who are dying should have the best care possible; this includes expert management of symptoms and support at all times. Care includes the adequate treatment of pain (see Chapter 16). Care also goes beyond the physical to psychological pain, induced by depression, anxiety, fear, and other unresolved emotional concerns that are just as strong and just as real. When emotional needs are not met, the total pain experience is intensified. Medication alone cannot relieve pain. Instead, empathic listening and allowing the person to verbalize his or her thoughts is an important intervention (see Chapter 4). If tears and sadness are present, gentleness of touch, closeness, and sitting near the person are helpful, when culturally appropriate. As an advocate, the gerontological nurse also makes sure that the medical care that is needed is received.

Caring for the dying also means helping the patient conserve energy. Dying calls for great amounts of energy to cope with the emotional and physical assault of illness on the body. How much can the individual do without becoming physically and emotionally taxed? What activities of daily living are most important for the person to do independently? How much energy is needed for the patient to be able to talk with visitors or staff without becoming exhausted? Only the person can answer these questions and the nurse can advocate for the person to be given the opportunity to do so; and in doing so, the patient is able to remain in better control and maintain composure.

Control

As one proceeds along the living-dying interval it often feels that control over one's life has been lost. The person is in the process of losing everything he or she has every known or would ever know. The potential loss of identity, independence, and control over body functions can lead to a sense of having lost control and self-esteem. The person may begin to feel ashamed, humiliated, and like a "burden." Control is the need to remain in a collaborative role relating to one's own living and dying and as active a participant in one's care as desired. The nurse can help the person meet these needs by taking every opportunity to return the control to the person and in doing so bolster the patient's self-esteem. Whenever possible the nurse can have the person decide when to groom, eat, wake, sleep, and so forth. The nurse never has the right to determine the activities of the individual, especially in relation to visitors and how time is spent.

Composure

In many cultures dying is an emotional activity—for the person and for those around him or her. The need for composure is that which enables the person to modulate emotional extremes as is appropriate within cultural norms. This is not to avoid the sadness; this is to have moments of relief. The nurse may use many of the countercoping techniques discussed earlier to help persons meet this need.

Communication

The need for communication is broad, from the need for information to make decisions to the need to share information. Although the type and content of communication that is acceptable to the person varies by culture, the nurse has a responsibility to make sure that the dying person has an opportunity for the communication he or she desires (see Chapter 3).

In a study of communication among the patient, family, and hospital staff about terminal illness, Glaser and Strauss (1963) identified four types: *closed awareness, suspected awareness, mutual pretense,* and *open awareness.* Each of these influences the work on the hospital unit and the care of the patient.

Closed awareness is described as "keeping the secret." Hospital staff and the family and friends know that the patient is dying, but the patient does not know it or knows and keeps the secret as well. Generally, caregivers invent a fictitious future for the patient to believe in, in hopes that it will boost the patient's morale. Although this happens less today because of legislation related to patients' rights, it still occurs. In some cultures it is expected.

In *suspected awareness*, the person suspects he or she is dying, but since it is not discussed it cannot be confirmed. Inquiries on the part of the person are indirect or avoided by others. Hints are bandied back and forth, and a contest ensues for control of the information.

Mutual pretense is a situation of "let's pretend." Everyone knows the patient has a terminal illness, but no one talks about it—real feelings are kept hidden.

Open awareness occurs when the patient, family, friends, nurses, and physicians openly acknowledge the eventual death of the patient. The patient may ask, "Will I die?" and "How and when will I die?"

The patient becomes resigned to dying, and the family grieves with the patient rather than for the patient. The nurse can encourage open awareness whenever possible while at the same time respecting the patient's culture. In some cultures, talking about an anticipated death is deemed helpful. In others, one can be aware of the dying but talking about it openly may be taboo.

Continuity

The need for continuity equates to preserving as normal a life as possible while dying and transcending the present by leaving a legacy for the future. Too often a dying patient can feel shut off from the rest of the world at a time when he or she is still capable of being involved and active in some way. Loneliness is the result of a loss of continuity with one's life. The nurse may ask about the person's life and those things most valued, and work with the family and the patient or resident on a plan to remain engaged in as many of the activities and past roles as possible. A father who watches a certain ballgame with his son every Sunday can continue to do this regardless of the need to be in a hospital, a nursing home, or an inpatient hospice unit. If the person is at home and is bedridden, it may make more sense to have the bed in a central area rather than in a distant room. Treating the person who is dying as an intelligent adult, holding a hand, or putting an arm around a shoulder if culturally acceptable says, "I care" and "You're not alone" and "You are important."

One approach people have taken to obtain continuity of their lives after death is in the establishment of legacies. Legacies can take many different forms and may range from memories that will live on in the minds of others to bequeathed fortunes. A grandmother who is likely to die before a favorite grandchild's wedding can create a legacy when she participates with planning, regardless of the age of the grandchild, thereby leaving an enduring and special legacy.

Closure

The need for closure corresponds to an opportunity for reconciliation and transcendence, the highest of Maslow's hierarchy. Reminiscence is one way of putting one's life in order, to evaluate the pluses and minuses of life. It is a means of resolving conflicts, giving up possessions, and making final good-byes. Learning to say "good-bye" today leaves open the possibility of many more "hellos." Pain and other symptoms that are not well controlled may interfere with this reconciliation, making appropriate interventions by the nurse especially important.

For some, closure means coming to terms with their spiritual selves, with Jesus, God, Allah, or Buddha. If the expressions of the patient have spiritual overtones, arranging for pastoral care may be offered but should never be done without the person's permission. The nurse can foster transcendence by providing patients with the time and privacy for self-reflection as well as an opportunity to talk about whatever they need to talk about, especially about the meanings of their lives and the meanings of their deaths.

Care, control, composure, communication, continuity, and closure create the borders necessary to complete the fabric of needs of the dying. Their influence is omnipresent in the other needs. Without them, the cloth can fray, and attempts to meet the needs will be limited.

The Family

The nurse is often present and supporting the family at the time of death and in the moments preceding it. Regardless of the age of the surviving family members, as spouse, partner, children, or friends, they too have needs, and nurses have a responsibility to care for them. Newly bereaved persons were asked what they had found most helpful (Richter, 1987). They most appreciated nurses who did the following:

▶ Kept me informed
▶ Asked how I was doing and offered support
▶ Put an arm around me when I cried
▶ Brought me food
▶ Knew my name
▶ Cried with me
▶ Brought a bed and encouraged me to stay in the room with my dying husband
▶ Told me to hold my husband's hand while he was dying
▶ Held my hand
▶ Got the chaplain for me
▶ Let me take care of my husband
▶ Stayed with me after their shift was over

Although these will not provide comfort to all, nor are all these behaviors always possible, they can be used as starting points.

DYING AND THE NURSE

Nurses are professional grievers. We invest time and caring, and if working with older adults, especially those who are frail and in acute and long-term care settings, we experience the death of patients and residents over and over again. Some consider the death of a patient as a failure, that they have "lost" the person they cared for; yet, when they are good deaths, they can be viewed as professional successes each time we share the special and very personal experience of providing safe conduct for elders while dying and gentle caring for their survivors. We can use the reminders of our own mortality as motivation to live the best we can with what we have. Nurses can seek support and give it to one another. As grievers, we too may need to tell the story of the dying, or the person, to those professionals around us, either in formal or informal support groups; and we must listen to those stories of our colleagues over and over again until they become part of the fabric of our colleagues' lives as well.

Caring for older adults requires knowledge of the grieving and dying processes as well as skills in providing relief of symptoms or palliative care. However, it is also acknowledged that working with the grieving or dying day in and day out is an art. The development of the art calls for inner strength and coping skills. The most important coping skills for nurses may be meaning-making and the ability to disengage (Desbiens and Fillion, 2007). The effective gerontological nurse has developed a personal philosophy of life and of death. Although this can and does change over time, it will help when times are difficult. Emotional maturity allows the nurse to deal with disappointment and postponement of immediate wants or desires. Maturity means that the nurse can reach out for help when needed. Finally, in order to provide comfort to grieving persons, nurses must be comfortable with their own lives or at least be able to set aside their own sadness and grief while working with the sadness and grief of others.

Palliative Care

Nurses routinely care for elders who have irreversible and progressive conditions, such as Alzheimer's disease and Parkinson's disease. Other elders have exhausted all treatment options or have decided that they want no further treatment for conditions such as cancer or end-stage heart or renal disease. A nursing home resident may elect to remain at the facility rather than return (ever) to a hospital, even if faced with an acute event, such as a myocardial infarction (MI) or stroke. They are receiving a type of care called *palliative care*, or that which focuses on comfort rather than cure, on the treatment of symptoms rather than disease, on quality of life left rather than quantity of life lived. *Open awareness* of dying is a requirement for hospice care (see following section); however, there is current (2007-2008) activity to incorporate other customs that are not based on such awareness for those preferring *mutual pretense* during the dying process, but are nonetheless in need of palliative care (Copp and Field, 2002). Palliative care comprises much of what is done in gerontological nursing and may indeed be the heart of caring. Some type of palliative care can be provided anywhere by anyone sharing these goals and skills.

The scope and specialty of palliative care has grown considerably over the years; research has been conducted, professional organizations have been formed, and standardized curricula have been developed. With the support of the American Association of Colleges of Nursing and City of Hope Medical Center a broad initiative was initiated in 1999 to train nurses through the End of Life Nursing Consortium (ANA-ELNEC) (www.aacn.nche.edu/ELNEC). It is hoped that by training nurses and faculty, nursing as a profession can provide the highest level of palliative care.

Whereas initially palliative care was the specialty of community-based hospices, specialized units and staff are now seen in long-term care and acute care facilities across the United States. Palliative care was originally not well reimbursed, but since a hospice benefit was added to Medicare Part A in the 1980s, some level of skilled palliative care is usually a covered service under most insurance plans (see Chapter 22).

Hospice

The term "hospice" refers to a formalized structure from which a significant amount of the palliative care in the United States is delivered. It gets its meaning from the medieval concept of hospitality in which a community assisted a traveler at dangerous points along his or her journey. Hospice has been a vehicle to help return nursing to its roots—as humane compassionate care, an ideal that has been the basis of nursing for centuries. The dying are indeed travelers—travelers along the continuum of life—and the community consists of friends; family; and specially prepared people to care, the hospice team.

The concept of the contemporary hospice was made famous by Dr. Cicely Saunders, founder of Saint Christopher's Hospice in London more than 30 years ago. Both for-profit and not-for-profit hospice organizations are now all over the United States and provide comprehensive and interdisciplinary care to persons assessed to be in the last 6 months of life. Under Medicare, a Hospice organization must provide medical, nursing, nursing assistant, chaplain, social work,

and volunteer support 24 hours per day. Additional services may include massage, music, art, and pet therapy and others. Hospices provide care not only to the dying but also to their families and friends through support before and after the death of loved ones.

The majority of hospice care is provided at home. The home becomes the primary center of care, provided by family members or friends, who are taught basic nursing care and how to administer the medication needed to provide comfort for their loved one who is dying. A growing number of in-patient hospice facilities exist as well. These have developed from home-based programs that have added free-standing, small in-patient facilities for those with symptoms that could not be managed at home and those without caregivers. Hospice nurses and others may also see patients who are residents in long-term care facilities and work with the staff to supplement care and provide expertise in symptom management. Long-term care facilities may also provide palliative care services guided by formal hospice principles. Pain control and the opportunity to die at home are the key ideas and activities that people associate with hospice services. In actuality, hospice represents much more. It supports and guides the family in patient care and ensures that the patient will not die alone and that the family will not be abandoned. Bereavement services for the family extend for a period of time on an emergency and regular basis after the death of the patient.

The Nurse's Role in Hospice Care

Palliative care nursing is the cornerstone of hospice care. The nurse provides much of the direct care and functions in a variety of roles: as staff nurse giving direct care, as coordinator implementing the plan of the interdisciplinary team or as executive officer responsible for clinical care, and as an advocate for humane care for persons who are dying and their families.

The American Nurses Association's *Standards and Scope of Hospice and Palliative Nursing Practice* (2002) enumerates the special skills, knowledge, and abilities needed by a nurse who provides end of life care:

1. Thorough knowledge of anatomy and physiology and considerable familiarity with pathophysiological causes of numerous diseases
2. Well-grounded skill in physical assessment and in various nursing procedures, such as catheterization and colostomy and traction care
3. Above-average knowledge of pharmacology, especially of analgesics, narcotics, antiemetics, tranquilizers, antibiotics, hormone therapy, steroids, cardiotonic agents, and cancer chemotherapy

4. Skill in using psychological principles in individual and group situations
5. Great sensitivity in human relationships
6. Personal characteristics such as stamina, emotional stability, flexibility, cooperativeness, and a life philosophy or faith
7. Knowledge of measures to comfort the dying in the last hours

The Hospice and Palliative Care Nurses Association provides guidance in end-of-life care. These guidelines bring gerontological theory, nursing concepts, and knowledge of medical management of acute and chronic conditions of elders together to provide the most sensitive and comprehensive care possible.

DECISION MAKING AT END OF LIFE

Decision making at the end of life has become a legal, ethical, medical, and personal concern. The lines between living and dying are blurred as a direct result of technological advances. This now allows ambivalence concerning whether death is to be delayed, fought or accepted.

The issue of who has the authority to make end-of-life decisions and for whom has been the subject of research, debate, and federal legislation. An adult is recognized as the decision maker; however, this assumption is based on a very Euro-American or Western perspective. Persons who are from non-Western traditions place less emphasis on the individual and more on the needs of the family or community (Mazanec and Tyler, 2003). Nurses have an obligation to know legal requirements in their jurisdictions and then work with the elder and the family to determine how these will fit with their cultural patterns and their needs as they relate to end-of-life decisions.

Advance Directives

Whereas people have always had opinions about their wishes, their right to refuse medical treatment was legislated in the United States by the Patient Self-Determination Act (PSDA) in 1990 and implemented in all states in 1991. Under the PSDA, the adult was recognized as the ultimate authority in the decision to forego life-sustaining treatment for himself or herself, rather than a physician or a health care agency. In other words, through the PSDA, adults were granted the legal authority to complete what are known as advance directives—or statements about their wishes, or directions to others—before the need for a decision arises.

These directives may be as detailed or as vague as desired, from "no treatment if I am terminally ill" to a breakdown of decisions about dialysis, antibiotics, tube feedings, cardiopulmonary resuscitation (CPR), and so on. Through the PSDA, any adult may also appoint another adult of his or her choosing to make decisions if he or she is unable to do so.

Two common forms of advance directives are known as living wills and durable power of attorney for health care (DPAHC), also called an advance health care directive (AHCD) (see Chapter 22). A living will is restricted to represent a person's wishes specific to the condition of a terminal illness. In most states a proxy may be appointed in a living will to speak on behalf of the person if he or she is unable to do so. In contrast, a person appointed in a DPAHC, called a health care surrogate, can speak for the other in all matters of health care. However, in some states the surrogate cannot make decisions related to withdrawal of life support. In many states, advance directives are legally binding documents that nurses, physicians, and health care institutions are required to respect. Both the proxy and the health care surrogate are expected to use what is known as *substituted judgment*. Substituted judgment means that the decision made on behalf of the other is believed to be the decision that he or she would make if able to do so.

All agencies in the United States that receive Medicare and Medicaid funds are mandated to disseminate PSDA information to their clients and inquire as to the existence of advance directives. Hospitals and long-term care facilities are responsible for providing written information at the time of admission about the individual's rights under law to both refuse medical and surgical care and to provide this decision in writing in advance. Health maintenance organizations (HMOs) are required to do the same at the time of member enrollment, as are home health agencies before the patient comes under the care of the agency. Hospices are obliged to inform patients of their self-determination rights on the initial visit. Providers (physicians and nurse practitioners) are encouraged but are not under obligation to provide this same information to their patients.

Although the exact format and signature (e.g., notarization) requirements vary from state to state, the PSDA is a federal mandate and applies to persons in all jurisdictions. There are several clearinghouses of related information, including www.fivewishes.com, where persons can obtain information relevant to their state and forms can be ordered or downloaded.

Although the nurse cannot provide legal information, she or he does serve as a resource person ready to answer many of the questions people have about end-of-life decision making. The nurse may be called not only to inquire about the presence of an existing advance directive, but also to ensure that the directive still reflects the person's wishes and advocate for the wishes to be followed. The nurse also has the responsibility to make sure that existing or newly created advance directives are available in the appropriate locations in the medical record (for information about advanced directive information by state see www.noah-health.org/en/rights/endoflife/adforms.html).

Euthanasia

The recognition of a patient's right to refuse life-sustaining medical measures renewed age-old questions over the patient's right to make decisions about the continuation of life. Some people, especially those who are suffering unremitting pain from a terminal illness, have ended their lives. Others have asked for assistance in accomplishing this in the most painless way possible (see Box 25-3).

In May 1992 the *Journal of the American Medical Association* reported that 73% of the general public in a large sample approved of some form of euthanasia. *Physician-assisted death, physician-assisted suicide, physician aid in dying*, and *passive* and *active euthanasia* are all terms that are heard. An example of physician-assisted suicide might be the physician providing the patient with sleeping pills and instructions about a lethal dose. This form is considered passive euthanasia because the physician has not administered the dose that results in death. The person who injects a lethal dose into a patient who voluntarily requested to be helped to die would be practicing active euthanasia, as in capital punishment.

In 1994 and again in 1997, voters in the state of Oregon passed the Death with Dignity Law, and Oregon became the first state in the United States to legalize physician-assisted suicide in the form of passive euthanasia (see the Legislative report found at www. leg.state.vt.us/reports/05Death/Death_With_Dignity_ Report.htm#Section1). This law enables an Oregon resident who is (1) a terminally ill adult for whom death is anticipated within 6 months, (2) a resident of Oregon and (3) able to make and communicate health care decisions, to obtain the assistance of a physician for the purpose of obtaining a dignified death at a time and in a manner of his or her choosing. The additional criteria required before the request can be granted are stringent and include one written and two oral requests at 15-day intervals followed by a 15-day waiting period to certify the person's desire to end his or her life. Two physicians must certify the diagnosis, the prognosis, the person's competency, and the voluntary nature of the request. The prescribing physician may request but not require that the person notify next-of-kin of the decision. The individual must be counseled on alternatives and receive counseling from a pharmacist. If these criteria are met, the patient's request is granted, and he or she may receive a prescription of a lethal dose of a medication from the physician. The person then decides if and when the dose is taken; it cannot be in the presence of the prescribing physician (State of Oregon 2007a). In 1998 the U.S. Attorney General tried various ways of preventing the enactment of this law; however, the voters' right to make this decision has been upheld. Legislation has been attempted in California, Hawaii, and Vermont, but has not succeeded (Pew Foundation, 2007a and 2007b). In 2008 a referendum to legalize physician-assisted suicide passed in the state of Washington, and it is anticipated that when enacted it will be similar to that of Oregon's. Physician-assisted suicide is permitted in the Netherlands and Belgium as well as Oregon (Pew Foundation, 2008).

The number of persons who have received lethal does of medications has increased steadily since 1998 to 85 persons in 2007. However, the number of persons who used their prescriptions has remained fairly steady since 2002, with a total of only 49 suicides since the law was inacted in 2007 (State of Oregon, 2007b). Instead of increasing the number of deaths to any significance, the impact of this law on the public has been an improvement in end-of-life care.

Box 25-3	Can I Help You?

As a nurse practitioner, I visited a nursing home resident. One day when checking on a woman with end-stage pulmonary disease, I asked, "Is there anything I can do for you at this time?" She responded quickly asking if I knew how she could reach Dr. Kevorkian*, a physician known for assisted suicide. I knew then that I had to be much more proactive in finding ways to make her more comfortable while she waited for death.

Kathleen Jett at 40

*See www.msnbc.msn.com/id/18974940.

Nurses have had strong opinions both for and against assisted, passive euthanasia. The American Nurses Association leaders as well as those from the End-of-Life Care Center at Johns Hopkins continues to examine this evolving issue. The nurse is involved in many end-of-life care situations because she or he is the primary care provider who implements the decisions of others around end-of-life care. However, such advice should not mean patients who want to end their lives should be abandoned.

Considerable confusion exists regarding terminology and interpretation of what effects the nurse's role may have. Many nurses believe that turning off the ventilator, turning off tube feedings, stopping intravenous fluids, or giving as much pain medication as is needed, even as directed by the patient, if the side effect is death, constitutes assisted suicide. Another perspective is that withdrawal of such devices is allowing natural death to occur, which is very different from actively doing something to cause death. Nurses individually and collectively must consider the implication of this for themselves and our profession.

KEY CONCEPTS

▶ Grief is an emotional and behavioral response to loss. Grief responses are individual; what is appropriate for a person from one ethnic group may be considered inappropriate by another.

▶ One never completely resolves grief. Instead, the individual incorporates the loss as a part of his or her life.

▶ Dying is a multifaceted, active process. It affects all involved: the one who is dying, the family, and the professional caregivers.

▶ The stages or phases of dying and the type of coping are not obligatory and do not prescribe the way one should die. Such expectations place an added burden on the one who is dying.

▶ The dying older adult is a living person with all the same needs for good and natural relationships with people as the rest of us.

▶ Hospice is both a concept and a health care program that focuses on care rather than cure and on the provision of comfort for the person who is dying and for significant others.

▶ Advance directives allow an individual control over life and death decisions by written communication and the appointment of a person (a proxy) to be the individual's advocate when he or she is not able to personally communicate his or her desires.

ACTIVITIES AND DISCUSSION QUESTIONS

1. Explore your response to being given a terminal diagnosis. What coping mechanisms work for you? With which awareness approach would you be comfortable?
2. Describe how you would deal with a dying person and his or her family when they are especially protective of one another.
3. Describe and strategize how you would bring up the topic of advance directives.
4. What advance directive is legally recognized in your state?
5. Describe how you would introduce the topic of dying with a patient who is critically ill and not expected to live.

RESOURCES

Websites

Association for Death Education and Counseling
www.adec.org

National Effort to Improve End of Life Nursing Care
www.aacn.nche.edu

National Hospice and Palliative Care Nurses Association
www.hpna.org

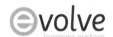

For additional resources, please visit evolve.elsevier.com/Ebersole/gerontological.

REFERENCES

American Nurses Association: *Standards and scope of hospice and palliative nursing practice,* Kansas City, Mo, 2002, The Association. Available at www.ana.org. Accessed 7/25/08.

Canavan K: ANA advises nurses not to participate in assisted suicide: RNs should consider implications of possible legalization, *Am Nurse* 28(4):8, 1996.

Chow A, Chan C, Ho S: Social sharing of bereavement experience by Chinese bereaved persons in Hong Kong, *Death Stud* 31(7):601-618, 2007.

Copp G, Field D: Open awareness and dying: the use of denial and acceptance as coping strategies by hospice patients. *Nurs Times Res* 7(2):118-127, 2002.

Coryell D: Good grief: healing through the shadow of grief, Rochester, Vt, 2007, Healing Arts Press.

Desbiens J, Fillion L: Coping strategies, emotional outcomes and spiritual quality of life in palliative care nurses, *Int J Palliat Nurs* 13(6):291-300, 2007.

Doka KJ: The spiritual crisis of bereavement. In Doka KJ, Morgan JD, editors: *Death and spirituality,* Amityville, NY, 1993, Baywood.

Doka KJ: Disenfranchised grief: new direction, challenges, and strategies for practice, Champaign, IL, 2002, Research Press.

Gerdner LA, Yang D, Cha D, Tripp-Reimer T: The circle of life, *J Gerontol Nurs* 33(5):20-31, 2007.

Giacquinta B: Helping families face the crisis of cancer, *Am J Nurs* 77(10):1585-1588, 1977.

Glaser BG, Strauss AL: *Awareness of dying,* Chicago, 1963, Aldine.

Glaser BG, Strauss AL: *Time for dying,* Chicago, 1968, Aldine.

Jett KF: *The loss response model,* Unpublished manuscript, 2004.

Kübler-Ross E: *On death and dying,* New York, 1969, Macmillan.

Lewis ID, McBride M: Anticipatory grief and chronicity: elders and families in racial/ethnic minority groups, *Geriatr Nurs* 25(1):44-47, 2004.

Mazanec P, Tyler MK: Cultural considerations in end-of-life care: how ethnicity, age and spirituality affect decisions when death is imminent, *Am J Nurs* 103(3):50-59, 2003.

Metzger PL, Gray MJ: End-of-life communication and adjustment: pre-loss communication as a predictor of bereavement-related outcomes, *Death Stud* 32(4):301-325, 2008.

National Cancer Institute (NCI): Culture and response to grief and mourning. 2006. Available at www.cancer.gov/cancertopics/pdq/supportivecare/bereavement/Patient/page10. Accessed 7/26/08.

Pattison EM: The experience of dying. In Pattison EM, editor: *The experience of dying,* Englewood Cliffs, NJ, 1977, Prentice-Hall.

Pew Foundation: *The right-to-die debate and the tenth anniversary of Oregon's death with dignity act.* October 9, 2007a. Available at http://pewforum.org/docs/?DocID=251. Accessed 7/25/08.

Pew Foundation: Oregon's death with dignity Law: 10 years later. October 10, 2007b. Available at http://pewforum.org/events/?EventID=155. Accessed 7/25/08.

Pew Foundations: Landscape evolves for assisted suicide. November 10, 2008. Available at http://pewforum.org/news/rss.php?NewsID=16905. Accessed 11/17/08.

Richter JM: Support: a resource during crisis of mate loss, *J Gerontol Nurs* 13(11):18-22, 1987.

Rodgers LS: Meaning of bereavement among older African American widows, *Geriatr Nurs* 25(1):10-16, 2004.

Starks H, Back AL, Pearlman RA et al: Family member involvement in hastened death, *Death Stud* 31(2):105-130, 2007.

State of Oregon: Death with dignity. Annual report—2007 summary, 2007a. Accessed 7/26/08 from www.oregon.gov/DHS/ph/pas/docs/Requirements.pdf.

State of Oregon: Annual report, 2007b. Available at www.oregon.gov/DHS/ph/pas/docs/year10.pdf. Accessed 7/26/08.

Taylor DH Jr, Kuchibhatla M, Ostbye T et al: The effect of spousal caregiving and bereavement on depressive symptoms, *Aging Ment Health* 12(1):100-107, 2008.

Ward L, Mathias JL, Hitchings SE: Relationships between bereavement and cognitive functioning in older adults, *Gerontology* 53(6):362-372, 2007.

Weisman A: *Coping with cancer,* New York, 1979, McGraw-Hill.

Weisman A: *The coping capacity: on the nature of being mortal,* New York, 1984, Human Sciences Press.

Worden JW: *Grief counseling and grief therapy: a handbook for mental health practitioners,* ed 4, New York, 2003, Springer.

Care Across
the Continuum

26

A mobile, youth-oriented society may find it difficult to fully comprehend the insecurity that elders feel when moving from one site to another in their later years. In addition to the stress of relocation and the initial anxiety of adapting to a new setting, elders typically move to ever more restrictive environments, often in times of crisis. This chapter discusses residential care options across the continuum with related implications for nursing practice. The major issues are the choice and control elders have about relocation, assistance provided to the elder in making personally appropriate choices, strategies to ease the transition between settings, and creation of environments that enhance care outcomes in whatever situation the elder is encountering.

RESIDENTIAL OPTIONS IN LATE LIFE

"Home" provides basic shelter, is a place to establish security, and is the place where one "belongs." It should provide the highest possible level of independence, function, and comfort. Most older people prefer to remain in their own homes and "age-in-place," rather than relocate, particularly to institutional living. The ability to age in place depends on appropriate support for changing needs so the older person can stay where he or she wants. Developing elder-friendly communities and increasing opportunities to "age in place" can enhance the health and well-being of older people. Many state and local city governments are assessing the community and designing interventions to enhance the ability of older people to remain in their homes and familiar environments. These interventions range from adequate transportation systems to home modifications and universal design standards for barrier-free housing. Local area agencies on aging are good sources of information on these kinds of programs. Figure 26-1 presents elements of an elder-friendly community.

With the aging of the baby boomers, architects are focusing on home design that adjusts to the changes that may accompany aging and allows people to stay in their homes safely even if they experience illness and functional decline. These new designs are being marketed as transgenerational or universal design and can benefit everyone, not just older people. Designs and modifications may include safety fittings in the bathroom, walk-in showers, wider doorways, remote-controlled devices for lights and window coverings, raised counter tops, polyurethane or cork flooring, and adjustable-height sinks.

Some older people, by choice or by need, move from one type of residence to another. A number of options exist, especially for those with the financial resources that allow them to have a choice. Residential options range along a continuum from remaining in one's own home; to senior retirement communities; to shared housing with family members, friends, or others; to residential care communities such as assisted living settings; to, for those with the most needs, nursing facilities (Figure 26-2). There are many different models of senior housing, and older people may seek assistance from gerontological nurses in choosing what kind of living situation will be best for them. It is important to be aware of the various options available in your local community.

Shared Housing

Shared housing among adult children and their older relatives has become a choice for many because of cultural preferences or need. The sharing may relieve the economic burdens of maintaining a home after widowhood or retirement on a fixed income. However, strong cultural influences predict the frequency of multigenerational residences. Among Asians, South Americans, and African Americans, it is often an expectation. Relocating from one's own home to the home of an adult child can have many benefits, but without adequate preparation it can also be stressful. Interventions to prevent relocation crisis are discussed later in the chapter. Box 26-1 presents some factors to consider when planning to add an older person to the household.

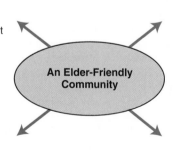

Addresses Basic Needs

- Provides appropriate and affordable housing
- Promotes safety at home and in the neighborhood
- Ensures no one goes hungry
- Provides useful information about available services

Optimizes Physical and Mental Health and Well-Being

- Promotes healthy behaviors
- Supports community activities that enhance well-being
- Provides ready access to preventive health services
- Provides access to medical, social, and palliative services

Promotes Social and Civic Engagement

- Fosters meaningful connections with family, neighbors, and friends
- Promotes active engagement in community life
- Provides opportunities for meaningful paid and voluntary work
- Makes aging issues a community-wide priority

Maximizes Independence for Frail and Disabled

- Mobilizes resources to facilitate "living at home"
- Provides accessible transportation
- Supports family and other caregivers

An Elder-Friendly Community

Fig. 26-1 Essential elements of an elder-friendly community. (*From Advantage Initiative, Center for Home Care Policy and Research, Visiting Nurse Service of New York [www.vnsny.org/advantage/]*).

Independence

Home ownership
Single-room occupation (SRO)
Condominium ownership
Apartment dwelling
Shared housing
Congregate lifestyles

**Independent to partial
dependence**

Retirement communities
Public housing complexes
Residence with family
Foster homes
Board and care
Residential homes
Continuing care retirement
   communities (CCRCs)

**Partial dependence
to complete dependence**

Nursing facilities
Skilled nursing facilities
Acute care facilities
Inpatient hospice care facilities

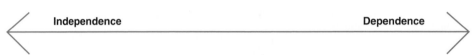

Independence ⟵⟶ Dependence

Fig. 26-2   Continuum of residential options based on level of assistance needed.

A variation of multigenerational housing has long existed in what has become known as "granny flats." These may be apartments added to existing homes or the construction of small housing units on family property with privacy as well as sharing of time and resources. Such arrangements allow families to be close enough to be of assistance if needed but to remain separate. They are practical and economical, and their production has continually expanded, particularly in Australia. In the United States, use of this model is minimal but existing "mother-in-law" cottages and apartments have served a similar purpose for many families for years.

Cohabitation or Group Homes

Another model of shared housing is that of opening homes to others. Older people often live in houses with ample space geared to family life, purchased in their young adult years. It is estimated that one half of the space is underused. Sharing a house can be easily implemented by locating, screening, and matching older people looking for houses to share with those who have them. The National Shared Housing Resource Center (NSHRC) has established subgroups nationally to assist individuals interested in home sharing. Those who have done so report feeling safer and less lonely. Studies on home sharing focus on the effects on well-being, finances, health, social life, and daily satisfaction. Most successful is the intergenerational model, in which an elder with a home locates a younger person to share the home. In each situation, the individuals must consider the following:
▶ Will men and women live together?
▶ Will the house include older peers only or people of all ages?

▶ Will there be equal or reciprocal exchange?
▶ Will the house provide temporary or permanent residence?
▶ Will residents sign an agreement form?
▶ Will residents respect privacy?
▶ What is the motivation for moving into a shared house: financial need, companionship, or services and assistance?

New Models of Community Care

PACE (Program for All Inclusive Care for the Elderly) is an alternative to nursing home care for frail older people who want to live independently in the community with a high quality of life. It provides a comprehensive continuum of primary care, acute care, home care, nursing home care, and specialty care by an interdisciplinary team. PACE is a capitated system in which the team is provided with a monthly sum to provide all care to the enrollees, including medications, eyeglasses, and transportation to care as well as urgent and preventive care. Participants must meet the criteria for nursing home admission, prefer to remain in the community, and be eligible for Medicare and Medicaid. Adult day services are also provided.

PACE is now recognized as a permanent provider under Medicare and a state option under Medicaid. More than two dozen sites serving Medicaid and dually-eligible patients currently are in operation nationwide. Approximately 17,000 persons are being served through the various sites. PACE has been approved by the U.S. Department of Health and Human Services (USDHHS) Substance Abuse and Mental

Box 26-1	Planning to Add an Older Person to the Household

Questions You Should Ask:
- What are the needs of the new member and of the family?
- Where will space be allotted for the new member?
- How will this new member be included in existing family patterns?
- How will responsibilities be shared?
- What resources in the community will assist in the adjustment phase?
- Is the environment safe for this new member?
- How will family life change with the added member, and how does the family feel about it?
- What are the differences in socialization and sleeping patterns?
- What are the older person's strong needs and expectations?
- What are the older person's skills and talents?

Modifications You Have to Make:
- Arrange semiprivate living quarters if possible.
- Regularly schedule visits to other relatives to give each family times of respite and privacy.
- Arrange adult day health programs and senior activities for the older person to help keep contact with members of his or her own generation. Consider how the older person will feel about giving up familiar surroundings and friends.

Discuss Potential Areas of Conflict:
- Space: especially if someone has given up his or her space to the older relative.
- Possessions: older people may want to move possessions into house; others may not find them attractive or may insist on replacing them with new things.

- Entertaining: times when old and young feel the need or desire to exclude the other from social events.
- Responsibilities and chores: the older person may feel useless if he or she does nothing and may feel in the way if he or she does something; young may feel that their position is usurped or may be angry if they are expected to wait on the parent.
- Expenses: increased cost of home maintenance, food, clothing, and recreation may not be shared appropriately.
- Vacations: whether to go together or alone; the young may feel uneasy not taking the older person out and resentful if they must.
- Child rearing: disagreement over child-rearing policies.
- Child care: grandparental babysitting may be welcomed by family and resented by older person; or if not allowed, older person feels lack of trust in capability.

Decrease Areas of Conflict by the Following:
- Respecting privacy
- Discussing space allocations
- Discussing the elder person's furnishings before move
- Making it clear in advance when social events include everyone or exclude someone
- Clearing decisions about household tasks—all should have responsibility geared to ability
- Paying a share of expenses and maintaining a separate phone reduces strain and increases feelings of independence

Health Services Administration (SAMHSA) as an evidence based model of care. Models such as PACE are innovative care delivery models, and continued development of such models are important as the population ages. More information about PACE models and outcomes of care can be found at www.cms.hhs.gov/QualityInitiativesGenInfo/10_PACE.asp and at www.npaonline.org/website/article.asp?id=4.

Adult Day Services

Adult day services are community-based group programs designed to provide social and some health services to adults who need supervised care in a safe setting during the day. They also offer caregivers respite from the responsibilities of caregiving. Most adult day

centers operate during normal business hours 5 days a week, but some offer services in the evening or on weekends. The three types of adult day centers are social (meals, recreation, some health-related services), medical-health (social activities and more intensive health and therapeutic services), and specialized (services provided only to specific care recipients such as those with dementia or developmental disabilities) (National Adult Day Services Association, 2008). On a recent visit to Scotland, one of the authors (T.T.) visited a day program designed to provide respite for people receiving hospice care.

Adult day services are an important part of the long-term care continuum, and more than 150,000 individuals receive care and services at an adult day center

(American Association of Homes and Services for the Aging [AAHSA], 2008). There are 34,000 centers in the United States, and 78% of them are operated on a nonprofit or public basis. Although most of these services are private pay, Medicaid covers the cost in some parts of the country. The national average daily rate is $61/day (includes 8 to 10 hours/day on average) compared to the average rate for home health aides of $19/hour. The average age of an adult day center care recipient is 72 and two thirds are women. Of adult day center recipients, 35% live with an adult child, 20% with a spouse, 18% in an institutional settings, and 3% with parents or other relatives, whereas 11% live alone (National Adult Day Services Association, 2008). Adult day services can assist older people to remain in the community and avoid unnecessary institutionalization. Local area agencies on aging are good sources of information about adult day services and other community-based options.

Senior Retirement Communities

Communities designed for elders are proliferating. Numerous combinations of single-family homes, apartments, activities, optional services, meals in the home, cafeterias, restaurants, housekeeping, golf, tennis, and security are available. In some cases, emergency services and health clinics are adjacent. These are all designed to make independent living feasible with the least effort on the part of the elder. Some senior communities are luxurious and have a wide range of physical and cultural amenities; others are simpler, providing only the basic necessities. Prices are consistent with the level of luxury provided and the range of services available.

Although the costs of the majority of senior communities are borne by the consumers, for elders with limited incomes, federally subsidized rental options are available in some areas of the country. Older adults benefiting from this option are assisted through rental housing subsidized by the U.S. Department of Housing and Urban Development (HUD). Although not all HUD housing is designated for senior living, Section 202 of the Housing Act, U.S. Department of Housing and Urban Development, approved the construction of low-rent units especially for elders. These units may also have provisions for health care, recreation, and transportation. There are more than 300,000 units of Section 202 affordable senior housing available in the United States. For each Section 202 affordable senior housing unit that is available, there are 10 eligible seniors on waiting lists for it. The average time an eligible senior is on the waiting list is 13.4 months (AAHSA, 2008). Under Section 8 of the Housing Act of 1983, tenants locate their own unit. Usually the tenant pays 30% of his or her adjusted gross income toward the rent, and HUD assists with supplementary vouchers to meet the fair market value of the rental.

An ideal public housing complex for low-income older adults will provide modern facilities, security, accessible services, privacy, and some entertainment and activities. An important consideration in planning low-cost housing units for older adults is the potential for evolution of services. Residents rarely move out, and as they age, their ability and independence are likely to decrease. Many cities across the country are developing model public housing for older people combining many of the elements noted in this section. This trend portrays a positive step in supporting elders who want to age in place, regardless of income.

Foster Care

Adult foster care is meant to provide assistive care in a homelike setting that will enhance function and quality of life and allow the elder to remain in a community-based setting. The operational definition of *adult foster care* is as follows: adult foster care offers a community-based living arrangement to adults who are unable to live independently because of physical or mental impairment or disabilities and are in need of supervision or personal care.

Homes providing foster care offer 24-hour supervision, protection, and personal care in addition to room and board. They may also provide additional services. Adult foster care serves a designated, small number of individuals (generally from one to six) in a homelike and family-like environment; one of the primary caregivers often resides in the home. A growing number of foster care homes are under corporate ownership, and in these situations, the home-like atmosphere tends to be lost. However, with state-regulated, outcome-oriented quality assurance strategies focused on achieving maximal function, autonomy, and social integration, adult foster care may fill a real need.

Residential Care Facilities

Residential care facility is the broad term for a range of nonmedical, community-based residential settings that house two or more unrelated adults and provide services such as meals, medication supervision or reminders, activities, transportation, or assistance with activities of daily living (ADLs). These kinds of facilities are for elders who need more care than is available in shared housing or for whom shared housing is not an option and nursing home care is not needed. Residential care facilities are known by more than 30 different names across the country, including *adult congregate facilities, foster care homes, personal care homes, homes for the elderly, domiciliary care homes, board and care homes, rest homes, family care homes, retirement homes*, and *assisted living facilities.*

Residential care facilities are the fastest growing housing option available for older adults in the United States. This kind of facility is viewed as more cost effective than nursing homes while providing more privacy and a homelike environment. Medicare does not cover the cost of care in these types of facilities. In some states, costs may be covered by private and long-term care insurance and some other types of assistance programs. The trend is growing for states to establish waiver programs to extend Medicaid services to this type of housing, but most residents of these types of facilities pay privately for their care. The rates charged and what services those rates include vary considerably, as do regulations and licensing.

Assisted Living. A popular type of residential care can be found in assisted living facilities (ALFs), also called *board and care homes* or *adult congregate living facilities* (ACLFs). There are 38,000 assisted living facilities in the United States, and more than 975,000 individuals live in assisted living residences (The National Center for Assisted Living, 2008). Assisted living is a residential long-term care choice for older adults who need more than an independent living environment can offer but do not need the 24 hours/day skilled nursing care and the constant monitoring of a skilled nursing facility.

The mean age of ALF residents is 85 years, and most are women (Box 26-2). Assisted living settings may be a shared room or a single-occupancy unit with a private bath, kitchenette, and communal meals, but all provide some support services. Assisted living provides security with independence and privacy, and it supports physical and social well-being with the health care supervision it provides.

Assisted living is more expensive than independent living and less costly than skilled nursing home care, but it is not inexpensive. Costs vary by geographical region, size of the unit, and relative luxury. The average monthly cost of living in an assisted facility is $2,969 (AAHSA, 2008). Most ALFs offer two or three meals per day, light weekly housekeeping, and laundry services, as well as optional social activities. Each added service increases the cost of the setting but also allows

Box 26-2	Profile of the Resident of an Assisted Living Facility

- 85 years old
- Female (76%)
- Needs help with at least two activities of daily living (ADLs)
  Bathing: 68%
  Dressing: 47%
  Toileting: 34%
  Transferring: 25%
  Eating: 27%
- Needs help with instrumental activities of daily living (IADLs)
  Housework: 91%
  Medications: 86%
- 50% have Alzheimer's disease or other dementia types of diagnosis
- Length of stay: 27 months
  34% move to a nursing facility
  37% die while a resident

Data from: National Center for Assisted Living: *Assisted living resident profile,* 2006. Available at www.ncal.org. Accessed 8/8/08.

for individuals with resources to remain in the setting longer, as functional abilities decline. Some states provide Medicaid reimbursement for a limited number of low-income seniors who live in modest ALFs, but generally the cost is borne by the consumer.

Many seniors and their families prefer ALFs to nursing homes because they cost less, are more homelike, and offer more opportunities for control, independence, and privacy. However, many residents of ALFs have chronic care needs and over time may require more care than the facility is able to provide. Services (e.g., home health, hospice, homemakers) can be brought into the facility, but some question whether this adequately substitutes for 24-hour supervision by registered nurses (RNs). Not every ALF has an RN or licensed practical–vocational nurse (LPN/LVN), and in most states, any skilled nursing provided by the staff other than nurse-delegated assistance with self-administered medication is prohibited. In the ALF there is no organized team of providers such as that found in nursing homes (nurses, social workers, rehabilitation therapists, pharmacists) (Wendel and Durso, 2006). Wallace (2003) noted that litigation involving ALFs is increasing related to understaffing, inability to meet residents' needs, inadequate staff training, lack of monitoring and medical supervision, and lack of communication with family about changes in residents' status.

With the growing numbers of older adults with dementia residing in ALFs, many are establishing dementia-specific units. It is important to investigate services available as well as staff training when making decisions as to the most appropriate placement for older adults with dementia. Continued research is needed on best care practices as well as outcomes of care for people with dementia in both ALFs and nursing homes. The Alzheimer's Association has issued a set of dementia care practices for ALFs and nursing homes (Alzheimer's Association, 2008) (www.ahca.org/quality/dementia_care_practice_recommendations_05.pdf), and an evidence-based guideline, *Dementia Care Practice Recommendations for Assisted Living Residences and Nursing Homes* (Tilly and Reed, 2008) is available at www.guideline.gov. Further information about dementia can be found in Chapter 21.

The Joint Commission and the Commission for Accreditation of Rehabilitation Facilities have published standards for accreditation of ALFs, but many people are advocating for more comprehensive federal and state standards and regulations. Advanced practice gerontological nurses are well suited to the role of primary care provider in ALFs, and many have assumed this role. The American Assisted Living Nurses Association has established a certification mechanism for nurses working in these facilities and has also developed a *Scope and Standards of Assisted Living Nursing Practice for Registered Nurses* (www.alnursing.org). Further research is needed on care outcomes of residents in ALFs and the role of unlicensed assistive personnel, as well as RNs, in these facilities. However, the nonmedical nature of ALFs is the primary factor in keeping costs down. Consumers are well advised to inquire as to exactly what services will be provided and by whom if an ALF resident becomes more frail and needs more intensive care. The National Center for Assisted Living provides a consumer guide for choosing an assisted living residence (www.longtermcareliving.com/assess/al/assisted8.cfm).

Continuing Care Retirement Communities.
Life care communities, also known as continuing care retirement communities (CCRCs), provide the full range of residential options, from single-family homes to skilled nursing facilities all in one location. Most of these communities provide access to these levels of care for a community member's entire remaining lifetime, and for the right price, the range of services may be guaranteed. Having all levels of care in one location

allows community members to make the transition between levels without life-disrupting moves. For married couples in which one spouse needs more care than the other, life care communities allow them to live nearby in a different part of the same community. This industry is maturing, and there are 1900 CCRCs in the United States, housing more than 745,000 older adults (AAHSA, 2008).

Most CCRCs are non-profit. They usually charge an entry fee ranging from $60,000 to $120,000, that covers and reflects the cost of the residence in which the member will live, the possible future care needed, and the quality and quantity of the community services. The average monthly cost of living in a not-for-profit CCRC is $2,672. Important to remember about these types of communities is that the residence purchased usually belongs to the community after the death of the owner. More information about life care communities is available from the American Association of Homes and Services for the Aging (AAHSA) (www.ahasa.org).

Population-Specific   Communities.
As the number of senior communities expands, older adults will have more options of moving somewhere that they find especially welcoming. These options include communities that emphasize a particular sport, like tennis or golf. Groups of people can also come together to form intentional communities, buying a cluster of home tracts and building in such a way to support their particular lifestyles or needs or personalities. Still others provide unique additional services, such as those in communities that specialize in providing residences for persons with, for example, a mental illness, alcoholism, or developmental disabilities.

Lesbian, gay, bisexual, and transgender (LGBT) seniors face several problems in housing in their older years. They often have little family support and may face discrimination in housing options. Many LGBT seniors say they do not feel welcome at traditional residential options. Those who wish to live together are discouraged from doing so by some organizations. Residential facilities and communities designed specifically for LGBT seniors are increasing in number across the country. Nurses should be aware of this heretofore invisible group of older adults who need access to welcoming resources. Chapter 23 discusses issues specific to LGBT seniors in more depth.

Nursing Homes.
Nursing homes are the settings for the delivery of around-the-clock care for those needing specialized care that cannot be provided elsewhere. When used appropriately, nursing homes fill an important need for families and elders. There are

16,100 certified nursing homes in the United States, and more than 1.4 million older adults reside in nursing homes. The majority of nursing homes are for-profit organizations, with only 31% being managed by non-profit organizations (AAHSA, 2008).

The settings called *nursing homes* most often include up to two levels of care: a *skilled nursing care* (also called *subacute care)* facility is required to have licensed professionals with a focus on the management of complex medical needs; and a *chronic care (*also called *long-term* or *custodial)* facility is required to have 24-hour personal assistance that is supervised and augmented by professional and licensed nurses. The settings that provide chronic care may include dementia-specific units and palliative care units. Often, both kinds of services are provided in one facility (see Chapter 2).

Residents of long-term facilities are predominantly women, 80 years or older, widowed, dependent in ADLs and instrumental activities of daily living (IADLs). More than 50% are cognitively impaired. Nursing homes now provide care for persons admitted under a range of circumstances and health conditions: persons recently discharged from hospitals; frail persons, many with dementia, who need custodial and skilled nursing care; and dying older persons who lack a caregiver or whose caregivers cannot meet their needs for care (Teno, 2002). Nursing homes are increasingly providing end-of-life care. Education in end-of-life care and development of new models of care provision are priorities in this setting. "Good nursing homes provide the essentials of end-of-life care: attention from people who have grown to love you, who care that you are comfortable, who work to help you keep your dignity and self-worth until the end. When a cure is not possible, they move beyond that to palliative care, controlling pain and symptoms while providing emotional and spiritual support. When it's done well, it's a similar experience to being surrounded by a loving family in your own home" (Jarvik and Collins, 2003) (see Chapter 25).

Costs of Care. Costs for nursing homes vary by geographical location, ownership, and amenities, but the average cost is $76,460 a year. The majority of the cost of care in nursing homes is borne by the individuals themselves (40%) and the state-federal Medicaid programs (49%). Medicare covers only the first 20 days of service that qualifies as skilled and rehabilitative and requires a significant copay for the next 80 days if needs for skilled care continue. Complex medical treatments (e.g., feeding tube, tracheostomy, intravenous [IV] therapy) and rehabilitation services such as occupational

therapy (OT), physical therapy (PT), or speech therapy (ST), are considered skilled care. Medicare does not cover the costs of care in chronic, custodial, and long-term units. For example, if the older person is in a skilled unit following surgical repair of a fractured hip, Medicare would cover the total cost for the first 20 days and a copayment would be required if skilled care needs continued, up to a maximum of 80 days. It would be unusual for a person to receive the total 80 days of coverage unless she or he had complex medical needs and treatments. If the older person was admitted to the nursing home because of a dementia diagnosis and the need for assistance with ADLs and maintenance of safety, Medicare would not cover the cost of care unless there was some skilled need. Medicaid does provide coverage for all levels of care. For many older people, the costs of nursing home care are excessive.

Concern is growing nationwide in connection with the financing of long-term care and the ability of the states and the federal government to continue to support costs through the Medicaid programs. The reimbursement levels of both Medicare and Medicaid do not cover actual costs, and there is fear that if further cuts are made, quality of care will be more drastically compromised. The increasing burden on Medicaid is unsustainable, and assuming present growth, Medicaid costs for long-term care will double by 2025 and increase fivefold by 2045 (AAHSA, 2008). AAHSA, in response to the nation's desperate need for a long-term care financing solution, has made recommendations for a model for future financing for long-term care (www.thelongtermcaresolution.org/problem.aspx). Health care coverage for people with long-term care needs is a major national issue that needs attention along with the growing numbers of uninsured individuals of all ages and the rising costs of care in this country.

The purchase of long-term care insurance is an option for some, and almost 30% of Americans over age 45 have purchased a policy. However, according to the AAHSA, only 1 in 5 individuals can afford this type of insurance and many more are screened out because of preexisting conditions. The average annual long-term care premium for people under 65 is $1337 and for those over 65 the annual cost is $2862. Estimates are that if every American purchased the best private coverage he or she could afford, Medicaid costs would still triple by 2045. Chapter 22 discusses Medicare, Medicaid, and long-term care insurance in more depth.

Regulations and Quality of Care. Nursing homes are one of the most highly regulated industries in the United States. Although nursing homes recognize the need to ensure quality, the lack of additional funding for legislated initiatives has left many nursing homes struggling to maintain quality and meet standards with few resources. Criteria and standards often create a bureaucratic structure and a punitive environment that challenges those caring for nursing home residents. Facilities are inspected frequently (minimally once a year) on an unannounced basis, any time of the day or night, to determine compliance with federal regulations and to investigate quality of care outcome indicators. Data from surveys, as well as facility outcomes of quality care indicators, are available to the public (www.cms.hhs.gov). A recent report, *Trends in Publicly Reported Nursing Facility Quality Measures* (American Health Care Association, 2008), provides data on quality measures related to physical condition, depression, physical functioning and weight loss, urinary systems, and post–acute care (www.ahca.org/research/oscar/trend_graph_facilities_qualitymeasures_200704.pdf).

The Omnibus Reconciliation Act (OBRA) of 1987 and the frequent revisions and updates are designed to improve the quality of resident care and have had a positive impact. Some of the requirements of OBRA and subsequent legislation include the following: comprehensive resident assessments (Minimum Data Set [MDS]), increased training requirements for nursing assistants, elimination of the use of medications and restraints for the purpose of discipline or convenience, higher staffing requirements for nursing and social work staff, standards for nursing home administrators, and quality assurance activities.

Regulations have also been created to protect the rights of the residents of nursing homes. Residents in long-term care facilities have rights under both federal and state law. The staff of the facility must inform residents of these rights and protect and promote their rights. The rights to which the residents are entitled should be conspicuously posted in the facility (Box 26-3). Also, the Long-Term Care Ombudsman Program is a nationwide effort to support the rights of both the residents and the facilities. In most states the program provides trained volunteers to investigate rights and quality complaints or conflicts. Each facility is required to post the name and contact information of the ombudsman assigned to the facility.

The Culture Change Movement in Nursing Homes. The public, as well as many health care professionals, hold a very negative view of nursing homes. Many older adults express that they would rather die than be "put into" a nursing home. If a move to a nursing

---

Box 26-3	Bill of Rights for Long-Term Care Residents

- The right to voice grievances and have them remedied
- The right to information about health conditions and treatments and to participate in one's own care to the extent possible
- The right to choose one's own health care providers and to speak privately with one's health care providers
- The right to consent to or refuse all aspects of care and treatments
- The right to manage one's own finances if capable, or to choose one's own financial advisor
- The right to be transferred or discharged only for appropriate reasons
- The right to be free from all forms of abuse
- The right to be free from all forms of restraint to the extent compatible with safety
- The right to privacy and confidentiality concerning one's person, personal information, and medical information
- The right to be treated with dignity, consideration, and respect in keeping with one's individuality
- The right to immediate visitation and access at any time for family, health care providers, and legal advisors; the right to reasonable visitation and access for others

NOTE: This list of rights is a sampling of federal and several states' lists of rights of residents or participants in long-term care. Nurses should check the rules of their own state for specific rights in law for that state.

---

home is necessary, families experience guilt and anxiety. Nursing homes are often blamed for all of the societal problems associated with the aging of our population and are not recognized as an integral part of the health care system. Daily, millions of dedicated caregivers in nursing homes are providing competent and compassionate care to very sick older people against great odds, for example, a lack of support, inadequate salaries and staff, inadequate funding, and lack of respect. It is time for their stories of care to be told, and it is time to recognize their needs for adequate and well-trained staff to do this very important work. "Care of the frail elderly and seriously ill persons is labor intensive and costly… in many nursing homes staff is assigned to more residents than they can properly care for. In situations where unrealistic workloads exist, resident needs are often unmet, raising the risk of harmful and costly complications. This frustrates those who feel responsible for the care of residents…Reasonable workloads are a necessary condition for quality care" (National Citizens' Coalition of Nursing Home Reform, 2001, p. 2; www.nccnhr.org/govpolicy/PF_461_2475_17942.cfm).

Although there are continued challenges and opportunities to improve care in nursing homes (and care in all settings for older adults) and in the fabric of the long-term care system, many nursing homes provide an environment that truly represents the best of caring and quality of life. The commitment and dedication of nursing home staff must be honored and supported. They have much to teach us about aging, nursing, and caring. Box 26-4 presents a description of caring themes expressed by nursing home caregivers in a recent study (Touhy et al, 2005).

Across the United States, the movement to transform nursing homes from the typical medical model into "homes" that nurture quality of life for older people and support and empower frontline caregivers is changing the face of long-term care. Begun by the Pioneer Network, a national not-for-profit organization that serves the culture change movement, many facilities are changing from a rigid institutional approach to one that is person-centered. "No matter how old, how sick, how disabled, how forgetful we are, each of us deserves to have a home—not an institution" (Baker, 2007; Baker as cited by Haglund, 2008, p. 8). The Eden Alternative, founded by Dr. Bill Thomas (www.edenalt.com), and the Wellspring Model developed by Wellspring Innovative Solutions in Seymour, Wisconsin (www.wellspringis.org) are examples of philosophies and programs of culture change.

The Eden Alternative is best known for the addition of animals, plants, and children to nursing homes. However, cats and dogs are not the heart of culture change. Truly transforming a nursing home requires involvement of all levels of staff and changes in values, attitudes, structures, and management practices. Some of the principles of culture change activities are as follows:

- ▶ Staff empowerment
- ▶ Resident involvement in decision making
- ▶ Individualized rather than routine task-oriented care
- ▶ Relationship building
- ▶ A sense of community and belonging
- ▶ Meaningful activities
- ▶ A homelike environment
- ▶ Increased attention to respect of staff and the value of caring

---

Box 26-4   How We Care: Voices of Nursing Home Staff

Responding to What Matters
Taking time to do the little things, competence, cleanliness, meeting basic needs, safe administration of medications, kindness and consideration

Caring as a Way of Expressing Spiritual Commitment
Spiritual beliefs led staff to long-term care and continue to motivate and guide the special care they give to residents; they reflect a spiritual commitment to caring for residents as expressed in the golden rule: "Do unto others as you would like done to you."

Devotion Inspired by Love for Others
Deep connection between staff and residents described as being like family, caring for residents as you would for your own mother or father, sharing of good and bad times, going out on a limb to be an advocate, listening and staying with residents when others had given up

Commitment to Creating a Home Environment
Nursing home is the resident's home, staff are guests in the home; the importance of cleanliness, privacy, good food, and feeling part of a family

Coming to Know and Respect Person as Person
Treating residents, families, and one another with respect and dignity, being recognized for the person you are, intimate knowing of likes and dislikes, individualized care

From Touhy T, Strews W, Brown C: Expressions of caring as lived by nursing home staff, residents, and families, *Int J Human Caring* 9(3):31, 2005.

Box 26-5 presents some of the differences between an institution-centered culture and a person-centered culture.

The Centers for Medicare and Medicaid (CMS) has endorsed culture change through initiatives such as Quality Improvement Organizations (QIOs) and the Advancing Excellence in America's Nursing Homes (www.nhqualitycampaign.org/). CMS has also released a self-study tool for nursing homes to assess their own progress toward culture change. The culture change movement is growing rapidly, and research is needed to

---

Box 26-5	Institution-Centered Versus Person-Centered Culture

Institution-Centered Culture

- Schedules and routines are designed by the institution and staff, and residents must comply.
- Focus is on tasks to be accomplished.
- Rotation of staff from unit to unit occurs.
- Decision making is centralized with little involvement of staff or residents and families.
- There is a hospital environment.
- Structured activities are provided to all residents.
- There is little opportunity for socialization.
- Organization exists for employees rather than residents.
- There is little respect for privacy or individual routines.

Person-Centered Culture

- Emphasis is on relationships between staff and residents.
- Individualized plans of care are based on residents' needs, usual patterns, and desires.
- Staff members have consistent assignments and know the residents' preferences and uniqueness.
- Decision making is as close to the resident as possible.
- Staff members are involved in decisions and plans of care.
- Environment is homelike.
- Meaningful activities and opportunities for socialization are available around the clock.
- There is a sense of community and belonging— "like family."
- There is involvement of the community— children, pets, plants, outings.

Adapted from The Pioneer Network: www.pioneernetwork.net. Accessed 8/8/08.

---

demonstrate costs, benefits, and outcomes (Rahman and Schnelle, 2008).

Making Nursing Home Decisions. Gerontological nurses are frequently asked for assistance in helping older adults and their families make decisions about choosing a nursing home. Gerontological nurse Marilyn Rantz and her colleagues have done extensive research and writing on the quality of care in nursing homes. *The New Nursing Homes: a 20-Minute Way to Find Great Long-Term Care* (Rantz et al, 2001) is an excellent resource. CMS provides a nursing home checklist on its website (www.cms.gov). The National Citizens' Coalition for Nursing Home Reform also provides resources for choosing a nursing home (www. nccnhr.org). Box 26-6 presents a guide to selecting a nursing home. CMS also provides a guide to comparing nursing homes across the United States based on data derived from quality indicator outcomes. Although this may be helpful, the data are basically derived from yearly nursing home survey data and may need considerable interpretation by health care professionals to be useful for consumers. The data may or may not be representative of the quality of the nursing home. The most appropriate method of choosing a nursing home is to personally visit the facility, meet with the director of nursing, observe care routines, discuss the potential resident's needs, and use a format such as the one presented in Box 26-6 to ask questions.

IMPROVING TRANSITIONS ACROSS THE CONTINUUM OF CARE

Older people have complex health care needs and often require care in multiple settings across the continuum. The current health care system is complex and poorly connected. Elders and their caregivers are vulnerable to experiencing serious quality of care concerns. Care transition refers to the movement of patients from one health care practitioner or setting to another as their condition and care needs change. Transitional care is a set of clinical and communication activities that should occur when patients move from one care setting to another. An older person may be treated by a family practitioner, hospitalized and treated by an intensivist, discharged to a nursing home and followed by another practitioner, and then discharged home or to a lesser care-intensive setting (e.g., ALF) where the family practitioner may or may not continue to follow him or her. Most health care providers practice in only one setting and are not familiar with the specific requirements of other settings. As a result, there are often significant misunderstandings and criticisms of care in the different settings across the continuum. As Barbara Resnick pointed out: "We can stop the finger pointing and start working together through the common transitions patients endure in our health care system. This will be a win-win situation for patients and providers alike" (2008, p. 154).

Transitions happen often, and there is increasing evidence that serious deficiencies exist for patients

Box 26-6   Selecting a Nursing Home

Central Focus
- Residents and families are the central focus of the facility

Interaction
- Staff members are attentive and caring
- Staff members listen to what residents say
- Staff members and residents smile at one another
- Prompt response to resident and family needs
- Meaningful activities provided on all shifts to meet individual preferences
- Residents engage in activities with enjoyment
- Staff members talk to cognitively impaired residents; cognitively impaired residents involved in activities designed to meet their needs
- Staff members do not talk down to residents, talk as if they are not present, ignore yelling or calling out
- Families are involved in care decisions and daily life in facility

Milieu
- Calm, active, friendly
- Presence of community, volunteers, children, plants, animals

Environment
- No odor, clean and well maintained
- Rooms personalized
- Private areas
- Protected outside areas
- Equipment in good repair

Individualized Care
- Restorative programs for ambulation, ADLs
- Residents well dressed and groomed
- Resident and family councils
- Pleasant mealtimes, good food, residents have choices
- Adequate staff to serve meals and assist residents
- Flexible meal schedules, food available 24 hours per day
- Ethnic food preferences

Staff
- Well trained, have high level of professional skill
- Professional in appearance and demeanor
- RNs involved in care decisions and care delivery
- Active staff development programs
- Physicians and advanced-practice nurses involved in care planning and staff training
- Adequate staff (more than the minimum required) on each shift
- Low staff turnover

Safety
- Safe walking areas indoors and outdoors
- Monitoring of residents at risk for injury
- Restraint-appropriate care, adequate safety equipment and training on its use

ADLs, Activities of daily living; *RNs,* registered nurses.

Adapted from Rantz MJ, Mehr DR, Popejoy L et al: Nursing home care quality: a multidimensional theoretical model, *J Nurs Care Qual* 12(3): 30-46, 1998.

undergoing transitions across sites of care. Individuals at high risk for transitional care problems include older people with multiple medical conditions or depression or other mental health disorders, isolated elders without family or friends, non-English speakers, immigrants, and low-income individuals (California HealthCare Foundation, 2007).

Approximately 23% of Medicare beneficiaries who are admitted to the hospital end up in another institution, typically a skilled nursing facility. Nineteen percent of Medicare beneficiaries are back in the hospital within 30 days. One-third admitted to hospitals end up making at least two transfers—such as home, hospital, skilled nursing facility, and back to the hospital or nursing home—within 30 days (Wilson, 2008). Transitions

during the course of hospitalization can also be problematic for older patients. Minimizing the number of transfers from unit to unit during a single hospitalization is associated with more consistent nursing care, fewer adverse incidents (e.g., nosocomial infections, falls, medication errors), shorter hospital stays, and lower overall costs (Kanak et al, 2008).

In light of shorter hospital stays and patients being discharged "quicker and sicker," models to improve transitional care will require continued attention. National attention to improving patient safety during transfers is increasing, and a growing body of evidence-based research provides data for design of care to improve transition outcomes. The Centers for Medicare and Medicaid Services (CMS) has begun several initiatives to improve transitions of care through the Quality Improvement Organizations (QIO). Improving transfer forms, developing evidence-based clinical performance measures, and implementing clinical performance improvement activities are examples of other activities being undertaken (Wilson, 2008). The Society of Hospital Medicine has begun a new quality improvement program to improve care transitions of older adults from the hospital setting (www.hospitalmedicine.org). Chapter 15 presents additional discussion of models to improve chronic care.

Nurse researchers Dorothy Brooten and Mary Naylor, and their colleagues, have significantly contributed to knowledge in the area of transitional care, and the quality cost model of transitional care is one of the NICHE models. Dr. Naylor is the Director of the NewCourtland Center for Transitions and Health at the University of Pennsylvania (www.nursing.upenn/chth/membership/). Nurses play a very important role in insuring the adequacy of transitional care, and many of the successful models involve the use of gerontological nurse practitioners and registered nurses in roles such as transition coaches and care managers (Naylor, 2002; Lagoe et al, 2005; Benedict et al, 2006; Coleman et al, 2006; Jablonski et al, 2007; Chalmers and Coleman, 2008; Francis, 2008; Hendrix et al, 2008; Luzinski et al, 2008; Trossman, 2008). Additional information on transitional care can be found at www.hartfordign.org/programs/niche/kit-cdp.html and www.nursing.upenn.edu/centers/hcgne/TransitionalCare.htm.

Relocation

One of the major stressors, and often a crisis for both the older person and his or her family, is relocation. Relocation to a long-term care facility is identified as one of the most stressful and one that many older people fear. With each move, if the adaptation is to be satisfying, one must begin to claim personal space by somehow placing one's stamp of individuality on the new surroundings. Because the older adult is particularly likely to move or be moved, the subject of relocation is significant. Nurses in hospitals, the community, and long-term care institutions frequently care for elders who have experienced relocation.

The first issue to address in any move is whether it is necessary and whether it will provide the least restrictive lifestyle appropriate for the individual. Questions that must be asked to assess the impact on the individual after a move are presented in Box 26-7. Nurses' concerns are with assessing the impact of

---

Box 26-7	Assessment of Relocation

- Are significant persons as accessible in the new location as they were before the move?
- Is the individual developing new and reciprocal relationships in the new setting?
- Is the individual functioning as well, better, or not as well in the new location? This determination cannot be made immediately, but this assessment must be done within at most 6 weeks of the move.
- Was the individual given options before the move?
- Was the individual given the opportunity to assess the new environment before making a decision to move?
- Has the individual been able to move important items of furniture and memorabilia to the new setting?
- Has a particular individual who is familiar with the environment been available to assist with orientation?
- Was the decision to move made hastily or with inadequate information?
- Does the new situation provide adequately for basic needs (food, shelter, physical maintenance)?
- Are individual idiosyncratic needs recognized, and is there an opportunity to actualize them?
- Does the new situation decrease the possibility of privacy and autonomy?
- Is the new living situation an improvement over the previous situation, similar in quality, or worse?

---

relocation and determining methods to mitigate any negative reactions.

Relocation stress syndrome is a nursing diagnosis describing the confusion resulting from a move to a new environment. Characteristics of relocation stress syndrome include anxiety, insecurity, altered mental status, depression, insecurity, loss of control, and physical problems (Iwasiw et al, 2003). An abrupt and poorly prepared transfer actually increases illness and disorientation. Research suggests that individuals are better able to meet the challenges of relocation if they have a sense of control over the circumstances and the confidence to carry out the needed activities associated with a move. Self-efficacy, defined as "the beliefs in one's capability to organize and execute the courses of action required to manage prospective situations" (Bandura, 1997, p. 2), may be an important variable in positive adjustment to a relocation. The Self-Efficacy

| **Box 26-8** | **Relocation Stress Syndrome** |

Relocation stress syndrome is a physiological and/or psychosocial disturbance as a result of transfer from one environment to another.

Defining Characteristics
Major
Change in environment or location
Anxiety
Apprehension
Increased confusion
Depression
Loneliness
Minor
Verbalization of unwillingness to relocate
Sleep disturbance
Change in eating habits
Dependency
Gastrointestinal disturbances
Increased verbalization of needs
Insecurity
Lack of trust
Restlessness
Sad affect
Unfavorable comparison of posttransfer and pretransfer staff
Verbalization of being concerned or upset about transfer
Vigilance
Weight change
Withdrawal

Related Factors
Past, concurrent, and recent losses
Losses involved with the decision to move
Feeling of powerlessness
Lack of adequate support system
Little or no preparation for the impending move
Moderate to high degree of environmental change
History and types of previous transfers
Impaired psychosocial health status
Decreased physical health status

Sample Diagnostic Statement
Relocation stress syndrome related to admission to long-term care setting as evidenced by anxiety, insecurity, and disorientation

Expected Outcomes
1. The resident will socialize with family members, staff, and/or other residents.
2. Preadmission weight, appetite, and sleep patterns will remain stable. If previous patterns were dysfunctional, more appropriate health patterns will develop.
3. The resident will verbalize feelings, expectations, and disappointments openly with members of the staff and/or family.
4. Inappropriate behaviors (e.g., "acting out," refusing to take medicines) will not occur.

Expected Short-Term Goals
1. The resident will become independent in moving to and from areas within the facility during the next 3 months.
2. The resident will react in a positive manner to staff effort to assist in adjusting to nursing home placement in the next 3 months.
3. The resident will express his or her thoughts or concerns about placement when encouraged to do so during individual contacts in the next 3 months.
4. During the next 3 months, the resident will not develop physical or psychosocial disturbances indicative of translocation syndrome as a result of the change in living environment.

Expected Long-Term Goals
1. The resident will verbalize acceptance of nursing home placement within the next 6 months.
2. The resident will indicate acceptance of nursing home placement through positive body language within the next 6 months.

Specific Nursing Interventions
1. Identify previous coping patterns during admission assessment. Clearly document these, and share the information with other staff members.
2. Include the resident in assessing problems and developing the care plan on admission.
3. Adjust for limitations in sensory-perceptual disturbances when planning care for residents. Visual disturbances necessitate special intervention to assist residents in finding their way around.
4. Staff members will introduce themselves when entering the resident's room, indicating the nature of their relationship with the resident. Example: "Hello, Mr. S. My name is Nancy. I'll be your nurse attendant today, helping you with your meals and your bath."
5. Each staff member providing care for the resident should make it a point to spend at least 5 minutes each day with new admissions to "just visit."

(Continued)

Box 26-8	Relocation Stress Syndrome—cont'd

6. Allow the resident as many opportunities to make independent choices as possible.
7. Identify previous routines for activities of daily living (ADLs). Try to maintain as much continuity with the resident's previous schedule as possible. Example: If Mr. S. has taken a bath before bed all of his life, adjust his schedule to continue that practice.
8. Familiarize the resident with unit schedules.
9. Encourage family participation through frequent visits, phone calls, and activity sessions. Be sure to let the family know schedules.
10. Establish familiar landmarks for the resident when leaving his or her room so that he or she can recognize areas more quickly.

11. Encourage family members to bring familiar belongings from home for the resident's room decorations.
12. Provide reorientation cues frequently. Example: "You are in the dining room. Your room is down the hall three doors just past the window."
13. Encourage the resident to talk about expectations, anger, and/or disappointments and the recent life changes that he or she has experienced.
14. Review the patient's medication list with the physician to verify the need for medications that might promote disorientation.
15. Provide for constructive activities. Initiate activity therapy consultation.

Relocation Scale (SERS), developed by Rossen and Gruber (2007), can be used to assess self-efficacy in individuals who are relocating, identify potential pre-relocation adjustment issues, and guide interventions to promote positive relocation outcomes.

To avoid some of the effects of relocation stress syndrome, the individual must have some control over the environment, preparation regarding the new situation, and maintenance of familiar situations to the greatest degree possible. Nurses must carefully assess and monitor older people for relocation stress syndrome effects. Working with families to help them plan relocations, understanding the effects of relocation, and implementing effective approaches are also necessary. It is important that some familiar and some treasured items accompany the transfer. Too often, elders arrive at long-term care institutions via ambulance stretcher from the hospital with nothing but a hospital gown. Everything familiar and necessary in their lives remains at the home they have left when they became ill. Even more distressing is when families or responsible parties sell the home to finance long-term care stays without the input of the elder. It is no wonder so many residents with dementia in nursing homes wander the hallways looking for home and for something familiar and comforting. Family members will need considerable support when an elder is moved into an institution. No matter what the circumstances, the family invariably feels that they have in some way failed the elder. These issues are discussed in more depth in Chapter 23. A summary of relocation stress syndrome and nursing

actions to prevent relocation stress during transition to long-term care are presented in Box 26-8. An evidence-based practice guideline, *Management of relocation in cognitively intact older adults* (Hertz et al, 2005) is available at www.guideline.gov.

IMPLICATIONS FOR GERONTOLOGICAL NURSING AND HEALTHY AGING

Throughout this chapter and the book we have offered many implications for gerontological nursing and healthy aging. Nurses with competence in care of older people will be in great demand as the population ages. Gerontological nurses have always assumed a leadership role in improving care for elders, ensuring fulfillment of all levels of needs on Maslow's hierarchy, and promoting healthy aging. Through their expertise, commitment, dedication, advocacy, and compassion, gerontological nurses who work with older adults in all settings will continue to be leaders in creating models that truly change the culture of existing systems. "How we as nurses move our aging society forward toward the middle of the 21st century will determine our character as we are no greater than the health of America" (Kagan, 2008, p. 102).

Perhaps our words in this book will provide you with the knowledge you need to fulfill this vision. Our hope is that you find as much joy and fulfillment as we have in our nursing of older adults. Irene Burnside (1980, p. 32) quoted Martin Buber when she wrote: "No one can say thank you the way an old person can." May you hear many thank you's in your practice.

KEY CONCEPTS

▶ A familiar and comfortable environment allows an elder to function at his or her highest capacity.

▶ Nurses must be knowledgeable about the range of residential options for older people so they can assist the elder and the family to make appropriate decisions.

▶ Nursing homes are an integral part of the long-term care system, providing both skilled (subacute) care and chronic, long-term, and palliative care. Projections are that this setting will provide increasing amounts of care to the growing numbers of older adults.

▶ Culture change in nursing homes is a growing movement to develop models of person-centered care and improve care outcomes and quality of life.

▶ Nurses play a key role in insuring optimal outcomes during transitions of care.

▶ The present long-term care system is fragmented, cost-prohibitive, difficult to access, and in need of major transformation to meet the needs of individuals of all ages in need of this type of care.

▶ Relocation has variable effects, depending on the individual's personality, health, cognitive capacities, sense of control, opportunities for choice, self-esteem, and preferred lifestyle.

ACTIVITIES AND DISCUSSION QUESTIONS

1. Identify three objects in your living space that are important to you, and explain why these are significant. Will you take these with you whenever you relocate?

2. Ask an older relative about the items or conditions in his or her home that make him or her feel secure and comfortable.

3. Discuss with this elder various moves he or she has made and how he or she felt about them.

4. How might the care needs of an older adult in assisted living, subacute care, and a nursing home differ? What is the role of the professional nurse in each of these settings?

5. Select three places listed in your phone book as retirement communities, and make inquiries regarding possible placement of an older adult parent. What questions did you ask? What is the cost? What are the provisions for health care? What types of activities and assistance are available? Which would you select for your grandmother and why?

6. In your experience in the acute care setting, what improvements would you suggest to improve transitions to other care settings? Discuss any experience you or your friends or family may have had with transitions after hospital discharge.

7. If you were the director of nursing, what would your nursing home be like (design, staffing, quality of care, training)?

RESOURCES

Organizations
Advancing Excellence in America's Nursing Homes
www.nhqualitycampaign.org/

The Eden Alternative
www.edenalt.com

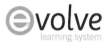

For additional resources, please visit evolve.elsevier.com/Ebersole/gerontological.

REFERENCES

Alzheimer's Association: *Quality Care Campaign,* 2008. Available at www.alz.org/we_can_help_quality_care.asp. Accessed 11/11/08.

American Association of Homes and Services for the Aging (AAHSA): *Aging services: the facts,* 2008. Available at www.aahsa.org/aging_services/default.asp. Accessed 7/12/08.

American Health Care Association: *Trends in publicly reported nursing facility quality measures,* July 2008, The Association. Available at www.ahcancal.org/research_data/trends_statistics/Documents/trends_nursing_facilities_quality_measures.pdf. Accessed 11/11/08.

Baker B: *Old age in a new age: the promise of transformative nursing homes,* Nashville, Tenn, 2007, Vanderbilt University Press.

Baker B, as cited in Haglund K: Closing keynote speaker found hope in changes benefiting residents and staff, *Caring Ages* 9(6):8, 2008.

Bandura A: *Self-efficacy: the exercise of control,* New York, 1997, W.H. Freeman.

Benedict L, Robinson K, Holder C: Clinical nurse specialist practice within an acute care for elders interdisciplinary model, *Clin Nurse Spec* 20(5):248-252, 2006.

Burnside I: Why work with the aged? *Geriatr Nurs* 2(3): 29-33, 1980.

California HealthCare Foundation: *Long-term care: improving care transitions project,* 2007. Available at www.chcf.org/topics/view.cfm?itemID=133512. Accessed 7/12/08.

Chalmers S, Coleman E: Transitional care. In Capezuti E, Swicker D, Mezey M et al, editors: *The encyclopedia of elder care,* ed 2, New York, 2008, Springer.

Coleman E, Fox P on behalf of the HMO Care Management Workgroup: One patient, many places: managing health care transitions. Part 1: Introduction, accountability, information for patients in transition, *Ann Long-Term Care* 12(9):25-32, 2004.

Coleman EA, Parry C, Chalmers S, Min SJ: The Care Transitions Intervention: results of a randomized controlled trial, *Arch Intern Med* 166(17):1822-1928, 2006.

Francis D: Iatrogenesis: the nurse's role in preventing patient harm. In Capezuti E, Swicker D, Mezey M et al, editors: *Evidence-based geriatric nursing protocols for best practice,* ed 3, New York, 2008, Springer.

Hendrix C, Heflin MT, Twersky J et al: Post-hospital clinic for older patients and their family caregivers, *Ann Long-Term Care* 16(5):20-24, 2008.

Hertz J, Rossetti J, Koren N, Robertson J: *Management of relocation in cognitively intact older adults,* Iowa City, IA, University of Iowa Gerontological Nursing Interventions Research Center, Research Dissemination Core, 2005. Available from www.guidelines.gov. Accessed 7/8/08.

Iwasiw C, Goldenberg D, Bol N, MacMaster E: Resident and family perspectives: the first year in a long-term care facility, *J Gerontol Nurs* 29(1):45-54, 2003.

Jablonski R, Utz S, Steeves R, Gray D: Decisions about transfer from nursing home to emergency department, *J Nurs Scholarship* 39(3):266-272, 2007.

Jarvik E, Collins L: "Living, and dying, in a nursing home: facilities fight stereotype as they try to provide attentive end-of-life care," January 30, 2003, Desert News Publishing. Available at http://deseretnews.com/article/content/mobile/1,5620,455028257,00.html?print?View=true. Accessed 7/12/08.

Kagan S: Moving from achievement to transformation, *Geriatr Nurs* 29(2):102-104, 2008.

Kanak MF, Titler M, Shever L et al: The effect of hospitalization on multiple units, *App Nurs Res* 21(1):15-22, 2008.

Lagoe R, Altwarg J, Mnich S, Winks L: A community-wide program to improve the efficiency of care between nursing homes and hospitals, *Topics Adv Prac Nurs EJournal* 5(2):2005.

Luzinski C, Stockbridge E, Craighead J et al: The community case management program: for 12 years, caring at its best, *Geriatr Nurs* 29(3):207-216, 2008.

Lyons W, Landefeld S: Improving care for hospitalized elders, *Ann Long-Term Care* 9(4):35-40, 2001.

Munroe D: Assisted living issues for nursing practice, *Geriatr Nurs* 24(2):99-105, 2003.

National Adult Day Services Association: *Adult day services: overview and facts,* 2008. Available at www.nadsa.org. Accessed 7/12/08.

National Center for Assisted Living: *What is assisted living,* 2008. Available at www.ncal.org/consumer/index.cfm. Accessed 7/12/08.

National Citizens' Coalition for Nursing Home Reform: *The nurse staffing crisis in nursing homes,* 2001. Available at http://www.nccnhr.org/govpolicy/PF_461_2475_17942.cfm. Accessed 11/11/08.

Naylor M: Transitional care of older adults. In Archbold P, Stewart B, editors: *Annual review of nursing research* 20, New York, 2002, Springer.

Omnibus Budget Reconciliation Act (OBRA) of 1987 (Public Law No. 100-203): Amendments 1990, 1991, 1992, 1993, and 1994, Rockville, Md, U.S. Department of Health and Human Services, Health Care Financing Administration.

Rahman A, Schnelle J: The nursing home culture change movement: recent past, present, and future directions for research, *Gerontologist* 48(2):142-148, 2008.

Rantz M, Popejoy L, Zwygart-Stauffacher M: *The new nursing homes: a 20-minute way to find great long-term care,* Lanham, Md, 2001, National Book Network.

Resnick B: Hospitalization of older adults: are we doing a good job? *Geriatr Nurs* 29(3):153-154, 2008.

Rossen E, Gruber K: Development and psychometric testing of the relocation self-efficacy scale, *Nurs Res* 56(4):244-251, 2007.

Teno J: Now is the time to embrace nursing homes as a place of care for dying persons, *Innovations End-of-Life Care* 4(2):2002. Available at www.edc.org/lastacts. Accessed 7/12/08.

Tilly J, Reed P, editors: *Dementia care practice recommendations for assisted living residences and nursing homes,* Washington, DC, Alzheimer's Association, 2008. Available at www.guideline.gov. Accessed 8/8/08.

Trossman S: Issues up close: care without gaps, *Am Nurse Today* 3(7):40-42, 2008.

Touhy T, Strews W, Brown C: Expressions of caring as lived by nursing home staff, residents, and families, *Int J Human Caring* 9(3):31, 2005.

Wallace M: Is there a nurse in the house? The role of nurses in assisted living: past, present and future, *Geriatr Nurs* 24(4):218-221, 235, 2003.

Wendel V, Durso S: A case study: challenges and issues caring for the older adult across the spectrum of settings, *J Nurs Practitioners* 2(9):600-606, 2006.

Wilson K: Panel reveals means to better transitions, *Caring for the Ages* 9(4):32, 2008.

Index

A

AACN. *See* American Association of Colleges of Nursing (AACN)

AARP, 387-388

Abnormal Involuntary Movement Scale (AIMS), 235, 416

Absorbent products for urinary incontinence, 142

Absorption pharmacokinetics, 220, 222

Abuse
alcohol and substance
acute alcohol withdrawal, 429
adverse drug effects with, 426
assessment, 426-428, 427b
gender and, 425-426
Healthy People 2010 goals, 407, 407b
interventions, 428-429, 428b
physiology of, 426
prescription medications used in, 429-430
prevalence, 424-425
elder
assessment of, 366, 366b, 367b, 373
gender and, 365, 365b
interventions, 366, 367b
mandatory reporting of, 366-367
National Elder Abuse Incidence Study, 371-372
perpetrators of, 365b
prevalence of, 364-365
prevention of, 367-368
signs of, 367b, 371-372
types of, 371-372
undue influence as, 366b

Accessory organs of the digestive system, 76

Acetaminophen, 222, 262, 267

Acquired immunodeficiency syndrome (AIDS), 400-401. *See also* Human immunodeficiency virus (HIV)

Actinic keratosis, 165, 166

Activities of daily living (ADLs)
assessment, 208-210, 210t, 216
chronic illness and, 241
dementia and, 343, 344-345
environmental safety and, 196-197
instrumental, 196, 201, 211b, 241, 457
residential care facilities and, 454-455, 455b
simplification strategies, 39b
urinary incontinence and, 137, 139
vision impairment and, 32-33

Activity theory of aging, 85

Actonel, 284

Actos, 278

Acupressure, 268

Acupuncture, 268

Acute alcohol withdrawal, 429

Acute care settings
description, 17-18
documentation in, 62-63
focus, 19b

Acute dystonia, 235

Acute grief, 437

Acute ischemia, 307

Acute myocardial infarction (AMI), 307

Acute pain, 261

Acute versus chronic illness, 242

Acyclovir, 262

ADLs. *See* Activities of daily living

Administration, medication, 232, 233b

Adult children and elders, 377, 386-387

Adult day services, 453-454

Advance directives, 62, 126, 446-447

Advanced-practice gerontological nurses (APGNs), 16-17

Adverse drug reactions (ADR), 226-228, 426

Advil, 267

Aeration, 207-208

African Americans
belief systems, 52
cultural awareness and, 50
dehydration in, 132
dementia and, 331
depression in, 417
diabetes in, 273
frailty syndrome among, 242-243
glaucoma and, 293
hair, 70
poverty among, 106
racism experienced by, 50-51
social exchange theory and, 87
vision impairments in, 32-33

Age-associated memory impairment (AAMI), 93-94

Ageism, 26
race and, 50-51

Agency for Healthcare Research and Quality, 268

Age-Related Eye Disease Study (AREDS), 297, 298b

Age-related macular degeneration (AMD), 296-298, 298b, 297f, 298f

Age-stratification theory of aging, 85-86

Agility and mobility, 180

Aging. *See also* Older adults
biological theories of, 67-68, 67b
bladder function changes with, 133-134
cardiovascular changes with, 71-72, 73b
chronic illness and, 240-241
cognition and, 91-95
cross-link theory of, 68
demographics, 1-3, 3f, 10, 48, 49
diabetes and, 277b
endocrine system changes with, 74-75
error theories of, 67
ethnicity and, 2-3, 3f
free radical theory of, 68
gastrointestinal system changes with, 75-76, 105
gender and, 2, 134, 243

Page numbers with "t" denote tables; those with "f" denote figures; and those with "b" denote boxes.